Palliative & End-of-Life Care

Clinical Practice Guidelines

SECOND EDITION

Feb 2011

Happy Birthday, maggie!
May this inspire you to
keep up the awesome
and compassionate care.
you are a wonderful
role model.
    Peace.
        Bttttner RN

Palliative & End-of-Life Care

Clinical Practice Guidelines

SECOND EDITION

Kim K. Kuebler, MN, RN, APRN-BC
Adult Nurse Practitioner
Private Practice
Savannah Georgia

Debra E. Heidrich, MSN, RN, CHPN, AOCN
Palliative Nurse Clinician
Bethesda North Hospital
TriHealth, Inc.
Cincinnati, Ohio

Peg Esper, MSN, RN, APRN-BC, AOCN
Nurse Practitioner, Medical Oncology
University of Michigan Comprehensive Cancer Center
Ann Arbor, Michigan

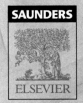

SAUNDERS

ELSEVIER

SAUNDERS
ELSEVIER

11830 Westline Industrial Drive
St. Louis, Missouri 63146

Notice

Nursing is an ever-changing field. Standard safety precautions must be followed, but as new research
and clinical experience broaden our knowledge, changes in treatment and drug therapy may become
necessary or appropriate. Readers are advised to check the most current product information
provided by the manufacturer of each drug to be administered to verify the recommended dose,
the method and duration of administration, and contraindications. It is the responsibility of the
appropriately licensed health care provider, relying on experience and knowledge of the patient,
to determine dosages and the best treatment for each individual patient. Neither the publisher nor
the editor assumes any liability for any injury and/or damage to persons or property arising from
this publication.

The Publisher

Previous editions copyrighted 2002, 2005

ISBN-13: 978-1-4160-3079-9
ISBN-10: 1-4160-3079-4

Executive Publisher: Barbara Nelson Cullen
Acquisitions Editor: Sandra Clark Brown
Developmental Editor: Sophia Oh Gray
Publishing Services Manager: Jeffrey Patterson
Project Manager: Mary G. Stueck
Senior Designer: Jyotika Shroff
Cover Designer: Jyotika Shroff

Working together to grow
libraries in developing countries

www.elsevier.com | www.bookaid.org | www.sabre.org

ELSEVIER   BOOK AID
International   Sabre Foundation

Printed in the United States of America

Last digit is the print number: 9 8 7 6 5 4 3 2

*This textbook is dedicated
to the memory of
my son, Jacob James,
whose spirit continues to live . . .*

K. Kuebler

CONTRIBUTORS

Jerald M. Andry, PharmD, MSc
Regional Medical Scientist
Boehringer Ingelheim Pharmaceuticals
Powell, Ohio
Chapter 27: Dyspnea

Jane M. Armer, PhD, RN
Director, Nursing Research
Ellis Fischel Cancer Center
Columbia, Missouri;
Professor, Sinclair School of Nursing
University of Missouri, Columbia
Columbia, Missouri
Chapter 30: Lymphedema

Elizabeth A. Ayello, PhD, RN, APRN, BC, CWOCN, FAPWCA, FAAN
President
Ayello, Harris, & Associates
Albany, New York;
Faculty, School of Nursing
Excelsior College
Albany, New York
Chapter 35: Ulcerative Lesions

Agnes Coveney, OSU, PhD
Director of Mission Integration
TriHealth
Cincinnati, Ohio
Chapter 5: Ethical Issues Surrounding Advanced Disease

Mellar P. Davis, MD, FCCP
Director of Research
Harry R. Horvitz Center for Palliative Medicine
Taussig Cancer Center
The Cleveland Clinic
Cleveland, Ohio
Chapter 2: Palliative and End-of-Life Care Perspectives

Shawn Davis, PharmD
Regional Medical Scientist
Boehringer Ingelheim Pharmaceuticals
Ridgefield, Connecticut
Chapter 27: Dyspnea

Suzanne W. Dixon, MPh, MS, RD
Vice President
Nutrition Product Development
P4 Healthcare, LLC
Portland, Oregon
Chapter 9: Nutrition

Peg Esper, MSN, RN, APRN-BC, AOCN
Nurse Practitioner, Medical Oncology
University of Michigan Comprehensive Cancer Center
Ann Arbor, Michigan
Chapter 1: The Advanced Practice Nurse in Palliative Care
Chapter 15: Malignancies
Chapter 17: Anxiety
Chapter 20: Cachexia and Anorexia
Chapter 25: Depression
Chapter 29: Hiccups
Chapter 32: Pain

Jennifer Fournier, RN, MSN, AOCN, CHPN
Clinical Nurse Specialist
Hospice Savannah, Inc.
Savannah, Georgia
Chapter 22: Cough

Michael J. Germain, MD
Associate Professor, Medicine
Tufts University
Boston, Massachusetts
Chapter 13: Chronic Kidney Disease

Phyllis A. Grauer, RPH, PharmD, CGP
President/Consultant
Palliative Care Consulting Group
Dublin, Ohio;
Assistant Clinical Professor
College of Pharmacy
The Ohio University
Columbus, Ohio
Chapter 7: Pharmacology

Debra E. Heidrich, MSN, RN, CHPN, AOCN
Palliative Nurse Clinician
Bethesda North Hospital
TriHealth, Inc.
Cincinnati, Ohio
  Chapter 3: The Dying Process
  Chapter 13: Chronic Kidney Disease
  Chapter 14: Neurological Diseases
  Chapter 15: Malignancies
  Chapter 17: Anxiety
  Chapter 18: Ascites
  Chapter 19: Bowel Obstruction
  Chapter 21: Constipation
  Chapter 26: Diarrhea
  Chapter 32: Pain

Roberta Kaplow, RN, PhD, CCNS, CCRN
Clinical Professor
Nell Hodgson Woodruff School
  of Nursing
Emory University
Atlanta, Georgia
  Chapter 33: Palliative Care Emergencies

Charles Kemp, FNP, FAAN
Senior Lecturer
Louis Herrington School of Nursing
Baylor University
Dallas, Texas
  Chapter 6: Spiritual Care Across Cultures

Kim K. Kuebler MN, RN, APRN-BC
Adult Nurse Practitioner
Private Practice
Savannah, Georgia
  *Chapter 1: The Advanced Practice Nurse
    in Palliative Care*
  *Chapter 2: Palliative and End-of-Life
    Care Perspectives*
  Chapter 11: Pulmonary Disease
  Chapter 23: Dehydration
  Chapter 27: Dyspnea

Louise P. Meyer, MS, ARNP, AOCN
Nurse Practitioner, Neuro-Oncology
Dartmouth-Hitchcock Medical Center
Lebanon, New Hampshire
  Chapter 28: Fatigue

Crystal Dea Moore, MA, MSW, PhD
Assistant Professor and Social Work
  Program Director
Skidmore College
Saratoga Springs, New York
  *Chapter 4: Advance Care Planning and
    End-of-Life Decision Making*
  Appendix A: Caregiver Resources

Marilyn O'Mallon, MSN, RN
Assistant Professor
Department of Nursing
Armstrong Atlantic State University
Savannah, Georgia
  *Appendix B: Clinician Resources and
    Assessment Tools*

James C. Pace, DSN, MDIV, APRN-BC, FAANP
Professor of Nursing and Coordinator,
  ANP-Palliative Care Program
School of Nursing
Vanderbilt University
Nashville, Tennessee
  *Chapter 1: The Advanced Practice Nurse
    in Palliative Care*
  Chapter 16: HIV/AIDS

Rhalene Gabuat Patajo, PharmD
Regional Medical Scientist
Boehringer Ingelheim Pharmaceuticals
Ridgefield, Connecticut
  Chapter 11: Pulmonary Disease

Kim Anne Pickett, MS, FNP
Nurse Practitioner
Focused Care Department
Hospice of Dayton
Dayton, Ohio
  Chapter 10: Cardiovascular Disease

Valarie A. Pompey, MS, APRN, BC, AOCNP
Oncology Nurse Practitioner
Michiana Hematology Oncology, PC
South Bend, Indiana
  Chapter 23: Dehydration
  Chapter 31: Nausea and Vomiting

Sheila H. Ridner, PhD, RN, ACNP
Research Associate in Nursing
School of Nursing
Vanderbilt University
Nashville, Tennessee
Chapter 30: Lymphedema

Joy E. Schank, MSN, RN, ANP, CWOCN
Adult Nurse Practitioner
Private Practice
Schank Companies
Himrod, New York
Chapter 35: Ulcerative Lesions

Carol L. Scot, MD
Medical Director
Sparrow Hospice and Palliative Care Services
Lansing, Michigan
Chapter 10: Cardiovascular Disease
Chapter 34: Pruritus

Pamela Sue Spencer, BA, RN, BSN, FNP
Family Nurse Practitioner, Primary Care
and Gastroenterology
Saginaw Veterans Administration
Saginaw, Michigan
Chapter 12: Hepatic Disease
Chapter 14: Neurological Diseases
Chapter 19: Bowel Obstruction

Catherine Vena, PhD, RN
Postdoctoral Fellow
Nell Hodgson Woodruff School of Nursing
Emory University
Atlanta, Georgia
Chapter 8: Sleep
Chapter 24: Delirium and Acute Confusion

REVIEWERS

Nancy M. Albert, MSN, RN, CCNS, CCRN, CAN
Director, Nursing Research
Division of Nursing
Clinical Nurse Specialist
George M. and Linda H. Kaufman Center
  for Heart Failure
The Cleveland Clinic Foundation
Cleveland, Ohio

Cynthia Reno Balkstra, MS, APRN, BC
Pulmonary Clinical Nurse Specialist
Pulmonary Center
St. Joseph's/Candler
Savannah, Georgia

Holly Brown, MSN, APRN, BC
Associate Faculty
Clinical Adult and Elder Health Department
Emory University
Atlanta, Georgia

Patricia C. Buchsel, RN, MSN, FAAN
Adjuvant Faculty
College of Nursing
Seattle University
Seattle, Washington

James M. Deshotels, SJ, APRN
Vice President for Mission
Daughters of Charity Services
  of New Orleans
New Orleans, Louisiana

Jan Frandsen, MSN, NP-C
Nurse Practitioner, Taussig Cancer Center
The Cleveland Clinic Foundation
Cleveland, OH

Kelli Gershon, APN, BC-PM
Advance Practice Nurse
Palliative Care
The University of Texas
M.D. Anderson Cancer Center
Houston, Texas

Lori A. Ladd, MSN, APRN, BC
Medical Liaison
Purdue Pharma
St. Louis, Missouri

John A. Mulder, MD
Clinical Faculty
Vanderbilt University
Nashville, Tennessee;
Chief Medical Officer
Alive Hospice, Inc.
Nashville, Tennessee

Carmencita M. Poe, RN, EDD, APRN-BC, OCN
Oncology Nurse Consultant
Poe Consulting
Little Rock, Arkansas

Jennifer Jean Seimens, RN, BSCN, BEd
Comcene Health Services
Home Care Nursing;
Thunder Bay Health Science Center
Sexual Assault/Domestic Violence Treatment
  Center
Thunder Bay, Ontario

James Varga, RPh, MBA
National Scientific Manager
Health Sciences and Systems: Respiratory
Boehringer Ingelheim Pharmaceuticals
Orlando, Florida

Patrick J. Vojta, PhD
Respiratory Medical Scientist
Boehringer Ingelheim Pharmaceuticals
Lafayette, Colorado

PREFACE

The evolution of palliative care in the United States has raised the bar of awareness and integrated the value and importance for advance practice nurses to apply evidence-based interventions in the care and management of patients with advanced disease. Palliative practices should be integrated into the traditional management of disease and not reserved for the imminently dying patient. Patients who live with symptomatic chronic disease experience interference with function and quality of life. It is the advance practice nurse who is able to offer the adult patient and family improved symptom management and provide an opportunity to optimize physical function. The advanced practice nurse is able to provide the patient and family a conduit of care from diagnosis until death by increasing the intensity of skilled palliative interventions as the disease progresses. This conduit of care includes continuity, collaboration, and coordination of services that are tailored to the disease and the patient.

This second edition will provide the clinician with current clinical information to support the multidimensional needs of the patient and family. Several new chapters have been added, covering topics including sleep, nutrition, pharmacology, communication, and cultural issues. The editors would like to acknowledge the interdisciplinary expertise of the contributors and reviewers. We wish to acknowledge with appreciation the support of our editors from Elsevier, Sandra Clark Brown and Sophia Oh Gray.

KK, DEH, PE

ACKNOWLEDGMENTS

To my mentor, my best friend, and my role model—my mother.

KK

Thank you to the patients, their family members,
and to my colleagues who have been my teachers.
Special recognition goes to
Bill, Bill, Emily, Glennis, Glenn, Bonnie, and Pam
for all of their encouragement and support over the years.
My work on this edition is especially dedicated to the memories of
William A. Heidrich, Jr., Gilbert Heidrich, and Kevin Heidrich.

DEH

To my husband and best friend Jerry for his love and encouragement,
my children Melissa and Tim whose smiles melt my heart,
and the many patients I have had the privilege to care for over
the years who have taught me how important it is
to try and make a difference in people's lives.

PE

FOREWORD

Coming to the end of one's life has always occasioned reflection, anguish, and spiritual growth. For most people the time near death holds its share of serious pain, isolation, and despair, as well as opportunities for transcendence, insight, and closure. But all too often in our modern era, the end of life has become an especially difficult part of life. In the past, the end of life usually came quite quickly; even 100 years ago, most people died of an infectious disease within a few days or weeks of contracting the illness. Most of us will die of a slowly progressive chronic illness or of the combination of a few such conditions. Many of us will die in old age, and we will have been disabled, sick, or dependent for some years. During that time our health care system will have performed scores of tests, provided myriad treatments, put forward specialists of all sorts—this is the same health care system that regularly loses records and patients, fails to support family caregivers, and runs up extraordinary costs.

It's not a pretty picture, but it can be so much better. We could figure out how to ensure reliable services for this, the neediest time of life. Every person living with eventually fatal illness could count on having good medical care, good symptom prevention and relief, continuity, planning for future issues, family support, sensitivity to the patient's and the family members' preferences, and support for living—all at a sustainable price. What would it take? First, it takes forging the will for reform. Second, it takes having excellent small systems that show us what can be done. Third, it takes a strategy that involves political realities as well as clinical performance.

Nursing is the natural home for much of this work. From Florence Nightingale to the present, monitoring quality and setting routines that achieve reliably high quality have been a special concern of nurses, and nurses manage many of the best programs in end-of-life care. Most hospice programs started with nursing, and care of the frail and demented rely predominantly on nurses and nurse management.

Serious chronic illness in old age has been the main way to live the last part of one's life for only a few decades. The society is still learning how to think about the experience: what to value and what to decry. It is evident that widespread overtreatment with medical interventions actually worsens the course, but so does abandonment. Most of the costs of health care over the lifespan are concentrated in the last few years. For those who live to the age of 85 years, half will live with cognitive failure. So much of what we do wrong is done because we still act as if the main target is a middle-aged man having a heart attack, who is in need of a hospital, surgeon, and emergency services. In truth, the main "consumers" of end-of-life care are older and sicker and they can survive for indefinite periods. Building care systems around the dominant "trajectories" of those last few years would require us to tailor services to match a short period of rapid decline, a longer course of episodic exacerbations and sudden dying, and a long period of decline.

Palliative and End-of-Life Care: Clinical Practice Guidelines takes up a broad array of practical insights and advice. The authors offer nurses anchor care arrangements that can reliably provide sustainable and excellent care for people living with serious and eventually fatal conditions.

Reform needs leaders with vision, insight, and commitment. Perhaps the readers of this book will be the leaders we need. Remember, if we don't get a workable and sustainable care system, we will eventually have to live through our own last years in the risky and unreliable arrangements we will have left in place.

Joanne Lynn, MD, MA, MS
Senior Scientist
RAND
Arlington, Virginia

FOREWORD

The publication of this edition of *Palliative and End-of-Life Care: Clinical Practice Guidelines* is evidence that Advanced Practice Nursing in palliative care is coming of age. The maturation and steady expansion of palliative advanced practice nursing is a hopeful trend within the field of palliative care. More importantly, the growing availability of advanced practice nurses (palliative nurse practitioners and clinical nurse specialists) with expertise in palliative care is sure to increase the quality of life of people living with frailty of advanced age or progressive illness as well as the well-being their families.

Palliative care is one area of health care progress in which nursing leadership should be impossible to ignore. As with other advances in public health attributable to nursing practice, there is risk that the important contributions of advanced practice nursing to palliative care will not receive the attention they deserve. Literally and metaphorically, nurses often practice behind drawn curtains. The intimate nature of nursing care demands the highest degrees of privacy. Furthermore, nurses tend to be understated about their work. This unassuming style persists among advanced practice nurses despite the independent and often central role they play in diagnosing and treating patients.

The past decade has witnessed rapid progress in the science and practice of palliative care and expansion of the delivery of palliative services. As this excellent new edition of *Palliative and End-of-Life Care: Clinical Practice Guidelines* goes to press, more than 1000 American hospitals have established clinical palliative care programs and the number of people referred to hospice programs in the United States continues to increase, topping one million annually. A virtual cornucopia of research has filled new and expanded palliative care specialty journals, and key articles have been published in top-tier medical and nursing journals. Palliative medicine has been formally recognized by the American Board of Medical Specialties, and fellowship programs are springing up in academic centers training a new generation of palliative specialists.

As a physician, I am proud of the contributions that doctors have made to the maturation of palliative care, yet I am mindful of the fundamental role nurses have played in its evolution. Although medicine in the modern age has been focused on uncovering and correcting the pathophysiology of disease, nursing has remained focused on the well-being of people living with illness, as well as their families. Hospice and palliative care emerged as correctives to the narrow focus on disease modification, reminding the medical establishment that it is not the disease that is our ultimate focus, but the person living with disease.

It is worth recalling that the late Dame Cicely Saunders, who is rightly credited with founding hospice care in the modern era, practiced as a nurse before becoming a physician. Explore the history of any hospice program in the United States and one is likely to discover a local nurse who became a charismatic champion of the needs of dying patients. Indeed, the fundamental values of nursing find full expression in palliative care.

In recent years, nurses with special training and expertise in palliative care have contributed in major ways to the expansion and maturation of palliative services and practice. As director of the Promoting Excellence in End-of-Life Care program of the Robert Wood Johnson Foundation, I have had the opportunity to witness this leadership first hand in pioneering programs across the United States. Nurse practitioners and clinical nurse specialists are often the lynchpins of young, innovative palliative care services, including those based in hospitals, medical ICUs, trauma units, dialysis centers, academic pediatric referral centers, nursing homes, and outreach clinics for underserved rural and urban populations. Working within clinical teams, palliative nurse practitioners and clinical nurse specialists typically perform the core clinical roles of assessing patients and families, diagnosing and treating underlying causes of symptoms and comorbid conditions, coordinating services and contributions from an interdisciplinary team, addressing psychosocial and spiritual distress, and guiding patients and families through the difficult work of life completion. In doing the hard work of caring, day in and day out, these advanced nurse clinicians have been breaking trail for an urgently needed, expanded field.

Advanced practice nurses specializing in palliative care exemplify both the science and art of nursing by coupling evidence-based knowledge and clinical skills with human values of respect, dignity, and loving care. As a discipline, these nurses embody the professional sophistication and pragmatism needed in today's social and health care environments. Collectively, advanced practice nurses represent an essential resource for meeting the needs of our society's ill, infirm and elderly members. This updated edition of *Palliative and End-of-Life Care: Clinical Practice Guidelines* is an outstanding resource for the teaching and practice of the current and coming generations of palliative advanced practice nurses.

Ira Byock, MD
Director of Palliative Medicine
Dartmouth-Hitchcock Medical Center
Lebanon, New Hampshire

CONTENTS

I GENERAL PRINCIPLES IN PALLIATIVE AND END-OF-LIFE CARE

  1 The Advanced Practice Nurse in Palliative Care, 3
     Kim K. Kuebler, James C. Pace, and Peg Esper

  2 Palliative and End-of-Life Care Perspectives, 19
     Mellar P. Davis and Kim K. Kuebler

  3 The Dying Process, 33
     Debra E. Heidrich

II IMPORTANT CONCEPTS IN PALLIATIVE AND END-OF-LIFE CARE

  4 Advance Care Planning and End-of-Life Decision Making, 49
     Crystal Dea Moore

  5 Ethical Issues Surrounding Advanced Disease, 63
     Agnes Coveney

  6 Spiritual Care Across Cultures, 75
     Charles Kemp

  7 Pharmacology, 85
     Phyllis A. Grauer

  8 Sleep, 111
     Catherine Vena

  9 Nutrition, 131
     Suzanne W. Dixon

III ADVANCED DISEASE MANAGEMENT

  10 Cardiovascular Disease, 153
      Carol L. Scot and Kim Anne Pickett

  11 Pulmonary Disease, 171
      Kim K. Kuebler and Rhalene Gabuat Patajo

  12 Hepatic Disease, 185
      Pamela Sue Spencer

  13 Chronic Kidney Disease, 191
      Michael J. Germain and Debra E. Heidrich

  14 Neurological Diseases, 201
      Debra E. Heidrich and Pamela Sue Spencer

  15 Malignancies, 215
      Debra E. Heidrich and Peg Esper

  16 HIV/AIDS, 233
      James C. Pace

IV   CLINICAL PRACTICE GUIDELINES

17   Anxiety, 245
Debra E. Heidrich and Peg Esper

18   Ascites, 259
Debra E. Heidrich

19   Bowel Obstruction, 269
Debra E. Heidrich and Pamela Sue Spencer

20   Cachexia and Anorexia, 279
Peg Esper

21   Constipation, 287
Debra E. Heidrich

22   Cough, 301
Jennifer Fournier

23   Dehydration, 315
Kim K. Kuebler and Valarie A. Pompey

24   Delirium and Acute Confusion, 327
Catherine Vena

25   Depression, 349
Peg Esper

26   Diarrhea, 361
Debra E. Heidrich

27   Dyspnea, 377
Kim K. Kuebler, Jerald M. Andry, and Shawn Davis

28   Fatigue, 395
Louise P. Meyer

29   Hiccups, 411
Peg Esper

30   Lymphedema, 417
Jane M. Armer and Sheila H. Ridner

31   Nausea and Vomiting, 431
Valarie A. Pompey

32   Pain, 447
Debra E. Heidrich and Peg Esper

33   Palliative Care Emergencies, 481
Roberta Kaplow

34   Pruritus, 503
Carol L. Scot

35   Ulcerative Lesions, 519
Elizabeth A. Ayello and Joy E. Schank

APPENDICES

A Caregiver Resources, 537
Crystal Dea Moore

B Clinician Resources and Assessment Tools, 541
Marilyn O'Mallon

Index, 551

UNIT I

GENERAL PRINCIPLES IN PALLIATIVE AND END-OF-LIFE CARE

THE ADVANCED PRACTICE NURSE IN PALLIATIVE CARE

Kim K. Kuebler, James C. Pace, and Peg Esper

■

Nursing is at the cornerstone in the care and management of patients living and dying from advanced disease. The advanced practice nurse who is either a clinical nurse specialist (CNS) or nurse practitioner (NP) has received additional education (graduate/doctoral) in areas related to medicine and advanced practice nursing. These areas include advanced knowledge and expertise in taking patient histories and performing physical examinations, ordering and interpreting diagnostics, and prescribing medications based on individual patient disease pathophysiology as well as pharmacokinetic, and pharmacodynamic metabolism. Differentiations between the CNS and NP are a result of educational preparation and focus, state practice acts, and specific practice settings, and are described in detail later in this chapter. The CNS and NP differ in their roles, and the majority of states within the United States identify these differing roles through state licensure and practice acts. For example, some states (e.g., Georgia) do not identify the CNS as an advance practice nurse and require registered nurse (RN) licensure without identifying an advanced practice title. In contrast, the majority of states in the United States require that the NP hold both an RN license and an NP license. Discussion on state-specific regulations is also described in further detail later.

A role-delineation study differentiating the CNS and NP was published by the American Nurses Association (ANA) and can be accessed at www.ana.org. The Oncology Nursing Society also completed a role-delineation study that differentiates the roles of the CNS and NP and has began to offer separate certification exams for these two roles (available at www.ons.org).

For the purposes of this chapter, the advanced practice nurse (APN) is identified as being either a CNS or an NP providing care and services to an adult patient population. It is with the understanding that the ANP is responsible for and has an active clinical management role in diagnosing, interpreting, and prescribing for individual patients in the palliative care setting. NPs are allowed to prescribe in all 50 states, whereas the CNS can currently prescribe in 30 states (available at www.nacns.org).

THE ROLE OF THE ADVANCED PRACTICE NURSE IN PALLIATIVE CARE

The APN who has undergone additional education in the care and management of adult patients is in an ideal position within the health care delivery team to ensure coordinated and continuous care for patients and families who are affected by chronic debilitating disease. While palliative care is appropriate for both adult and pediatric patients, the focus in this text is the adult patient and APNs who provide care to this patient population. APNs can serve as the conduit for the patient and family as they traverse the multiple dimensions associated with advanced disease. These dimensions include symptom burden, functional capabilities, communication patterns, and the psychoemotional and spiritual issues that interfere with quality of life.

The APN's ability to perform comprehensive physical evaluations, order and interpret diagnostics, and prescribe appropriate medications while receiving reimbursement allows this clinician to become a valuable and important member in the patient's plan of care (Kuebler, 2003). The APN can be instrumental when initiating palliative interventions throughout the patient's disease trajectory (from diagnosis until death), reducing symptoms and promoting a seamless care model that reduces a fragmentation of care (Davis, Walsh, LeGrand, et al., 2002; Kuebler, 2003). It is the coordination and continuous care provided by the APN throughout the disease course that can help to reduce patient abandonment and isolation from within the healthcare system.

APNs not only provide comprehensive palliative care in a continuous and coordinated fashion but can do this by offering the patient and family compassion along with skilled assessment, interventions, and ongoing evaluation throughout the course of advanced disease until death. This clinician meets the discipline recommendations in palliative care as defined by the World Health Organization (1990):

- Substantial body of knowledge
- Recognized skill sets requested in consultation and clinical practice
- Evidence-based practice, a result of disseminated research data in peer review publications
- Development of professional organizations
- Growing number of APNs seeking training and additional education in the field
- Extensive bibliography

Davis and colleagues (2002) have further identified essential skills necessary for palliative care clinicians to include effective communication, informed decision making, competent management of clinical complications, symptom control, psychological care, care of the dying, and coordination of care (Davis et al., 2002). The APN who integrates palliative interventions into the patient's plan of care is able to incorporate these skills into practice. The APN is able to provide the patient with his or her advanced knowledge of pathophysiology, pharmacology (pharmacodynamic and pharmacokinetic metabolism), and the ability to use appropriate evidence-based interventions (Kuebler, 2003). The APN who is in a collaborative practice arrangement with a physician is able to manage the complex needs of the patient by ordering and interpreting diagnostics, prescribing appropriately, and identifying prognostic indicators that help to set the stage for caring conversations that may shift the goals of care from curative to palliative. The APN is able to identify, support, and make the appropriate referrals that address the multidimensional needs of the patient and family within communities (Kuebler, 2003).

DIFFERENTIATING THE ROLES OF THE ADVANCED PRACTICE NURSE

Today is an exciting time for APNs who are defining and influencing the care of individuals, families, and communities as well as nursing care delivery systems. Most healthcare systems acknowledge four major APN "specialties." The certified registered nurse anesthetist (CRNA), the certified nurse midwife (CNM), the clinical nurse specialist (CNS), and the nurse practitioner (NP). Each and every advanced practice specialty draws from the rich history of the discipline of nursing while addressing a different societal need for health care. For purposes of discussions related to palliative care, this section (and chapter) address the description and differentiation of the CNS and NP roles.

The Clinical Nurse Specialist

The CNS is an RN with a graduate degree (master's or doctoral degree) leading to preparation as a CNS. The CNS specializes in a particular care setting (critical care, home care, community care) as well as in a specific disease or health issue (diabetes, medical-surgical, pulmonary, trauma). The CNS is deemed a clinical expert in the application of theoretical principles and research-based knowledge in regard to this chosen area of specialization in setting and practice. The CNS's scope of practice is generally defined as encompassing three distinct spheres of influence (Lyon, 2005):
1. Patient/family (direct care)
2. Nursing personnel (advancing the practice of nursing)
3. Organizational/network of care (advancing the organizational management of care)

Practice is usually designated as within a specified interdisciplinary team (e.g., oncology services) or a particular service within an institutional setting (e.g., nursing services or department of internal medicine). Most often, it is the employer that defines the nature and scope of the CNS's sphere of influence, provides and funds the position either totally or in part, and determines how specific outcomes are to be evaluated and by whom. The National Association of Clinical Nurse Specialists (NACNS) (2004) statement on clinical nurse specialists practice and education defines the core competencies for the CNS in each of these core spheres. Additional direct and indirect care aspects of the CNS include indirect roles as consultant-liaison, staff advocate, peer educator, change agent, policy analyst, patient educator, product evaluator, researcher (to include contributing scholarship to the literature), supervisor, mentor, and community advanced practice nurse (Hawkins & Thibodeau, 2000). Currently, there is a shortage of CNSs across the country. During the 1990s, many hospitals and academic centers were pressured to downsize or eliminate CNS positions as a result of reductions in reimbursables to hospitals, the increased costs of care, and the "nonreimbursable" nature of many, if not most, CNS roles (Hawkins & Thibodeau, 2000).

Current challenges for APNs who function in CNS roles include the absence of standardized credentialing requirements for CNS practice that allow for uniformity across state lines. This has led to differing philosophies regarding the educational preparation for the CNS, a defined scope of practice (despite the development of core CNS "competencies"), whether a "second" license is needed for an expanded scope of practice to include prescriptive authority in some states, and how to ensure competence in specialty areas of practice where no current examination exists. There is an evolving need for the CNS to continue to contribute to the literature to support advance nursing practice with a focus on specific disease and care settings, outcomes evaluation based on nursing interventions (best practices) in patient care, and the systematic evaluation of evidence-based innovations in nursing practice. These contributions support the valuable role of the CNS and the impact that they can make on patient care (Lyon, 2005).

The Nurse Practitioner

NPs are usually defined by a specified patient population: family NP (FNP), adult NP (ANP), gerontology NP (GNP), women's health NP (WHNP), psychiatric-mental health NP (PMHNP), acute care NP (ACNP), and pediatric NP (PNP). NP curricula share certain core content areas (advanced pathophysiology, pharmacotherapeutics, advanced health assessment, research and theory development, role development) and then explore pertinent specialty content according to designated populations of need and interest. It is generally recognized that the primary activities/functions of the NP include screening, physical and psychosocial assessment by means of taking health histories and performing physical examinations, patient care management to include follow-up when deviations from the norm are detected, continuity of care, health promotion, problem-centered services related to diagnosis, identification and mobilization of resources, health education, and patient and group advocacy (Hawkins & Thibodeau, 2000). A key component of these functions is the management of pharmacologic therapeutics in all 50 states across all therapeutic specialties and in all locales (Towers, 1991) (Box 1-1). APN curricula are challenged to emphasize quality of care, financial as well as time-based productivity, evidence-based outcomes, and practice cost outcomes, while contributing to equity of care (Allan, 2005). Current challenges include the need to develop practice models that create effective evidence-based interventions for populations differing in terms of ethnicity, culture, gender, and geographic location.

Box 1-1	**Examples of Core Nurse Practitioner Competencies**

- Assists consulting physician with treatments and/or examinations
- Consults with physician regarding history, physical examination, assessment, and/or plan of care as needed and as required by protocol (protocol manual on file and duly signed by all parties)
- Dictates or writes clinic notes and any needed discharge summary
- Makes rounds with or in consultation with sponsoring physician
- Obtains health history and performs physical examinations
- Provides health counseling and guidance and instructions to patients regarding diet, medications, disease education, exercise, discharge plans, and follow-up care
- Performs procedures/treatments in consultation with physician with appropriate documentation of same
- Writes or issues orders that are authenticated by both NP and consulting physician
- Determines diagnostics and procedures necessary to augment physical findings and interprets laboratory, radiographic, and clinical data in planning the course of management
- Prescribes medications for patients according to the approved formulary and/or protocol (state dependent)
- Takes call for specified periods of time with physician backup and responds to emergencies within his or her professional limitations

For the past decade, there has been discussion related to singular titling of advanced practice roles with analysis of the commonalities and differences between the CNS and NP. Such titling takes into consideration educational preparation, regulatory issues to include core competencies, certifications, and state–related/defined practice allowances. By 1995, the umbrella "APN" title was accepted as nomenclature for the CNS, NP, CNM, and CRNA designations. The exclusive designation of one title that defines one entity in advanced nursing practice where CNS and NP roles are merged in some way awaits determination.

THE MACMILLAN NURSE

The historical and positive role that the Macmillan nurse has demonstrated throughout the British communities can easily be applied to that of the American APN providing palliative care. Macmillan nurses are posted throughout the United Kingdom; they are highly respected for their palliative care skills and in many ways are the public face of specialist palliative care in the United Kingdom (Skilbeck & Seymour, 2002).

The Macmillan nurse's key role is to influence patient care by providing direct and indirect services. Indirect services involve strategic and policy-making activities (e.g., administrative, legislative) that influence patient care. They accomplish this by empowering and supporting primary care providers by advising on and assessing the development of patient care plans and clinical practice and through teaching and education (Macmillan Cancer Support, 2006). Direct care offered by Macmillan nurses is at the request of primary care providers and usually occurs when individual patients present with complex problems that would require specialist nurse intervention in the management and planning of their care (Macmillan Cancer Support, 2006). The focus of this role is clinical expertise, education, research, and management, contributing to multidisciplinary activities in various settings (e.g., hospital, long-term care, community home care) (Jack, Oldham, & Williams, 2003).

The Macmillan nurse is a CNS who is required to demonstrate a range of abilities that include expertise in and knowledge of advanced disease management and clinical leadership skills that enable other health care professionals to develop palliative expertise. Effective and therapeutic communication skills are required to ensure that their knowledge and skills are passed on to primary care providers (Macmillan Cancer Support, 2006).

A study that evaluated Macmillan nursing outcomes in patients with advanced cancer (n = 26) revealed that Macmillan nurses provided important assistance to patients by facilitating clinical discussion between patient and physician during medical consultations. They participated in co-coordinating actions resulting from those discussions and navigating the patient and his or her family through the healthcare system (Corner, Halliday, Haviland et al., 2003). It was pointed out in this study that Macmillan nurses spent more time with patients and their caregivers, answering questions, explaining medical terminology, and assisting patients to feel more secure about their treatment and what was happening to them—along with understanding the rationale behind specific diagnostics and whether further investigations were necessary and/or how to understand the results of these findings. Macmillan nurses often serve as the intermediary between the medical treatment team and the patient (Corner et al., 2003).

The described role of the Macmillan nurse can be easily applied to the role of the APN in various care settings. However, the NP with a distinct medical management role in palliative care could also benefit by applying attributes used to describe the role of the Macmillan general practitioner (GP). The Macmillan GP is a primary care physician specially trained in palliative care (Macmillan Cancer Support, 2006).

The Macmillan GP in the United Kingdom serves as a facilitator to improve the care of patients with cancer by providing collaborative practice with physicians in primary, oncology, and palliative care settings (Macmillan Cancer Support, 2006). Aspects of this role that can be applied to the APN in palliative care include the following (Macmillan Cancer Support, 2006):

- Being an APN in active practice for at least 3 years, with clinical experience in managing patients with cancer and palliative care needs
- Showing an active interest in oncology and palliative care with a good understanding and awareness of the emerging cancer and palliative care evidence and strategies nationally and internationally
- Demonstrating interest in education and training in palliative care
- Having comprehensive interpersonal, communication, and presentation skills
- Working as a member of the multiprofessional (interdisciplinary) team, appreciating different roles and responsibilities of the team
- Maintaining skills and knowledge in cancer, internal medicine, and palliative care

Lessons Learned from Macmillan Nurses

The presence of palliative care in the United States is predominantly in the setting of end-of-life care—the APN's valuable role in this area of health care is not well understood, with little or no data to support the positive outcomes that can occur between the APN, patient, and family. Palliative care in general, and in nursing specifically, has been accompanied by a preoccupation with questions regarding the benefits that may arise from referral to a palliative care service, or to a nurse specialist, despite the long history of advocating outcomes in nursing research (Corner, Clark, & Normand, 2002). This may come from the analogy of medicine's evidence-based practice, which attempts to measure the impact of disease management on indicators of health outcomes (Corner et al., 2002). Therefore, the role of the APN in palliative care should reflect a genuine preoccupation with demonstrating the effectiveness of the care provided by APNs or whether a specialized palliative care service is of value (Corner et al., 2002). Macmillan nurses have been able to articulate and successfully demonstrate the value of their role in the care and management of patients living with and dying from advanced disease through clinical outcomes. APNs may consider applying the Macmillan nurse framework and the collection of clinical outcomes in their role as a palliative care provider in the United States. As APNs collaborate and clarify their roles in the provision of palliative care, they can aim to apply the best evidence to practice that can help to further inform and influence the development of policy and practice in palliative nursing. Clinical outcomes that will come from this role can further be used to correlate with conventional evidence to provide the best care for the patient and his or her family (Corner et al., 2002).

THE ROLE OF THE ADVANCED PRACTICE NURSE WITHIN THE INTERDISCIPLINARY TEAM

Ideally, all APNs work in team settings where a pooling of talent between and among a variety of professional staff members contributes to the holistic care of patients and families. APNs function independently in terms of their appointed roles and licensure stipulations but contribute interdependently with other team members to ensure seamless and comprehensive healthcare services across systems. The paradigm of the interdisciplinary team (IDT) is "we" where this pool of talent, knowledge, and skills contributes to gains in quality and productivity. Healthcare experts who are members of an IDT might include other medical providers (e.g., MD, NP, CNS, physician assistants [PAs], pharmacists, dietitians, RNs, social workers, occupational and rehabilitation specialists, chaplains, ancillary support service personnel, and community health care personnel). Serving as a team player necessitates functioning with maturity—respecting other professionals, sharing roles and responsibilities, promoting a spirit of cooperation and respect, and abandoning antagonism and conflict (the "us" versus "them" mentality as opposed to a needed spirit of cooperation and respect) (Venegoni, 2000).

Unfortunately, current reimbursement patterns foster the model where a single clinician is reimbursed without considering the skills and services rendered by additional providers or the specified needs of individuals and families. Changes in reimbursement patterns that provide for team-practice reimbursement rates are under consideration by certain payers. Such reimbursement mechanisms would identify substitutive services (where multidisciplinary clinicians offer the same services), supplemental services (multidisciplinary clinicians offer a core set of services plus additional or supplements), and complementary services (where multidisciplinary clinicians offer different services). Using this model, reimbursement is tied to *services* rather than to the discipline of the provider (Davis & Gilliss, 1998). It is therefore important for APNs who integrate unique provider skills into the care and management of patients in many therapeutic areas to collect the important outcomes data that demonstrate comprehensive, collaborative, coordinated, and cost-effective care.

THE ROLE OF THE ADVANCED PRACTICE NURSE IN DIVERSE SETTINGS

Data from the ANA place the number of advanced practice nurses in the United States at just under 100,000 (ANA, 2005). Approximately 58,000 APNs are certified through the American Nurses Credentialing Center (2005). The body of APNs is made up of NPs, CNSs, CNMs, and CRNAs. The American Medical Association estimates that there will be more than 106,500 NPs in the United States in 2006 (Heitz & Van Dinter, 2000). A greater emphasis has been placed on the integration of palliative care within the healthcare arena as a general construct, and the role of the APN in this setting has become an area of increased interest, focus, and research.

Nurses are in a unique position to provide interventions into the cascade of symptoms that patients often experience along the continuum of heath and illness, from birth until death. APNs with additional education and experience are even more uniquely qualified to have an impact on the care of these patients. The role of the APN is being addressed in legislative settings nationwide. Over 250 bills have been introduced in state legislatures across the country that address the practice of APNs, and approximately 20 bills have been enacted at the time of this writing (ANA, 2005).

Specifically focusing on the role of the NP, it is clear that these clinicians have found a place in almost every healthcare setting. This provides NPs with multiple opportunities to facilitate palliative care interventions. An example is the NP providing services for patients with end-stage renal failure. Many of these patients die before receiving hospice services—a result of chronic dialysis and an unwillingness to accept hospice care for fear of relinquishing ongoing dialysis. The NP in this setting has many challenges, which include the physical, spiritual, emotional, psychosocial, and ethical domains of providing care. It is important that these professionals have the resources available to address and meet the palliative care needs of this patient population. Currently, however, it is not uncommon for limited attention to be given to palliative care issues within established practice guidelines and protocols for chronic, life-limiting illnesses (Emnettm, Byock, & Twohig, 2002; Mast, Salama, Silverman et al., 2004).

The oncology NP can demonstrate a unique role in providing palliative care. Depending on the size and type of setting, the NP's day is filled with the urgent complaints made by patients experiencing symptoms related to therapy, managing clinical trials, and coordinating treatment plans. It is not uncommon, however, for this clinician to integrate palliative interventions into the management of patients receiving "noncurative" therapies. Many institutions do not have the luxury of an inpatient palliative care service or a palliative consultation service. As these patients move from aggressive therapy to treatments that are purely supportive, the NP has the opportunity to create seamless transitions for patients and their families. The NP can participate in the responsibility of managing the care of patients admitted to home hospice care—this intervention provides the patient with valuable continuity and coordination of care.

Regardless of the setting within which the APN practices, there are many opportunities for taking the lead to ensure quality palliative care for patients and their families. This need has been reiterated in the Clinical Practice Guidelines for Quality Palliative Care (National Consensus Project for Quality Palliative Care, 2004).

PROTOCOLS AND GUIDELINES: WHAT ARE THEY?

Guidelines

Guidelines are statements developed to provide practitioners and patients with information to assist in decision making regarding healthcare choices for specific clinical situations. They represent the culmination of experience, literature reviews, and state-of-the-art practice typically agreed on by consensus panels (Emanuel, Alexander, Arnold et al., 2004).

The ANA Social Policy Statement, revised in 1996, defined the four essential features of nursing practice (ANA, 1996a), to consider when developing practice guidelines:

- Attending to the full range of human experiences and responses to health and illness, without restriction—differing from the problem-focused approach
- Integrating objective data with knowledge gained from an understanding of the patient's or group's subjective experience

- Applying scientific knowledge to the processes of diagnosis and treatment
- Providing a caring relationship that facilitates health and healing

The ANA also maintains that "advanced practice registered nurses integrate education, research, management, leadership, and consultation into clinical roles, and they function in collegial relationships with nursing peers and other professionals and individuals who influence the health environment" (ANA, 1996b).

These elements of basic and advanced nursing practice are intermingled throughout specific clinical guidelines to improve the quality of life for those patients with a life-limited diagnosis (English & Yocum, 1998). While many APNs practice independently, many state regulations require a collaborative practice arrangement, written or verbal, agreed on between an APN and a physician. Palliative care often presents clinicians with challenges outside of the scope of practice and expertise of many nurses. It is therefore important for the APN to identify possible interdisciplinary resources, including a physician versed in palliative medicine along with other members of the interdisciplinary team, to address and support the multiple needs of the patient living with chronic debilitating disease.

These nursing elements encourage the APN to define and develop specific guidelines with a collaborative physician. A carefully developed practice agreement that includes practice guidelines between the APN and collaborating physician allows the APN to practice independently within the scope of nursing practice and without the need to adhere to a rigid, preset course of action. The APN has the ability to use his or her level of expertise, scope of practice, and continued relationship with the patient and family to provide individualized and compassionate care.

Protocols

Protocol is typically used within diplomatic circles but can also be applied to a variety of venues. Scientists have long used the term to define experiment or research designs. The dictionary defines *protocol* as a "correct code of conduct" (Yahoo Education, 2005).

In applying this definition to the APN's practice, it can be used as an agreed-on set of expectations that are carried out when performing a specific procedure or task or managing a specific disease and/or symptom. As previously mentioned, the APN's scope of practice is determined by the specific state practice act, institutional mandates, or both. Collaborative practice agreements (discussed later in this chapter) may also specify how protocols are utilized and incorporated into daily clinical practice.

The Use of Guidelines and Protocols in Clinical Decision Making

Guidelines and protocols should permit the practitioner to incorporate the use of sound clinical judgment when providing individualized patient care, as opposed to rigid adherence to a step-by-step process. A rigid "cookbook" approach to symptom management does not take into account the individual situation and the resultant needs and responses of the patient. The pharmacological management of frequently occurring symptoms in a patient with end-stage disease requires careful assessment, individualized sequential trials of therapy, and ongoing evaluation and monitoring. The management of any symptom requires patience, experience, and ongoing education with the patient and family. While this is true in all clinical situations, it is especially important in palliative and end-of-life care. Applying algorithms specific to an individual symptom such as pain, dyspnea, or delirium may not necessarily produce the desired outcome. While the use of algorithms and care maps should not be discouraged, careful attention should be given to individual patient and family variations, their responses, and the context of care.

Guidelines can help to facilitate care toward best known practices, based on the current evidence. They serve to decrease the variability in care and to improve quality (Emanuel et al., 2004; O'Connor, 2005). It is important to update clinical guidelines or protocols with the integration of current evidence-based interventions. Maintaining an ongoing knowledge of the current research provides the APN with state-of-the-art interventions (evidenced-based practice). The use of guidelines and protocols that incorporate proven therapies benefits patients in everyday practice without sole reliance on personal intuition or anecdotal experiences.

The APN in palliative care is exploring ways and means to embrace evidence-based practice with a model of practice that includes clinical state, setting, circumstances, research evidence, patient preferences, healthcare resources, and clinical expertise. APNs practice from guidelines and protocols that should be tied into the growing body of science that is defining and promoting the field of palliative medicine.

STATE PRACTICE GUIDELINES

Each state's individual nurse practice act determines the specific scope of practice for the APN. State nursing practice acts define the role and responsibilities for practicing APNs to include the following (Berry & Kuebler, 2002; Buppert, 1999; Kuebler & Moore, 2002):
- Participate in a collaborative practice arrangement with a physician
- Practice under specific protocols and/or guidelines or practice agreements regarding specific diagnosis, evaluation, and management of disease
- Licensure requirements and specialty certifications
- Prescribing responsibilities (prescriptive authority), the need for delegated prescribing, or whether there is a need for the APN to obtain a DEA (Drug Enforcement Agency) provider number
- Ability to obtain reimbursement under state Medicaid programs

The rules governing APN practice routinely come from the state board of nursing (Buppert, 1999). Often, the board of medicine is also involved in APN practice guidance. To learn about specific state rules, access the state board of nursing or seek information from the state nursing association. The American Academy of Nurse Practitioners (AANP) is a valuable resource for this information and can be accessed at www.aanp.org.

Collaborative Practice Arrangement

The Centers for Medicare and Medicaid Services (CMS) in 1998 amended the definition of collaboration to read as follows:

> Collaboration involves systemic formal planning and assessment and a practice arrangement that reflects and demonstrates evidence of consultation, recognition of statutory limits, clinical authority, and accountability for patient care, according to a mutual

agreement that allows the physician and the nurse practitioner to function as independent as possible (*Federal Register*, 1998).

Successful collaboration requires a re-thinking of the traditional medical hierarchical model of practice (Lysaught, 1986). In a collaborative practice arrangement, the APN and the physician can focus on a holistic approach to patient care. Collaborators are partners and not substitutes for one another who agree to ongoing participation in the patient's plan of care (Berry & Kuebler, 2002; Lysaught, 1986). Figure 1-1 provides an example of a collaborative practice arrangement between an independent NP and a collaborating physician.

It is important to note that regardless of specific state practice acts that do or do not require a collaborative practice arrangement, in order for the APN to submit for a federal Medicare reimbursement provider number, a physician must be identified in the application process. A consulting and supportive physician relationship provides medical direction in the event that the APN's clinical decision making occurs outside the scope of his or her practice (Buppert, 1999).

Delegate Prescriptive Authority

Currently in the United States, more than half of the states allow NPs to prescribe schedule II medications. Some of these states require a delegated authority, meaning that the collaborative physician delegates prescribing practices to the NP. Other states may limit prescribing practices to certain medication schedules (Kuebler, 2003). An example of a delegated prescribing arrangement is given in Figure 1-2.

REIMBURSEMENT ISSUES

The legislation that provided authorization for APNs to receive direct reimbursement for the provision of reimbursable Medicare services was passed under the Balanced Budget Act of 1997 and became effective in January 1998 (AANP, 2004). Since this time, ANPs have been providing reimbursable care for patients covered under Medicare Part B providers. Prior to this legislation, care was provided exclusively by physicians (AANP, 2004). Under this law, APNs may provide, order, and refer patients under their own PIN (personal identification number) and UPIN (universal provider identification number). The bill states that the services of the APN cannot be restricted by site and/or geographical areas. Under this new legislation, APNs are no longer limited to billing under the "incident to" clause, which suggests that the APN practice exclusively with an attending physician and provide clinical practice for stable follow-up patients, excluding any new patients or returning patients with a new problem (AANP, 2004). The incident-to billing arrangement will reimburse the collaborative physician at 100% reimbursement, whereas NPs who bill under their own PINs receive 85% of what physicians bill under the same reimbursable codes.

The PIN and UPIN numbers for all physicians and practitioners are being replaced by the NPI (national provider identifier). The objective for establishing an NPI is to assign a unique provider number to each provider of health care services. This will eliminate the need to use multiple numbers for billing and insurance purposes (Towers, 2004). It is anticipated that this new identification system will be used

Collaborative Care Concepts Inc.
COLLABORATIVE PRACTICE AGREEMENT
BETWEEN MD and NP

MISSION STATEMENT

Collaborative Care Concepts Inc. treats each individual patient with compassion, respect and individuality. We provide expert care and services based upon individual needs and resources. Clinical decision-making is done by placing each patient and family at the center of care and determined upon patient goals. Our services support the patient and family in collaboration with the healthcare team in providing comprehensive care. We strive to provide continuity and advocacy for all of our patients and their families while improving quality of life.

COLLABORATIVE PRACTICE ARRANGEMENT

Collaboration involves systemic formal planning, assessment and a practice arrangement that reflects and demonstrates evidence of consultation, recognition of statutory limits, clinical authority and accountability for patient care, according to a mutual agreement that allows the physician and the nurse practitioner to function independently as appropriate.

RESPONSIBILITIES OF THE ADULT NURSE PRACTITIONER (NP)

- Works in collaboration with MD
- Provides high-quality primary and palliative health care services within the accepted standards of the American Nurses Association and certified by the American Nurses Credentialing Center
- This includes:
  - Performs a comprehensive history and physical examination
  - Directs diagnosis/treatment of episodic and chronic health problems
  - Orders and interprets diagnostic studies pertinent to the patient's diagnosis
  - Refers to appropriate health care providers, such as home health care and/or physician specialists
  - Performs health screening and immunizations
  - Provides health care education and counseling
  - Performs follow-up for continuity of care
  - Provides home visits
  - Offers first-line response for common life-threatening injuries and acute illnesses
  - Maintains records and appropriate sharing/transfer information when clients are referred or transferred to another health care provider
  - Participates in publications, presentations and research to improve both education and improved quality of life for the patient with advanced illness

PROVISION FOR REFERRAL AND CONSULTATION

Upon consultation or referral the NP will provide a comprehensive physical examination, obtain a history and physical and collaborate with the patient's healthcare provider - when consulting on palliative interventions. The NP is responsible for obtaining and documenting consultations and care plan in the patient record.

Consultation options consist of telephone physician contact, referral to a clinic, physician's office, the acute care system or the local emergency room. Options are selected based upon the urgency and complexity of the presenting problem. If the NP is unsure of the appropriate disposition he or she is to consult with the collaborative physician regarding this matter. Referrals to medical specialists or other community health care providers are made by the NP should this be necessary.

Figure 1-1 Sample collaborative practice agreement.

RESOLUTIONS OF DISAGREEMENT BETWEEN NP AND MD

Should a disagreement arise between the NP and the collaborating physician regarding diagnosis and/or treatment, one or more of the following means may be used to resolve the disagreement:
- Refer to the current literature appropriate to the area in question
- Consult with other physicians and/or NPs

RESPONSIBILITES OF THE COLLABORATING PHYSICIAN

The responsibilities will include:
- Collaboration between MD and NP to provide primary and palliative health care services by following mutually approved protocols and/or reference texts that support evidenced based practice interventions.
- Delegate's prescriptive authority within the guidelines set by the Georgia Department of Licensing and Regulation of Health Care Professionals. Writes for schedule II medications as needed.
- Periodically review patient records, provide medical direction if needed and provide continuity to patients and their families should they require acute medical assessment and/or hospitalization.
- Be available for telephone and/or interactive consultation as needed.

Signature _____ Date _____
                MD

Signature _____ Date _____
                NP

Figure 1-1, cont'd Sample collaborative practice agreement.

throughout healthcare in compliance with the Health Insurance Portability and Accountability Act of 1996 (HIPAA) and regulations related to the transportability of provider data among various systems (Towers, 2004). Initiated on May 23, 2005, all healthcare providers can apply for their NPI; information on the process to obtain an NPI is available at http://nppes.cms.hhs.gov. As of July 1, 2005, a hard-copy application was made available (obtain at Web site provided). The requirement for use of the NPI in reimbursement transactions is planned for May 23, 2007, for individual

This is an agreement between Dr _____ and NP_____, that this agreement provide the NP with delegated prescriptive authority to prescribe medications for the management of specific diseases and any associated symptoms. This agreement is based upon state specific requirements. Class two medications are not considered appropriate for the NP within the state of Michigan. Therefore, I request that all requests for schedule II medication are made directly with me to meet patient need and demand. The prescribing of all medications is based upon current evidence to support the best patient outcome. Differences in agreement are covered under the collaborative practice agreement.

MD _____ Date _____

NP _____ Date _____

Figure 1-2 Delegated prescriptive authority.

providers and May 23, 2008, for small businesses (Towers, 2005). More valuable information about reimbursement can be obtained from the AANP Web site (www.aanp.org).

Medicare Prescription Drug Improvement and Modernization Act

The Medicare Prescription Drug Improvement and Modernization Act (MMA), better known as the Medicare Prescription Bill, included significant language influencing NP practice. After 2006, Medicare recipients without pharmaceutical coverage may want to enroll in the voluntary Medicare Endorsed Pharmaceutical Discount Programs made available through specific pharmacies and pharmaceutical companies (Towers, 2005). The APN may want to become familiar with the various options to explore with individual patients. An important component of this legislation is in the provision of direct reimbursement for serving in the capacity as primary provider for patients who are enrolled in the Medicare Hospice Benefit or in Medicare reimbursed skilled home care. Currently, NPs are not able to directly admit patients into hospice care (this requires two physicians who designate a limited prognosis of 6 months or less) or into the services of skilled home care. The NP, however, is able to seek reimbursement when providing services that reflect primary care management (Towers, 2005).

CONCLUSION

It is the APN who can provide the coordination and comprehensive care management that are often lacking for the patient and his or her family living with a chronic or life-limiting disease. APNs who provide services to adult patients can easily integrate their knowledge and skills into the assessment, management, and evaluation of symptoms that accompany advanced disease from diagnosis until death in multiple settings. Identifying and managing the multidimensional needs of the patient and family make the APN a unique professional on the health care delivery team who is able to collaborate with other providers, make appropriate referrals (psychosocial, spiritual, individual specialists), and engage the patient and family in meaningful conversations that include care options and modifications in advance care planning.

APNs who integrate palliative interventions throughout the trajectory of disease can help the patient and family to better understand prognostic indicators that may suggest a needed shift in care from curative to palliative in nature. It is this coordination of care and patient and family familiarity with the APNs that supports a reduction in a fragmented and less costly care delivery. Lack of coordination comes at a high cost, and it is in the delivery and the collection of palliative clinical outcomes that the APN can demonstrate value within the current reimbursement structure.

APNs have the potential to define, demonstrate, and differentiate their roles and influence patient outcomes when palliative care is utilized. Applying the best evidence and collecting important outcome data that identify patient quality of life through functional capabilities, reduction in symptom burden, access to supportive services, and cost effectiveness will make this provider a leader in the provision and practice of palliative care.

Box I-2	Additional Resources

Agency for Healthcare Research and Quality
www.ahrq.gov

Agency for Healthcare Research and Quality National Guideline Clearinghouse
www.guideline.gov

American Academy of Nurse Practitioners
www.aanp.org

American College of Nurse Practitioners
www.nurse.org/acnp/index.shtml

Federal Register **rules and updates**
www.epa.gov/earth1r6/6en/w/offshore/permit11021998.pdf

National Association of Clinical Nurse Specialists
www.nacns.org

Nurse Practitioner Central
www.npcentral.net

Reimbursement realities for advanced practice nurses
www.nursing.umn.edu/professional/reimbursement

REFERENCES

Allan, J. (2005). *The nurse practitioner: A look at the future.* In J. Stanley (Ed.). *Advanced nursing practice* (2nd ed., pp. xxviii-xxx). Philadelphia: Davis.

American Academy of Nurse Practitioners. (2004). *Medicare reimbursement fact sheet.* Washington, DC: Author, Office of Health Policy. Retrieved May 14, 2006, from www.aanp.org.

American Nurses Association. (1996a). *A social policy statement.* Washington, DC: American Nurses Publishing.

American Nurses Association. (1996b). *Scope and standards of advanced practice registered nursing.* Washington, DC: American Nurses Publishing.

American Nurses Association. (2005). *Government affairs—Summary of state legislation related to APRNs.* Retrieved August 10, 2005, from www.nursingworld.org/member/gova/aprns05.cfm.

American Nurses Credentialing Center. (2005). *Frequently asked questions about ANCC certification.* Retrieved August 18, 2005, from www.nursingworld.org/ancc/certification/certfaqs.html.

Berry, P. & Kuebler, K. (2002). The advanced practice nurse in end-of-life care. In K. Kuebler, P. Berry, & D. Heidrich, D. (Eds.). *End-of-life care clinical practice guidelines* (pp. 3-14). Philadelphia: Saunders.

Buppert, C. (1999). State regulation of nurse practitioner practice. In Buppert, C. (Ed.). *Nurse practitioner's business practice & legal guide* (pp. 104-110). Gaithersburg, Md.: Aspen.

Corner, J., Clark, D., & Normand, C. (2002). Evaluating the work of the clinical nurse specialists in palliative care. *Palliat Med, 16,* 275-277.

Corner, J., Halliday, D., Haviland, J., et al. (2003). Exploring nursing outcomes for patients with advanced cancer following intervention by Macmillan specialist palliative care nurses. *J Adv Nurs, 41,* 561-574.

Davis, L. & Gilliss, C. (1998). Primary care and advanced practice nursing: Past, present, and future. In C.M. Sheehy & M.C. McCarthy (Eds.). *Advanced practice nursing: Emphasizing common roles* (pp. 114-136). Philadelphia: Davis.

Davis, M., Walsh, D., LeGrand, S. (2002). End-of-life care: The death of palliative medicine [Editorial]. *J Palliat Med, 5,* 813-814.

Emanuel, L., Alexander, C., Arnold, R.M., et al. (2004). Integrating palliative care into disease management guidelines. *J Palliat Med, 7,* 774-783.

Emnettm J., Byock, I., & Twohig, J.S. (2002). *Pioneering practices in palliative care.* Publication produced by Promoting Excellence in End-of-Life Care. Retrieved July 26, 2005 from www.promotingexcellence.org/apn.

English, N. & Yocum, C. (1998). *Guidelines for curriculum development on end-of-life and palliative care in nursing education.* Arlington, Va.: National Hospice and Palliative Care Organization.

Federal Register. November 2, 1998, 63(211).

Hawkins, J. & Thibodeau, J. (2000). Advanced practice roles in nursing. In J. Hawkins & J. Thibodeau (eds.). *The advanced practice nurse* (5th ed., pp. 7-40). New York: Tiresias.

Heitz, R. & Van Dinter, M. (2000). Developing a collaborative practice agreement. *J Pediatr Health Care, 14,* 200-203.

Jack, B., Oldham, J., & Williams, A. (2003). A stakeholder evaluation of the impact of the palliative care clinical nurse specialist upon doctors and nurses, within an acute hospital setting. *Palliat Med, 17,* 283-288.

Kuebler, K. (2003). The palliative care advanced practice nurse. *J Palliat Med, 6,* 707-714.

Kuebler, K. & Moore, C. (Eds.). (2002). *The Michigan advanced practice nursing palliative care self-training modules.* Lansing, Mich.: Michigan Department of Community Health: Module Nine.

Lyon, B.L. (2005). Clinical nurse specialists: Current challenges. In J. Stanley (Ed.). *Advanced nursing practice* (2nd ed., pp. xxv-xxviii), Philadelphia: Davis.

Lysaught, J. (1986). Retrospect and prospect in joint practice. In Steel, J. (Ed.). *Issues in collaborative practice* (pp. 15-33). Orlando, Fla.: Grune & Stratton.

Macmillan Cancer Support. Retrieved May 14, 2006, from www.macmillian.org.uk.

Mast, K.R., Salama, M., Silverman, G. K. (2004). End-of-life content in treatment guidelines for life-limiting diseases. *J Palliat Med, 7,* 754-773.

National Association of Clinical Nurse Specialists (NACNS). (2004). *Statement on clinical nurse specialist practice and education.* Harrisburg, Pa.: Author. Retrieved May 14, 2006, from www.nacns.org.

National Consensus Project for Quality Palliative Care. (2004). National Consensus Project for Quality Palliative Care: Clinical practice guidelines for quality palliative care, executive summary. *J Palliat Med, 7,* 611-617.

O'Connor, P.J. (2005). Adding value to evidence-based clinical guidelines. *JAMA, 294,* 741-743.

Skilbeck, J. & Seymour, J. (2002). Meeting complex needs: An analysis of Macmillan nurses' work with patients. *Int J Palliat Nurs, 8,* 574-582.

Towers, J. (2004). Medicare Modernization Act (MMA): *Are you utilizing its provisions?* (September, pp. 5-6) Washington, DC: American Academy of Nurse Practitioners, Academy Update Office of Health Policy.

Towers, J. (2005). *National provider identifier implementation begins* (June, p. 8). Washington, DC: American Academy of Nurse Practitioners, Academy Update Office of Health Policy.

Venegoni, S.L. (2000). Healthcare delivery systems and environments of care. In J.V. Hickey, R.M. Ouimette, & S.L. Venegoni (Eds.), *Advanced practice nursing: Changing roles and clinical applications* (2nd ed., pp. 151-174). Philadelphia: Lippincott Williams & Wilkins.

World Health Organization. (1990). *Cancer pain relief and palliative care* (p. 804). Technical Report Series. Geneva: Author.

Yahoo Education. (2005). *Definitions.* Retrieved August 10, 2005, from http://education.yahoo.com/reference/dictionary/entry/protocol.

CHAPTER 2

PALLIATIVE AND END-OF-LIFE CARE PERSPECTIVES

Mellar P. Davis and Kim K. Kuebler

∎

CURRENT TRENDS

The April 21, 2005, cover story from *USA Today* touted that the "U.S. is getting old fast, seniors will out number school-age children in many states by 2030, the Census Bureau says in a report out today. That promises to intensify the political tug-of-war between young and old for scarce resources" (El Nasser, 2005). This article reviewed the recent population predictions by the U.S. Census Bureau that identified which states will have the largest elderly population growth over the next 25 years. "As you reach the end of life the last year or last two years—the use of medical care is very intense" (Cauchi, 2005, p. 3A). Most states are worried about access and utilization of state Medicaid funding as the Baby Boomers age and place more healthcare demands upon limited resources. Another front page article printed in the February 24, 2005 *USA Today* reported, "Health care tab ready to explode, costs could be 19% of total economy by 2014" (Appleby, 2005). Growth in healthcare spending will outpace economic growth through the next decade. By 2014, the nation's spending for healthcare will equal $11,045 per person, up from $6,423 per person in 2005 (Appleby, 2005).

Yet another news release from June 15, 2005, reports that older Americans are less willing to sacrifice physician/hospital choice to save costs (Cassil, 2005). Elderly Americans are much less willing than are working-age Americans to limit their choice of physicians and hospitals to save on out-of-pocket medical costs (Cassil, 2005). The U.S. Department of Health and Human Services (DHHS) has projected that, by 2013, the enrollment share of Medicare managed care plans will increase by 30% from the current level of 12% (Cassil, 2005).

These newsworthy reports parallel the issues that will affect the care of patients living with chronic disease over the next several decades. By 2030, for the first time in history the old will outnumber the young; by 2010, the oldest of the Baby Boomers will reach the age of 65. Not only will there be an increase in older people, but also more people will be living longer with chronic disease (DHHS, 2002; Lynn & Adamson, 2003). Currently, the leading causes of death in the United States are cancer, heart disease, stroke, chronic obstructive pulmonary disease, and dementia (DHHS, 2002; Lynn & Adamson, 2003). Chronic diseases are symptomatic, are progressive, and can interfere with the patient's functional ability and quality of life.

It is here where palliative care can help to support the care of symptomatic patients, improve quality of life, and provide care options that focus on comfort versus cure in a disease that is no longer curable. Palliative care clinicians understand the importance of partnering with traditional care and offering to serve as the conduit between all providers while maintaining patient and family goals of care and providing the coordination, continuity, and cost-effective care that is often lacking in this patient population.

Because the majority of the palliative care programs have been initiated in the oncology setting, this has restricted palliative interventions into the management of chronic debilitating nonmalignant diseases (Kuebler, Lynn, & Von Rohen, 2005). Patients with other diseases such as heart failure and emphysema can also benefit by the knowledge and skills of the palliative care clinician and the comprehensiveness and reliability of palliative care programs (Kuebler et al., 2005). This chapter provides a historical overview of the field of palliative care. It briefly touches on the definitions associated with *supportive, palliative, end-of-life*, and *hospice care*. The advanced practice nurse (APN) providing services to the patient and family who are facing a limited prognosis is in an ideal position to apply the philosophy of palliative care to the care of the patient from diagnosis until death and to recognize when to consider supportive services such as hospice care.

DIFFERENTIAL TERMS AND HISTORICAL PERSPECTIVES

Preceding World War II, the specialty of oncology was divided into surgery, immunology, and endocrinology (Seymour, Clark, & Winslow, 2005). The majority of patients, however, often presented with advanced malignancy; the availability of palliative treatments within the traditional care system were rare, and prescribed opioids were limited for fear of hastening death, precipitating addiction, and producing euphoria (Seymour et al., 2005).

During this era, suffering at the end of life was perceived as a test of spiritual and psychological character. There were a few community-based studies during this time, highlighting the degree of suffering in individual patients. Despite patient suffering, the investigators did not recommend a change in policy or an evaluation of or change in practice patterns (Seymour et al., 2005). Some studies recommended that prescribers consider earlier use of opioids but do so with trepidation (Seymour et al., 2005). Peer reviewed papers found in medical publications during this time that documented the physical, mental, and emotional distress associated with dying generated limited, if any, medical interest in the care of the dying patient (Hinton, 1963).

History of Cancer Pain Management

The modern techniques to manage cancer pain were developed in the 1950s and 1960s and primarily focused on a biomedical approach versus the patient-centered holistic approach common today. The biomedical philosophy was based on the belief that there is a linear relationship between pain and the patient's perception of his or her pain (Seymour et al., 2005). Pain was often viewed as an indicator of disease, and little attention was given to the patient's complaint of pain and how it interfered with quality of life. Physicians focused on disease management as opposed to the patient's perception of his or her symptoms (Seymour et al., 2005). Dr. Wall, a pioneer in the field of pain management, cleverly articulated the approach to symptom management during this time as the following: "In the course of this new direction, symptoms were placed on one side as a sign post along a highway which was driven towards the intended destination. Therapy directed at the sign post was denigrated and dismissed as merely symptomatic" (Wall, 1986, p. 1). Therefore, the frequent use of cordotomy, rhizotomy, and myelotomy was preferred and sought as a means of relieving pain, with opioids often held until the very end of life.

BEGINNING WINDS OF CHANGE

In 1958, Cicely Saunders from the United Kingdom and John Bonica from the United States simultaneously participated in separate prospective observational studies of patients living with and dying from advanced disease and their medical management. These investigators identified two common myths held by healthcare providers caring for this patient population regarding the management of cancer-related pain (Meldrum, 2005; Wall, 1997):

- Opioids are inevitably addicting.
- Opioids should be administered only with long dosing intervals.

Saunders and Bonica, however, regarded pain and suffering as an integral part of the daily responsibilities of the physician and nurses providing patient care. These pain management leaders took the initial and controversial stance that opioids were essential in the successful management of cancer-related pain (Meldrum, 2005; Seymour et al., 2005). Saunders' first publication in 1958 outlined a philosophy of care that highlighted a holistic, multidimensional, patient-centered approach to pain and symptom management. This philosophy of care continues to provide the framework on which the hospice and palliative care movement is built. This care model includes the following key concepts (Seymour et al., 2005):

- The role of the physician should be to accompany the dying patient.
- All caregivers involved in the patient's care should enter into and help to support the patient's inner resources for his or her comfort.
- Physicians and nurses should apply the knowledge and science accumulated from evidence-based research and practice to provide relief and comfort for the dying patient and his or her family.

St. Christopher's Hospice

Saunders' initial work began at St. Joseph's Hospice in London in 1958 and continued for 7 years. During this time, Saunders recorded detailed regimens of oral and regular opioid treatments, developed symptom management protocols when newly developed medications became available, listened and recorded conversations with patients, traveled, lectured, and authored extensively on the importance and value of opioid interventions in the management of cancer-related pain (Saunders, 2001). On one of her many trips to the United States, she became acquainted with Dr. Raymond Houde from Memorial Sloan-Kettering Cancer Institute in New York City. Houde had designed and participated in many clinical crossover trials involving various opioids in the management of cancer-related pain (Meldrum, 2005). Saunders embraced the value of rigorous research designs and positive clinical outcomes associated with research trials that could promote the selection and utilization of opioid medications in the management of patients with cancer pain. She then brought opioid research to St. Joseph's Hospice and later to St. Christopher's, both designated as demonstration sites. The positive research findings further confirmed Saunders' assertions regarding the effective and safe use of routine opioids in the management of cancer-related pain (Meldrum, 2005).

The initial collaborative opioid studies took place between St. Christopher's Hospice in the United Kingdom and Memorial Sloan-Kettering in the United States. Their combined published papers within the peer reviewed literature became the cornerstone in the foundation to the first World Health Organization (WHO) guidelines on cancer care management in 1982 (Meldrum, 2005).

This new approach to pain management through the utilization of opioids revealed that the methods used for pain control were simple and widely transferable from patient care settings, including the home environment (Saunders, 2001). St. Christopher's became a preeminent clinically based, multidiscipline educational program. Clinicians often took sabbaticals at St. Christopher's to become skilled and knowledgeable about the care and management of patients living with and dying from advanced malignancies. Many of the initial clinicians from St. Christopher's took their newfound skills into the development of the earlier programs such as the Connecticut Hospice, Calvary Hospital, and the Royal Victoria Hospital in Montreal, Canada (Saunders, 2001).

St. Christopher's Hospice, located in London, opened in 1967 with 54 patients, a 16-bed residential wing for the elderly, child care for the staffs' children, a chapel for spiritual care, and planned bereavement services. Home care for home-bound patients began in 1969 and soon became the dominant focus of care (Saunders, 2001). As St. Christopher's became recognized and sought after in the care of ill cancer patients, the inpatient-to-outpatient ratio became 1:10 (Saunders, 2001).

Palliative Medicine

The successful demonstration projects initiated at St. Joseph's Hospice and St. Christopher's led to the establishment of palliative medicine as a medical subspecialty in 1987. Practitioners in New Zealand, Australia, and the United Kingdom took the lead in establishing this medical specialty (Saunders, 2001). Palliative medicine today is a direct result of Saunders' international travels, strong basic and clinical research studies, disseminated data, collaboration among multiple disciplines, and application of the reigning philosophy of "living until you die" (Saunders, 2001).

Saunders' efforts, however, were not without several pitfalls that occurred along the road of hospice and palliative medicine development. The elitism, perfectionism, and protests from "conventional" care providers delayed and alienated important links to the palliative medicine movement (Saunders, 2001). The initial focus of palliative medicine was predominantly on cancer care, which further led to delays in accepting the challenges associated with other diseases such as human immunodeficient virus/acquired immunodeficiency syndrome (HIV/AIDS), chronic heart failure, chronic obstructive pulmonary disease, and amyotrophic lateral sclerosis. Today, however, these diseases have been integrated into the overview of palliative medicine.

CHALLENGES TO THE FUTURE OF PALLIATIVE MEDICINE

The ongoing reductionism and subspecialization that originates from Western medicine in the twenty-first century will challenge the ability to maintain the "whole person" concept of care. The explosion of HIV/AIDS in developing countries will prompt an urgent need to shorten the gap in basic palliative care between developed and developing countries (Saunders, 2001). There is a need to standardize palliative practices, and the routine utilization of psychometrically valid and reliable symptom assessment and quality of life instruments can help to identify outcomes for patients who receive palliative interventions. Palliative care clinicians could learn from Saunders' original methods of listening, recording, observing, and measuring specific interventions. Palliative care clinicians should develop the skills and knowledge that are associated with appreciating and understanding the spiritual, social, and psychologic stress that patients experience with a life-limiting disease—and the impact that this has on the family or loved ones.

Current Palliative Care Trends

There is much activity to develop, validate, and promulgate symptom guidelines. This work is often derived from academic centers and transferred to community-based practices. However, these guidelines should be portable, simple, affordable, and effective. Palliative services should be considered as an extension of care to all patients with advanced disease and not reserved for the dying (Davis, Walsh, LeGrand et al., 2002). Palliation should begin prior to the end of life. This concept has been endorsed by the WHO revised definition of palliative care (Sepulveda et al., 2002): whereas palliative care

> ... is applicable early in the course of disease, in conjunction with other therapies that are intended to prolong life, such as chemotherapy or radiation therapy, and includes those investigations needed to better understand and manage distressing clinical complications (WHO, 2002).

Often, the aims that palliative care offer to the patient and family differ from the aims of treatment used in curative care (Widder & Glawisching-Goschnick, 2002). Clinicians, however, should consider integrating palliative interventions into the traditional disease-modifying plan of care. For example, discussions with the patient and his or her family that describe and discuss disease-modifying therapies should also include descriptions of and discussions on the integration of palliative interventions that can be used to improve the patient's symptom profile and quality of life (Kuebler et al., 2005). Therefore, disease-modifying care (curative care) and palliative care can and should occur simultaneously and routinely. This allows clinicians to modify the course of disease management whenever possible by increasing the intensity of palliative interventions when the patient becomes symptomatic and all medical therapeutics in reversing underlying pathophysiology have been exhausted (Kuebler et al., 2005).

DEFINITION OF TERMS

Palliative care, supportive care, end-of-life, and *hospice care* are terms that are frequently used interchangeably. Yet, hospice and end-of-life care are distinctly different from the others. While hospice and end-of-life care are always a part of palliative care and/or supportive care, the reverse is not always true (Kuebler et al., 2005). The following discussion identifies the differences and similarities associated with these terms.

Supportive Care

The cure for cancer remains below 50% for all patients who present with cancer, and cancer accounts for more than 25% of all deaths in the United States (Browner & Carducci, 2005). Therefore, the evaluation and successful management of symptoms that accompany malignancy can help to define how well the patient lives with his or her disease (Cherny, Catane, & Kosmidis, 2003). Supportive care and its associated interventions are often used concurrently with traditional disease management to effectively manage the symptoms associated with a diagnosis of cancer or other advanced diseases (Cherny et al., 2003). *Supportive care* has been defined as optimizing comfort, improving function, maintaining social support, and minimizing the adverse effects of antitumor therapy during active cancer treatments (Cherny et al., 2003).

The National Institute for Clinical Excellence (NICE) guidelines in supportive and palliative care identified and described 13 characteristics associated with supportive care (Box 2-1). The rationale associated with defining these supportive care characteristics includes the following (Thomas & Richardson, 2004) points:

- There is a wide variation in the quality of care from institution to institution.
- Services are not universally available.
- The needs of patients often go unrecognized throughout the course of disease.
- Supportive services are generally multidisciplinary and there is a lack of interprofessional communication and coordination.

Box 2-1	**Key Elements to Supportive Services (National Institute for Clinical Excellence Model)**

1. Coordination of care
2. Patient views and values are ascertained during the development of supportive services
3. Face-to-face communication
4. Information that includes options at each pathway of care and free information services (verbal, written, or video) sensitive to culture, education, spiritual, and language needs
5. Psychological supportive services
6. Social supportive services
7. Spiritual supportive services
8. Palliative care services (general)
9. Specialists in palliative care services
10. Rehabilitation services
11. Complementary services
12. Social services for families and caregivers
13. Workforce development for supportive and palliative services

Data from Cherny, N. (2003). European Society of Medical Oncology (ESMO) joins the palliative care community. *Palliat Med, 17*, 475-476.

Supportive and palliative care services are by no means components of or exclusive of one another. Both are "highly patient-oriented approaches and dependent on each other like Siamese twins and each are important in the education and clinical practice of optimal comprehensive cancer care" (Senn & Glaus, 2002). Supportive care is perhaps the least well-defined label given to the treatment of symptoms and palliation (Kuebler et al., 2005). The supportive care label in oncology includes therapies that support patients through antineoplastic therapies. Supportive care specialists have made notable strides in the management of treatment related complications, including chemotherapy-induced nausea and vomiting, mucositis, growth, factors for myelosuppression and anemia, and bisphosphonates for bone-related complications (Body, 2003; Desai & Demetri, 2005; Gralla et al., 2005; Senn & Glaus, 2002).

Antibiotic transfusion services and psycho-oncology, although older in existence than "target-specific" supportive therapies, are nonetheless important for good supportive care. Finally, nutrition support provided for those who have lost weight due to lack of calories rather than for cancer cachexia should be considered as part of supportive services (MacDonald, 2003).

Palliative Care in Palliative Medicine

Palliative medicine is the medical subspecialty within internal medicine that combines supportive care with the medical management of disease-modifying therapy (Byock, 2000). Seven skill sets have been identified to successfully provide palliative medicine; they include the following (Davis et al., 2002):

- Effective communication
- Patient-centered decision making appropriate for the stage of disease and condition of the patient
- Management of cancer or nonmalignant disease complications
- Symptom control
- Psychosocial and spiritual care
- Care of the dying (end-of-life care)
- Coordination of care and continuity

Palliative care (the practice of palliative medicine) is not a time-confined but rather a goal-oriented and patient-centered care delivery model (Davis et al., 2002). Palliative medicine is preventive in that early interventions prevent and improve poorly managed pain and other symptoms, improve communication patterns between patient and providers, reduce a discontinuous or fragmented care approach, and reduces psychosocial or spiritual suffering that is amplified if left untreated in the dying process (Davis et al., 2002; MacDonald, 2003). Palliative medicine has become a recognized subspecialty with a substantial body of peer-reviewed literature, a growing number of physicians entering the field, ongoing clinical research, and disseminated data (Davis et al., 2002).

The WHO's first definition of palliative care appeared in 1990, and the modified version of this definition was published in 2000. The 1990 definition emphasizes control of symptoms but identifies the potential for earlier application of the principles of palliative care, whereas the current definition stresses the preeminence of the prevention of suffering achieved through either eliminating the anticipated causes of suffering (e.g., use of bowel hygiene when placing patients on opioid therapies) or treating the cause of distress at onset to prevent or slow progression (e.g., development of delirium, increased pain, or functional loss) (MacDonald, 2005).

The palliative philosophy of care, as embraced by the Last Acts Palliative Care Task Force (2004), The National Hospice and Palliative Care Organization (NHPCO, 2006), WHO (2002), and the Center to Advance Palliative Care (CAPC, 2006), includes the following elements:

- Provides relief from pain and other distressing symptoms, reducing the symptom burden
- Identifies death as a normal process, neither hastened nor postponed
- Recognizes that the dying process is profoundly individualized and occurs within the dynamics of the family
- Enhances the quality of life by recognizing and integrating interventions for the physical, psychological, social, and spiritual dimensions of the patient
- Utilizes the multidisciplinary team to address the multiple needs of the patient and family; this includes bereavement counseling if needed
- Enhances quality of life and may positively influence the course of disease
- Applies evidence-based practice to support appropriate interventions that improve patient quality of life

Palliative Care Programs

"For a health care system whose essential motivation is based on curing the sick, the treatment of the chronically ill is not very satisfying ... there is a paradox of everyone agreeing on the importance of research and prevention, yet continuing to increase disproportionately the amount spent on treating existing illness," wrote the Canadian government in a report (Lalonde Report, 2004). The accelerating population of the aging are living longer with advanced (chronic) disease; this has created an impetus in both Canada and the United States in placing most of the health care resources on the treatment of fatal conditions, which in many instances could have been prevented (MacDonald, 2005). The demonstration of palliative care has never come at a more important time. Oncology settings have set the stage for palliative care programs. As more programs develop across the United States, there is an increasing need for standards and competencies that will promote the best care possible. The integration of palliative medicine into comprehensive cancer centers in the United States not only is a requirement for being identified as a center of excellence but has been successfully accomplished (Ahmedzai et al., 2004).

A WHO Demonstration Project, the Harry R. Horvitz Center for Palliative Medicine at the Cleveland Clinic Foundation, is a comprehensive integrated program that includes hospice consultation services, an outpatient clinic, acute care inpatient services, hospice and home care services, and hospice inpatient services (Walsh, 2001). The Cleveland Clinic palliative medicine program assumes primary care management for the patient while undergoing chemotherapy or radiation therapy. The advantages include (1) multiple points of access and day-to-day assessment and management prevent untoward symptoms; (2) expertise for these complex and often highly symptomatic patients; and (3) reduction in the patient's symptom burden, which improves quality of life and reduces the cost associated with seeking multiple providers (Lagman & Walsh, 2005).

Palliative services should be evaluated by the same standards economically, administratively, and philosophically as any other medical service. The net financial impact of an acute medicine unit can be the same as that of an oncology unit (Davis, Walsh, & Nelson, 2001; Lagman & Walsh, 2005). Other palliative medicine programs aside from the Cleveland Clinic Program include the M. D. Anderson Cancer Center, which was initiated in 1999 and opened an inpatient unit in 2003. Other programs, such as those of Northwestern University, University of Wisconsin, and the National Cancer Institute, among others, are active and integrated into a comprehensive cancer center. These programs are dedicated to (1) hospitalwide service with consultation, (2) physicians trained in palliative medicine, (3) multidisciplinary care, (4) continuity, (5) strong commitment to educating clinicians in palliative medicine, and (6) research and desire to advance the discipline of palliative care (CAPC, 2006; Lagman & Walsh, 2005).

The CAPC (2006) has developed standardized aspects of palliative care that have been endorsed by multiple national organizations, and these standards may be considered in any setting adapting a palliative medicine program.

Similarities and Differences

As a result of the palliative medicine centers of excellence, national professional organizations/associations, and federal and state attention to this needed area of medicine—a new standard of care has been determined that integrates palliative interventions into traditional medicine. This mixed management model combines the benefit of palliative and/or supportive care with traditional (curative) care and is focused on treatments for comfort, individual coping, and maintaining quality of life (Bomba, 2005; Browner & Carducci, 2005; Byock, 2000; Choi & Billings, 2002). This model has been extended to nonmalignant life-limiting disease such as heart failure, pulmonary obstructive disease (COPD), and others (Davis et al., 2005; Hauptman & Havranek, 2005; Pantilat & Steimle, 2004) This new paradigm provides for the continuum to range from aggressive curative care to comfort care, and allows for parallel management from diagnosis to death—supporting coordination, continuity, and cost effectiveness (Browner & Carducci, 2005).

The term *palliative medicine*, however, should not be used synonymously or confused with end-of-life care. To "broadcast that palliative care is about caring for the dying simply reinforces (that the physician should only refer patients) when they are actively dying" (Woodruff, 2002). *End-of-life care* is a quantitative term that excludes the purpose of care and fails to recognize the skill sets inherent in good palliative medicine (Davis et al., 2002). *End-of-life care* is a term that does not adequately describe the patients who have a high case mix index with complex problems requiring the skills for effective palliation. It advertises interest in only the imminently dying and encourages a discontinuous rather than a parallel or mixed care model (Davis et al., 2002).

When patients and their families have exhausted all treatments to reverse the life-limiting disease and all therapies modifying the disease have failed, the patient who has not received palliative care prior to this cross in the road may be highly distressed and symptomatic. Because the patient is close to the end of his or her life, he or she may be referred to an end-of-life care specialist. If Saunders describes optimal palliative services as encouraging patients to "live until they die," then the term *end-of-life services* does little to promote this.

HOSPICE AND END-OF-LIFE CARE

Florence Wald, dean at the School of Nursing at Yale University, New Haven, Connecticut, is considered the mother of the American hospice movement. In 1963, she invited Saunders to give a series of lectures throughout the communities of New Haven. These lectures and associated conversations lead to a seminal event and establishment of The Connecticut Hospice in 1974 (Saunders, 1999). Since this time, Wald's observations have been apropos to the current structure of hospice care. "Hospices grew throughout the nation first as a grass roots healthcare reform effort. Later healthcare and governmental planners became increasingly convinced of the financial as well as the quality of life benefits. Consumers grew to understand that they had the right to influence the quality of their remaining life. Ethical and philosophical values regarding self-determination, family and staff support, dignity, and interdisciplinary team responsibility lead to the change in perception of what patients and families should receive from healthcare providers" (Foster & Corless, 1999, p. 12).

Many of Wald's beliefs and her advocacy for end-of-life care can be associated with the European Society of Medical Oncologists' core principles in end-of-life care (2003) (Box 2-2).

In the 1994 Standards of a Hospice Program of Care, the National Hospice and Palliative Care Organization (NHPCO) defined *hospice care* as a model of palliative care in a defined group of people. "Hospice offers palliative care to all terminally ill

---

Box 2-2	European Society of Medical Oncology Core Principles for End-of-Life Care

 1. Respect the dignity of both the patient and caregivers.
 2. Be sensitive to and respectful of the patient's and family's wishes.
 3. Use appropriate measures (therapeutically) that are consistent with the patient's wishes.
 4. Make alleviation of pain and other symptoms a high priority.
 5. Recognize that good care of the dying person requires quality medical care but also entails services that are family and community based to address psychological, social, and spiritual as well as religious problems.
 6. Offer continuity with the primary physician and/or oncologist if the patient so desires.
 7. Advocate access to therapies that are expected to improve the patient's quality of life and ensure that the patient who chooses alternatives to nontraditional treatments is not abandoned.
 8. Provide palliative and hospice services.
 9. Respect the patient's right to refuse treatment (or assigned surrogates may authorize refusal of treatment when the patient cannot participate).
10. Respect the physician's professional responsibility to discontinue burdensome and ineffective therapies with consideration for both patient and family preference.
11. Promote clinical and evidence-based research in the end-of-life care.

From Cherny, N.I., Catane, R., & Kosmidis, P. (2003). ESMO takes a stand on supportive and palliative care. *Ann Oncol,* 14, 1336, by permission of Oxford University Press.

people and their families regardless of age, gender, nationality, race, creed, sexual orientation, disability, diagnosis, availability of a primary care, or ability to pay" (NHPCO, 1994, pp. 39-74). The prevailing precept of hospice care is that dying is a normal stage in the lives of individuals and families (Last Acts Palliative Care Task Force, 1997).

When the Medicare hospice benefit was adopted by the U.S. Congress in 1982 to support the development of hospice care, an appropriate length of hospice service was thought to be 6 months. However, patients currently enrolled rarely reach a 6-month hospice admission, with the average length of stay now less than 30 days (Byock, 2000). In 1994, the medium length of stay in hospice was 26 days, and in 1998, it was 19 days (Lynn, 2001; NHPCO, 1994). The 6-month survival criteria could be interpreted as "virtually all patients with this condition would be dead" or it would be reasonable to assume that someone in this condition would have less than 6 months to survive (Lynn, 2001).

Failure to optimize length of hospice service is related to attitudes, beliefs, and misperceptions. A few of the barriers that are associated with late referral into hospice care include a public perception that end-of-life and palliative care reflects the care of a loved one who is actively dying and a belief that most patients will enter into hospice care a few days prior to death and often with a loss of function (low Karnofsky Performance Score [40 or lower]), progressive disability, and limited ability to provide self-care, all of which rapidly worsen prior to death (Lynn, 2001). Hospice, a valuable service for the patient and family at the end-of-life, includes:

1. Home care services (which are the most common)
2. Hospice teams within hospitals
3. Hospice units within hospitals
4. Hospices with hospital affiliations
5. Freestanding hospices (autonomous)

Some hospices will have several of these elements within their programs (Abyad, 1994). Independent programs with full home care services are likely to be the most innovative in practice. However, sound home care programs remain the essential element to all hospices (Abyad, 1994). The goal of hospice is to allow patients to die with dignity, comfort, and pain and symptom control within their own home. The structure of the interdisciplinary team within hospice differs compared with that within palliative programs. A registered nurse with advanced training in physical assessment, pain control, and symptom management provides much of the day-to-day care, and the physician is the advisor and supervisor of care. The hospice nurse must be skilled in family care and provide specialized services such as wound care, intravenous medications, and catheter insertions (Perron & Schonwetter, 2001). The social worker is trained in counseling the dying patient and family. Chaplains provide spiritual support and religious services. Volunteers provide a multitude of functions such as sitting with the patient to allow families to have respite time to run errands or providing some domicile help for families. Medicare requires that 5% of patient care be delivered by trained volunteers. For hospice interdisciplinary work to be effective, communication within an interdisciplinary meeting is required (usually once weekly). Family meetings are arranged depending on need. Communication with the attending (nonhospice) physician who has been involved in care is maintained and is particularly important if there are changes in therapeutics (Perron & Schonwetter, 2001).

Hospices may need to assist with alternate placement of patients when home care is no longer possible or when temporary admission to an inpatient hospice or palliative medicine unit is warranted because symptoms are not well controlled or families are exhausted. These respite or symptom admissions are covered by the Medicare Hospice Benefit. The Medicare Hospice Benefit that provides a per diem reimbursement is not adjusted to case mix but must cover all medications, durable medical equipment, and visits made to the home by the various disciplines involved in the patient's care.

THE FUTURE OF PALLIATIVE AND END-OF-LIFE CARE

The future and growth of palliative medicine are largely determined by its acceptance within the traditional medical model. Legislative changes may influence the manner in which this is achieved—reimbursement criteria are evaluated based on patient prognosis and/or prognostic indicators. It is safe to say that in this era, health care costs cannot keep rising faster than the gross domestic product (Appleby, 2005). The focus of palliative care on preventing symptoms, coordinating care services, reducing unnecessary diagnostics or expensive therapeutics, and offering ongoing conversations with the patient and his or her family about changes in the disease and shifts in the plan of care can only be considered a valuable service to patient, family, and society.

The APN is in an ideal position to facilitate early conversations with a patient and family and to ensure ongoing and updated advance care planning, especially when the patient experiences an acute exacerbation of the disease, which reduces his or her functional capacities. The APN is able to recognize when along the disease trajectory to initiate and integrate palliative interventions, increase the intensity of interventions, and make referrals for alternate support for the patient and family. The APN who is skilled and knowledgeable about the pathophysiology of disease, the impact of specific symptoms, and their appropriate management can become a vital member of the patient's health care team and help to support the patient to "live until they die."

REFERENCES

Abyad, A. (1994). The hospice movement: Growth as an alternative, not integrated movement. *Medical Interface, 7*, 129-132.

Ahmedzai, S.H., Costa, A., Blengini, C., et al. (2004). A new international framework for palliative care. *Eur J Cancer, 40*, 2192-2200.

Appleby, J. (Thursday, February 24, 2005, front page cover). Health care tab ready to explode: costs could be 19% of economy by 2014. *USA Today*.

Body, J.J. (2003). Effectiveness and cost of bisphosphonate therapy in tumor bone. *Cancer, 97(3 Suppl.)*, 859-865.

Bomba, P.A. (2005). Enabling the transition to hospice through effective palliative care. *Case Manager, 16*, 48-52.

Browner, I. & Carducci, M.A. (2005). Palliative chemotherapy: Historical perspective, applications, and controversies. *Semin Oncol, 32*, 145-155.

Byock, I. (2000). Completing the continuum of cancer care: Integrating life prolongation and palliation. *CA: Cancer J Clin, 50*, 123-132.

Cassil, A. (2005). *Older Americans less willing to sacrifice physician-hospital choice to save costs: Findings suggest Medicare managed care plans will face challenges in enrolling seniors.* Washington, DC: The Center for Studying Health System Change, news release. Retrieved May 14, 2006, from http://hschange.org/CONTENT/746/?PRINT=1.

Cauchi, R. (April 21, 2005). U.S. is getting old fast. *USA Today*, 3A.

Center to Advance Palliative Care (CAPC). Retrieved May 14, 2006, from www.capc.org.

Cherny, N.I., Catane, R., & Kosmidis, P. (2003). ESMO takes a stand on supportive and palliative care. *Ann Oncol, 14,* 1335-1337.

Choi, Y.S. & Billings, J.A. (2002). Changing perspectives on palliative care. *Oncology, 16,* 515-522.

Davis, M.P., Albert, N.M., & Young, J.B. (2005). Palliation of heart failure. *Am J Hosp Palliat Care, 22,* 211-222.

Davis, M.P., Walsh, D., LeGrand, S.B., et al. (2002). End-of-life care: The death of palliative medicine? *J Palliat Med, 5,* 813-814.

Davis, M.P., Walsh, D., LeGrand, S.B., et al. (2005). An inter-institutional comparative analysis by all patient revised-diagnosis related group and case mix index. *J Support Oncol, 3(4)* 313-316.

Davis, M.P., Walsh, D., & Nelson, K.A. (2001). The business of palliative medicine: management metrics for an acute-care inpatient unit. *Am J Hosp Palliat Care, 18,* 26-29.

Department of Health and Human Services. (2002). *Healthy people 2010. Objectives for improving health (Part A).* Washington, DC: United States Department of Health and Human Services, Disease Prevention and Health Promotion.

Desai, J. & Demetri, G.D. (2005). Recombinant human erythropoietin in cancer-related anemia: an evidence-based review. *Best Pract Res Clin Haematol, 18,* 389-406.

El Nasser, H. (April 21, 2005). U.S. is getting old fast. *USA Today,* 3A.

Foster, Z. & Corless, I.B. (1999). Origins: An American perspective. *Hospice J, 14,* 913.

Gralla, R.J., Roila, F., Tonato, M., Multinational Society of Supportive Care in Cancer, American Society of Clinical Oncology, Cancer Care Ontario, Clinical Oncological Society of Australia; European Oncology Nursing Society, European Society of Medical Oncology, National Comprehensive Cancer Network, Oncology Nursing Society, & South African Society of Medical Oncology. (2005). The 2004 Perugia Antiemetic Consensus Guideline process: Methods, procedures, and participants. *Support Care Cancer, 13,* 77-79.

Hauptman, P.J. & Havranek, E.P. (2005). Integrating palliative care into heart failure. *Arch Intern Med, 165,* 374-378.

Hinton, J. (1963). The physical and mental distress of the dying. *Q J Med, 32,* 120.

Kuebler, K., Lynn, J., & Von Rohen, J. (2005). Perspectives in palliative care. *Oncol Nurs, 21,* 2-10.

Lagman, R. & Walsh, D. (2005). Integration of palliative medicine into comprehensive cancer care. *Semin Oncol, 32,* 134-138.

Lalonde Report (2004). *Report on the health of Canadians.* Retrieved May 14, 2006, from www.phac-aspc.gc.ca/ph-sp/phdd/report/1996/chap1e.htm.

Last Acts Palliative Care Task Force. (1997). Precepts of palliative care. *J Palliat Med, 1,* 109-112.

Lynn, J. (2001). Serving patients who may die soon and their families: the role of hospice and other services. *JAMA, 285,* 325-332.

Lynn, J. & Adamson, D. (2003). *Living well at the end of life: Adapting health care to serious chronic illness and old age.* Arlington, Va.: RAND Publication, RAND Health White Paper.

MacDonald, N. (2003). Nutrition as an integral component of supportive care. *Oncology, 17(Suppl. 2),* 8-10.

MacDonald, N. (2005). Modern palliative care: An exercise in prevention and partnership. *Oncol Nurs, 21,* 69-73.

Meldrum, M. (2005). The ladder and the clock: Cancer pain and public policy at the end of the twentieth century. *J Pain Symptom Manage, 29,* 41-54.

National Hospice and Palliative Care Organization (NHPCO). (1994). Standards of a hospice program of care. *Hospice J, 9,* 39-74.

National Hospice and Palliative Care Organization (NHPCO). Retrieved May 14, 2006, from www.nhpco.org.

Pantilat, S.Z. & Steimle, A.E. (2004). Palliative care for patients with heart failure. *JAMA, 291,* 2476-2482.

Perron, V. & Schonwetter, R. (2001). Hospice and palliative care programs. *Primary Care: Clinics in Office Practice, 28.*

Saunders, D.C. (1999). Origins: International perspectives, then and now. *Hospice J, 14,* 17.

Saunders, C. (2001). The evolution of palliative care. *J Royal Soc Med, 94,* 430-432.

Senn, H.J. & Glaus, A. (2002). Supportive care in cancer–15 Years thereafter. *Support Care Cancer, 10,* 8-12.

Sepulveda, C., Marlin, A., Yoshida, T., et al. (2002). Palliative care: The world health organization's global perspective. *J Pain Symptom Manage, 24,* 91-96.

Seymour, J., Clark, D., & Winslow, M. (2005). Pain and palliative care: The emergence of new specialties. *J Pain Symptom Manage, 29,* 2-13.

Thomas, R. & Richardson, A. (2004). The NICE guidance on supportive and palliative care–Implications for oncology teams. *Clinic Oncol, 16,* 420-424.

Wald, F. (1997). Hospice past to future. In Stack J (Ed.). Death and the quest of meaning (essays in honor of Herman Feifel). North Vale, N.J.: Jason Aronson Publishers.

Wall, P.D. (Ed.) (1986). Editorial. *Pain, 25,* 1-4.

Wall, P.D. (Ed.) (1997). The generation of yet another myth on the use of narcotics. *Pain, 73,* 121-122.

Walsh, D. (2001). The Harry R. Horvitz Center for Palliative Medicine (1987-1999): development of a novel comprehensive integrated program. *Am J Hospice Palliat Care, 18,* 239-250.

Widder, J. & Glawisching-Goschnick, M. (2002). The concept of disease in palliative medicine. *Medical Health Care Philosophy, 5,* 191-197.

Woodruff, R. (2002). The problem of definitions. *Prog Palliat Care, 10,* 17.

World Health Organization (WHO), National Cancer Control Programmes. (2002). *Policies and managerial guidelines* (2nd ed). Geneva: Author.

CHAPTER 3

THE DYING PROCESS

Debra E. Heidrich

■

"How people die remains in the memories of those who live on."
Dame Cicely Saunders

■

As diseases progress and death nears, the focus, goals, and rhythm of care change. A decline in physical functioning is often the first indication that a patient is entering the terminal phase of life (Gauthier, 2005). Functional decline usually occurs 4 to 5 months before death in persons with malignant diseases and approximately 3 to 4 months before death in persons with organ failure. Frail persons in long-term care settings tend to have a slow decline in function over the last 12 months of life (Lunney, Lynn, Foley et al., 2003). As physical function declines, the number of medical disciplines directly providing care to the patient often decreases as the individual becomes too weak for an office or clinic visit. And, the number of informal caregivers (i.e., family and friends) increases as the patient becomes increasingly dependent on others for care. The physical and emotional demands of caring for a loved one at end-of-life can be overwhelming. It is during this time that patients and family members need the expertise and support of a palliative or hospice care program.

At the time patients and families need consistency, follow-through, and a feeling of connection, they may—and rightly so—feel increasingly distant from the relationships with their health care providers. It is during this time that the advanced practice nurse (APN) can provide valuable continuity by facilitating home care resources and by providing consultation and support via telephone contact and/or home care visitations.

The terminal phase is not simply a continuation of the previous care (Furst & Doyle, 2003). Symptoms often change at end-of-life. Disease-specific symptoms may intensify (e.g., dyspnea in pulmonary malignancy), others subside, and new symptoms may appear. The prevalence of symptoms at end-of-life as reported in the literature varies with the study setting, patient population, data collection tool, and timing of data collection in relation to patients' deaths (Table 3-1).

Mercadante, Casuccio, and Fulfaro (2000) evaluated 370 home-based patients with advanced cancer and showed that the peak of opioid consumption, symptom frequency, and symptom severity correlated with poor functional status. Symptoms of nausea, vomiting, dry mouth, gastric pyrosis (heartburn), and diarrhea decreased as performance status declined, whereas dyspnea, drowsiness, weakness, and confusion tended to increase and to peak at the lowest levels of functional status.

The author would like to acknowledge Patricia H. Berry, Julie Griffie, and Kate Ford Roberts for their contributions that remain unchanged from the first edition of this textbook.

TABLE 3-1 ■ Symptom Prevalence at End of Life

Author	Setting/Population	No. of Subjects	Anxiety or Worry	Anorexia	Constipation	Concentration Difficulties	Confusion/Delirium	Depression/Feeling Sad	Drowsy	Dry Mouth	Dyspnea	Fatigue/Lack of Energy	Nausea and Vomiting	Pain
Klinkenberg, Willems, van der Wal, et al., 2004	After-death survey of relatives of older adults	270	31	—	—	—	36	28	—	—	50	83	25	48
Kutner, Kassner, & Nowels, 2001	Hospice staff from 16 hospices rating of patient symptoms	348	43	63	39	60	—	51	61	34	48	83	24	76
Tranmer, Heyland, Dudgear, et al., 2003	Interviews of hospitalized patients near end-of-life	135	70	52	39	44	—	53	70	81	62	84	44 Nausea 25 Vomiting	63
Hickman, Tilden, & Tolle, 2001	Family members of persons who died in a hospital	103	26	53	30	—	—	43	59	60	65	67	—	59
Hall, Schroder, & Weaver, 2002	Chart audit noting symptoms in last 48 hours of life in long-term care settings	185	—	—	—	—	29	—	—	—	62	—	—	44

Data from Klinkenberg, M., Willems, D.L., van der Wal, G., et al. (2004). Symptom burden in the last week of life. *J Pain Symptom Manage, 27(1),* 5-13; Kutner, J.S., Kassner, C.T., & Nowels, D.E. (2001). Symptom burden at the end of life: Hospice providers' perceptions. *J Pain Symptom Manage, 21(6),* 473-480; Tranmer, J.E., Heyland, D., Dudgeon, D., et al. (2003). Measuring the symptom experience of seriously ill cancer and noncancer hospitalized patients near the end of life with the Memorial Symptom Assessment Scale. *J Pain Symptom Manage, 25(5),* 420-429; Hickman, S.E., Tilden, V.P., & Tolle, S.W. (2001). Family reports of dying patients' distress: The adaptation of a research tool to assess global symptom distress in the last week of life. *J Pain Symptom Manage, 22(1),* 565-574; and Hall, P., Schroder, C., & Weaver, L. (2002). The last 48 hours of life in long-term care: A focused chart audit. *J Am Geriatr Soc, 50(3),* 501-506.
—, Not reported in the study

In another study, Klinkenberg, Willems, van der Wal et al. (2004) identify seven symptoms most often reported in the literature at end-of-life: fatigue, pain, dyspnea, depression, anxiety, confusion, and nausea and/or vomiting. Family caregivers were queried to identify the presence of these symptoms during the last week of their loved ones' lives and to rate the frequency, severity, and burden associated with each symptom experienced by their loved ones. Seventy-five percent of patients had two or more of these symptoms in the final week of life (range = 0 to 7; mean, 2.7). All seven symptoms were perceived by caregivers as burdensome to patients, with fatigue being the most burdensome, followed by pain, anxiety, dyspnea, depression, nausea/vomiting, and confusion. While studies of this nature are often difficult to generalize across settings and populations, it is clear that patients at end-of-life are at risk and experience multiple symptoms that create significant burdens and interfere with quality of life.

Although psychosocial symptoms are common in the dying patient, they are often not adequately evaluated or managed (Georges, Onwuteaka-Philipsen, van der Heide et al., 2005). Depression and anxiety (or anxiety-related symptoms such as nervousness, worry, or irritability) are included in most studies of symptom prevalence. The issues of loss, grief, isolation, sexual dysfunction, disturbed self-concept, spiritual distress, loneliness, and concerns about caregiver burden are less often assessed, yet these issues are no less important than physical symptoms. Georges et al. (2005) noted that a peaceful death is impeded by feelings of anxiety and loneliness.

Seriously ill patients queried about the importance of selected attributes to quality end-of-life care identified the following as the five most important concepts (Steinhauser, Christakis, Clipp et al., 2000):

- Freedom from pain
- Being at peace with God
- Presence of family
- Being cognitively aware
- Having treatment choices honored

Providing multidimensional care is essential at the end of life—including optimal physical care (e.g., pain relief), spiritual care, psychosocial care, and ongoing communication regarding advance care planning. Patients and families who were asked to identify the most important aspects of a physician's skills when providing end-of-life care identified emotional support more often than medical competence (Wenrich, Curtis, Ambrozy et al., 2003).

Careful evaluation of all symptoms is necessary throughout the course of a patient's care, including the last days and hours of life. Ideally, interventions are aimed at addressing and relieving the underlying cause rather than treating the outward symptom. For example, restlessness related to the discomfort from urinary retention is best relieved with catheterization rather than the introduction of a benzodiazepine. The underlying cause is not always readily identifiable or treatable; in these circumstances, interventions are directed to lessen the uncomfortable symptom.

The APN is in an ideal position to anticipate, evaluate, and monitor for physical and psychosocial symptoms. Providing the patient and family with the appropriate education about what to expect based on the disease process can reduce the anxiety and fear that often accompany "not knowing." For example, dyspnea, respiratory secretions, cough, and pain are expected symptoms in the patient with metastatic lung cancer. Teaching the patient and family what to expect and how to address these symptoms when they do occur makes it less likely that these events will be perceived as "crises."

It is important to realize that each situation is unique and that the patient and family often ascribe meaning to their experiences based on their own perspectives. For each patient and family, psychological, spiritual, cultural, and family issues converge and contribute to the end-of-life experience, no two of which are alike.

With few exceptions, the health care team has only one chance to "get it right" when caring for patients and families at end-of-life (Berry & Griffie, 2005). Excellent palliative care received in the months prior to death is not remembered if physical and psychosocial symptoms are not optimally addressed in the dying process (Furst & Doyle, 2003). This point was emphasized by Dame Cicely Saunders when she stated, "How people die remains in the memories of those who live on."

CARE AT END-OF-LIFE

Patients nearing death are often weak, fragile, and less tolerant of physical and psychosocial stress. It is during this time that palliative interventions intensify and the focus on restorative care decreases. The goals of care are to prevent and appropriately manage symptoms and to support quality of living throughout the dying process.

Medications

During the dying process, the APN should evaluate all medications that the patient is taking and consider discontinuing medications that are not required to promote comfort (Ellershaw & Ward, 2005). The clinician must discuss with the patient and family why specific medications are no longer necessary. Without an appropriate explanation, the discontinuation of medications may appear to the patient or family as a death-hastening intervention. Medications such as antihypertensives, antidepressants, laxatives, antiulcer drugs, anticoagulants, long-term antibiotics, iron preparations, and vitamin supplements that are no longer essential may be discontinued. Medications such as steroids, replacement hormones, hypoglycemics, diuretics, antiarrhythmics, and anticonvulsants should be evaluated for efficacy and usefulness in the management of the disease and symptoms; those that are no longer beneficial for patient comfort may be discontinued (Furst & Doyle, 2003). It is important for the APN to understand how to successfully taper certain medications (e.g., antidepressants, steroids, hormones, benzodiazepines, and anticonvulsants) to avoid the discomforts associated with abrupt withdrawal.

Some patients are able to swallow until a few hours before they die, whereas others are unable to swallow for weeks or days before death occurs. Alternate routes of administering medications, including sublingual, buccal, rectal, subcutaneous, and intravenous, may be considered. Some individuals consider certain routes objectionable (e.g., rectal, subcutaneous). Discussing these various routes with the patient and family and assessing their willingness and ability to use these routes are important considerations when planning care.

Dehydration

Patients should be encouraged to maintain oral fluid intake for as long as possible. As death approaches, however, patients are often unable to take in adequate fluid by mouth. There is considerable debate regarding the use of nonoral hydration at the end of life and no consensus on the single best approach to care (Fainsinger, 2005). It is essential for the APN to assess the potential risks and benefits of artificial hydration while aiming to maintain comfort, prevent complications, and avoid unnecessary or distressing procedures (see Chapter 23). Key considerations when determining the role of nonoral hydration include the following (Fainsinger, 2005):

- Expressed wishes of the patient or surrogate decision-maker regarding the use of hydration
- Patient-defined goals that can be influenced by hydration
- Symptom burden that may be improved by withholding hydration (e.g., fluid overload) or providing hydration (e.g., delirium)
- Burden to patient and caregivers of maintaining nonoral hydration
- Family distress concerning withholding hydration/nutrition

When in doubt, a time-limited trial of nonoral hydration while vigilantly monitoring for improvement or uncomfortable effects is appropriate.

A dry mouth is not necessarily an indicator that the patient needs rehydration (Furst & Doyle, 2003). Patients should be encouraged to keep the mouth moist by sipping cold water, allowing ice chips to melt in the mouth, or eating sorbet (lemon flavoring is refreshing and stimulates saliva). As an alternative, water or normal saline (1 teaspoon of salt in a quart of water) can be sprayed into the mouth using a sprayer bottle or an atomizer. Artificial saliva preparations are available in liquids, sprays, and gels and can be applied to the oral mucosa. Water-soluble lubricants, such as KY Jelly or Surgilube, can be used to keep lips and gums moist. Careful evaluation of the oral mucosa is necessary to assess for lesions or signs of infection.

Signs and Symptoms of the Imminent Dying Process

With few exceptions, there are predictable signs and symptoms that signal that death is nearing. The clinician can use these symptoms as a guide to help the patient and family plan for the death and to clarify with family members their desires and needs at the time of death.

Asthenia

As weakness increases, the patient may progress from a bed-to-chair activity level to being completely bed-bound. Joints may become stiff and add to discomfort (Ferris, von Gunten, & Emanuel, 2003; Moneymaker, 2005). Unless movement makes the patient more uncomfortable or agitated, caregivers should be taught gentle passive range-of-motion exercises and interventions to prevent skin breakdown, such as turning schedules and the use of air mattresses (see Chapter 28).

Pain

In the dying process, a new pain may develop and chronic pain may increase in intensity, decrease in intensity, or remain the same (Pitorak, 2003). As renal function declines, some medications will remain in circulation longer or their active metabolites (e.g., morphine-3-glucuronide and morphine-6-glucuronide) may accumulate. The need to adjust analgesic doses or schedules should be evaluated throughout the dying process (see Chapter 32). Not all patients have pain, and some with mild pain may not need or desire significant intervention.

Changes in Mentation

In the days to weeks before the patient dies, he or she may doze frequently, even in the middle of conversations, and total sleeping time increases (Moneymaker, 2005). The patient may progress from being sleepy to lethargic to obtunded to semicomatose to comatose (Ferris et al., 2003). It is important to not "test" for the level of consciousness with an uncomfortable stimulus, such as a sternal rub; document the level of arousal when the patient's name is called or with a gentle shaking of the shoulder. Not all patients proceed through this progressive decline in their level of consciousness; some remain conscious up until the final 10 to 15 minutes of life.

A short attention span or difficulty processing information becomes more common as death approaches. Keeping sentences or questions short and allowing time for the patient to process both the question and the response to the question may assist with communication. The APN must evaluate if the difficulty in concentration is an early sign of delirium and, if present, treat it appropriately (see Chapter 24).

Agitation or delirium at end-of-life can be caused by physical discomfort, emotional and spiritual distress, medications, or dehydration. The APN should assess for any conditions or medications that might contribute to delirium and treat them appropriately based on the cause and the patient's proximity to death. One factor that may contribute to delirium in the final days or hours of life is sudden discontinuation of specific medications, such as analgesics and anxiolytics, by caregivers "because the patient didn't ask for them." Withdrawal from nicotine can be managed with a transdermal nicotine patch, and a benzodiazepine may be required to treat the delirium associated with alcohol withdrawal. Unresolved emotional or spiritual issues may also contribute to agitation and should be evaluated.

Circulatory Changes

Initially, the patient may become tachycardic as the body tries to compensate for the decreased cardiac output. However, over time the heart rate begins to slow (Moneymaker, 2005; Pitorak, 2003). This change can be used to signal that death is approaching and to help the family acknowledge that death is imminent.

With the decreased cardiac output, the skin may become cool and clammy. The patient often appears pale but may initially be flushed (Moneymaker, 2005; Pitorak, 2003). The skin may change from being uniformly pale to varying shades of red, blue, and purple. The soles of the feet, knees, ankles, and elbows are first to develop a blotchy, mottled appearance. Venous blood pools in dependent areas of the body, such as the sacrum and lower back (Ferris et al., 2003; Moneymaker, 2005; Pitorak, 2003).

Decreased Urine Output

Reduced blood flow to the kidneys causes a decrease in urine production. In addition, the patient's fluid intake is generally decreased, which also contributes to this syndrome. As awareness decreases, the patient may experience urinary retention or incontinence (Ferris et al., 2003; Moneymaker, 2005; Pitorak, 2003). A lack of urine output does not mean that there is no urine in the bladder. A thorough physical examination is necessary to identify a distended bladder, which may contribute to discomfort and possible agitation. Intermittent catheterization may be warranted in patients who are positive for urinary retention, and the decision to provide ongoing catheterization should be considered on an individual basis.

Changes in Breathing Patterns

As the chest wall muscles weaken, breathing may be shallow with an increase in the respiratory rate (Ferris et al., 2003). Patients who experience tachypnea and dyspnea should be properly evaluated, and the appropriate interventions should be initiated (i.e., opioids, bronchodilators, anxiolytics, etc.) (see Chapter 27).

Declining cardiac and respiratory function often precipitates hypercapnia. Over time, the brain becomes less responsive to the rising carbon dioxide levels, resulting in irregular breathing patterns, which are commonly known as Cheyne-Stokes respirations (Ferris et al., 2003; Moneymaker, 2005). Supplemental oxygen does not alter this symptom, and patients may find masks or cannulas uncomfortable. However, pulmonary patients who have lived many years with supplemental oxygen may continue to find comfort in knowing that they have their oxygen. Family members may find watching the progressive lengthening of apnea particularly distressing and may require additional interdisciplinary support during this time.

Saliva and oropharyngeal secretions may accumulate in the upper airway, leading to gurgling respirations, often called the "death rattle" (Ferris et al., 2003). Suctioning is rarely helpful as the secretions tend to reaccumulate and the irritation of the catheter may stimulate additional secretions. Yankauer suctioning may be an uncomfortable experience for the patient, especially if he or she is dyspneic (Furst & Doyle, 2003). An alternate approach is to reposition the patient by rolling to a side-lying position or raising the head of the bed. If position changes are ineffective, consider the use of anticholinergics (e.g., scopolamine or hyoscyamine) via the sublingual, buccal, subcutaneous, or transdermal route (Furst & Doyle; Pitorak, 2003). It is important to note that anticholinergics do not affect existing secretions; therefore, earlier initiation is paramount in treating this symptom. It is also important to identify whether the patient's existing medications have anticholinergic properties (e.g., chlorpromazine, prochlorperazine, bronchodilators). Adding additional anticholinergics may lead to xerostomia and, if coupled with the drying effects of opioids, may precipitate discomfort. Anticholinergics can also lead to sedation and confusion, particularly in the dehydrated elderly patient. Teaching caregivers the importance of good oral care will ensure comfort. The APN should consider being proactive about medicating appropriately to help reduce the incidence of noisy respirations, especially in patients with an underlying cardiac and pulmonary diagnosis.

Decreased Interest in Food Intake

Although many factors contribute to diminished nutritional intake throughout the disease progression, physical weakness at end-of-life often contributes to dysphagia (Ferris et al., 2003). It is hoped that the advantages and disadvantages of artificial nutrition have been discussed throughout the course of the patient's care. At this time, the APN can reinforce that artificial nutrition during the dying phase often does not contribute to physical comfort or prolong life (Strasser, 2003). This can be an emotionally charged issue and should be met with supportive guidance for the patient and family. At times, cultural or emotional considerations make it appropriate to consider a trial of nutritional augmentation to support the patient and family. The patient and family should be made aware of the limited time associated with a "trial" and to assess and evaluate for any untoward side effects.

Nearing Death Awareness

Callanan and Kelley (1993) defined *nearing death awareness* as a special knowledge about the process of dying that reveals what dying is like and what is needed in order to die peacefully. Patients may describe or discuss being in the presence of someone not alive, seeing a place, knowing or choosing when death will occur, preparing for travel or change, needing reconciliation, being held back, or having symbolic dreams. While not universal, these experiences are common and it is helpful to discuss nearing death awareness with patients and families to help to normalize these experiences. Some of these experiences may be spiritually and emotionally comforting to the patient and his or her caregivers.

Inability to Close Eyes

Patients may lose the ability to close their eyes completely when asleep, which can be very disturbing to family members. This occurs most often in patients with significant fat and muscle wasting from cachexia. The loss of the retro-orbital fat pad allows the eye to fall farther back into the eye socket, and sometimes the eyelids are not long enough to cover the additional distance back as well as all of the conjunctiva, leaving part of the conjunctiva visible while the patient sleeps (Ferris et al., 2003). Maintain eye moisture with artificial tears, eye lubricants, normal saline drops, or a moist cloth covering the eyes.

Changes in Sensory Perception

Visual acuity may decline and there may be increased sensitivity to bright light (Berry & Griffie, 2005). Bright lights, including ceiling lights or bright sunshine through a window, should be avoided. It is believed that patients are able to hear even when they are unable to respond during the final days and hours. The APN should encourage caregivers to talk to the patient in a soft voice and/or to play music that the patient enjoys. And family members should be cautioned to not have conversations "over" the patient or say anything that they do not want the patient to hear.

CARING FOR THE CAREGIVERS

Preparing the patient and family for the death event and the time immediately after death is an important intervention for the APN. An open and caring discussion of what to anticipate in the dying process reduces the incidence of fear and apprehension. These discussions provide the APN with the opportunity to evaluate the caregiver's ability to support the patient through the dying process and to make plans for any additional caregiver support or a transfer to a different care setting, as appropriate, when death approaches.

Caring for a dying loved one can be exhausting. However, many family members report that despite the physical, financial, and emotional tolls of providing this care, the experience is extremely rewarding, and many view it as a final act of love. Others may be overwhelmed by, or unable to perform, the amount of physical care required or they may be unable to emotionally cope with the situation. Options for care include hiring additional caregivers (when financially feasible), transfer to a long-term care setting or residential hospice setting, and use of hospice continuous home care or hospice acute medical care (when medically justified).

Transfer from the home setting may lead to feelings of guilt in the caregivers, especially if the patient communicated a desire to die at home. Some guilt may be assuaged by reinforcing that the most important goal is to keep the patient as comfortable as possible and that the family's decision to transfer the patient is indeed in the best interest of the patient.

Family members may not be confident that they will be able to identify when death has occurred. The APN can provide the family with education on what to expect at the time of death. This includes cessation of breathing and heart rate, dilated and fixed pupils, and the potential for bowel and bladder incontinence when rectal and bladder sphincters relax. Caregivers should know who to notify at the time of death to initiate the official death pronouncement and to make arrangements for transport of the deceased to the funeral home or elsewhere. The clinician should verify that the caregivers have the appropriate contact information. Likewise, the family should have an understanding that in the event that an ambulance is called, the emergency medical services personnel are often required to attempt resuscitation unless there is an accepted "do not resuscitate" order—this varies from state to state.

CARE AT THE TIME OF DEATH

If present at the time of death, clinicians have a unique opportunity to support the family, care for the body, and facilitate the initial process of grieving. Gentle, reverent care of the body after death conveys to the family the clinician's care and concern for the person who has died. Ideally, the APN has previously discussed any important rituals for care of the body after death and has developed plans that respect special cultural and religious rituals (see Chapter 6). The clinician present at the time of death confirms these plans and contacts the appropriate funeral home personnel, religious leader, or lay personnel from the religious/cultural society.

Family members are often bewildered and need gentle guidance about what to do next (Kissane, 2003). Activities that assist in the early process of grieving include:

- Listening to the family as they reminisce about the deceased person's life and/or dying
- Facilitating religious rituals by notifying a clergy or pastoral care worker
- Allowing the family time alone with the body as desired
- Allowing the family to participate in the care of the body as desired

The degree of involvement in the care of the body by family members will vary with cultural or religious backgrounds and personal preferences. Activities such as combing hair or helping to dress the patient in other clothes should be encouraged. Children may be included, depending on circumstances and their maturity. Prepare those caring for the body that when the body is turned, air may escape from the lungs, causing a "sighing" sound.

If only one family member is present at the time of death, the clinician should ask about other family members or friends who can be called to be present with the bereaved or accompany him or her home. Family members may want time to say their good-byes to their loved ones in ways that are meaningful to them, including talking to the deceased, saying prayers, or telling stories reminiscent of the deceased.

Clinicians should become familiar with the local laws regarding death pronouncement and notification, especially when it occurs outside of a health care institution. In some states, registered nurses or APNs can sign death certificates; in others, nonphysician clinicians report the absence of vital signs to physicians, who make the official pronouncement over the telephone; and in others, the funeral home is required to transport the body to an emergency department for death pronouncement. The need to notify the coroner's office of a home death also varies from one municipality/county to another. The APN must know these laws and procedures to ensure a smooth transition from home to funeral home.

CARE OF THE BEREAVED

Bereavement care is an essential part of a comprehensive palliative care program (National Consensus Project for Quality Palliative Care, 2004). The APN plays an important role in anticipating grief reactions, providing support for the bereaved, and recognizing those responses that may indicate complicated grieving and making appropriate referrals.

Providing bereavement care requires an understanding of the normal grieving process and the tasks of grief work. Grief is a normal and expected reaction to a loss; family members will grieve the loss of their loved ones. One role of the APN is to reinforce that grieving is a healthy, necessary process that individuals must go through to be able to move on in their lives. Clinicians should validate as normal the manifestations that the bereaved may be experiencing. Normal manifestations of grief are listed in Box 3-1.

In addition to knowing the normal responses to grief, it is helpful for those working with the bereaved to understand the tasks of the grieving process. The following four tasks of mourning must be accomplished for a satisfactory conclusion to the work of bereavement (Worden, 1982):

- Accept the reality of the loss
- Work through the pain of grief
- Adjust to the environment in which the deceased is missing
- Emotionally relocate the deceased and move on with life

This last task is the most difficult. It involves finding a place for the dead in the grievers' emotional lives that allows them to go on living effectively in the world. The grieving process takes time and energy.

The first year of bereavement is the most intense—the first birthdays, holidays, and anniversaries without the deceased, as well as the anniversary of the death, can be very difficult. The length of mourning, however, is proportional to the strength of the

Box 3-1	Manifestations of Grief*		
Psychological	**Social**	**Somatic**
Numbness	Restlessness or	Appetite disturbances
Confused/unsure	inability to sit still	Sleep disturbances
what to do	Painful inability to initiate	Crying
Disbelief	and maintain organized	Sighing
Sadness	patterns of activity	Lack of strength
Anxiety (mild to panic)	Social withdrawal	Physical exhaustion and
Anger		lack of energy
Guilt		Feeling that "something
Acute feelings of separation		is stuck in the throat"
and yearning		Heart palpitations
Searching or calling out for		Shortness of breath
the deceased		Nervousness or tension
Dreaming about the deceased		Loss of sexual desire or
Seeing, hearing, or feeling the		hypersexuality
presence of the decreased		

Data from Rando, T.A. (1984). *Grief, dying and death: Clinical interventions for caregivers.* Champaign, Ill.: Research Press Co.

*All of these are normal manifestations of grief. However, if any exist for long periods of time or at a high level of intensity, consider a consult to evaluate for a complicated grief reaction.

attachment to the lost person (Kissane, 2003). Palliative care and hospice bereavement programs generally follow families for 13 months after a death to provide support through this time. Table 3-2 identifies interventions to assist persons with the grieving process.

Mourning the loss of a spouse is among the most intense and may continue for years. Spouses tend to play multiple roles in each other's lives, including friend, confidante, lover, partner, and source of emotional and financial support (Dutton & Zisook, 2005). Therefore, the loss of a spouse represents multiple losses to the individual.

Most persons adapt to bereavement successfully, and it can even be associated with improved coping, personal growth, and a new appreciation for life (Dutton & Zisook, 2005). However, in a minority of the population, grief can be complicated. If any of the "normal" responses to grief are extremely intense or protracted, it may indicate a psychiatric disorder such as clinical depression, anxiety disorder, alcohol and/or other substance abuse, psychotic disorder, or post-traumatic stress disorder (Kissane, 2003). Referral to trained counselors, psychologists, or psychiatrists may be indicated.

Professional and nonprofessional caregivers from the health care system also experience grief when the patients they care for die. The grief of staff may be more intense when a patient has been under their care for a long period of time or when dealing with multiples losses. Bereavement support for staff, through self-care, support groups, and individual counseling, is essential.

TABLE 3-2 ■ Interventions for Grieving Persons

Task	Interventions
Accept reality of the loss	Listen actively without judgment.
	Encourage gentle exploration of what the future may look like without the deceased.
	Assess and encourage the development of social support systems.
	Encourage time with the body of the deceased at the time of death.
	Offer ample opportunity to repeat the story of the death; listen patiently and attentively.
	Normalize feelings through personal contacts and written materials regarding grief and loss.
	Avoid the use of platitudes.
	Attend the funeral or visitation if possible; send a personal letter or card to the family.
	Respect survivor's feelings without judgment.
Work through the pain of grief	Assist in identifying manifestations of grief and normalize them.
	Assist the survivor in placing a meaning on the death.
Adjust to the environment in which the deceased is missing	Assist the survivor in further identifying the meaning of the loss in practical terms.
	Provide practical assistance with developing needed skills.
	Advise the survivor to minimize change and to grieve where things are familiar.
Emotionally relocate the deceased and move on with life	Provide a nonjudgmental and supportive ear as the survivor explores this task.
	Validate and normalize feeling associated with moving the thoughts and memories of the deceased to an effective place that allows for a reinvestment in life.
	Encourage attendance at grief and loss support or educational groups.

Data from Worden, J.W. (1991). *Grief counseling and grief therapy: A handbook for the mental health practitioner* (2nd ed.). New York: Springer.

CONCLUSION

APNs play an important role in the care of patients and families near death and afterward. The goals of care at this time are the provision of a comfortable dying for the patient, a positive experience for the family, and effective grieving for the bereaved. In order to accomplish these goals, the APN should evaluate and manage the physical, psychosocial, emotional, and spiritual symptoms in the days and weeks leading up to a patient's death—while anticipating grief reactions and providing support to loved ones after the death event.

REFERENCES

Berry, P.H. & Griffie, J. (2005). Planning for the actual death. In B.R. Ferrell & N. Coyle (Eds.). *Textbook of palliative nursing* (2nd ed., pp. 561-580). New York: Oxford University Press.

Callanan, M. & Kelley, P. (1993). *Final gifts: Understanding the special awareness, needs, and communications of the dying.* New York: Bantam Books.

Dutton, Y.D. & Zisook, S. (2005). Adaptation to bereavement. *Death Studies, 29(10),* 877-903.

Ellershaw, J. & Ward, C. (2005). Care of the dying patient: The last hours or days of life. *BMJ, 236(1),* 30-34.

Fainsinger, R. (2005). *Non-oral hydration in palliative care. Fast facts and concepts #133.* End-of-Life Physician Resource Center. Retrieved May 14, 2006, from www.eperc.mcw.edu/fastFact/ff_133.htm.

Ferris, F.D., von Gunten, C., & Emanuel, L.L. (2003). Competency in end-of-life care: Last hours of life. *J Palliat Med, 6(4),* 605-613.

Furst, C.J. & Doyle, D. (2003). The terminal phase. In D. Doyle, G. Hanks, N. Cherny, & K. Calman (Eds.). *Oxford textbook of palliative medicine* (3rd ed., pp. 1119-1133). New York: Oxford University Press.

Gauthier, D.M. (2005). Decision making near the end of life. *J Hospice Palliat Nurs, 7(2),* 82-90.

Georges, J.J., Onwuteaka-Philipsen, B.D., van der Heide, A., et al. (2005). Symptoms, treatment, and "dying peacefully" in terminally ill cancer patients: A prospective study. *Support Care Cancer, 13(3),* 160-168.

Kissane, D.W. (2003). Bereavement. In D. Doyle, G. Hanks, N. Cherny, et al. *Oxford textbook of palliative medicine* (3rd ed., pp. 1137-1151). New York: Oxford University Press.

Klinkenberg, M., Willems, D.L., van der Wal, G., et al. (2004). Symptom burden in the last week of life. *J Pain Symptom Manage, 27(1),* 5-13.

Lunney, J.R., Lynn, J., Foley, D.J., Lipson, S., & Guralnik, J.M. (2003). Patterns of functional decline at the end of life. *JAMA, 289(18),* 2387-2392.

Mercadante, S., Casuccio, A., & Fulfaro, F. (2000). The course of symptom frequency and intensity in advanced cancer patients followed at home. *J Pain Symptom Manage, 20(2),* 104-112.

Moneymaker, K.A. (2005). Understanding the dying process: Transitions during final days to hours. *J Palliat Med, 8(5),* 1079.

National Consensus Project for Quality Palliative Care. (2004). *Clinical practice guidelines for quality palliative care.* Brooklyn, N.Y.: Author.

Pitorak, E.F. (2003). Care at the time of death. *Am J Nurs, 103(7),* 42-52.

Steinhauser, K.E., Christakis, N.A., Clipp, E.C., et al. (2000). Factors considered important at the end of life by patients, family, physicians, and other care providers. *JAMA, 284(19),* 2476-2482.

Strasser, F. (2003). Eating-related disorders in patients with advanced cancer. *Support Care Cancer, 11(1),* 11-20.

Wenrich, M.D., Curtis, R., Ambrozy, D.A., et al. (2003). Dying patients' need for emotional support and personalized care from physicians: Perspectives of patients with terminal illness, families, and health care providers. *J Pain Symptom Manage, 25(3),* 236-246.

Worden, J.W. (1982). *Grief counseling and grief therapy: A handbook for the mental health practitioner.* New York, Springer.

UNIT II

IMPORTANT CONCEPTS
IN PALLIATIVE AND
END-OF-LIFE CARE

ADVANCE CARE PLANNING AND END-OF-LIFE DECISION MAKING

Crystal Dea Moore

■

Advance care planning is a collaborative process among patients, family members, and health care professionals whereby patients clarify their goals, values, and preferences for future medical treatment (Tulsky, 2005). As part of the advance care planning process, patients may choose to complete advance directives, which are legal documents that specify treatment preferences (e.g., living will), and formally appoint decision-making surrogates (e.g., durable power of attorney for health care). Patients, family members, and health care professionals can have both unique and shared goals related to advance care planning and advance directive completion (Kolarik, Arnold, Fischer et al., 2002). For example, increased communication about patient treatment preferences can be an objective for all three groups. For patients, advance care planning provides an opportunity to increase knowledge about and perceived control over the dying process. Families can learn about patient preferences related to end-of-life care, which can inform the decision-making process. Decreasing conflict with family members and decision-making surrogates about patient treatment plans can be an outcome desired by health care providers. Appropriate and thoughtful advance care planning can serve numerous interests.

This chapter seeks to describe strategies to promote advance care planning and broad issues in surrogate decision making in end-of-life care. Challenges to the process are addressed, and communication strategies to meet these challenges are described. Specific suggestions to help clinicians begin and maintain discussions about patient values and goals and descriptions of the legal documents used to record patient preferences are offered. Finally, issues specific to surrogate decision making are discussed. This chapter is intended to be a practical guide to the advance care planning process for clinicians.

THE ADVANCE CARE PLANNING PROCESS

The advance care planning process can be a challenging endeavor for numerous and complex reasons. The challenges associated with engaging patients and families in meaningful discussions about goals, values, and future treatment preferences can be mitigated through the development of communication strategies that promote honesty, trust, rapport, and respect. Health care professionals can be integral to initiating and maintaining discussions about patients' relevant goals and values that provide the context for treatment preferences and care plans at the end-of-life.

Challenges in Advance Care Planning

Given clinical and human realities, there are numerous factors that can hinder the advance care planning process, including health care system influences, deficient communication skills, and various psychological barriers. Meaningful advance care planning discussions are borne out of a trusting relationship between the patient and clinician, something that takes time to nurture and cultivate. Health system issues, including professional time limitations on visits with patients and families, and patient engagement with multiple providers can impede a professional's capacity to build rapport and trust (Kolarik et al., 2002; Tulsky, 2005). Clinicians may lack specific training in communication skills and the willingness to broach and maintain discussions about potentially sensitive, emotionally charged issues with patients and families. The overuse of medical jargon can also interfere with patient education, comprehension, and meaningful, clear discussions (Limerick, 2002; Reisfield & Wilson, 2003). Finally, patients and families may be reticent to ask clarification questions, not wanting to appear ignorant or to step outside the expected role of the "good patient."

Psychological barriers, including fear and anxiety, can also influence the quality of advance care planning discussions. Clinicians may be concerned about causing psychological harm or destroying patient and family hope through frank discussions about diagnosis and prognosis (Morrison, 1998; Steinhauser, Christakis, Clipp et al., 2001). Patients and families can also become emotionally stressed during discussions that convey bad or sad news, and their abilities to process and respond to information can be limited. Finally, patients, families, and clinicians all have a set of unique experiences related to illness and dying, and those previous experiences can influence expectations about and willingness to address such issues in the present, thereby affecting communication quality (Lee, Back, Block et al., 2002; Moore, 2005a). Despite these challenges, clinicians can develop communication strategies to engage patients and families in the advance care planning process.

Communication Strategies for Advance Care Planning

The development of a trusting relationship with patients and families is integral to high-quality medical care, especially at end-of-life (Tulsky, 2005). The quality of the patient-clinician relationship trust and rapport can be enhanced by encouraging patients to share their concerns and questions using active listening, demonstrating respect, talking in an honest and straightforward manner, being sensitive when delivering difficult news, and maintaining engagement about advance care planning issues with the patient and family throughout the disease process (Moore, 2005b; Quill, 2000; Tulsky, 2005; Wenrich, Curtis, Shannon et al., 2001). Encouraging questions and open discussion of concerns is facilitated by active listening skills. Active listening and avoiding the tendency to interrupt can give patients and families the sense that the clinician truly cares and is invested in understanding their perspectives.

Active listening involves the use of open-ended questions and appropriate reflection back about the content of the speaker's message. For example, to begin a dialogue, a provider can ask an open-ended question such as, "What do you understand about your illness at this point?" (Moore, 2005a; Norlander & McSteen, 2000; Tulsky, 2005). This can provide an assessment of the patient's knowledge base about the illness and any salient concerns he or she may currently have. Once an open-ended question is posed, it is important to allow sufficient time for patients to respond and to avoid the tendency to interrupt. To ensure that the message content is understood and convey that the provider is really listening, reflecting the main ideas and feelings of the patient's statement can be helpful. For example, a clinician may say in response to a patient's dialogue, "You're really concerned about the side effects of your current medication, but you are afraid that if you don't take the drug, your condition will worsen. Let's talk about some options." Reflection used in conjunction with open-ended questions can help clinicians learn about what is most important to their patients and promote patient-centered care.

Some advance care planning discussions can be emotionally charged, and providers need to develop skills that manage this affect (Tulsky, 2005). Discussions fraught with emotion are often difficult for providers. Not all concerns uncovered during palliative care discussions have solutions (e.g., finding meaning in the illness experience, fear of dying, being overwhelmed with caregiving responsibilities). Whether or not such painful emotions are expressed, many patients and families coping with advanced illness experience them regardless, and opening up dialogue about difficult emotions can reduce the isolation they are apt to feel (Lo, Quill, & Tulsky, 1999). Lo and colleagues (1999) remind clinicians that they "do not have sole responsibility for responding to the patient's suffering" (p. 747). Referring troubled patients and families to a social worker, psychologist, member of the clergy, or another mental health professional can be helpful and appropriate.

When patients and families do become emotional, Tulsky (2005) suggests that providers:

1. Acknowledge the affect (e.g., "Making these decisions is not easy. This must be overwhelming.")
2. Identify loss (e.g., "It must be hard thinking about what kind of care you want when your condition gets worse. I know how much you value your independence.")
3. Legitimize feelings (e.g., "Many patients in your situation become sad thinking about these decisions. I think that is normal under the circumstances.")
4. Offer support (e.g., "I will be here for you throughout your treatment.")
5. Explore ("You said that you were scared about the future. What scares you the most?")

Direct discussion and validation of emotion without false reassurance or premature advice giving can be effective in diffusing emotionally charged clinical discussions.

Trust and respect are further cultivated when providers communicate in a straight-forward and honest, yet sensitive, manner. Evidence suggests that a vast majority of patients want to be fully informed about their illness and what to expect about their physical condition (Jenkins, Fallowfield, & Saul, 2001; Steinhauser et al., 2001; Wenrich et al., 2001). In one study, patients and family members ranked honest and straightforward discussion as one of the most important aspects of patient-provider communication in end-of-life care (Wenrich et al., 2001). They wanted physicians to be willing to discuss dying and to balance honesty and sensitivity. This is a formidable challenge to providers in palliative care but one that is important to quality advance care planning discussions. The Wenrich study indicated that poor communication "[s]temmed from being too blunt, not picking an appropriate time and place to provide bad news, and giving the sense that there was no hope" (p. 872).

One way of balancing hope and honesty in the context of ongoing advance care planning discussions is to frame discussions with patients in terms of 'hoping for the best yet preparing for the worst' (Back, Arnold, & Quill, 2003). Patients' hopes can be discussed while anticipation of and preparation for future health states and treatment scenarios are explored. Such discussions can start by clinicians articulating hope and preparation early in the course of treatment and then revisiting the topic throughout the disease trajectory. Patients can be asked, "Could you tell me more about what you are hoping for? That will help me do a better job for you" and "What are your concerns if things do not go as we hope?" (Back et al., 2003). Supporting and validating the patient's hopes, fears, and other emotions that result from such discussions are important. It is also important to note that what patients and families hope and prepare for can change during the disease trajectory. For example, during the early stages of the disease, hope may be invested in cure. As the disease progresses and attempts at cure show little success, providers can explore other hopes of the patient and family and what preparations need to be made.

Finally, it is important that health care professionals be aware of their nonverbal behavior and the context in which communication occurs with patients and families. Self-awareness of one's nonverbal communication is the first step in making needed changes. Practitioners should assess how they carry themselves when interacting with patients and families. Do they have an open posture that invites discussion (e.g., avoiding crossed arms)? Do they make appropriate and consistent eye contact? Environmental issues, such as privacy and avoiding outside interruptions, need to be considered, particularly when sensitive issues are addressed. The setting and the manner in which a message is conveyed can be powerful and have the potential to affect overall communication quality. Box 4-1 provides suggestions related to rapport-enhancing communication strategies.

Box 4-1	Rapport-Enhancing Verbal and Nonverbal Communication Strategies
Verbal Strategies	**Nonverbal Strategies**
Use open-ended questions to explore patient concerns.	Give patient undivided attention.
Paraphrase the content of the patient's communication using some of the patient's own words.	Avoid multitasking.
	Directly face the patient at eye level.
	Avoid distracting mannerisms.
	Maintain an open posture.
Validate patients' and family members' feelings.	Lean forward.
	Maintain appropriate eye contact.
Summarize broad themes during the interaction.	Be sensitive to and aware of cultural differences in nonverbal behavior.
Deliver diagnostic and prognostic information sensitively and with empathy.	Develop self-awareness about one's own nonverbal behaviors and what they communicate to others.
Assess preferences for receiving medical information.	
Avoid the use of medical jargon.	

From: Moore, C.D. (2005a). Advance care planning. In K.K. Kuebler, M. Davis, & C.D. Moore (Eds.). *Palliative practices: An interdisciplinary approach.* St. Louis: Elsevier Mosby.

Values Clarification and Discussion of Goals

Advance care planning unfolds over time in the context of the clinical relationship. Through the use of open-ended questions, active listening skills, and documentation of discussions, health care professionals can assist patients in clearly elucidating their values and goals that can ultimately inform end-of-life care. Patients may choose to document their treatment preferences and choices for decision-making surrogates in a formal advance directive, but the advance care planning process is as important (possibly more important) as the advance directive document itself in shaping end-of-life decision making and medical care (Kolarik et al., 2002; Lo, 2004; Tulsky, 2005).

As previously suggested, assessing the patient's understanding of his or her illness can help the health care professional better understand the patient's knowledge base and suggest areas for further patient education. It is also important to assess how much the patient wants to know about the illness; although most patients want full information about their condition (Jenkins et al., 2001; Wenrich et al., 2001), not all patients do. Cultural issues may influence this aspect of advance care planning, with some cultural groups preferring not to have direct discussions about diagnosis and prognosis, especially when the outlook is grim (Chan, 2004; Van Winkle, 2000; Yeo & Hikoyeda, 2000). The patient's preferences in this area can be assessed by directly asking, "How much do you want to know about your illness?" and "Who should we involve in these discussions?" Some patients from diverse backgrounds may only want their family to be involved in discussion about diagnosis and prognosis. Clinicians should educate themselves about cultural traditions of groups with whom they are likely to interact.

Assessment of patient goals can help inform current and future treatment planning. Care plans can be developed that facilitate the patient and family's short- and long-term goals. What does the patient want to accomplish in his or her life? This can range from living long enough to participate in an important family event (e.g., wedding or graduation) to managing symptoms well enough so that the patient can finish his family genealogy for his loved ones. At certain points in the disease trajectory, cure can also be a patient goal, and curative treatment plans should be developed and implemented. Regardless of patient goals, clinicians can help patients attempt to realize their aspirations through agreed-upon treatment plans; as patients' conditions change, health care providers can provide education, information, and recommendations and help patients reevaluate their plans.

Developing an understanding of patient values, or the principles, ideas, or qualities deemed worthwhile, can help clinicians deliver appropriate patient-centered care. Including family members and decision-making surrogates in the process of values clarification can lead to better-informed decision-makers and, it is hoped, decisions made by surrogates that are congruent with patient wishes. For some families, advance care planning conversations are not easy discussions to have. Patients and family members alike may be reticent to discuss such issues due to the emotions they can evoke. Clinicians can assist by initiating such discussions during medical encounters that address hopes and plans for the future and what makes life worthwhile for the patient. Patients can be asked to elaborate on what makes life worthwhile for them and to explain what terms such as "quality of life" mean. Various tools have been developed to help guide such discussions, including *Making Medical Decisions* (American Association of Retired Persons, 1996), *Five Wishes* (Commission on Aging with Dignity, 1998), *Talking About Your Choices* (Choice in Dying, 1996), and *Your Life, Your Choices* (Pearlman, Starks, Cain et al., 2001). Effective advance care planning discussions include those individuals who will potentially make decisions on behalf of the patient.

Another fruitful area for discussion related to patients' values is the topic of their personal experiences with others' illness, dying, and death. Patient expectations related to one's own disease process can be highly influenced by witnessing significant others coping with advanced illness and dying. Clinicians can ask patients if anyone close to them has died of disease and what that experience taught them about death and dying, thereby providing further opportunity to learn about patient values. For example, a patient may say of a loved one, "She was in such pain at the end. If that would happen to me, I want a lot of medication to control the pain" or "He was alone when he died. Dying alone must be horrible." These statements give considerable insight into personal values that are relevant to palliative care.

Finally, spirituality and existential issues figure prominently in how patients cope with advanced disease and dying. People struggle to make sense of their illness experience, and their construction of meaning can affect their emotional states and compliance with treatment. Clinicians can learn how the patient is making meaning of their disease by asking, "What thoughts have you had about why you got this illness at this time?" (Lo et al., 1999). In addition, spirituality and religious beliefs can influence choices that patients and families make about medical care. Health care professionals can accommodate these beliefs in the context of treatment by finding out if the patient has any beliefs that should be taken into consideration by the health care team.

Exploring patient values and goals can help clinicians develop patient-centered care plans. Inclusion of family and decision-making surrogates in the advance care planning process when possible can decrease potential conflict among the patient, family, and health care team. Completing advance directives as part of this process has been demonstrated to ease the burden of the decision-making process for the surrogate (Davis, Burns, Rezac et al., 2005; Tilden, Tolle, Nelson et al., 2001). Suggested questions to help initiate and maintain advance care planning discussion are listed in Box 4-2.

ADVANCE DIRECTIVES

Karen Ann Quinlan, Nancy Cruzan, and Terri Schiavo are names of individuals who highlight the importance of advance directive completion prior to a crisis. All three women's lives were cut short by some unexpected tragedy, and due to legal wrangling over their end-of-life treatment, their families paid a high emotional price and their dying processes were subject to lengthy court battles. These cases spurred ethical debates over a patient's right to refuse life-sustaining treatment, the role of the family in end-of-life decision making, and medicine's technological imperative. In response, numerous public policies related to end-of-life decision making were formulated. One such piece of legislation, the Patient Self-Determination Act (PSDA) of 1990 (P.L. 101-508, § 4206), was the first federal statute to focus on the right of adult patients to refuse life-sustaining medical treatment. The PSDA mandates that health

Box 4-2	**Suggested Questions for Advance Care Planning Discussions**

PATIENT UNDERSTANDING OF ILLNESS

- What do you understand about where things stand right now with your illness? (Lo et al., 1999)
- What do you know about your treatment options?

PATIENT PREFERENCES REGARDING INFORMATION DELIVERY

- How much do you want to know about your illness?
- Who would you like to be present during such discussions?

CONSIDERATIONS IN CHOOSING DECISION-MAKING SURROGATES

- Who would you want to make decisions for you if something happened and you were unable to make decisions about your care?
- Have you spoken with this person about being your decision-maker? Have you discussed your wishes with him or her?
- Have you informed other important people in your life about your choice of decision-maker?
- How well do you think this person can deal with any disagreements others may have about your wishes?
- If you anticipate any disagreements, what do you think is the best way to address this?
- To what extent do you want your family/loved ones to have input in decisions that are made about your health care?
- How important is it that your family as a whole agree with the decisions that are made on your behalf?

PATIENT GOALS

- What is important for you to accomplish at this point in your life?
- As you think about the future, what is most important to you (what matters the most to you)? (Lo et al., 1999)
- What are your hopes/fears for the future?
- If you were to die sooner rather than later, what would be left undone? (Quill, 2000)
- What type of legacy do you want to leave your family/loved ones? (Lo et al., 1999)

PATIENT VALUES

- What makes life worth living? (Quill, 2000)
- What would have to happen for your life to not be worth living?
- What nourishes your spirit?
- How do you feel about quality versus quantity of life?
- What are your thoughts about pain control? Would you want your pain controlled even if it meant that you might not be as alert?

PERSONAL EXPERIENCES WITH ILLNESS, DEATH, AND DYING

- Has anyone close to you died of an illness? What happened? What was it like for you?
- What other significant losses have you experienced?
- What would you consider a "good death"?

Continued

Box 4-2	**Suggested Questions for Advance Care Planning Discussions—cont'd**

SPIRITUALITY/EXISTENTIAL ISSUES

- What thoughts have you had about why you got this illness at this time? (Lo et al., 1999)
- Is faith (religion, spirituality) important to you in this illness and has it been important to you at other times in your life? (Lo et al., 1999)
- Would you like to explore religious/spiritual matters with someone? Do you have someone to talk to about these things? (Lo et al., 1999)
- Do you have any spiritual/religious beliefs that should be taken into consideration by your health care providers?

care organizations that receive federal health care dollars must inform patients about their rights to formulate advance directives, provide community and staff education about the documents, and maintain policies pertaining to advance directives.

The passage of the PSDA, patient and family concern regarding use of life-sustaining technology, and medical professionals' concern for patient welfare and legal liability resulted in a plethora of research on end-of-life decision making and advance directives during the 1990s. The seminal study was the $30 million SUPPORT study (The Study to Understand Prognoses and Preferences for Outcomes and Risks of Treatment), designed to investigate and improve end-of-life decision making and reduce the frequency of prolonged and painful death (SUPPORT Principal Investigators, 1995). This study suggested that clinical outcomes (e.g., timing of do-not-resuscitate [DNR] orders, time spent in the intensive care unit) were relatively uninfluenced by the presence of an advance directive in the patient's chart. Literature in the field has evolved to focus on the process of advance care planning instead of advance directive documents (e.g., Karel, Powell, & Cantor, 2004; Norlander & McSteen, 2000; Prendergast, 2001; Quill, 2000; Tulsky, 2005). For clinicians who work with patients with advanced illness, the message is clear—advance directives, executed without appropriate, timely, meaningful, and inclusive advance care planning discussions, are not a means to patient-centered, holistic care at end-of-life.

Every state has legislation that governs the implementation and execution of written advance directives, and it is imperative that clinicians thoroughly acquaint themselves with their state policies. The Web site for Compassion and Choices provides copies of advance directive forms for each state that can be downloaded (compassionandchoices.org/ad). Typically, advance directives take on three forms: oral directives, a written instructional directive (e.g., living will or health care directive), and a durable power of attorney for health care (health care proxy in some states) (Lo, 2004). In addition, 37 states have statutes that grant family members, in a stated order of priority, the right to make medical decisions for incapacitated patients in the absence of advance directives (Hosay, 2003). Advance directives are firmly rooted in the principle of patient self-determination and the notion of extended autonomy; even when patients are unable to express their preferences, their individual choices can be given voice via a written document or a decision-making surrogate who is familiar with their wishes.

Oral directives consist of discussions that patients have with family members, loved ones, and health care professionals about end-of-life treatment preferences. More common than written directives (Emanuel, Barry, Stoekler et al., 1991; Lo & Steinbrook, 2004), such discussions may not meet the "clear and convincing" evidentiary standard required by some advance directive statutes such as those in New York and Missouri (Lo, 2004). In any discussions that patients have with health care providers, it is important that the substantive content regarding relevant goals, values, and stated treatment preferences be recorded in the patient's record for future reference and to enhance communication about patient preferences among multiple providers.

Living wills are documents that explicitly state patient treatment preferences. Most commonly, treatments to be avoided at end-of-life are explicated (e.g., no artificial nutrition or hydration), but the documents can also specify types of desired treatments (e.g., adequate pain control medication). Living wills generally specify treatment preferences related to DNR orders, life-sustaining therapies including mechanical ventilation, feeding tubes, antibiotics, hemodialysis, and pain control (Quill, 2000). Estimates indicate that fewer than 25% of U.S. adults have a written advance directive (Emanuel et al., 1991; Hanson & Rodgman, 1996; Lo, 2004; Salmond & David, 2005), and the literature enumerates numerous potential problems with the living will. For example, the language used may be vague and hard to interpret (Happ, Capezuti, Strumpf et al., 2002; Lynn, 1991); patients may be hardpressed to anticipate all medical scenarios and may write directives that do not suit their best interests under certain circumstances (Lo, 2004; Lynn, 1991); the documents may not be available when needed (Tulsky, 2005); discussions about end-of-life treatment preferences are uncommon among patients and providers (Lo, 2004); and clinicians may not provide care as indicated in the written directive (Teno, Licks, Lynn et al., 1997).

On the other hand, a living will promulgated from a thoughtful and appropriate advance care planning process may indeed be helpful. As previously discussed, evidence suggests that advance directives have the potential to reduce family stress and decrease regret over medical decisions made on behalf of the patient (Davis et al., 2005; Tilden et al., 2001). A written document may also be helpful if there is family conflict about the course of treatment, if there is disagreement between the patient and health care providers, or when a patient wants to appoint someone outside of the definition of the traditional family (e.g., friend, same-sex partner) (Tulsky, 2005).

In addition to completing a living will, capacitated patients may choose to officially appoint a health care proxy or decision-making surrogate. Documenting one's choice for a decision-making surrogate has been described as being "more flexible and comprehensive than a living will" (Lo, 2004, p. 317). Decision-making surrogates are able to assess current medical realities in the context of the patient's stated preferences to (theoretically) arrive at medically sound decisions that honor the patient's wishes. It is important that patients thoughtfully choose a decision-making surrogate. In helping patients to choose a proxy, clinicians can ask, "Who would you want to make decisions for you if something happened and you were unable to make decisions about your care?" If the patient has someone in mind, it can be important to determine if the decision-making surrogate has been informed about the choice: "Have you spoken with this person about this? Have you informed other important people in your life that this is your wish?"

Patients should think about choosing a surrogate decision-maker who is able to cope with potential conflict. Patients can be asked, "How well do you think this person can deal with any disagreements others may have about your wishes? If you anticipate any disagreements, what do you think the best way is to address this?" Some patients may wish to choose more than one surrogate; for example, a patient may appoint an alternative decision-maker in the event the main surrogate is unable to be present. Other patients may want the family as a unit to make decisions by consensus; this should be clarified among the patient and the family. Under such circumstances, the appointment of a family spokesperson can help to streamline the communication process with the health care team and decrease confusion.

When patients complete advance directives, they should be informed that they are free to change the documents at any time. Advance care planning discussions do not end when a living will or durable power of attorney for health care has been completed. Discussions about end-of-life treatment wishes should be revisited if there is a significant change in the patient's condition or life circumstances. Patients can and do change their minds about end-of-life treatment, especially when there are significant changes in their health status. If patients do change their advance directives, the old copies should be destroyed and replaced with updated documents. Medical records should reflect the most recent version, and other health care professionals involved in the patient's care should be made aware of the status of the changes. Decision-making surrogates should receive the most current copy of the documents as well.

Although not an advance directive, clinicians should be aware of the POLST (Physician Orders for Life Sustaining Treatment) form used in various states and locales across the country to assist health care professionals in honoring the end-of-life care wishes of patients. The POLST translates a patient's advance directive into a set of physician's orders on a standardized form that documents end-of-life treatment preferences. This set of physician orders is intended to be portable across medical settings and increase the likelihood that a person's end-of-life care wishes will be implemented. The POLST form was developed in Oregon in 1991 and is also used in West Virginia and Washington, as well as in parts of Wisconsin, Pennsylvania, New York, Utah, New Mexico, Michigan, Georgia, and Minnesota (Hickman & Newman, 2005). Evaluation research indicates that the POLST is effective in promoting end-of-life medical care that is congruent with patient wishes (Lee, Brummel-Smith, Meyer, Drew et al., 2000; Meyers, Moore, McGrory et al., 2004; Tolle, Tilden, Nelson et al., 1998). More information about the POLST can be found at www.polst.org.

SURROGATES, FAMILIES, AND END-OF-LIFE DECISION MAKING

When patients are unable to make their own medical decisions, clinicians routinely rely on significant others to guide the decision-making process. Working with patients' family members as decision-making surrogates is a routine aspect of delivering palliative care. The responsibility of surrogate decision making usually falls to the family because of their intimate and longstanding knowledge of the patient's goals, values, preferences, and best interests. The family is seen as being most concerned with the patient's welfare and thus is expected to make decisions in the patient's best interest

(Buchanan & Brock, 1989; Chan, 2004). Through the appointment of an *informed proxy*, patient self-determination is extended in the face of decisional incapacity. To realize this goal of extended patient autonomy, surrogates and family members are routinely called on to use the *substituted judgment* standard, one of the predominant legal approaches adopted by the courts that regulate the termination of medical treatment of an incapacitated patient (Rhoden, 1988).

This standard mandates that medical decisions for an incapacitated patient be made as that patient would have made them for himself or herself if able and requires that the decision-maker be objective (Buchanan & Brock, 1989; Rhoden, 1988). Substituted judgments can be guided by the content of a living will or previously stated oral directives. As previously discussed, a majority of patients do not complete written documents, and even if a patient does have a living will, a surrogate may be called on to make decisions that are not directly addressed by the document. Thus, surrogates may be required to infer the patient's treatment predilections from their knowledge of the patient's character, goals, and values. This process entails a certain amount of imagination and deduction on the part of the surrogate while requiring him or her to be objective, uninfluenced by personal emotions and biases.

The other predominant legal standard that is used by surrogates to arrive at decisions to terminate life-sustaining treatment is the *best interests* standard. This standard weighs the burdens of the patient's life in the current state against the benefits of continuing life in that state (Buchanan & Brock, 1989). In order to terminate treatment, the burdens of artificially prolonging a life must clearly and significantly outweigh its benefits. The standard is used when there is little, if any, information about the patient's treatment preferences, and it calls for an objective judgment as to what best serves the patient's interests. This objectivity is described in a document produced in 1987 by the New York State Task Force on Life and the Law as "a judgment that is consistent with what most people would decide for themselves under the same circumstances" (Collopy, 1999, p. 41).

The aforementioned judgment standards are assumed to be rational methods of making end-of-life treatment decisions for a significant other (Chan, 2004). In the real world of end-of-life care and surrogate decision making, it is doubtful that most surrogates purely and rationally use either the substituted judgment or best interests standard when arriving at decisions (Berger, 2005; Chan, 2004; Moore, Sparr, Sherman et al., 2003). It has been argued that the distinction between the best interests and substituted judgment standards is not entirely clear (Rhoden, 1988). Substituted judgment requires a consideration of the patient's character, values, past preferences, and history to make medical decisions that are congruent with what the patient would have wanted; is it possible for a surrogate to make such judgments objectively without one's personal biases (e.g., love and concern for the patient) affecting the decision? The best interests standard asks the surrogate to consider only the patient's current condition in order to make a decision that best serves the patient's current medical interests; how can one appropriately arrive at a decision that promotes the patient's current interests without considering the patient's past and making judgments about quality of life concerns (Moore et al., 2003)?

These points illuminate the complexities and difficult realities that clinicians face when developing and implementing end-of-life treatment plans and further emphasize the importance of advance care planning discussions that include the family and/or significant others. When coping with an advanced illness, family members of patients are deeply affected, and their concern, love, and interests are likely to influence the end-of-life decision-making process; this reality runs contrary to the rationality assumed by the substituted judgment and best interests standards. In addition, patients are often concerned about being a burden on their families at end-of-life. Some patients want their family and decision-making surrogates to consider the interests of the collective when making medical decisions on their behalf (Chan, 2004; Moore et al., 2003). Patients can be deeply concerned as to how treatment decisions affect the well-being of the family (Berger, 2005).

It can be posited that the patient's and family's interests are "often indistinct, mutual, and reciprocal" (Berger, 2005, p. 3), and this emphasis on the interdependence of the individual and family is seen among various cultural groups. This is not to say that the family's interests should be paramount to or even be given equal weight with the patient's interest in all cases but rather that honoring patient's wishes can include consideration of the decision's impact on the collective. As part of the advance care planning process, providers can address this issue with patients: "What do you want your surrogate to consider when he or she makes medical decisions for you?" "How much input do you want your family to have in decisions that are made about your care?" Other questions to assess the impact of the illness on the patient's family from the perspective of the patient include "How is your family handling your illness?" (Quill, 2000) and "What are your loved one's fears about your illness? What are their hopes?" (Moore, 2005a). Clinicians may choose to pose the same types of question to family members. These discussions can help health care professionals better understand family dynamics and the degree to which the family is considering the patient's interests as well as their own in the context of end-of-life decision making.

CONCLUSION

The ultimate goals of the advance care planning process are to facilitate self-determined life closure and to help patients have a "good death." Realizing these goals requires effort on the parts of patients, clinicians, and family members to communicate openly, honestly, and consistently. All patients have a unique past and present, values and goals that are meaningful to them, connections to others, and futures that can unfold in ways that finish the narration of their life in a coherent and consistent manner. To perceive patients in this way acknowledges them as a person, not just as a patient with a collection of signs and symptoms. Health care professionals who partner with patients, surrogates, and family members in the advance care planning process can help to ensure that a patient's personhood is honored in the last phase of life.

REFERENCES

American Association of Retired Persons. (1996). *Making medical decisions: Questions and answers about health care powers of attorney and living wills*. Washington, DC: Author.

Back, A., Arnold, R.M., & Quill, T.E. (2003). Hope for the best, and prepare for the worst. *Ann Intern Med, 138(5)*, 439-444.

Berger, J.T. (2005). Patients' interests in their family members' well-being: An overlooked, fundamental consideration within substituted judgments. *J Clin Ethics, 16(1),* 3-10.

Buchanan, A.E. & Brock, D.W. (1989). *Deciding for others: The ethics of surrogate decision making.* New York: Cambridge University Press.

Chan, H.M. (2004). Sharing death and dying: Advance directives, autonomy, and the family. *Bioethics, 18(2),* 87-103.

Choice in Dying. (1996). *Whose death is it anyway? Talking about your choices.* New York: Author.

Collopy, B.J. (1999). Autonomy in long term care: Some crucial distinctions. *Gerontologist, 28(Suppl.),* 10-17.

Commission on Aging with Dignity. (1998). *Five wishes.* Tallahassee, Fla: Author.

Davis, B.A., Burns, J., Rezac, D., et al. (2005). Family stress ad advance directives: A comparative study. *J Hospice Palliat Nurs, 7(4),* 219-227.

Emanuel, L., Barry, M., Stoeckle, J., et al. (1991). Advance directives for medical care: A case for greater use. *New Engl J Med, 324,* 889-895.

Hanson, L.C. & Rodgman, E. (1996). The use of living wills at the end of life: A national study. *Arch Intern Med, 13(156),* 1018-1022.

Happ, M.B., Capezuti, E., Strumpf, N.E., et al. (2002). Advance care planning and end-of-life care for hospitalized nursing home residents. *J Am Geriatr Soc, 50(5),* 829-835.

Hickman, S. & Newman, J. (2005). *National POLST paradigm initiative.* Retrieved August 25, 2005, from www.ohsu.edu/polst/docs/POLST_nppi.pdf?

Hosay, C. (2003). The need to educate nursing home administrators about variations in state legislation affecting patients' rights to refuse treatment. *Illness, Crisis Loss, 11(2),* 148-161.

Jenkins, V.A., Fallowfield, L.J., & Saul, J. (2001). Information needs of patients with cancer: results from a large study in UK cancer centres. *Br J Cancer, 84,* 48-51.

Karel, M.J., Powell, J. & Cantor, M.D. (2004). Using a values discussion guide to facilitate communication in advance care planning. *Patient Educ Couns, 55(1),* 22-31.

Kolarik, R.C., Arnold, R.M., Fischer, G.S., et al. (2002). Objectives for advance care planning. *J Palliat Med, 5(5),* 697-704.

Lee, M.A., Brummel-Smith, K., Meyer, J., et al. (2000). Physician Orders for Life-Sustaining Treatment (POLST): Outcomes in a PACE program. *J Am Geriatr Soc, 48(10),* 1219-1225.

Lee, S.J., Back, A.L., Block, S.D., et al. (2002). Enhancing physician-patient communication. *Hematology,* 464-483.

Limerick, M. (2002). Communicating with surrogate decision-makers in end-of-life situations: Substitutive descriptive language for the healthcare provider. *Am J Hospice Palliat Care, 19(6),* 376-380.

Lo, B. (2004). Advance care planning. *Am J Geriatr Cardiol, 19(6),* 316-320.

Lo, B., Quill, T.E. & Tulsky, J.A. (1999). Discussing palliative care with patients. *Ann Intern Med, 130(9),* 744-749.

Lo, B., & Steinbrook, R. (2004). Resuscitating advance directives. *Arch Intern Med, 164,* 1501-1506.

Lynn, J. (1991). Why I don't have a living will. *Law Med Health Care, 19(1-2),* 101-104.

Meyers, J., Moore, C.D., McGrory, A., et al. (2004). Physician Orders for Life-Sustaining Treatment Form: Honoring end-of-life directives for nursing home residents. *J Gerontol Nurs, 30(9),* 37-46.

Moore, C.D. (2005a). Advance care planning. In K.K. Kuebler, M. Davis, & C.D. Moore (Eds.). *Palliative practices: An interdisciplinary approach.* St. Louis: Elsevier Mosby.

Moore, C.D. (2005b). Communication issues and advance care planning. *Semin Oncol Nurs, 21(1),* 11-19.

Moore, C.D., Sparr, J., Sherman, S., et al. (2003). Surrogate decision-making: Judgment standard preferences of older adults. *Soc Work Health Care, 37(2),* 1-16.

Morrison, M.F. (1998). Obstacles to doctor-patient communication at the end of life. In M.D. Steinberg & S.J. Youngner (Eds.). *End-of-life decisions, A psychosocial perspective* (pp. 109-136). Washington, DC: American Psychiatric Press.

Norlander, L. & McSteen, K. (2000). The kitchen table discussion: A creative way to discuss end-of-life issues. *Home Healthc Nurse, 18(8),* 532-539.

Patient Self-Determination Act of 1990, P.L. 101-508, § 4206m 104 Stat. 1388.

Pearlman, R.A., Starks, H., Cain, K., et al. (2001). *Health Services Research and Development: Your life, your choices, 2003.* Retrieved May 16, 2006, from www.hsrd.research.va.gov/publications/internal/ylyc.htm.

Prendergast, T.J. (2001). Advance care planning: Pitfalls, progress, promise. *Crit Care Med, 29(2)*, 34-39.

Quill, T.E. (2000). Initiating end-of-life discussions with seriously ill patients: Addressing the "elephant in the room." *JAMA, 284(19)*, 2502-2507.

Reisfield, G.M. & Wilson, G.R. (2003). Ambiguity in end-of-life communications. *J Termin Oncol, 2(2)*, 61-66.

Rhoden, N.K. (1988). Litigating life and death. *Harvard Law Review, 102*, 375-446.

Salmond, S.W. & David, E. (2005). Attitudes toward advance directives and advance directive completion rates. *Orthop Nurs, 24(2)*, 117-125.

Steinhauser, K.E., Christakis, N.A., Clipp, E.C., et al. (2001). Preparing for the end of life: Preferences of patients, families, physicians, and other care providers. *J Pain Symptom Manage, 22(3)*, 727-737.

SUPPORT Principal Investigators. (1995). A controlled trial to improve care for seriously ill hospitalized patients: The study to understand prognoses and preferences of outcomes and risks of treatments. *JAMA, 274*, 1591-1598.

Teno, J.M., Licks, S., Lynn, J., et al. (1997). Do advance directives provide instructions that direct care? *J Am Geriatr Soc, 45(4)*, 508-512.

Tilden, V.P., Tolle, S.W., Nelson, C.A., et al. (2001). Family decision-making to withdraw life-sustaining treatments from hospitalized patients. *Nurs Res, 50(2)*, 105-115.

Tolle, S.W., Tilden, V.P., Nelson, C.A., et al. (1998). A prospective study of the efficacy of the physician order form for life sustaining treatment. *J Am Geriatr Soc, 46(9)*, 1097-1102.

Tulsky, J.A. (2005). Beyond advance directives: Importance of communication skills at the end of life. *JAMA, 294(3)*, 359-365.

Van Winkle, N.W. (2000). End-of-life decision making in American Indian and Alaska Native Cultures. In K. Braun, J. Pietsch & P. Blanchette (Eds.). *Cultural issues in end-of-life decision making* (pp. 127-144). Thousand Oaks, Calif.: Sage.

Wenrich, M.D., Curtis, J.R., Shannon, S.E., et al. (2001). Communicating with dying patients within the spectrum of medical care from terminal diagnosis to death. *Arch Intern Med, 161*, 868-874.

Yeo, G. & Hikoyeda, N. (2000). Cultural issues in end-of-life decision making among Asians and Pacific Islanders in the United States. In K. Braun, J. Pietsch & P. Blanchette (Eds.). *Cultural issues in end-of-life decision making*. Thousand Oaks, Calif.: Sage.

CHAPTER 5

ETHICAL ISSUES SURROUNDING ADVANCED DISEASE

Agnes Coveney

■

The most painful sight we ever confront is that of beauty yielding to impermanence.
– Arthur Frank, At the Will of the Body: Reflections on Illness (1991)

■

The core purposes of clinical practice are to attend to the person in need, to ameliorate suffering, and to promote the achievement of human good, both for the individual patient and for the community. In assuming the social role and profession, the advanced practice nurse (APN) publicly professes to undertake a fundamental obligation in the caring relationship between professional and patient. The ethical basis of that relationship is the clinician's good faith and motivation to avoid harm. Ethical decision making expresses the moral obligation underlying medical care—to protect the dignity and welfare of the often vulnerable other. Thus, in collaborative goal setting, choices support the person's total well-being and are based on clinical evidence. O'Rourke (2000) describes human well-being and the goods of human life as "preserving life, seeking the truth, loving our families, generating and nurturing future generations, and forming communities with other people." The APN caring for persons in late-stage chronic illness or in a critical exacerbation of a disease state navigates, with patients, families, and the interdisciplinary care team, the trajectory of advanced disease and ensures ethical treatment decisions based on the totality of the patient. This chapter examines the ethical issues in advanced disease and end-of-life care.

The ethical framework for the clinical approach to advanced disease and end-of-life care is one of comfort and dignity in advanced disease and during the last phase of life. A good death, as defined by the Institute of Medicine's Committee on Care at the End of Life, is "one that is free from avoidable distress and suffering for patients, families and caregivers; in general accord with patients' and families' wishes; and reasonably consistent with clinical, cultural and ethical standards" (Della Santina & Bernstein, 2004). Ethical dilemmas or conflicts arise with disagreement over treatment goals. With timely advance care planning, clear explanations of condition and prognosis, and well-documented discussions about goals of care, all measures that support patient rights and quality care, the clinician can reduce or prevent ethical crises for the family and the care team (Lynn & Goldstein, 2003; Teno, 2001). Palliative care allows clinicians in geriatric medicine to continue to offer treatments rather than dismissing the patient or ruling out care with curative intent (Emanuel, 2004). With their emphasis on the relief of suffering, assistance with pain and symptom management, and ongoing communication to articulate and fulfill the mutually agreed-upon goals of care, palliative care and hospice care constitute ethical medicine.

PATIENT SELF-DETERMINATION AND INFORMED CONSENT

The ethical principle of self-determination requires that a person is accorded the freedom to make decisions for himself or herself, yet it is not completely accurate to operate from the image of an independent self with no obligation to consider the needs and interests of other persons. While *self-determination* is defined as "respecting the decision making capacities of autonomous persons," it is also true that persons exist in multiple relationships (Beauchamp & Childress, 2001). The total treatment decision, of which informed consent is a part, also takes into account the patient's aspirations and goals, as well as the interrelated functions of the person—physiological, psychological, social, and spiritual (O'Rourke, 2000).

Enacted in 1991, the Patient Self-Determination Act creates the foundation for the patient's exercise of decision-making authority. The law was prompted in part by highly publicized legal cases involving life-sustaining or life-prolonging treatment decisions for patients unable to express their wishes. It was also prompted by the advances in medical technology that made such life-sustaining treatment possible (Ulrich, 1999). The legal standards of informed consent and confidentiality arise from the ethical principle of self-determination. In the process of informed consent, the patient is given, in language that he or she can understand, a description of the intervention, treatment or medication, its purpose, anticipated outcome, its risks and benefits, and any alternatives to the treatment. Medical practices, home care, nursing homes, and hospitals honor confidentiality and privacy policies governing the sharing of a patient's medical and financial information.

PATIENT–HEALTH CARE PROFESSIONAL RELATIONSHIP

The APN meets patients and families in moments of vulnerability and limiting health conditions. The inequality of medical knowledge in the patient-professional relationship requires the APN to respect the integrity of the patient. Beyond rule following, the ethic of the patient-professional relationship entails a degree of altruism as well as particular virtues or characteristic motives deep within the person (Pellegrino & Thomasma, 1988). Many worthy characteristics are discussed in the arena of virtue ethics. Beauchamp and Childress (2001) suggest five central virtues—compassion, discernment, trustworthiness, integrity, and conscientiousness. The moral virtues, instilled in upbringing and functioning deep in a person's character, become habitual ways of responding and acting ethically. Just as the experienced APN uses clinical assessment skills habitually, almost unconsciously, the virtues as ethical habits are implemented without having to be consciously recalled and intentionally put into action.

The ethic of the patient-professional relationship is further defined by two related principles—*nonmaleficence*, avoiding the causation of harm, and *beneficence*, a group of norms prescribing actions for the good of the patient (Beauchamp & Childress, 2001). Acting for the patient's good, the APN considers, concurrently, the clinical condition and the patient as a unique person living in interdependent relationships. Moreover, the APN does not act as a neutral technician, abandoning moral stance and values system when patient and family demands go against sound medical judgment or ethical principles. The APN should seek assistance when conflicts in treatment or care plan goals threaten the integrity of clinician clinical judgment and ethical principles. Additionally, because it is subjective, the motivation of acting in the patient's best interest should be checked and tested by seeking the view of a colleague or the review of the treatment goals with an institutional ethics committee.

Finally, the honesty inherent in the patient-professional relationship entails not avoiding the communication of difficult truths about diagnosis and prognosis to the patient and family. Marked by care and empathy, such conversations empower the patient and family with information needed for decisions and good-byes. Within the ethic of the patient-professional relationship, the APN discerns with the patient and family a course of care that supports the whole person with advanced disease.

DECISIONAL CAPACITY

The APN caring for patients in advanced disease seeks to determine whether the patient, in the present moment, understands the medical choices and their consequences. Legal determinations of competency introduce a complex process in which a professional in psychiatry or psychology evaluates the patient and attests to competency, using a strict clinical and legal framework. It may be more practical and it is acceptable, in cases of fluctuating capacity, to consider an alternative approach, decisional capacity (Robbins, 1996). Rather than applying the standard tests for orientation, the assessment of decisional capacity weighs the patient's ability to understand the information relevant to the decision and its consequences (Ulrich, 1999). When the patient lacks decisional capacity, decisions made on behalf of the patient promote the convergence of the patient's interests and the clinician's medical knowledge. In cases involving the more formal determinations of competency, and for assistance in the regulations and policy governing related determinations of next-of-kin and guardianship, the APN should utilize resource persons in the institution and community, including social workers, legal counsel, and agencies specializing in elder service and protection (Curtis, 2004).

SURROGATE DECISION MAKING

The APN and physician call on surrogate decision-makers when a patient is incapable of making a treatment decision or has not formulated a living will or advance directive. Generally, the order of precedence in surrogates is as follows: the durable power of attorney for health care, anyone specified by the patient, a legal guardian with specific authority to make medical decisions, the spouse, children of age, and parents (Robbins, 1996). In one approach for surrogate decision making, substituted judgment, surrogate decision-makers attempt to decide as the patient would have decided if he or she were capable. In this approach, the surrogate decision-maker must have some knowledge of the desires and values of the patient and, most important, what constitutes the patient's own understanding of well-being (O'Rourke, 2000). The patient's advance directives and past statements and choices help reveal patient wishes. In another approach, best interests, the surrogate decision-maker makes a decision for the patient when there is no information about the patient's wishes, determining what course of action best supports the welfare of the patient. Clinicians, after providing information on the patient's condition and prognosis, should ask the family what they think their loved one would have wanted and should explain to the family what will be done in terms of comfort measures (Shannon, 2001). When surrogate decision-makers are unaware of or unsure of the patient's wishes, the decision should be made based on the patient's best interests, not on what the surrogate would do if in such a situation. Clinicians should seek the assistance of pastoral care, social workers, and other institutional resources when the surrogate's decision is counter to the patient's best interests and is influenced by subjective aspects such as grief and fear.

ADVANCE DIRECTIVES

Ideally as part of advance care planning, advance directives outline the patient's wishes for medical care and are formulated when the patient is still competent. (Advance care planning is discussed more fully in Chapter 4.) These legal documents support the moral authority of the patient's family or surrogates to decide on behalf of the person. In the absence of advance directives, an informed family or a surrogate, with the physician and APN, may withhold life-sustaining treatment, based on the patient's preferences and clinical condition. In the best case, the patient has communicated his or her wishes and intent to family members, to a surrogate decision-maker, or to a power of attorney for health care. Although advance directives vary from state to state, the living will generally outlines a person's wishes about life-prolonging treatment and artificially provided nutrition and hydration. In the health care power of attorney advance directive, the patient has named the person who will speak for him or her and carry out the patient's wishes. Either document becomes effective when the patient lacks decisional capacity. These directives also allow that, in the presence of a terminal or permanent vegetative state, life-sustaining treatments may be withheld. A *terminal condition* is generally defined as a condition caused by disease, illness, or injury that is irreversible, incurable, and untreatable. A further requirement may entail that two physicians attest to and document the terminal condition. The opportune time for the documentation of advance directives is in an office visit or on admission to an extended care facility, prior to crisis situations. Turning points in the patient's advanced disease are opportunities to review goals and advance directives in consideration of the total condition and well-being of the patient (Della Santina & Bernstein, 2004). The physician and APN hold the trust and respect of the patient and family and can encourage the completion of such documents, normalizing the discussion of advanced illness and death and helping families and patients move beyond fear and avoidance of mortality (Quaglietti, Blum, & Ellis, 2004).

WITHHOLDING AND WITHDRAWING TREATMENT

Withholding a treatment entails a decision against instituting that treatment or therapy. Withdrawing a treatment concerns a decision to stop and possibly remove the treatment. For this discussion, treatments include those understood as life sustaining or life prolonging—cardiopulmonary resuscitation, artificial nutrition and hydration, ventilatory support, and dialysis—as well as other interventions not generally classified as such—vasopressors, intravenous fluids, and antibiotics. Although it is a common misapprehension, there is no moral or legal distinction between decisions to withhold and withdraw treatment. Both decisions concern changing the goals of care when the treatments that no longer modify disease are ineffective and unwanted by the patient, a process that most often occurs over time rather than during one meeting or conversation (Derse, 2005). To make either decision ethically requires a careful weighing of several factors, including the patient's condition and prognosis and the ability of the treatment to reverse the terminal progression of the disease, to alleviate suffering and reduce burden, and to support or weaken the patient's total well-being, including the patient's ability to pursue the goods of life (Panicola, 2001).

Regulatory emphasis on caloric intake and the rehabilitative function of nursing homes causes some facilities to resist allowing the patient or family to withhold or withdraw tube feeding (Miller, Teno, & Mor, 2004). Elderly residents may lack decision-making capacity, and there may be no family, friends, or surrogates with knowledge of the resident's life and preferences (Lynn, 1989). It is important for the APN to become familiar with the facts rather than operate out of a fear of liability and from unsupported assumptions about whether a treatment can be foregone or withheld (Meisel, Snyder, & Quill, 2000).

Withdrawing a treatment may occur after a time-limited trial of the intervention. Due to the difficulty in predicting life expectancy in advanced disease and the unpredictable course of noncancer illness, a time-limited trial is a helpful approach when establishing treatment decisions (Miller et al., 2004). A time-limited course of the therapy should be considered in the presence of benefit; and, in the absence of benefit, the patient, family, and clinician agree to discontinue therapy after establishing a set time-frame (O'Rourke, 2000).

Technological innovations in medicine offer clinicians a means to guide their patients through a medical crisis to a return to health. The message implicit in medical advances, the technological imperative, asserts that if a medical innovation is available, it must be used. Thus, medical advances constitute weighty decisions for the patient and family in the situation of advanced disease and end of life. The burden of treatment decisions for families and patients grows even heavier as they struggle to determine whether the treatment offered thus far is sufficient and when it is acceptable to forego the medical technology available. In decisions to withhold or withdraw treatment, it is important to recall that the goal of medicine is an optimally functioning human being whose interdependent functions—physiological, psychological, social, and spiritual or creative—further the fulfillment of the purpose of life (O'Rourke, 2000).When treatments cannot achieve those goals, it ethically acceptable to withhold or withdraw them. Palliative care provides the clinician the ability to offer tangible comfort and alleviation of symptoms, replacing unnecessary and unhelpful measures.

WEIGHING BENEFITS AND BURDENS

In weighing the benefits and burdens of care and treatments, the clinician, patient, and family consider whether the burdens of treatment outweigh the benefits. Does the continued use of the treatment or diagnostic test constitute a burden or benefit?

Do the burdens of the intervention outweigh the benefits? Will the treatment reverse the course of the illness and return the patient to previous well-being? Will the treatment allow the patient to enjoy the things enjoyed previously, including awareness of and pleasure in relationships? Because clinicians differ on what they consider to be ordinary treatment, the assessment of ordinary versus extraordinary treatment is not as helpful as is the consideration of benefits and burdens. The benefits and burdens principle is used within a moral framework of embracing life as a value while, at the same time, recognizing that life is not an absolute good (O'Rourke, 2000). Life is to be enjoyed as a gift, yet there are limits to what must be done to sustain life in the context of advanced disease and end-of-life care (Sheehan, 2001). In the context of advanced disease and terminal condition, it is permissible to forego measures that entail excessive burden—pain, suffering, and expense—to the patient or family and when those measures will create unwanted side effects and will not improve condition or outcome.

MEDICAL FUTILITY

For this discussion, *futile treatment* is treatment that is unable to reverse the course of the disease and that offers no hope of benefit. Because families sometimes insist on futile treatment, a well-developed process for timely, ongoing communication within the team and with the family can prevent conditions that lead to demand for futile treatment—family feelings of a loss of control, insufficient information to keep pace with the patient's condition, and a lack of information on what is possible to achieve given the patient's situation (Hamel & Panicola, 2003). Sound medical judgment, rather than family demands and court decisions, should determine what treatment is appropriate and what therapy is offered and is not offered. Futile treatments prolong the eventuality of death, fuel unrealistic hope, counter the goals of medicine, and frustrate health care team members (O'Rourke, 2000). Giving in to unrealistic demands for treatment puts the medical profession in jeopardy of losing its essential responsibility for patient well-being. To approach treatment decisions with an excessive fear of legal liability risks the weakening of the professional ethic and the transfer of clinical decision making to the courts. Measures that limit clinician vulnerability to legal challenge include clear documentation, explicit rationales for a course of treatment, adherence to policy and processes, and involvement of institutional resources such as the ethics committee (Robbins, 1996).

A crucial ethical distinction in cases of medical futility is that of fatal pathology, an illness or condition that will cause death if not addressed by means of medical intervention or surgery. In withholding or withdrawing a life-sustaining treatment, the patient suffering from a fatal pathology dies of the underlying disease that rendered them unable to breathe, eat, or process bodily waste. In such a case, the person died of the inexorable course of the disease. The withholding or withdrawing of the treatment does not constitute a new cause of death; instead death follows its natural course (O'Rourke, 2000). Clinical judgment determined that the treatment would not further the total well-being of the patient, including the physical and spiritual dimensions (Paris, 1998). To make such a determination requires knowledge of the patient's overall outlook, respect for the patient's dignity, and recognition of the imminence or nearness of death, rendering the treatment ineffective.

CLINICAL LEADERSHIP

In the patient-professional relationship, the patient and family rely on the clinician's medical knowledge regarding what treatments will and will not benefit the patient. The physician has the competence to make medical decisions and the responsibility to come to decision making having already determined what is and is not medically appropriate and what will not be offered based on what is within the bounds of good medical practice (O'Rourke, 2000; Sheehan, 2001). Using the clinical leadership approach, the health care professional accepts the responsibility for his or her share of the clinical decision, ruling out inappropriate choices, explaining that based on his or her medical judgment and years of clinical experience, the treatment will not benefit the patient and may even harm the patient. Patients and families consent to the clinician's determination that the treatment is not indicated; they are not asked to choose to forego a beneficial treatment. Contrary to assumptions in the field, no legal or ethical mandate exists requiring physicians to offer families all conceivable treatments (Hamel & Panicola, 2003). Even if a patient or family requests an outcome of continued physiological function, if the patient is unable to pursue the goods of life, the family request does not legitimate the pursuit of that outcome. This is especially true when the demand for futile treatment necessitates ongoing medical care affecting the use of medical resources (O'Rourke, 2000).

The fiduciary ethical claim in the patient-professional relationship necessitates trust and respect for the vulnerability of the patient. In the approach of clinical leadership, the physician offers guidance, empowering the patient to help himself or herself (Pellegrino & Thomasma, 1988). A core competency for the clinician is the ability "to guide the transition from curative and palliative goals of treatment to palliative goals alone," basing the plan on outcomes evidence and clinical judgment (Surgeons' Palliative Care Workgroup, 2003). APNs and physicians in the care team should guard against paternalism or unilateralism by seeking independent opinions from physicians, ethics consultants, chaplains, or pastoral care staff on whether treatment can achieve the therapeutic goal. Open discussion of the proposed plan of care can also assess the strength of data and clinical experience to support an assessment of the futility of the treatment (Curtis, 2004). The clinician must be able to understand family grief, their wish to keep the patient alive by any means and cost, and their often unrealistic hope in the technological advances of medicine.

THE PRINCIPLE OF DOUBLE EFFECT

Pain management in the terminal phase of advanced disease is guided by the principle of double effect. The principle makes ethical distinctions among intentions and consequences, particularly those consequences that are anticipated (O'Rourke, 2000). Thus, an act that brings about two foreseen effects, one good and the other adverse, is not always morally prohibited (Beauchamp & Childress, 2001). The motivation pursuing a good effect, such as managing pain in the terminal phase, may bring about two results—the intended effect of pain relief as well as an unwanted but foreseen side effect, the suppression of respiration. In the context of terminal conditions, the distinction of motive and wanted and unwanted effects is essential in assessing the morality of the act. Guided by this principle, high doses of opioids and sedatives may be ordered by the physician when the intention is to relieve suffering and not to cause the patient's death. The dose must be the lowest dose that effects relief of symptoms. The patient must be in a terminal condition, the need to relieve suffering must be urgent, and there must be consent of the patient or surrogate decision-maker. For further conditions to the principle and guidance on the appropriate context and application of the principle of double effect, see Lo and Rubenfeld (2005).

Thorough documentation of the clinician's intentions is essential, including indications for the administration of analgesics and sedatives (Truog, Cist, Brackett et al., 2001). Guidelines such as clinical parameters and dosage indications are necessary in the use of sedative agents for the management of pain and symptoms in dying patients. The APN has a crucial role in providing family education in the dying process—what the patient feels and does not feel—and in understanding the role and intent of palliative sedation, which is to provide comfort and alleviation of symptoms, not to cause or hasten death (Foley, 2001).

COMMUNICATION AND MEDIATION

A review of findings from the Study to Understand Prognosis and Preferences for Outcomes and Risks of Treatments (SUPPORT) revealed that treatment preferences of seriously ill patients are poorly understood and unknown to physicians, family, and surrogates (Covinsky, Fuller, Yaffe et al., 2000). The last three decades of publicly debated medical ethics cases concerning disagreement over life-sustaining treatments involve family disputes, the limits of medicine, and intrusion by society into the personal nature of medical care (Dresser, 2005). Communication and mediation skills of the APN, the care team, or other resource persons support ethical care and patient advocacy, assisting patients and families in navigating the decisions of advanced disease and end-of-life care.

Patients and families appreciate clinicians' sensitive and candid communication. Families want clinicians who do not shy away from discussions about death (Curtis & Patrick, 2001; Twohig & Byock, 2004). Time spent listening increases family satisfaction. Consensus in the care team prevents the communication of conflicting messages to the patient and family. Effective goal setting and treatment decisions made with the patient and family seek to understand what quality of life would be important to the patient after treatment (Curtis, 2004). Proactive communication may successfully circumvent a latent family conflict, arising in the highly charged arena of death or medical crisis, that threatens to derail the meticulously established, condition-appropriate care plan.

Protocols for communication and decision making are summarized by Morrison and Meier (2004). Weissman (2004) offers a case review outlining a structured approach to decision making for patients in the acute, terminal phase of advanced disease. Scripting in open-ended questions intended to assist the patient and family articulate goals, hopes, and questions is provided by Tobin and Larson (2000). Phrasing for the clinician in introducing prognosis and treatment options, including hospice care, is reviewed in Pantilat and Steimle (2004). Several case reviews and investigations in the medical literature provide invaluable insights into the essential element in ethical treatment decisions, clear, sensitive, and timely clinician communication (Bradley, Hallemeier, Fried et al., 2001; Emanuel, Fairclough, Wolfe et al., 2004; Hallenbeck, 2005; Larson & Tobin, 2000; Quill, 2000; Rabow, Hauser, & Adams, 2004; Roter, Larson, Fischer et al., 2000; von Guten, Ferris, & Emanuel, 2000; Wenrich, Curtis, Ambrozy et al., 2003).

Religion often influences treatment decisions in the circle of health professionals and family surrounding the patient with advanced disease. An active faith life can bring stability, acceptance, and transcendent hope to patients and families. For some faith traditions, belief in life after death is held in balance with the value of life. Yet, the care team, acutely aware of the burdens of aggressive treatment in the last stage of life, may find themselves in disagreement with patients and families insisting on aggressive treatment. The basis for such a choice on the part of the family may be a strongly held religious conviction involving hope in a miracle, faith in technology to bring about a cure, or a view that physical life is to be maintained no matter the cost. Recourse to a theological argument or stance may also be the means of stating grief (Brett & Jersild, 2003). In such cases, the APN would do well to seek the assistance of a chaplain, social worker, or spiritual advisor in the community known to and respected by the family (Mosley, Silveria, & Door, 2005). (Chapter 6 offers a more extensive investigation of the topics of culture and religion.)

The APN, physician, and team rely on each other as sounding boards when the solution to an ethical dilemma or family conflict seems too clouded by their own emotions or opinions. The institutional ethics committee provides deliberation with others who are not involved in the case but are experienced in ethical decision making, in a collaborative discernment of the issues and solutions. Ethics committees are generally advisory and are involved in case review and consultation, clarifying the medical problem, and obstacles to communication; at times, they make specific recommendations (Ross, Glaser, Rasinski-Gregory et al., 1993). Bioethics mediation, as a resource for the APN and care team, combines ethical consultation approaches with the skills of mediation, helping the parties in a conflict discover reasonable solutions and options in achieving the goals of care (Dubler & Liebman, 2004).

JUSTICE

Justice norms consider the fair distribution of benefits, risks, and costs (Beauchamp & Childress, 2001). In the Judeo/Christian tradition, it means ensuring that basic needs are provided for the poor (Kammer, 1991). Because health is necessary to the pursuit of the goals of human life as it is lived in community, health care is a public good. Although some may be reluctant to cite cost considerations, American health care is affected by the sum of decisions and practices in every arena of medical care and medical industry. Assessments vary on the amount of health care spending in the last stage of illness, but these costs are significant when weighed against other social goods (Curtis, 2004; Miller et al., 2004). Limits for health care spending are outlined in managed care plans, payer limits, and institutional policies and processes to contain costs (e.g., hospital formularies), but these piecemeal cost controls are unable to check total spending. While it is true that clinicians act as advocates for their patient and bedside rationing is not appropriate, it is also true that, in the aggregate, the inappropriate use of costly technology drives up the cost of health care. In contrast, unpaid family caregivers incur significant financial costs, sometimes must leave employment, and may risk a depletion of savings. Virtually invisible in the official economy, the economic value of unpaid family caregiver contribution and cost for the approximately 27.6 million families in this situation is estimated at $196 billion (Hauser & Kramer, 2004). A just resolution of the problem of the equitable distribution and cost controls in American health care would require a national dialogue and a rough consensus on what would constitute a "decent minimum" of health care and what "equal access" to health care would require (Beauchamp & Childress, 2001). Justice is an important ethical consideration as it calls for a broader view of the common good in contrast to individual needs and wants.

CONCLUSION

It is not easy to navigate the diminishment of advanced illness, the frailty of old age, and death. The last stages require a letting go, a personal ethos of surrender and dispossession. The health care team sustains the patient through the crises, ethical dilemmas, and decision points. An ethic of empathy and professionalism mark the way clinicians prepare the patient and family for the passage of advanced disease and death. Although life experiences vary, the APN's personal awareness and acceptance of mortality, influence the way the clinician plots a course through end-of-life decisions with patients. In the end, formal obligations of fidelity in the patient-professional relationship are translated into the human expression of faithfulness to the vulnerable other, the patient and family journeying through advanced disease.

REFERENCES

Beauchamp, T.L. & Childress, J.F. (2001). *Principles of biomedical ethics* (5th ed.). New York: Oxford University Press.

Bradley, E.H., Hallemeier, A.G., Fried, T.R., et al. (2001). Documentation of discussions about prognosis with terminally ill patients. *Am J Med, 111*, 218-223.

Brett, A.S. & Jersild, P. (2003). "Inappropriate" treatment near the end of life: Conflict between religious convictions and clinical judgment. *Arch Intern Med, 163*, 1645-1649.

Covinsky, K.E., Fuller, J.D., Yaffe, K., et al. (2000). Communication and decision-making in seriously ill patients: Findings of the SUPPORT project. *J Am Geriatr Soc, 48 (Suppl.)*, S187-S193.

Curtis, J.R. (2004). Communicating about end-of-life care with patients and families in the intensive care unit. *Crit Care Clin, 20*, 363-380.

Curtis, J.R. & Patrick, D.L. (2001). How to discuss dying and death in the ICU. In J.R. Curtis & G. Rubenfeld (Eds.). *Managing death in the intensive care unit* (pp. 85-102). New York: Oxford University Press.

Della Santina, C. & Bernstein, R.H. (2004). Whole-patient assessment, goal planning, and inflection points: their role in achieving quality end-of-life care. *Clin Geriatr Med, 20*, 595-620.

Derse, A.R. (2005). Limitation of treatment at end-of-life: Withholding and withdrawal. *Clin Geriatr Med, 21*, 223-238.

Dresser, R. (2005). Schiavo's legacy: The need for an objective standard. *Hastings Center Report, 35*, 20-22.

Dubler, N.N. & Liebman, C.B. (2004). *Bioethics mediation: A guide to shaping shared solutions.* New York: United Hospital Fund.

Emanuel, E.J., Fairclough, D.L., Wolfe, P., et al. (2004). Talking with terminally ill patients and their caregivers about death, dying, and bereavement. *Arch Intern Med, 164*, 1999-2004.

Emanuel, L.L. (2004). Palliative care I: Providing care. *Clin Geriatr Med, 20*, xi-xiii.

Foley, K.M. (2001). Pain and symptom control in the dying ICU patient. In J.R. Curtis & G. Rubenfeld (Eds.). *Managing death in the intensive care unit* (pp. 103-125). New York: Oxford University Press.

Frank, A. (1991). *At the will of the body: Reflections on illness.* New York: Houghton Mifflin.

Hallenbeck, J. (2005). Palliative care in the final days of life. *JAMA, 293,* 2265-2271.

Hamel, R.P. & Panicola, M.R. (2003). Are futility policies the answer? *Health Prog, 84,* 21-24.

Hauser, J.M. & Kramer, B.J. (2004). Family caregivers in palliative care. *Clin Geriatr Med, 20,* 671-688.

Kammer, F. (1991). *Doing faith justice.* Mahwah, N.J.: Paulist Press.

Larson, D.G. & Tobin, D.R. (2000). End-of-life conversations: Evolving practice and theory. *JAMA, 284,* 1573-1578.

Lo, B. & Rubenfeld, G. (2005). Palliative sedation in dying patients. *JAMA, 294,* 1810-1816.

Lynn, J. (1989). Elderly residents of long-term care facilities. In J. Lynn (Ed.). *By no extraordinary means: The choice to forgo life-sustaining food and water* (pp.163-179). Bloomington, Ind.: Indiana University Press.

Lynn, J. & Goldstein, N.E. (2003). Advance care planning for fatal chronic illness: Avoiding commonplace errors and unwarranted suffering. *Ann Intern Med, 138,* 812-818.

Meisel, A., Snyder, L., & Quill, T. (2000). Seven legal barriers to end-of-life care: Myths, realities, and grains of truth. *JAMA, 284,* 2495-2501.

Miller, S.C., Teno, J.M., & Mor, V. (2004). Hospice and palliative care in nursing homes. *Clin Geriatr Med, 20,* 717-734.

Morrison, R.S. & Meier, D.E. (2004). Palliative care. *N Engl J Med, 350,* 2582-2590.

Mosley, K.L., Silveria, M.J., & Door Goold, S. (2005). Futility in evolution. *Clin Geriatr Med, 21,* 211-222.

O'Rourke, K. (2000). *A primer for health care ethics: Essays for a pluralistic society* (2nd ed.) (pp. 16-19). Washington, DC: Georgetown University Press.

Panicola, M.R. (2001). Withdrawing nutrition and hydration. *Health Prog, 82,* 28-33.

Pantilat, S.Z. & Steimle, A.E. (2004). Palliative care for patients with heart failure. *JAMA, 291,* 2476-2482.

Paris, J.J. (1998). Hugh Finn's right to die. *America, 197,* 13-15.

Pellegrino, E.D. & Thomasma, D.C. (1988). *For the patient's good: The restoration of beneficence in health care.* New York: Oxford University Press.

Quaglietti, S., Blum, L., & Ellis, V. (2004). The role of the adult nurse practitioner in palliative care. *J Hospice Palliat Nurs, 6,* 204-214.

Quill, T.E. (2000). Initiating end-of-life discussions with seriously ill patients. *JAMA, 284,* 2502-2507.

Rabow, M.W., Hauser, J.M., & Adams, J. (2004). Supporting family caregivers at the end of life. *JAMA, 291,* 483-491.

Robbins, D.A. (1996). *Ethical and legal issues in home health and long-term care: Challenges and solutions.* Gaithersburg, Md.: Aspen.

Ross, J.W., Glaser, J.W., Rasinski-Gregory, D., et al. (1993). *Health care ethics committees: The next generation.* Chicago: American Hospital Publishing.

Roter, D.L., Larson, S., Fischer, G.S., et al. (2000). Experts practice what they preach: A descriptive study of best and normative practices in end-of-life discussions. *Arch Intern Med, 160,* 3477-3485.

Shannon, S.E. (2001). Helping families prepare for and cope with a death in the ICU. In J.R. Curtis & G. Rubenfeld (Eds.). *Managing death in the intensive care unit* (pp. 165-182), New York: Oxford University Press.

Sheehan, M.N. (2001). Feeding tubes: Sorting out the issues. *Health Prog, 82,* 22-27.

Surgeons' Palliative Care Workgroup. (2003). Office of promoting excellence in end-of-life care: Surgeons' Palliative Care Workgroup report from the field. *J Am Coll Surg, 197,* 661-686.

Teno, J.M. (2001). Advance care planning in the outpatient and ICU setting. In J.R. Curtis & G. Rubenfeld (Eds.). *Managing death in the intensive care unit* (pp. 75-82), New York: Oxford University Press.

Tobin, D.R. & Larson, D.G. (2000). *Advanced illness coordinated care program: Training manual.* Altamont, N.Y.: The Life Institute Press.

Truog, R.D., Cist, A.F., Brackett, S.E., et al. (2001). Recommendations for end-of-life care in the intensive care unit: The Ethics Committee of the Society of Critical Care Medicine. *Crit Care Med, 29,* 2332-2348.

Twohig, J.S. & Byock, I. (2004). Aligning values with practice. *Health Progress, 85,* 27-33.

Ulrich, L.P. (1999). *The patient self-determination act: Meeting the challenges in patient care.* Washington, DC: Georgetown University Press.

von Guten, C.F., Ferris, F.D., & Emanuel, L.L. (2000). Ensuring competency in end-of-life care: Communication and relational skills. *JAMA, 284,* 3051-3057.

Weissman, D.E. (2004). Decision making at a time of crisis near the end of life. *JAMA, 292,* 1738-1743.

Wenrich, M.D., Curtis, R., Ambrozy, D.A., et al. (2003). Dying patients' need for emotional support and personalized care from physicians. *J Pain Symptom Manage, 25,* 236-246.

CHAPTER 6

SPIRITUAL CARE ACROSS CULTURES

Charles Kemp

■

The purpose of palliative care is to relieve suffering in all dimensions of human life. Stated with greater precision, the purpose of palliative care is to facilitate an internal and external physical, psychosocial, cultural, and spiritual environment in which there is increased opportunity for a good death (dying), which may be seen as one in which reconciliation with God (or spirituality), self, and others occurs (Kemp, 1999). In this construct, symptom management (especially the physical environment) is a means to an end, not the *raison d'être* of palliative care.

DEFINITIONS AND CONCEPTS

- *Spirituality* is the incorporation of a transcendent dimension in life.
- *Religion* is an organized effort, usually involving ritual and devotion, to manifest spirituality. "Organized" does not necessarily imply group efforts; individual ritual and devotion are integral to all major world religions.
- *Faith* is the acceptance without objective proof, of something, such as God.
- *Culture* is "the learned and shared beliefs, values, and lifeways of a designated or particular group that are generally transmitted intergenerationally and influence one's thinking and action modes" (Leininger, 2002).
- *Cultural competence* is the ability to "perform and obtain positive clinical outcomes in cross-cultural encounters" (Lo & Fung, 2003, p. 162).
- *Spiritual care competence* may be defined in a like manner: the ability to "perform and obtain positive clinical outcomes" in spiritual care encounters (Lo & Fung, 2003, p. 162).

Spiritual and cultural issues, characteristics, and needs are often intertwined and difficult to separate. In other cases, they may have little connection with one another and sometimes one is of greater importance than the other (Kemp & Rasbridge, 2004).

The incorporation of these concepts into the complex matrix of care for a person who is dying and her or his family enhances the opportunity for a good death—however one might define "good death." The question then becomes, how does one incorporate these concepts into the care or, how does one *perform* such care? There are no universals in being able to provide the care. Unlike the use of opioid and adjuvant medications to treat pain, clear guidelines in providing culturally and spiritually competent care are difficult to establish on the shifting sands of individual differences in patients and caregivers, cultural and language barriers, religious and spiritual variables, changes in physical condition, and the myriad other factors affecting the patient and family.

As with the treatment of physical symptoms, failure also occurs in providing spiritual care and/or cross-cultural care. In postmodern society, radically different spiritual and cultural realities exist, and their intersection in, for example, the palliative care setting, is not always a success story. Spiritual care based on one faith (or on spirituality without a specific religious foundation) may not connect in any way with a person of a nonsyncretic faith such as evangelical Christianity or Islam (Narayanasamy, 2004a). Likewise, failure may accompany attempts to reach across the cultural chasm between a postmodern, high-tech culture and a traditional culture of the developing world. A myriad of individual, familial, systemic, gender, cultural, and other reasons for failure exist. Regardless of success or failure, working toward rapport and manifesting respect for all aspects of the patient's life and being are essential qualities of health care.

There are, however, *care-enhancing factors* that have at least the potential to enhance the opportunity for a good death. For the sake of clarity these are considered separately here, but as with Yalom's "curative factors" for group psychotherapy, they are intricately interdependent, part of a dynamic process, and of varying value in various situations and at various stages of the process (Yalom, 1995). The most straightforward way to use these care-enhancing factors is to operationalize them one by one or several at a time *over time* in providing palliative care. For example, clinical competence in physical care would be operational from the beginning of a particular care situation, as would nonjudgmental acceptance of the person receiving care. However, at the outset of care, the advanced practice nurse (APN) may lack cultural or spiritual care competence specific to the patient. This factor would be operationalized as the APN gains specific cultural competence or competence related to the patient's religion. The term "over time" recognizes that the APN may require time to acquire or implement some factors and that the patient may not immediately (or ever) recognize that a factor is present, that the APN is accepting of the patient's past, religion, or other aspects of the self.

CARE-ENHANCING FACTORS

Clinical Competence in Physical Care

Competent physical care is the first and an essential step in providing care in all human dimensions. While there may sometimes be exceptions (e.g., spiritual factors may transcend physical suffering), it is nearly always necessary to first or at least concurrently address physical issues (Kemp, 1999). The challenge for the APN is to maintain his or her physical care competencies and to apply evidence-based practice to the dynamics of palliative care. A rapid acquisition of new competencies may be required in the care of a patient with a diagnosis or problems such as an unusual paraneoplastic syndrome, cutaneous manifestation of a less common cancer, or other problem with which the APN is less familiar. Likewise, new and specific cultural or spiritual care competencies may need to be acquired.

Cultural Care Competence

As cited earlier, Lo and Fung's definition of *cultural competence* is the ability to "perform and obtain positive clinical outcomes in cross-cultural encounters" (2003, p. 162).

Within this broad competence are two more specific competencies:

- *Generic* cultural competence is "knowledge and skills applicable to any patient or community cross-cultural encounter" and is gained principally through ongoing mindful experience in cross-cultural encounters (Kemp, 2005). At least in part, such knowledge and skills include attributes such as those noted later (see Care-Enhancing Interventions).
- *Specific* cultural competence is "knowledge and skills applicable to patients and communities from specific cultural backgrounds" and is gained through study, investigation, and experience in working with specific cultures (Kemp, 2005, p. 45). It is important to recognize (1) how one's own culture influences one's perceptions (positive and negative) of other cultures and (2) that culture-specific knowledge is only a starting point to understanding individuals from that culture.

Spiritual Care Competence

As with cultural competence, *spiritual care competence* may be defined as the ability to "perform and obtain positive clinical outcomes" in patient care encounters that involve spiritual matters such as spiritual despair (or spiritual strength); similarly, there are two basic components in spiritual care competence (Lo & Fung, 2003, p. 162):

- *Generic* spiritual care competence is knowledge and skills applicable to any patient spiritual care encounter and is gained principally through ongoing mindful experience in spiritual care encounters. "Mindful" refers to participant-observer interactions The APN should remain aware of the effects of her or his care on patients and of personal reactions to patients in these situations—in terms of both individual patients and any patterns of effect(s).
- *Specific* spiritual care competence consists of knowledge and skills applicable to patients and communities from specific religious or faith backgrounds. Specific competence is gained through study, investigation, and experience in working with people from specific religions. It is important for the APN to recognize that (1) a person's own faith background influences that person's perceptions (positive and negative) of other faiths and (2) faith- or religion-specific knowledge is only a starting point for understanding individuals from that faith background.

Religion and faith are often highly charged or controversial topics. In some cases, books and other resources are attempts to justify the author's position, positive or negative, about the topic, especially when writing about faiths other than the author's. While it is impossible for most health professionals to read the scripture of every world religion, it will benefit professionals and their patients to be familiar with *primary scriptural sources* and commentary on faiths with which there is contact (e.g., practitioners who care for Muslim patients will benefit from reading the *Qur'an* and related commentary).

Care-Enhancing Interventions

The following discussion of care-enhancing factors is based on the idea of the existence of basic human needs that generally hold true across cultures and time. The factors/human needs as explicated here are not definitive, that is, there are authors who have noted more, fewer, or slightly different needs, but these are likely acceptable to most practitioners. Care-enhancing factors include the patient experiencing (and the APN promoting) the following (Bartel, 2004; Galek, Flannelly, Vane et al., 2005; Maslow, 1998; Narayanasamy, 2004b; Yalom, 1995):

- Self-actualization or growth and fulfillment
- Meaning
- Hope
- Relatedness (spiritually, to God, deity or deities, higher power; culturally, to culture)
- Forgiveness or acceptance
- Transcendence

Religion, faith, and culture offer answers or guidance to varying extents to answers to these issues. A lack (partial or complete) in religion, faith, or culture may result in difficulties for the patient in addressing these issues. Such a lack also, of course, guides the APN in providing care.

Self-Actualization or Growth and Fulfillment

Self-actualization or growth and fulfillment may be viewed as integral to spiritual growth. Indeed, in the discussions below, self-actualization or growth and fulfillment are implicit in almost every category of care-enhancing factors. In this section, however, the discussion is focused more on cross-cultural care.

Maslow (1998) was clear that self-actualization is the realization of the full human and preexistent potential of a person—which is not dissimilar to the purposes of palliative care given above. For the vast majority of humankind, self-actualization is not a state a person reaches and remains in. Rather, it is a process of progress mostly toward a higher state of being with all the shortcomings inherent in being human.

Assessment and Interventions

Tripp-Reimer, Brink, & Saunders (1984) published a definitive short cultural assessment tool, which is adapted here. Readers may note numerous potential connections to both spiritual issues (e.g., what do you think caused your problem?) and insights into individual or family issues in the context of palliative care (e.g., what problems has your sickness caused you or your family?):

- What do you think caused your problem?
- Do you have an explanation for why it started when it did?
- What does your sickness do to you; how does it work?
- How severe is your sickness? How long do you expect it to last?
- What problems has your sickness caused you or your family?
- What do you fear about your sickness?
- What kind of treatment do you think you should receive?
- What are the most important results you hope to receive from the care team?

Applying the questions to what one already knows about the patient—for example, a Mexican migrant worker who is Catholic, separated from family, depressed, and in pain—should generate at least a preliminary care plan related to the patient's spiritual and cultural beliefs.

Recalling that self-actualization is a *process of progress*—it can be seen that working through problems, reinforcing strengths, answering questions, applying spiritual and other care-enhancing factors, and practicing acceptance of the patient and his culture lead toward this process of progress. The patient's experience may thus trend toward increased insight, connection, and sense of acceptance—and concomitantly, decreased pain in all or most spheres of being.

Finding or Searching for Meaning

The search for meaning is central in life and in the process of dying. In a strictly personal sense, this search may include a review of life and its events, fulfillments, inadequacies, positive aspects, and mistakes and an exploration of how to live the remaining days of life. In a broader, yet still personal sense, the search for meaning may also include the meaning of dying, human existence, and suffering (Buckley & Herth, 2004; Kemp, in press; Parker-Oliver, 2002).

Assessment and Interventions

Although patient behavior may offer clues to whether meaning (or its negative, meaninglessness) is an issue, direct assessment is usually the best way to (1) discover if meaning or meaninglessness or both are issues and, (2) if meaning is not an issue, build on or reinforce the presence of meaning as a strength. Direct assessment includes questions (Kemp, in press; Narayanasamy, 2004b) such as the following:

- "What gives you a sense of meaning or purpose in life—now or in the past?" Looking at present and past may yield insight into existing spiritual or cultural issues that have their basis in the past (e.g., a refugee who was an influential or important person in her or his homeland may exist in a state of meaninglessness and powerlessness in the present).
- "If you had your life to live over again, what would you want to be different?" The answers to this and other such questions are likely to be given over time as the patient has time to remember and reflect. This question is in some respects psychosocial in nature, but in other respects it is linked to spiritual issues in that it looks to the meta-question, "Is there judgment in the universe, and if there is, will I be found wanting?" (see Forgiveness or Acceptance).
- "What does it mean to you that this (e.g., end-of-life, suffering, and so on) is happening?" Religion, faith, and culture all may provide answers, and in some cases the answers may be problematic for the patient, such as when dying and suffering are perceived as punishment for sins.

In general, intervention focuses on supporting the patient on her or his journey through the issues related to these questions. Often, there is a reluctance to face mistakes or fears in life either with another person or even within oneself. At the same time, however, there may also be the recognition that this is the last chance to look back and perhaps find resolution. The central role of the APN in the patient's search for meaning is to support and accept the person and be willing to listen to difficult thoughts and feelings. Often, the regrets are the common mistakes made in life, such as dishonesty and deceptions. In some cases, the story is more difficult, such as being a victim of sexual abuse (or an abuser).

Box 6-1	Note on Evangelism

Many Christians believe that anyone who is not a Christian will go to hell. This presents a potential for conflict among the APN (who does not wish for the patient to go to hell), the patient (who does not have the same belief and does not wish to change religions), and the institution (few Western health care institutions support attempts to change the faith of patients). In most cases, Western institutional policies on patient rights are sufficient to prevent conflict around religious and faith issues. Comforting the APN who is in this situation, Christian scripture is clear on the question of how one treats the afflicted (without respect to the other person's faith): "I was hungry and you fed me … I was sick and you looked after me …" (Matthew 26: 35-36). Islam is also strongly evangelistic, but assignment to heaven or hell is based solely on whether a person is or is not a believer.

Cultures permeated by religion usually provide a religious or spiritual answer to these questions. Cultures that are not strongly religious provide fewer answers. In some cases, such as strongly religious Theravada Buddhist cultures, for example, the culture and religion do not place a high value on meaning or reasons why. Instead, the focus is more on accepting what is (see Forgiveness and Acceptance). The question of why may be answered in several religiously oriented cultures, such as Muslim or Hindu, as either the will of God or fate, neither of which is open to intervention except in terms of acceptance. In all cases, the intervention remains supporting the patient as she or he works through these sometimes difficult questions.

Experiencing Hope

In terminal illness, hope for a good outcome shifts from hope for cure to hope for a good death (although some hope for cure commonly coexists). In a few unfortunate cases, the loss of hope for a cure means the loss of all hope and a state of despair. Although the varieties of hope are as varied as the patients who are hoping, hope for a good death often includes hope for symptoms being managed with minimal suffering, living fully within the constraints of the illness, reconciliation (with self, others, and God), a good future for survivors, and life after death (Duggleby & Wright, 2004; Kemp, 1999; Little & Sayers, 2004).

Assessment and Interventions

As with meaning, a direct approach to understanding the patient's sense of hope is often the best means of assessment, for example, "Let's talk about hope, Mr. Simpson. Given your condition, what do you hope for?" A common answer to this question may elicit a humorous or wry response, which often includes the hope "to not die."

- *Hope for symptoms being managed/minimal suffering.* This area is usually focused on physical care and, as has been previously discussed, is a primary concern. There may be no greater comfort to patient or family than a health team that vigorously and competently works to relieve pain, dyspnea, nausea, and the other physical symptoms that may accompany the illness.
- *Hope for living as fully as possible.* The hope for a full life within the context of terminal illness includes, but is not limited to, maintaining as much independence

and control as is possible (including dying at home), maintaining or even increasing connections with loved ones, and maintaining or increasing connections with religion and faith (Buckley & Herth, 2004; Tang, 2003).

■ *Hope for reconciliation with self, others, and God* was noted earlier to be central to the purposes of palliative care (indeed, to human existence) and may be approached as follows:

▶ Reconciliation with self is addressed through exploration of the question of how life was lived in relation to what might have been. In a spiritual sense, reconciliation with self can be seen as self-realization and may be achieved through spiritual practice, study, or grace.

▶ Reconciliation with others is focused on healing relationships with loved ones. Regardless of culture or religion, there are patients with highly conflicted or even toxic relationships (such as when there was extreme abuse) and reconciliation is not always possible. When this is the case, the goals of care shift toward understanding and acceptance.

▶ Reconciliation with God presupposes (as do these other reconciliations) a previous relationship or "re" conciliation. The prior relationship might be seen as one in earlier years *or* as one that was always there, whether in consciousness or not. It is not uncommon for people who enter into a deep relationship with God or a state of enlightenment to say something such as, "It was like I came to myself [see Reconciliation with Self] and realized these were things I had always known."

How are these reconciliations achieved? First, it must be recognized that these cannot be conferred by another. However, it is realistic to offer the hope that they are possible. One of the underlying, but not always expressed, questions in terminal illness is, "Can I do this?" The question may even be assumed by the APN, who might ask the patient, "Are you wondering if you can do this?" Or simply say to the patient, "You know, you can do this. You can go through this tough time and may even find there is more to learn in life" (Kemp, in press).

■ As with the hope to live, hope for a good future for survivors is not always realistic. Among older patients, the death of one spouse often means a significant drop in income and a diminishment of social or other resources. In the case of a survivor with a disability such as mental illness, the future prospects may be markedly less when a loved one dies. On the other hand, reconciliation leaves a lasting positive memory (Duggleby & Wright, 2004).

■ Hope for life after death, through either survival of the soul or transmigration of the soul, is a tenet in all major world religions, at least one of which is connected

---

Box 6-2

A little over a month before he died, the famous atheist Jean-Paul Sartre declared that he so strongly resisted feelings of despair that he would say to himself, "I know I shall die in hope." Then, in profound sadness, he would add, "But hope needs a foundation." (Lugt, 1995).

to some extent with every culture. Here, the role of religion and faith in palliative care settings is obvious (although certainly not limited to the issue of life after death) (Kemp, 1999).

Spiritual Relatedness

Relatedness in a spiritual sense is to God or some approximation of what would be considered as God, such as deity, higher power, and so on, and/or relatedness to religion or religious practice—not relatedness to other people (Kemp, in press; Narayanasamy, 2004b). As noted earlier, to at least some extent all cultures (although not all political systems) support religion and faith. Of course not everyone believes in God, and a lack of belief in God does not mean a bad death—whether among atheists or those whose religion does not have a god. In a formal sense, Buddhism denies the presence of God, but in a practical sense, the concept of God or deity is very much alive in the practice and devotion of many Buddhists.

Assessment and Interventions

Two questions that are helpful in terms of spiritual connectedness are, "Talk about what you believe in" and "Talk about what you believe about God or in religion." Simply the opportunity to explicate and explore beliefs is enormously therapeutic in most cases.

In some instances, there is a negative view of religion and little or no relationship with God. It is helpful to determine when the negative view or relationship began because often there is a particular incident when a person felt failed by religion or faith. Exploration of such a situation may uncover a desire to return to an earlier, more positive view or relationship. Means of promoting a positive view or relationship are centered on creating or encouraging a therapeutic milieu that encourages spirituality and religion, regardless of patients' faiths or cultures. This includes

- Individual staff members manifesting values consistent with spirituality—working in a loving, caring, respectful, accepting, and diligent manner
- Supporting patients and families in exploring and explicating their own beliefs
- Enabling prayer and religious ceremonies or rituals consistent with the patient's religion and culture

People from "other cultures"—especially refugees and immigrants—may feel a strong sense of aloneness, especially at end-of-life. They are likely to be deeply touched by any attempt to reach across barriers or gaps between cultures. Being respectful and accepting of others is, of course, fundamental to cultural competence.

Forgiveness or Acceptance

A fundamental question at end-of-life is, "Is there judgment, and if so, how will I be judged?" Every major world religion says, unequivocally, yes, there is judgment and provides details on how one is judged. Judgment in the monotheistic religions (Judaism, Christianity, and Islam) is final and includes the possibility of forgiveness or punishment (or, in some cases, an intermediate state). In the case of Hinduism and Buddhism, how one lives determines the state in which one is reborn, and because there is an endless cycle of deaths and rebirths until enlightenment is achieved, there is no final judgment or forgiveness. The focus among Hindu or Buddhist patients would then be on acceptance of how life was lived rather than on forgiveness.

Assessment and Interventions

As with the question of relatedness with God or a higher power, assessment is part of the intervention, that is, the opportunity to explicate and explore beliefs and concerns regarding forgiveness or acceptance. A powerful question that goes to the heart of the issue is, "What do you think will happen to you?" (Narayanasamy, 2004b, p. 1143).

A therapeutic milieu that encourages spirituality and religion, regardless of patient faith or culture, is critical to intervention. Being accepting of patients as individuals, of their faiths, and of their cultures is probably the most important intervention. Acceptance is an individual characteristic of the APN but also may be an institutional value.

Although experienced as offenses against God, in many situations the acts of commission or omission for which people seek forgiveness were against people, either others and/or self (it is often easier to be forgiven by others than by oneself). No lay person or health professional can confer forgiveness, nor can clergy except as a representative of God, but acceptance and thus, indirectly, forgiveness can be manifested. Being accepted by another is an important first step on the journey toward being forgiven.

Transcendence

Transcendence is going beyond oneself or one's circumstances—even going beyond the awesomeness of death. In several places in this chapter it has been noted that in life, things happen. In every life there are losses and mistakes, and in some respects life is painful and sad. How can a person go beyond the losses, mistakes, and sadness of life and thus come to redefine life, death, and relationships?

Assessment and Interventions

A person who has transcended the pain of life and awesomeness of death will generally lack anxiety, anger, or depression and will manifest peace and harmony, especially with respect to relationships with self, others, and God or faith. If there is any doubt, one could note the absence of conflict and presence of peace, and ask the patient if those perceptions are accurate, followed by something to the effect of, "Talk about how you feel or what is going on with you (and how did you get to this place?)."

Elisabeth Kübler-Ross' (1969) final stage in dying is termed *acceptance*, but it might also be seen as transcendence. In Kübler-Ross' construct, the patient worked through denial, anger, bargaining, and depression to reach a state of acceptance; indeed, working through these stages (or, more accurately, states of mind) tends to increase the likelihood of, but not necessarily lead to, acceptance or transcendence. The same holds true for the care-enhancing factors presented here: the presence of self-actualization, meaning, hope, relatedness, and forgiveness or acceptance in a person's life increases the likelihood of, but does not lead directly to, transcendence.

Transcendence is not acquired by a set of behaviors or interventions. It is a great blessing that may or may not last. One can only give thanks.

CONCLUSION

The critical issues in providing competent spiritual care across cultures are

- Understanding that the ultimate purposes of end-of-life care are *reconciliation* with God (or spirituality), self, and others
- Acquiring general and specific knowledge of cultures, religions, and the common end-of-life problems
- Being accepting of faiths, cultures, and the people who find meaning in them
- Being willing to work through processes of care and to not always achieve success

REFERENCES

Bartel, M. (2004). What is spiritual? What is spiritual suffering? *J Pastor Care Counsel, 58,* 187-201.

Buckley, J. & Herth, K. (2004). Fostering hope in terminally ill patients. *Nurs Stand, 17,* 33-41.

Duggleby, W. & Wright, K. (2004). Elderly palliative care cancer patients' descriptions of hope-fostering strategies. *In J Palliat Nurs, 10,* 352-359.

Galek, K., Flannelly, K.J., Vane, A., et al. (2005). Assessing a patient's spiritual needs: A comprehensive assessment. *Hol Nurs Pract, 19,* 62-69.

Kemp, C.E. (1999). *Terminal illness: A guide to nursing care* (2nd ed.). Philadelphia: Lippincott.

Kemp, C.E. (2005). Cultural issues in palliative care. *Semin Oncol Nurs, 21,* 44-52.

Kemp, C.E. & Rasbridge, L.A. (2004). *Refugee and immigrant health.* Cambridge: Cambridge University Press.

Kemp, C.E. (2005) Spiritual care in terminal illness. In B. Ferrell & N. Coyle (Eds.). *Oxford textbook of palliative nursing* (2nd ed.). New York: Oxford University Press.

Kübler-Ross, E. (1969). *On death and dying.* New York: MacMillan.

Leininger, M. (2002). Transcultural nursing and globalization of healthcare: Importance, focus, and historical aspects. In M. Leininger & M.R. McFarland (Eds.). *Transcultural nursing* (3rd ed.). New York: McGraw-Hill.

Little, M. & Sayers, E.J. (2004). While there's life … hope and the experience of cancer. *Soc Sci Med, 59,* 1329-1337.

Lo, H.-T. & Fung, K.P. (2003). Culturally competent psychotherapy. *Can J Psychiatr Nurs, 48,* 161-170.

Lugt, H.V. (1995). *The triumph of hope. Our Daily Bread.* Retrieved July 27, 2005, from www.rbc.org/odb/odb-04-17-95.shtml.

Maslow, A. (1998). *Toward a psychology of being* (3rd ed.). Hoboken, N.J.: Wiley.

Narayanasamy, A. (2004a). Commentary on J. MacLaren, A kaleidoscope of understandings: Spiritual nursing in a multi-faith society. *J Adv Nurs, 45,* 457-464.

Narayanasamy, A. (2004b). The puzzle of spirituality for nursing: A guide to practical assessment. *Br J Nurs, 13,* 1140-1144.

Parker-Oliver, D. (2002). Redefining hope for the terminally ill. *Am J Hospice Palliat Care, 19,* 115-120.

Tang, S.T. (2003). When death is imminent: Where terminally ill patients with cancer prefer to die and why. *Cancer Nurs, 26,* 245-251.

Tripp-Reimer, T., Brink, P.J., & Saunders, J.M. (1984). Cultural assessment: Content and process. *Nurs Outlook, 32,* 78 82.

Yalom, I.D. (1995). *The theory and practice of group psychotherapy* (4th ed.). New York: Basic Books.

CHAPTER 7

PHARMACOLOGY

Phyllis A. Grauer

■

Judicious prescribing of medication requires an understanding of the principles of pharmacology. Pharmacology is the study of the drug, the body's effect on the drug, and the drug's effect on the body. Variability in drug response occurs among individuals and populations, including those of different age groups and ethnic backgrounds and those with concurrent disease states and concomitant drug therapies; hence, drug dosage regimens must be individualized. These variations in response are attributed to many factors; however, they can be categorized into two major areas of study: *pharmacokinetics* and *pharmacodynamics*. Figure 7-1 illustrates the principles of pharmacokinetics and pharmacodynamics.

Clinical *pharmacokinetics* examines the effects of the body on a drug, specifically absorption, distribution, metabolism, and excretion of drugs. Factors that influence these processes include the following:

- How quickly a drug is *absorbed* into the blood and how different dosages affect that absorption
- How the drug is *distributed* into organs or tissues of the body and to the site of action
- How the body *metabolizes* the drug and whether the drug is changed by the body into an active or inactive compound
- How long it takes the body to *metabolize* and eliminate half of the drug (the drug's half-life)
- How long it takes the drug to be *excreted* from the body

Pharmacodynamics is the study of the body's reaction to drugs. This area of pharmacology evaluates the body's response to pharmacological, biochemical, physiological, and therapeutic effects of a drug. Basically, pharmacodynamics is the study of the activity of drugs on receptor sites within the body resulting in a clinical effect.

Of note, "pharmacogenomics" is an emerging area of study. The focus of pharmacogenomics is the identification of variations in the human genome (a total gene complement) that affect the response to medications. Advances in pharmacogenomics may permit drugs to be tailor-made for individuals and adapted to each person's genetic makeup. Although environment, diet, age, lifestyle, and state of health all can influence a patient's response to specific medications, understanding an individual's genetic makeup is thought to be key in creating personalized drugs that would provide patients greater efficacy and safety. Because of the infancy and complexity of pharmacogenomics, it is beyond the scope of this chapter.

For the clinician, rational incorporation of the principles of pharmacology into therapeutic decision making will result in achieving the desired therapeutic outcome while preventing adverse drug events and promoting optimal symptom management.

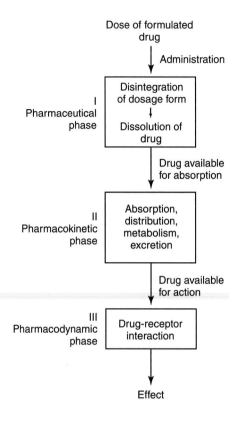

Figure 7-1 Drug pharmacology progression through pharmacokinetic and pharmacodynamic phases. (From Kuebler, K.K., Davis, M.P., & Moore, C.D. [2005]. *Palliative practices: An interdisciplinary approach.* St. Louis: Elsevier Mosby, Figure 4-1.)

UNDERSTANDING PHARMACOKINETIC PARAMETERS

Once a drug enters the circulatory system, it is distributed to tissues, reabsorbed into the bloodstream, and then eliminated from the body. Pharmacokinetic parameters define the factors that affect drug concentration within the human body over time.

Routes of Administration

A myriad of factors affect the dosage and matrix used in medications that influence the drug's delivery to the specific site of action. These factors include the drug's ability to penetrate barriers (i.e., the wall of the gastrointestinal tract and skin), the stability of the drug in acid environments such as the stomach (pH 2), the degree of tissue irritation when the drug is administered intramuscularly or subcutaneously, and the fraction of drug that is inactivated by the first pass through the liver. Table 7-1 describes the most common routes of administration.

It is important to note that there are several determinants associated with oral medication use that may interfere with the drug's absorption from the gastric mucosa. These determinants include dissolution, gastric emptying time, intestinal motility, drug interactions in the gut lumen, and passage through the gut wall. Box 7-1 outlines these in further detail.

At the end of life when patients are unable to swallow and/or a parenteral route is unavailable, many drugs used for the treatment of symptoms in palliative care can be

TABLE 7-1 ■ Characteristics of Various Routes of Administration

Route	Characteristics
Oral (PO)	Drug must be dispersed in solid dosage form to permeate the gastrointestinal lining and enter circulatory system.
	Most is absorbed in small intestine, where there is less acidic environment.
	Rate of absorption is dependent on gastric emptying and intestinal motility.
	Extent of absorption is dependent on drug's ability to permeate gastrointestinal lining and enter circulatory system.
	Drug enters portal circulation, passes through liver, and therefore is subject to hepatic extraction and metabolism.
	Drugs inactivated by acidic environment of stomach are typically enteric coated to prevent contact with stomach acid. Once the drug enters the less acidic environment of small intestine, the enteric coating dissolves, allowing drug to be dispersed and then absorbed.
	Extended-release drugs use various forms of pharmaceutically prepared release mechanisms so drug is released from oral dosage form over time.
Sublingual (SL)	This route avoids contact with acidic stomach environment.
	Drug is absorbed through mucosa under the tongue and enters bloodstream through numerous capillary beds.
	Much drug that is absorbed sublingually bypasses the liver.
	There is greater lipophilicity of drug and more is completely absorbed sublingually.
Rectal (PR)	Rectal mucosa is fed by blood vessels that pass through liver and by blood vessels that avoid portal circulation.
	Percent of drug absorbed through each system depends on where drug is placed in rectum.
	Many drugs administered rectally have erratic and often unpredictable absorption.
	Do not administer drugs dependent on constant serum concentration within a narrow therapeutic range (e.g., phenytoin, digoxin, warfarin).
Transdermal (TD)	Skin is the body's strongest barrier against absorption of toxins from environment into systemic circulation.
	Few drugs will penetrate skin and be absorbed into subcutaneous capillary beds.
	Extent of absorption is dependent on lipophilicity and drug's molecular structure.
	Amount absorbed is determined by surface area to which it is applied.
	Drugs administered topically for systemic absorption are best formulated in predetermined patch sizes (e.g., fentanyl TM patch).
Intravenous (IV)	Drug has rapid onset of action.
	Rate-limiting step is time it takes to reach site of action and produce therapeutic effect.
	Only soluble drugs are able to be administered by IV injection.
	Drugs administered IV are not affected by first-pass liver extraction and inactivation.
Intramuscular (IM)	Rate at which a drug is absorbed from muscle into bloodstream is dependent on type of diluent used to prepare drug formulation.
	Oil-based drugs are typically absorbed more slowly that those in aqueous solution.
	Drug is not affected by first-pass liver extraction and inactivation.
Subcutaneous (SC)	Route is used for drugs that are not irritating to surrounding tissue and where volume of drug product administered does not typically exceed 2 ml of fluid.
	Type of formulation used should determine how rapidly drug is absorbed into capillary walls and enters circulatory system.
	Drug is not affected by first-pass liver extraction and inactivation.

Continued

TABLE 7-1 ■ Characteristics of Various Routes of Administration—cont'd

Route	Characteristics
Intraspinal	Some drugs that act on the central nervous system can be administered epidurally and intrathecally. Route often allows for decreased dosage requirements and localized action, reducing intensity of adverse effects. Route can be used for opioids and other adjuvant pain medications such as local anesthetics.
Inhalation (INH)	Drug is generally absorbed rapidly if particles are small. Multidose inhalers require good administration technique in order to deliver drug through bronchial tree to alveolar bed for absorption. Nebulizer administration of drug is less dependent on technique and is more efficacious in patients who are weak and debilitated (although absorption is less).
Topical (TOP)	Route is typically intended to exert action locally and considered to avoid systemic absorption. Sites of action include skin, eyes, nose, ears, and vaginal and rectal tissues.

Data from Olson, J (2003). *Clinical pharmacology made ridiculously simple* (2nd ed.). Miami, Fla: MedMaster.

Box 7-1   Factors Affecting Drug Absorption from the Gut

DISSOLUTION

- Physical/chemical properties of the drug
- Crystal size and form
- Excipients (e.g., tablet fillers such as lactose)
- Dosage forms (enteric coated, sustained-release formulations)
- pH of the stomach and intestines

GASTRIC EMPTYING RATE

- Stability of the drug in an acid pH
- Solution or solid dosage forms (liquids and small particles empty more quickly)
- Presence of food or antacids
- Drugs (opioids and anticholinergics slow emptying time, metoclopramide increases emptying time)
- Disease (autonomic nervous system abnormalities such as Parkinson's disease)
- Intestinal interactions in the gut
  - Formation of complexes (tetracyclines and divalent metal compounds, e.g., Al^{2+})
  - Absorption (ion exchange resins, cholestyramine)
  - Food (i.e., dairy products, proteins) (many antibiotics)

PASSAGE THROUGH THE GUT WALL

- Physical/chemical characteristics of the drug (quaternary ammonium compound, vancomycin)
- Metabolism by enzymes in the intestinal endothelium

Modified from Birkett, D.J. (2003). *Pharmacokinetics made easy*. North Ryde, Australia: McGraw-Hill Australia Pty. Ltd., Table 5-1, p. 36.

given via alternative routes of administration. Although there is a lack of published information and controlled studies regarding these alternate routes of administration, knowledge of the characteristics of the drug, including lipophilicity, molecular weight, and pK_a, can help the pharmacist predict whether a drug is likely to be absorbed via a particular route. Literature supports both benzodiazepines such as lorazepam and diazepam and certain opioids such as methadone and fentanyl as being well absorbed into the sublingual capillaries, whereas morphine is absorbed to a much lesser extent through the sublingual mucosa (Akinbi & Welty, 1999; Weinberg, Inturrisi, Reidenberg et al., 1988). The majority of the effect of morphine, as well as that of oxycodone and hydromorphone, occurs when the sublingually administered drug trickles down the esophagus and is absorbed by the gastrointestinal tract (Akinbi & Welty, 1999; Weinberg et al., 1988). Methadone administered rectally has a more rapid onset of action than does oral methadone, making it a feasible alternative when the oral and parenteral routes are not options (Dale, Sheffels, & Kharasch, 2004). Knowledge of the extent of absorption through each route of administration is imperative in order to appropriately guage the dose of medication (Katzung, 2003). The quantitative measure of the absorption of a drug into the circulation is known as the drug's *bioavailability*.

Bioavailability

The bioavailability of a drug is the fraction of the administered dose that reaches the systemic circulation. For example, the bioavailability of an intravenous injection is 100% (Birkett, 2003), whereas bioavailability will vary for other routes of administration depending on factors that affect the extent of absorption into the circulatory system and first-pass hepatic metabolism. The measurement that determines absolute bioavailability is called the *area under the curve (AUC)*. This measurement is determined by calculating the AUC of the plasma concentration plotted over time (Birkett, 2003) (Figure 7-2).

The bioavailability of a specific drug is the determinant of the dosage and is equivalent to the drug administered via various routes of administration. For example, chronic use of morphine administered orally has a bioavailability of around 20% to 30% of the parenteral dose (100% bioavailability) (Doyle, Hanks, Cherny et al., 2005). This means that a patient who has been receiving 10 mg of morphine intravenously will require approximately 30 mg of morphine orally to achieve the same analgesic effect as experienced from the intravenous dose (American Pain Society, 2003).

Drugs are considered bioequivalent when the extent and rate of absorption are similar and there is no difference between the therapeutic and adverse effects. A generic drug company, for example, that manufactures a drug in the same dosage form as a brand-name product will often use the AUC bioavailability data when comparing the two drugs. For a generic drug to be considered equivalent to the brand drug, the bioavailability must be similar to that of the brand product (USDHHS-FDA, 2006). The *Electronic Orange Book* is an online publication of the U.S. Department of Health and Human Services Food and Drug Administration that lists approved drug products and their therapeutic equivalence evaluations.

Therapeutic Range

Therapeutic range is defined as the plasma concentration that occurs between the concentration of drug needed to achieve the desired pharmacological effect and the

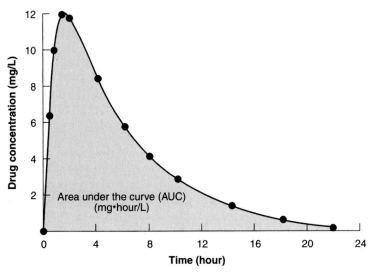

Figure 7-2 Measurement of clearance. (From Birkett, D.J. [2003]. *Pharmacokinetics made easy.* North Ryde, Australia: McGraw-Hill Australia Pty. Ltd., Figure 1-2.)

concentration where adverse effects are observed (Figure 7-3). For some drugs, this range is narrow, and for other drugs, it is wide. The narrower the range, the more monitoring is needed to prevent adverse drug effects or clinical misadventures. Some monitoring is done based on plasma drug concentrations (e.g., gentamicin, theophylline, and digoxin). Other drug monitoring is done by measuring physiological changes that are caused by the drug (e.g., measuring international normalized ratio for Coumadin [warfarin] and thyroid-stimulating hormone for levothyroxine).

Volume of Distribution

Once the drug is absorbed into the systemic circulation, it is distributed throughout the body. The apparent volume of distribution (V_D) is a measure of where the drug goes once it is completely distributed throughout the body (Table 7-2). It is the ratio of the fraction of drug unbound to protein in the plasma to the fraction of unbound drug in the tissue, and it is expressed as liters per kilogram (L/kg). The volume of distribution is also determined by the strength of binding of the drug to plasma proteins in relationship to the strength of binding to tissue components. If a drug is highly bound by tissue and not by blood, it will allow most of the drug to be held in the tissues of the body and little will be held within the blood. In this case, the drug will have a large volume of distribution. The V_D is measured by plotting the logarithm of the plasma concentration against time. The result is a straight line that can be extrapolated back to zero (Birkett, 2003). The plasma concentration at zero time (C_0) divided by the dose equals the volume of distribution:

$$V_D = \frac{C_0}{\text{dose}}$$

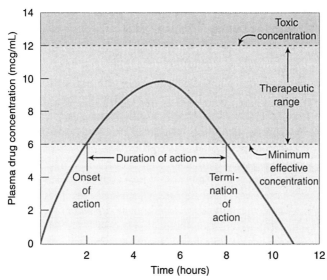

Figure 7-3 Single-dose drug administration: pharmacokinetic values for this drug are as follows: onset of action = 2 hours; duration of action = 6 hours; termination of action = 8 hours after administration; peak plasma concentration = 10 mcg/mL; time to peak drug effect – 5 hours; $t_{1/2}$ = 4 hours. (From Adams, M.P., Josephson, D.L., & Holland, L.N. [2005]. *Pharmacology in nursing: A pathophysiologic approach.* © 2005, pp. 53, 54. Reprinted by permission of Pearson Education, Inc., Upper Saddle River, N.J.)

TABLE 7-2 ■ Examples of Volumes of Distribution (V_D) and Half-life ($t_{1/2}$)

Drug	V_D (L/kg)	V_D/70 kg (L)	$t_{1/2}$ (hr)
Morphine	3.3 (3-4)	230	2-4 (Immediate release)
Lorazepam	1.3	91	12-16
Diazepam	1.1	77	20-50
Chlorpromazine	20	1400	2 (30)*
Haloperidol	20	1400	20
Fentanyl	6	420	2–4 (IV), 17 (TD)
Methadone	4 (1-8)	280	7-59
Warfarin	7 (6-7)	490	20-60
Digoxin	7 (6-7)	490	37-48

Data from Lexi-Comp Online. (2006). Retrieved March 30, 2006, from www.lexi.com.
*Biphasic elimination: initial (terminal).

Loading Doses

A loading dose (LD) can be used when attempting to achieve a rapid concentration of a specific drug. The volume of distribution is the pharmacokinetic parameter used when calculating an LD of a drug. For example, if a drug has a V_D of 40 liters (L) and the desired concentration (c) is 10 mg/L, then a loading dose to achieve that concentration is 400 mg:

$$LD = V_D \times (c)\ 400\ mg = 40\ L \times 10\ mg/L$$

It is important for the clinician to understand that the administration of an LD will decrease the time it takes to achieve a desired concentration and will not decrease the time it takes to reach steady-state (Birkett, 2003).

Half-Life

The half-life $(t_{1/2})$ is identified by the time it takes for the plasma concentration and the amount of drug within the body to fall by half after it has undergone absorption and distribution. Half-life is the reciprocal function of the elimination rate constant. The half-life and elimination rate constant are determined by both clearance (CL) and V_D (Urso, Blardi, & Giorgi, 2002) (Figure 7-4). Half-life determines the duration of action after a single dose of a drug and the amount of time required to reach steady state with constant dosing.

The therapeutic concentration range, also known as the therapeutic window, is the drug concentration range where most patients will have a therapeutic effect with the least amount of adverse effects. In general, the usual therapeutic range and drug effect are proportional to the logarithm of drug concentration. Therefore, drug effect after a single dose usually declines in a linear relationship over time. Notwithstanding, a number of mechanisms result in a dissociation of the usual relationship between drug concentration and effect. Changes in volume of distribution due to dehydration of overhydration and changes in renal or liver function are examples of factors that will affect the drug concentration–and–effect relationship.

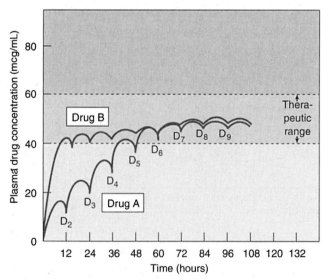

Figure 7-4 Multiple-dose drug administration; drug A and drug B are administered every 12 hours; drug B reaches the therapeutic range faster, because the first dose is a loading dose. (From Adams, M.P., Josephson, D.L., & Holland, L.N. [2005]. *Pharmacology in nursing: A pathophysiologic approach.* © 2005, pp. 53, 54. Reprinted by permission of Pearson Education, Inc., Upper Saddle River, NJ.)

Steady State

Steady state occurs when the rate of drug administered is equal to the rate of elimination from the body. It generally takes *three to five drug half-lives* to reach *steady state*. For example, when immediate-release morphine ($t_{1/2}$ ≈4 hours) is administered routinely every 4 hours, steady state is achieved within 24 hours. For a drug with a longer half-life, such as methadone ($t_{1/2}$ ≈20 to 35 hours), steady state is achieved in approximately 6 to 10 days (Lugo, Satterfield, & Kern, 2006).

Drug concentrations are often measured as unbound plasma drug concentrations rather than as whole blood concentrations. With oral and intermittent dosing, once the steady state has been achieved, despite a fluctuation in drug doses, the amount of drug administered will equal the amount of drug eliminated. This results in an average drug concentration that is equal to an intravenous infusion (Olson, 2003).

With intermittent dosing, when the dosing interval is equal to the half-life of the drug, the result is about a two-fold fluctuation in drug concentration over the dosing interval. In cases where the drug is administered orally and at an interval that is not equal to the drug's half-life, the degree of plasma concentration fluctuation over the dosing interval is determined by both the absorption rate and the relationship of the dosing interval to the half-life. Although a drug may be at steady state, if the dose is changed, it again will take three to five half-lives to reach a new steady state. Conversely, upon discontinuation of a dose, it takes four half-lives to eliminate 94% of the drug from the body (Birkett, 2003; Olson, 2003).

Dosing Intervals

To achieve a sustained systemic blood level of medication that has a short half-life and a narrow therapeutic window, drugs are often formulated in an oral sustained-release matrix. Morphine is an example of a drug that is available in an immediate-release form (i.e., on administration, the entire dose is available to be absorbed and distributed to the site of action) and in a sustained-release format where systemic blood levels are available for 8, 12, and 24 hours after ingestion of a single-unit dose. When morphine is administered as an immediate-release dose, it is typically dosed at an interval close to its half-life (i.e., every 4 hours) to maintain a constant therapeutic systemic level. Sustained-release morphine has the same half-life and clearance as immediate-release morphine. The sustained-release matrix formulation is designed to gradually release drug, resulting in a fraction of morphine available for absorption and distribution. Consequently, altering the sustained-release matrix through crushing, for example, will destroy the delayed absorption property and result in a bolus of the entire dosage, leading to loss of a sustained serum concentration and potentially toxicity (Olson, 2003).

Clearance

Medication clearance (CL) is the most important pharmacokinetic property of a drug. It is the measure of the efficiency of irreversible elimination of the drug from the systemic circulation and is expressed as the volume of blood cleared of unchanged drug per unit of time. Furthermore, it is the sum of drug clearance from systemic circulation, which includes the body's vital organs. CL determines the steady-state concentration of a drug for a given dose rate.

When a drug is administered at a continuous intravenous infusion rate (k_0), the steady-state concentration (C_{ss}) is determined by the quotient of k_0 and CL:

$$C_{ss} = \frac{k_0}{CL}$$

However, if a drug is administered intermittently, as in the case of oral dosing, C_{ss} is determined by

$$C_{ss} = \frac{F(D/\tau)}{CL}$$

where F is the fraction of the dose absorbed into the systemic circulation, D is the dose of the drug, and τ is the dosage interval.

It is important for the clinician to note that the clearance of a drug can be altered by several factors, including liver and kidney insufficiency, changes in protein and tissue binding, and the concomitant administration of other medications.

Linear Pharmacokinetics

Once a drug is in the body, the process of elimination begins. The majority of drugs are eliminated by "first-order," or linear, pharmacokinetics. This process of elimination is exponential or logarithmic (Figure 7-5). As an example of linear pharmacokinetics, when a dose is doubled from 200 mg/day to 400 mg/day, the patient's serum drug concentration also doubles (Birkett, 2003).

Multiple Compartment Distribution of Drugs

A drug within the systemic circulation is distributed to the body's tissues at a rate and extent that are dependent on tissue perfusion and the ease with which it can pass through the lipid membranes of the cells. Tissues in the brain, liver, kidneys, and heart are highly perfused, whereas skeletal muscle and fat are less perfused, making distribution to these tissues much slower. The rate at which the drug is distributed from or to the site of action, in most cases, determines the onset and duration of action from its pharmacological effect (Birkett, 2003).

Distribution depends on the following four factors:

1. *Blood flow:* Tissues with the highest blood flow receive the drug first.
2. *Protein binding:* Drugs that are bound to plasma proteins do not cross lipid membranes.
3. *Lipid solubility:* The more lipid soluble a drug is, the more rapidly it is distributed to other tissues.
4. *Degree of ionization:* Only ionized (polar) drugs can cross cell membranes.

Protein Binding

To a greater or lesser extent, the majority of medications bind to plasma proteins. The major drug binding proteins in plasma are albumin, α_1-acid glycoprotein (AAG), and lipoproteins. It is the unbound drug within the bloodstream that is free to distribute throughout the tissues of the body and to the site of pharmacological activity. Unbound drug is also that portion of total plasma drug that is available for metabolism and excretion. In general, clearance of high-extraction-ratio drugs is high—a result of

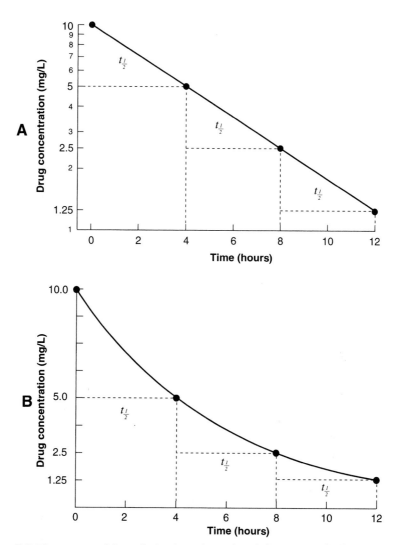

Figure 7-5 Time course of drug elimination. First order of elimination of a drug with a half-life of 4 hours plotted on (**A**) a linear scale and (**B**) a semilogarithmic scale. The plasma concentration falls by half each half-life. (From Birkett, D.J. [2003]. *Pharmacokinetics made easy*. North Ryde, Australia: McGraw-Hill Australia Pty. Ltd., Figure 3-1.)

low protein binding; conversely, clearance of low-extraction-ratio drugs is dependent on the amount of protein binding. More highly bound drugs have a longer duration of action and a lower volume of distribution.

If a drug is highly protein bound, proportionally larger doses are required to achieve the desired therapeutic effect compared with a drug that has minimal protein binding (Birkett, 2003). Problems occur, for example, when drug B is administered and is in competition with drug A for the protein binding site. The result is an increase in the amount of free drug A. This is particularly important with drugs that are highly protein bound. If a drug is 97% bound to albumin and there is a 3% reduction in binding due to displacement by another drug, then the free drug concentration doubles from 3% to 6%. However, if a drug is 70% bound and there is a 3% reduction in binding, the increase in free drug will make little difference (70% to 73%) (Birkett, 2003).

Warfarin is an example of a drug that is highly protein bound and has a narrow therapeutic window. Displacement of warfarin from plasma protein by other drugs can be extremely dangerous and requires careful monitoring. Changes in protein binding are important when interpreting the results of therapeutic drug monitoring in medications where total rather than unbound concentrations are measured (Birkett, 2003; Davis, 2005).

Lipid Solubility

When considering the administration of diazepam in a patient who is having a seizure, the anticonvulsant effect of the diazepam occurs very quickly but wears off within a few hours. Yet the diazepam can remain in the body for several days. In this case, diazepam is rapidly absorbed into the systemic circulation where it is carried to "vessel-rich" organs—principally, the brain. After several minutes, the drug is redistributed to other tissues (fat, muscle, etc.), and the concentration within the brain decreases, allowing another seizure to possibly occur. In this setting, diazepam has been redistributed into other compartments within the body.

A graphic description of this phenomenon would be to illustrate a rapid fall in blood concentration, a plateau, and then an insidious gradual decline. The initial phase is the rapid redistribution, or alpha, phase. The plateau is the equilibrium phase (where blood concentration equals tissue concentration). The gradual decline, or beta, phase is reflective of the elimination phase, when the blood and tissue concentrations fall in tandem. This process describes a two-compartmental model (Birkett, 2003).

When the log concentration is graphed versus time and the alpha and beta elimination line can be extrapolated back to the y axis, the point where each line intersects the y axis at zero time is $[c]_0$, the theoretical point representing the concentration that would have existed at the start if the dose had been instantly distributed (dose/V_D). From this new straight line, one can determine how long it takes for the concentration to drop by 50%—the elimination half-life. Likewise, a similar process can be performed on the alpha phase: the redistribution half-life. Log concentration is an important concept, yet the reality is that most medications are more complicated than this and require sophisticated calculations (Birkett, 2003; Katzung, 2003).

Drug Ionization

Highly ionized drugs cannot pass through lipid membranes, whereas unionized drugs can freely cross the membrane. For example, morphine is highly ionized but fentanyl is not. Consequently, fentanyl has a faster onset of action, as a result of its ability to rapidly cross lipid membranes. The degree of ionization depends on the pK_a of the drug and the pH of the local environment. The pK_a refers to the pH at which 50% of the drug is ionized. Most drugs have either a weak acid or a weak base. Acids are ionized at a high pH (i.e., in an alkaline environment). Bases are ionized within an acidic environment (low pH). For a weak acid, the more acidic the environment, the less ionized is the drug, and it can easily cross lipid membranes. Consider a drug that at an acid pK_a is 50% ionized; if two pH points are added to this (more alkaline), it becomes 90% ionized and will result in slower absorption. If the pH is reduced by two units, it becomes 10% ionized (more acidic) and can cross the lipid membrane readily. With weak bases, the opposite effect occurs (Birkett, 2003).

Local anesthetics are an example of weak bases: the closer the pK_a of the local anesthetic to the local tissue pH, the more unionized is the drug. This is why lidocaine (pK_a 7.7) has a faster onset of action than bupivacaine (pK_a 8.3). If the local tissues are alkalinized (e.g., by adding bicarbonate to the local anesthetic), then the tissue pH is brought closer to the pK_a, and the onset of action is accelerated.

DRUG CLEARANCE FROM THE BODY

The clearance of specific drugs can occur through excretion into the urine, gut, sweat, or expired air and/or through metabolic conversion into a different compound (metabolites), which often occurs in the liver. The sum of these processes equals total body clearance, and physiological clearance is determined through the following factors:
1. Blood flow to the organ that metabolizes (liver) or eliminates (kidney) the drug
2. Efficiency of the organ in extracting the drug from the bloodstream

Renal Clearance of Drugs

Renal drug clearance is identified as the net result or the addition of drug and/or its metabolites into the urine via (1) passive glomerular filtration *plus* (2) active tubular secretion *minus* (3) drug reabsorption from the urine into the blood through passive tubular reabsorption (Birkett, 2003).

Glomerular filtration occurs when drugs passively diffuse from the blood into the nephron by perfusion across the capillaries of Bowman's capsule. Small nonionic drugs pass more readily, whereas those medications that are bound to proteins cannot pass through capillaries into the urine. The rate of glomerular filtration depends in part on blood pressure.

Tubular secretion is an active transport process (requires energy) where drugs are secreted into the nephron tubule from the efferent arteriole. This process involves carriers or transporters that bind to the drug. The size and charge of the drug are less important. There are at least two active secretion mechanisms in the proximal tubule—one for anions and one for cations. Drug interactions occur due to competition of anions for anion transporters and cations for cation transporters. Active tubular secretion is saturable, which can lead to nonlinear kinetics (see pp. 94 and 95).

Passive tubular reabsorption occurs when drugs diffuse from the nephron tubule back into the systemic circulation. This process is influenced by urine flow rate, lipid solubility, and the degree of ionization (urine pH and drug pK_a) of the drug in the tubular fluid. As with glomerular filtration, small nonionic drugs reabsorb more readily. Changing or altering the pH of the urine can influence the degree of reabsorption.

All mechanisms are reduced equally in renal dysfunction, so renal drug clearance decreases in proportion with creatinine clearance. The need to adjust drug doses in renal dysfunction depends on the fraction excreted unchanged (f_e), the therapeutic

TABLE 7-3 ■ Effects of Renal Failure and Dialysis on Opioids

Opioid	Renal Failure	Dialysis
Morphine	Avoid → Glucuronide metabolites cause neuroexcitability and accumulate	Parent drug and metabolites are removed by dialysis Watch for rebound as drug from central nervous system reequilibrates
Hydromorphone	Caution → Less effect of glucuronide metabolite accumulation than with morphine	Parent drug partially removed by dialysis, no data on metabolites
Oxycodone	Insufficient data → Anecdotal data of central nervous system depression	Avoid; no data
Codeine	Do not use → Active metabolite accumulates	Do not use
Methadone	Appears safe → In GFR >10 mL/min, some recommend decrease in dose	Parent drug is not dialyzed and metabolites are inactive
Fentanyl	Probably safe	Not dialyzed

Data from Dean, M. (2004). Opioids in renal failure and dialysis patients. *J Pain Symptom Manage, 28,* 497-504.

index of the drug, and the presence of active or toxic metabolites. Table 7-3 illustrates the impact of renal failure and dialysis on opioid use.

Hepatic First-Pass Clearance

Many drugs are extensively metabolized by the liver. Drugs administered orally are delivered from the gut to the portal vein in the liver. The liver extracts a portion of the administered drug, leaving less drug available to distribute to the site of action. Morphine, for example, is a drug that exhibits extensive first-pass elimination. To achieve the same therapeutic effect, the dose of oral morphine must be three times the intravenous dose (Birkett, 2003; Doyle et al., 2005).

The systemic bioavailability of a drug after oral administration is determined by the extent of absorption into the portal circulation and first-pass extraction by the liver. The extraction ratio of a drug is measured from 0 (no drug is removed on the first pass through the liver) to 1.0 (the drug is completely removed from the circulation on the first pass through the liver). Drugs that enter the liver for the first time through the portal system and are extensively and irreversibly removed by the liver have high extraction ratios (Birkett, 2003). The extent of first-pass hepatic extraction is a major determinant of the bioavailability of high–, but not low–, hepatic extraction ratio drugs and is a major source of variability in drug response for high–hepatic extraction ratio drugs. The degree of hepatic extraction determines the appropriate route of drug administration, the effects of liver disease, specific drug interactions, and the correlation between oral and intravenous doses.

Factors Affecting Hepatic Clearance of Drugs

Hepatic extraction of drugs is determined by the following three parameters (Table 7-4):
1. Fraction of drug unbound in plasma
2. Intrinsic activity of the metabolizing liver enzymes
3. Liver blood flow (normal liver blood flow = 90 L/min)

TABLE 7-4 ■ Factors Affecting Hepatic Clearance

Extent of Liver Clearance	Examples of Drugs	Blood Flow (≈90 L/hr)	Intrinsic Clearance (0 to 1.0)	Protein Binding (0% to 100%)
High	Propranolol Lidocaine Morphine	Greatly dependent	Little to no dependence	Little to no dependence
Intermediate	Acetaminophen Desipramine Nortriptyline	Moderately dependent	Moderately dependent	Moderately dependent
Low	Warfarin Diazepam Carbamazepine	Little to no dependence	Greatly dependent	Greatly dependent

Modified from Birkett, D.J. (2003). *Pharmacokinetics made easy.* North Ryde, Australia: McGraw-Hill Australia Pty. Ltd., Table 4-2, p. 31.

For low–hepatic extraction ratio drugs (drugs that are not extensively removed from the portal circulation), the hepatic systemic clearance is determined by protein binding and enzyme activity. For high–hepatic extraction ratio drugs, hepatic clearance is determined by hepatic blood flow. The systemic clearance of metabolized drugs with intermediate hepatic extraction ratios is affected by all three processes.

DRUG METABOLISM

The majority of medications require biotransformation or metabolism before they can be excreted from the human body. In general, this metabolism results in a drug that is more polar and water soluble. Metabolism can render a drug either active or inactive, and in some cases, drug metabolism will transform an inactive or less active drug (prodrug) into a more active medication. An example can be found when codeine is metabolized into morphine, which is a more potent opioid agonist than the parent drug, codeine. Most metabolism occurs in the liver, although metabolism can occur in other tissues (kidneys, brain, skin, blood, lungs, and gastrointestinal tract). Medications are usually transformed by two types of metabolic reactions: phase I and phase II reactions. Phase I (nonsynthetic) reactions convert the parent drug through oxidation, reduction, or hydrolysis to a more polar form. Phase II (synthetic) reactions conjugate the drug with a group such as glucuronic acid, glycine glutamine, sulfate, methyl, or acetate to create a hydrophilic conjugate that is able to be renally excreted (Olson, 2003).

Morphine is extensively metabolized by phase II glucuronidation to morphine 3-glucuronide (M3G) (55%) and morphine 6-glucuronide (M6G) (10%). Although M6G has been shown to have analgesic activity, M3G has no beneficial action and is thought to be responsible for neurotoxic side effects (hyperalgesia, allodynia, and myoclonus), particularly in high doses and in patients with renal insufficiency (Davis, Varga, Dickerson et al., 2003; Dean, 2004). There appears to be significant individual variability in the degree of glucuronidation that would explain why some patients can tolerate higher doses of morphine than others without experiencing adverse side effects (Holthe, Klepstad, Zahlsen et al., 2002).

Ten percent of oxycodone is metabolized by phase I *O*-demethylation via the CYP450 enzyme CYP2D6 to oxymorphone and the inactive metabolite noroxycodone by *N*-demethylation. Although oxymorphone is 14 times as potent as oxycodone, the contribution of oxymorphone to analgesia is considered to be of no consequence. Renal insufficiency does decrease elimination of oxycodone and its metabolites, but the impact is less significant than that of morphine (Davis et al., 2003).

Drug metabolism is determined by the affinity of the drug for the enzyme (K_m) and the velocity of the reaction (V_{max}). The equation for enzyme drug reaction is

$$CL_{int} = \frac{V_{max}}{K_m}$$

The velocity (V_{max}) of the conversion of drug to metabolite depends on the quantity of the enzyme, the enzyme structure, and drug interactions (Birkett, 2003).

CYTOCHROME P450 ENZYMES

The cytochrome system is responsible for the majority of drug metabolism. Variations in drug clearance (up to 10-fold) can occur between individuals as a result of genetic enzyme polymorphisms that regulate enzyme activity in the cytochrome P450 (CYP) enzyme system. The most predominant cytochrome enzymes involved in drug metabolism include CYP3A4, CYP2D6, CYP1A2, CYP2C9, and CYP2C19. These enzymes account for 90% of drug metabolism. Based on liver mass, the fractions of total cytochrome isoforms are approximately 30% CYP3A4, 20% CYP2C9, 13% CYP1A2, and 1% to 5% CYP2D6 (Birkett, 2003; Ingelman-Sundberg, 2001). A vast number of medications are metabolized by a handful of cytochrome enzymes. These enzymes have wide drug specificity. In addition, some drugs are metabolized by several different cytochrome enzymes. Many drugs that are frequently used in palliative care are affected by the CYP450 enzymes and result in potentially dangerous drug interactions. Methadone, for example, is metabolized primarily by CYP3A4 but also by CYP2D6, CYP1A2, CYP2C9, and CYP2C19. Several drugs can activate or *induce* enzyme metabolism. When this occurs, substrate drugs that are metabolized by the induced enzyme are metabolized more rapidly, resulting in a decrease in blood levels in the body and possible reduction in the therapeutic effect. Cigarette smoke can also induce CYP1A2. A patient who is stabilized on methadone and quits smoking may experience symptoms of methadone toxicity (Davis & Walsh, 2001). Likewise, enzymes can be *inhibited* by competitive (reversible) or noncompetitive (irreversible) drug binding to the enzyme active site, thereby preventing further drug metabolism. Noncompetitive inhibition can be reversed by a generation of a new enzyme. The tricyclic antidepressant desipramine competitively inhibits CYP2D6, resulting in increased desipramine plasma levels when administered with methadone (Davis & Walsh, 2001). A substrate drug that is metabolized by an enzyme that is inhibited by another drug will result in decreased metabolism leading to higher serum drug concentrations and possible toxicity. Table 7-5 lists drugs that are substrates, inducers, and inhibitors of CYP enzymes.

Interpatient difference in the degree of activity of CYP enzymes is extensive. Age and ethnicity also factor into these variations. Individual genetic influence and polymorphism are major topics of research (Ingelman-Sundberg, 2001).

TABLE 7-5 ■ Cytochrome P450 (CYP) Enzyme Family

CYP1A2

Substrates   Amitriptyline, caffeine, clomipramine, clozapine, cyclobenzapine, imipramine, methadone, metoclopramide, mirtazapine, olanzapine, propranolol, riluzole, *R*-warfarin, theophylline, zileuton

Inducers   Amobarbital, butabarbital, charcoal-broiled beef, cigarette smoke, cruciferous vegetables, mephobarbital, mexiletine, omeprazole, pentobarbital, phenobarbital, phenytoin, secobarbital

Inhibitors   Cimetidine, ciprofloxacin, diltiazem, enoxacin, erythromycin, fluoxetine, fluvoxamine, grapefruit juice, mexiletine, norfloxacin, paroxetine, sertraline, verapamil, zileutin

CYP2C9

Substrates   Amitriptyline, carvedilol, celecoxib, diclofenac, flurbiprofen, fluvastatin, glimepiride, ibuprofen, imipramine, irbesartan, losartan, montelukast, naproxen, phenytoin, piroxicam, tolbutamide, torsemide, *S*-warfarin, zarfirlukast

Inducers   Butabarbital, carbamazepine, mephobarbital, pentobarbital, phenobarbital, rifampin, rifapentine, secobarbital

Inhibitors   Amiodarone, cimetidine, fluconazole, fluvastatin, metronidazole, miconazole, ritonavir, sulfamethoxazole, trimethoprim, zafirlukast, zileutin

CYP2C19

Substrates   Amitriptyline, citalopram, clomipramine, diazepam, imipramine, lansoprazole, mephenytoin, omeprazole, pentamidine, phenytoin, propranolol, *R*-warfarin

Inducers   Phenytoin, rifampin

Inhibitors   Felbamate, fluoxetine, fluvoxamine, ketoconazole, omeprazole

CYP2D6

Substrates   Amitriptyline, captopril, carvedilol, chlorpromazine, clomipramine, clozapine, codeine, desipramine, dextromethorphan, dihydrocodeine, diphenhydramine, encainide, flecanide, fluoxetine, haloperidol, hydrocodone, hydromorphone, imipramine, loratadine, maprotiline, methadone, metoprolol, mexiletine, mirtazapine, nortriptyline, ondansetron, oxycodone, paroxetine, perphenazine, propafenone, propranolol, risperidone, ritonavir, sertraline, thioridazine, timolol, tolterodine, tramadol, trazodone

Inducers   Bromocriptine, cimetidine, clarithromycin, cyclosporine, danazol, diltiazem, ergotamine, erythromycin, ethinyl estradiol, fluconazole, fluoxetine, fluvoxamine, gestodene, grapefruit juice, indanivir, itraconazole, ketoconazole, miconazole, midazolam, nefazodone, nicardipine, nifedipine, omeprazole, paroxetine, progesterone, propoxyphene, quinidine, ritonavir, sertraline, testosterone, troleandomycin, valproic acid, verapamil, zafirlukast, zileutin

Inhibitors   Amiodarone, cimetidine, diltiazem, fluoxetine, fluvoxamine, haloperidol, paroxetine, propafenone, quinidine, sertraline, thioridazine, tramadol, tricyclic antidepressants

CYP3A4

Substrates   Acetaminophen, alfentanil, alprazolam, amitriptyline, amlodipine, amprenavir, astemizole, atorvastatin, buspirone, carbamazepine, cerivastatin, citalopram, clarithromycin, codeine, cyclosporine, dapsone, delavirdine, dexamethasone, diazepam, diltiazem, disopyramide, donepezil, efavirenz, erythromycin, ethinyl estradiol, felodipine, fentanyl, finasteride, haloperidol, imipramine, indinavir, isradipine, itraconazole, ketoconazole, lansoprazole, lidocaine, loratadine, losartan, lovastatin, methadone, midazolam, mirtazapine, montelukast, nefazodone, nelfinavir, nicardipine, nifedipine, nimodipine, nisoldipine, pimozide, prednisone, propafenone, quetiapine, quinidine, quinine, repaglinide, rifabutin, ritonavir, saquinavir, sertraline, sibutramine, sildenafil, simvastatin, sufentanil, tacrolimus, tamoxifen, terfenadine, testosterone, theophylline, tolterodine, toremifene, triazolam, troleandomycin, valproic acid, verapamil, *R*-warfarin, zileuton, zolpidem

Modified from Dipiro, J.T., Talbert, R.L., & Yee. G.C., et al. (2005). *Pharmacotherapy: A pathophysiologic approach* (6th ed.). New York: McGraw Hill, pp. 1624-1625, Table 87–5.

Continued

TABLE 7-5 ■ Cytochrome P450 (CYP) Enzyme Family—cont'd

CYP3A4—cont'd

Inducers	Amobarbital, butabarbital, carbamazepine, clarithromycin, dexamethasone, ethosuximide, isoniazid, nafcillin, pentobarbital, phenobarbital, phenytoin, primidone, rifabutin, rifampin, rifapentine, troglitazone
Inhibitors	Cyclosporine, cimetidine, diltiazem, erythromycin, fluconazole, fluoxetine, grapefruit juice, ketoconazole, midazolam, nifedipine, paroxetine, progesterone, propoxyphene, sertraline, testosterone

NONLINEAR PHARMACOKINETICS

In linear pharmacokinetics, doubling the dose of drug given usually results in doubled serum drug concentration at a steady state, because the drug elimination rate is proportional to the drug concentration in the blood. There are some drugs that do not follow this rule. Instead of the serum concentration of the drug increasing proportionally with an increase in the amount of drug given, the serum concentration may be either more or less than expected.

When the drug-metabolizing enzymes or renal active secretion processes become saturated, a larger-than-expected increase in drug concentration (both total and unbound) may be seen with increased dose of drug. After the point of saturation is reached, even a small increase in dosage rate can result in a large increase in drug concentration and consequent toxicity. This is known as Michaelis-Menten kinetics (Birkett, 2003).

When the dosage of a low-clearance drug is increased, saturation of protein-binding sites can cause a less-than-expected increase in total drug concentration. Although the concentration of unbound drug increases because there are no protein-binding sites available for the drug, clearance of the drug (based on the unbound portion of the drug) increases, resulting in a less-than-expected change in the overall steady-state concentration of drug (Birkett, 2003).

Therapeutic Drug Monitoring

Some drugs require therapeutic drug monitoring of serum concentration to maintain a target concentration range. By maintaining the drug concentration within these parameters, optimal therapeutic affect will be achieved and drug toxicity can be avoided. However, drug concentrations need to be interpreted in the context of the clinical features of the patient. Interpreting drug concentration information and making drug regimen adjustments depend on obtaining accurate information about both the timing and the handling of the serum sample and about patient-specific factors that influence drug disposition. Very few drugs that are used for symptom control in palliative care require monitoring of serum concentrations. However, those drugs that remain necessary for patient comfort and have narrow therapeutic ranges, such as digoxin, theophylline, and phenytoin, may need to be monitored as the patient's condition changes (e.g., weight loss or dehydration) to avoid toxicity.

PHARMACODYNAMICS

Drugs exert their pharmacodynamic action at three different levels: cellular, organism or individual, and population levels (Olson, 2003).

Cellular Pharmacodynamics

At the cellular level, drugs produce their action at specific receptor sites. Receptors are typically proteins or glycoproteins that reside on the cell surface, on an organelle within the cell, or in the cytoplasm of the cell in finite numbers. Hence, the effect of the drug at the therapeutic dose plateaus either before or at the point of receptor saturation. Once a drug binds to the receptor, one of several actions is likely to occur:

1. Ion channel is opened or closed (e.g., calcium or sodium channels).
2. Biochemical messengers called "second messengers" are activated. These secondary messengers initiate a series of chemical reactions within the cell, which transfer the signal stimulated by the drug. These messengers include compounds such as cyclic adenosine monophosphate, cyclic guanosine monophosphate, calcium, and inositol phosphates.
3. Normal cellular function, such as DNA synthesis, bacterial cell wall production, and protein synthesis, is physically changed.
4. A cellular function is "turned on" or "turned off" (activated or deactivated) (Olson, 2003).

Furthermore, drug response is dependent on both the *affinity* of the drug for its receptor and the drug's *efficacy* once it is bound to the receptor.

The drug's affinity to a receptor refers to the strength with which it binds to a receptor. At steady state, equilibrium exists between the amount of drug that is bound to receptors and drug that is free. Drugs can dissociate from a receptor after they have been bound to the receptor. The *dissociation constant* (K_D) of a drug is the measure of its affinity for a particular receptor and is the concentration of drug required to achieve a 50% receptor occupancy. The higher the affinity of a drug to a receptor, the less likely it is to dissociate from the receptor. Several classifications are used to identify receptor activity and include the following.

Agonists

Drugs that alter the physiology of a cell are referred to as *agonists*. Typically, the change in cell function does not occur until a minimum number of receptors are occupied. Agonists can further be classified based on their degree of activity at the receptor level (Olson, 2003).

- *Strong agonist.* If a maximal effect is exerted when only a small fraction of receptors on the cell are occupied, the drug is considered a *strong agonist.* Morphine is an example of a strong opioid agonist.
- *Weak agonist.* Conversely, if a greater number of receptors must be occupied in order to produce the same effect as a strong agonist, the drug is considered to be a *weak agonist.* Propoxyphene is considered to be a weak opioid agonist.
- *Partial agonist.* If all the receptors are occupied by a drug, yet the maximum desired effect is still not achieved, the drug is considered to be a *partial agonist.* An example of a partial opioid agonist is butorphanol.

Antagonists

Antagonists inhibit or block responses caused by agonists (Olson, 2003).

- *Competitive antagonists.* Drugs that compete with agonists for the receptor site are known as *competitive antagonists.* While the receptor site is occupied by an antagonist, an agonist cannot bind to the receptor because it appears to have less affinity for the receptor than does the antagonist. As the dose of the agonist increases, it can be overcome by the antagonist when binding to any additional receptor sites and reclaim the receptor site from the antagonist at equilibrium. Therefore, competitive antagonists are considered to be *surmountable.* Naloxone is an example of a competitive opioid antagonist.
- *Noncompetitive antagonists.* Drugs that bind to sites other than the receptor sites where an agonist binds are known as noncompetitive antagonists. Once an antagonist is bound to a receptor site, it changes the configuration of the agonist receptor site and renders it unrecognizable by the agonist. This type of antagonism is *insurmountable.* Angiotensin II receptor blockers are examples of noncompetitive antagonists of angiotensin II.
- *Irreversible antagonist.* These agents are nonequilibrium competitive antagonists that compete for the same receptor site that an agonist does; however, they are insurmountable. That is, they cannot be displaced by increased doses of an agonist, as is the case with competitive antagonist agents. Phenoxybenzamine is an irreversible α_1-antagonist.

Antagonism of therapeutic effect is a result from processes that are unrelated to receptor binding sites and is further described.

- *Physiological antagonism.* Antagonism of therapeutic activity that can occur when two drugs have unrelated mechanisms of action but produce opposite effects. The cholinergic agent urecholine decreases urinary retention, while oxybutynin, an anticholinergic drug, causes urinary retention and therefore physiologically antagonizes the action of urecholine.
- *Antagonism by neutralization.* Drugs that bind to one another when administered at the same time and render both drugs inactive can cause antagonism by neutralization. Aluminum hydroxide, for example, when administered with tetracycline, inactivates tetracycline.

ORGANISM PHARMACODYNAMICS

Unlike receptor site pharmacodynamics, organism pharmacodynamics identifies the observations that are made regarding the activity of drugs in an individual or organism. Various terms are used to reflect observations at this level (Olson, 2003):

- *Efficacy* refers to the degree of drug that is able to produce a maximum effect. For example, an antilipidemic drug (drug A) may decrease low-density lipoproteins (LDL) by 30% at the maximum dose, whereas another antilipidemic agent (drug B) lowers LDL by only 20% at the maximum dose. In this case, drug A is more efficacious in lowering LDL than drug B (Olson, 2003).
- *Potency* signifies the amount of drug required to produce a given response. When comparing parenterally administered opioid analgesics, hydromorphone 1.5 mg

produces the same amount of analgesia as morphine 10 mg. Therefore, hydromorphone is more potent than morphine (Olson, 2003).

POPULATION PHARMACODYNAMICS

Several definitions are used to describe the behavior of drugs and how they interface within the general patient population. These definitions are further described (Olson, 2003).

- *Effective concentration 50%* (EC_{50}) is the concentration of drug that produces the desired therapeutic effect in 50% of the population. In general, drug doses should range between EC_{20} and EC_{80}.
- *Lethal dose 50%* (LD_{50}) is the concentration of drug that causes death in 50% of the population.
- *Therapeutic index* is calculated by dividing the LD_{50} by the EC_{50}. It is used to identify the measure of safety of a specific drug.
- *Margin of safety* is the margin or difference between the therapeutic and lethal dose of a specific drug.

PHARMACODYNAMIC AND PHARMACOKINETIC PROPERTIES

Age

The incidence of adverse drug reactions (ADRs) is directly related to the number of medications a patient is taking and the presence of concomitant diseases. What is considered a "therapeutic burden" can occur at any age; however, the presence of older age and the physiological changes that occur in the body (i.e., reduced organ function) can increase the risk of medication misadventures (Abernethy, 1999). The geriatric population is at risk due to multiple disease states and their impact on the pharmacokinetic and pharmacodynamic responses to drug therapy. The rate of ADRs in older adults (older than 65 years) is two to three times higher than that of younger adults. It is estimated that 20% of all hospital admissions of geriatric patients are due to unrecognized ADRs (Turnheim, 2003, 2004).

The effect of aging on pharmacokinetic parameters varies. In general, both aging and pharmacokinetic properties determine the extent of absorption after oral administration of medication is unchanged by the aging process. However, transdermal administration of medication may be altered in older patients. In order to achieve the optimal systemic effects from transdermal medication, the drug must diffuse across the stratum corneum and enter the microcirculation within the dermal layers. There are alterations in skin features that affect transdermal delivery in the aging, such as drying of the stratum corneum, changes in lipid composition of the skin, and decrease in dermal capillaries. The chemical composition of the drug determines the effect age will have on absorption. Lipophilic drugs tend to be absorbed to a lesser extent in elderly than in younger patients. Fentanyl is an example of a lipophilic drug that has shown to have decreased absorption in the elderly (Cusack, 2004; Turnheim, 2003).

As patients age, their body fat tends to increase while lean body mass decreases. Frequently, elderly patients become more dehydrated due to decreased fluid intake, diuretic medications, and reduced appetite. Changes in plasma protein in the elderly are small but can be more pronounced if the patient is severely ill or malnourished. All these factors can alter the volume of distribution of drugs. Alternately, changes in transport mechanisms in tissues such as the small intestine and the kidney can also affect drug distribution and elimination (Cusack, 2004).

Liver function and its composition incur minimal changes with age, even though the liver size and blood flow decrease. Synthetic phase 2 metabolism (glucuronidation, acetylation, and sulfation) has not been shown to be altered in the elderly. However, phase 1 CYP metabolism may vary with age. Genetic polymorphism of enzymes may be one explanation for these changes (Cusack, 2004). Alteration in renal drug elimination does occur in the elderly. Glomerular filtration changes with aging are thought to be due to structural changes within the nephron. The Cockcroft-Gault formula for determining creatinine clearance includes age in calculation along with gender, serum creatinine, and body weight as follows:

$$\text{Creatinine clearance (mL/min)} = \frac{(140 - \text{age}) \times \text{Body weight (kg)} \times 0.85 \text{ for women}}{\text{Serum creatinine (mg/dL)} \times 72}$$

Age can also alter renal tubular function. Renal tubular transport of organic bases does not appear to be changed, but renal tubular organic acid transport declines with age (Cusack, 2004).

Pharmacodynamic changes that occur with age impact the effects of drugs in the elderly patient. These changes occur both at the receptor level and as a result of homeostatic changes. Elderly patients tend to have a decrease in dopamine D_2 receptors. This can lead to an increased incidence of extrapyramidal symptoms from dopamine antagonist drugs. Downregulation of β-adrenoceptors from increased norepinephrine release results in a reduced response from β-adrenergic agonists. Likewise, β-blockers produce less antihypertensive activity, probably due to lower renin levels in the geriatric patient. Decreased cholinergic neurons and receptors in the elderly most likely explain why anticholinergic drugs can cause increased confusion (Turnheim, 2003).

Drug-induced orthostatic hypotension occurs at a 5% to 33% incidence in the elderly population. Homeostatic mechanisms for counterregulating blood pressure in response to changes in position progressively decrease in the aging patient. This is potentiated by drugs that decrease either blood pressure or vascular volume. The result is an increased risk of falls (Turnheim, 2004).

Elderly patients are often sensitive to centrally acting drugs; therefore, it is important for the clinician to consider reducing initial doses by 50% (Turnheim, 2003). This heightened sensitivity is a direct result of a reduction in brain size and a decrease in the number of neurons and synapses (Turnheim, 2003).

An increased awareness of physiological changes that occur with aging should alert the clinician to use caution when determining which drug and what dose to use in the elderly patient. Typically, when adjusting medication doses in the elderly, it is prudent to "start low and titrate slowly."

Gender

Females have a larger volume of distribution of lipophilic drugs compared with men, because women typically have a higher percentage of body fat (Craft, 2003).

Reduced activity of CYP3A and CYP2D6 in women leads to an increase in bioavailability of drugs that are metabolized by these enzymes. Therefore, clearance of drugs like oxycodone, desipramine, sertraline, and oxycodone (CYP2D6) can be reduced compared with males, so dosages for women may be less (Davis et al., 2003; Schwartz, 2003). Men tend to have greater renal function, such as glomerular filtration and tubular secretion, than women relative to corrected body size (Schwartz, 2003). Glucuronidation (influencing, among others, acetaminophen) is diminished in females (Schwartz, 2003). Gender-related differences in drug metabolism may lead to ADRs and drug-drug interactions. Although these gender differences are of note (10% to 30% difference), other factors such as age and disease states have greater influence on pharmacokinetics than gender (Schwartz, 2003).

Ethnicity

Whites, Asians, and African Americans have varying amounts of CYP2D6, CYP2C9, and CYP2C19, resulting in variations in drug interactions and rates of metabolism of drugs metabolized by these families of enzymes (Davis & Walsh, 2001). A number of palliative medications are influenced by this, such as diazepam, phenytoin, and warfarin (Bjornsson, Callaghan, Einolf et al., 2003).

Smoking and Alcohol Consumption

Cigarette smoking increases the metabolism of specific drugs that are substrates of CYP1A2, whereas alcohol increases metabolism of drugs that are substrates of CYP2E1. If changes occur in use or amount of alcohol or cigarettes, affected drug dosages may need to be adjusted. Methadone is an example of a drug where metabolism is influenced by the chronic use of alcohol and cigarette use (Davis & Walsh, 2001). If a patient discontinues the use of alcohol or cigarettes while prescribed methadone, it is likely that the patient will experience increased side effects (e.g., sedation) from an elevation in methadone levels. If this occurs in a terminally ill patient, it is important that the clinician does not mistakenly attribute this as the dying process.

Disease State

Disease states can dramatically influence the pharmacokinetics and pharmacodynamics of drugs. Depending on the disease state, any number of circumstances can occur. In patients who are malnourished (e.g., a patient with a malignancy), drugs that are highly protein bound will have an increase in free drug resulting in possible toxicity. Diabetic patients may experience an exacerbation of hyperglycemia due to use of corticosteroids. Drugs that are primarily metabolized by the liver (e.g., acetaminophen, morphine) should be used cautiously or avoided completely in patients who have end-stage liver failure. Oxycodone elimination half-life increases threefold (13.9 hours) in end-stage liver disease, necessitating reduced doses or extended dose intervals (Davis, Walsh, LeGrand et al., 2002). Extensive edema or ascites, for example, may result in third spacing of hydrophilic drugs, such as digoxin, leading to decreased serum concentrations and increased half-life. Renal failure has a profound effect on most opioids. Table 7-6 lists considerations in opioid dosing as it relates to renal failure.

TABLE 7-6 ■ **Glomerular Filtration Rate (GFR) and Dosage**

Morphine		Methadone		Oxycodone		Hydromorphone	
GFR (mL/min)	Dosage (% of Normal)	GFR (mL/min)	Dosage (% of Normal)	GFR (mL/min)	Dosage (% of Normal)	GFR (mL/min)	Dosage (% of Normal)
20-50	75	20-50	100	>60	100	>60	100
10-20	50	10-20	100	30-60	?	30-60	50
10	25	10	59	<30	? Reduce	<30	25

Data from Dean, M. (2004). Opioids in renal failure and dialysis patients. *J Pain Symptom Manage, 28,* 497-504.

POLYPHARMACY

Polypharmacy has many definitions. Most commonly, it is defined in the outpatient setting as the concomitant ingestion of four or more medications. Perhaps a more appropriate definition is the prescription, administration, or use of more medications than are clinically indicated in a given patient. This definition avoids enumeration of medications and recognizes that unnecessary adverse events can be the result of one unnecessary medication. Polypharmacy has distinct subgroups. Appropriate polypharmacy is when a patient is on several medications but each is appropriately indicated. In this case, decreasing the number of medications would not be beneficial. Inappropriate polypharmacy is when a patient is taking more medications than are necessary (Rollason & Vogt, 2003). The prevalence of polypharmacy increases with age. Two-thirds of persons over the age of 70 take between two and four medications, and one-fifth take five or more medications. The incidence of ADRs increases exponentially as the number of medications taken increases. The risk of drug-drug interactions approaches 100% when patients take eight or more medications (Rollason & Vogt, 2003). These interactions can include increased or decreased efficacy due to synergistic effects or competitive activity. Failure to recognize significant drug interactions may result in undertreatment or overdosing (Bernard & Bruera, 2000). The clinician should consider ongoing and careful monitoring for effectiveness and appropriateness of prescribed medications.

PRINCIPLES OF GOOD PRESCRIBING

When considering prescribing a medication for a patient
- Identify *patient*-related pharmacokinetic and pharmacodynamic factors.
- Identify *drug*-related pharmacokinetic and pharmacodynamic factors.
- Identify desired therapeutic outcome.
- Anticipate adverse effects and drug-drug interactions.
- Implement monitoring strategies.

REFERENCES

Abernethy, D.R. (1999). Aging effects on drug disposition and effect. *Geriatr Nephrol Urol, 9,* 15-19.
Adams, P.A., Josephson, D.L., & Holland, L.N. (2005). *Pharmacology for nurses: A pathophysiologic approach.* Upper Saddle River, N.J.: Pearson Prentice Hall.

Akinbi, M.S. & Welty, T.E. (1999). Benzodiazepines in the home treatment of acute seizures. *Ann Pharmacother, 33,* 99-102.

American Pain Society (2003). *Principles of Analgesic Use in the Treatment of Acute Pain and Cancer Pain.* Glenville, Ill.: American Pain Society.

Bernard, S.A. & Bruera, E. (2000). Drug interactions in palliative care. *J Clin Oncol, 18,* 1780-1799.

Birkett, D.J. (2003). *Pharmacokinetics made easy.* North Ryde, Australia: McGraw-Hill Australia Pty. Ltd.

Bjornsson, T.D., Callaghan, J.T., Einolf, H.J., et al., & Pharmaceutical Research and Manufacturers of America Drug Metabolism/Clinical Pharmacology Technical Working Groups. (2003). The conduct of in vitro and in vivo drug-drug interaction studies: A PhRMA perspective. *J Clin Pharmacol, 43,* 443-469.

Craft, R.M. (2003). Sex differences in drug- and non-drug-induced analgesia. *Life Sci, 72,* 2675-2688.

Cusack, B.J. (2004). Pharmacokinetics in older persons. *Am J Geriatr Pharmacother, 2,* 274-302.

Dale, O., Sheffels, P., & Kharasch, E.D. (2004). Bioavailabilities of rectal and oral methadone in healthy subjects. *Br J Clin Pharmacol, 58,* 156-162.

Davis, M. (2005). Pharmacology. In K.K. Kuebler, M.P. Davis, & C.D. Moore (Eds.). *Palliative practices: An interdisciplinary approach.* St. Louis, Elsevier Mosby.

Davis, M.P., Varga, J., Dickerson, D., et al. (2003). Normal-release and controlled-release oxycodone: Pharmacokinetics, pharmacodynamics, and controversy. *Support Care Cancer, 11,* 84-92.

Davis, M.P. & Walsh, D. (2001). Methadone for relief of cancer pain: A review of pharmacokinetics, pharmacodynamics, drug interactions and protocols of administration. *Support Care Cancer, 9,* 73-83.

Davis, M.P., Walsh, D., LeGrand, S., et al. (2002). Symptom control in cancer patients: The clinical pharmacology and therapeutic role of suppositories and rectal suspensions. *Support Care Cancer, 10,* 117-138.

Dean, M. (2004). Opioids in renal failure and dialysis patients. *J Pain Symptom Manage, 28,* 497-504.

Doyle, D., Hanks, G., Cherny, N., et al. (2005). *Oxford textbook of palliative medicine* (3rd ed.). New York: Oxford University Press.

Holthe, M., Klepstad, P., Zahlsen, K., et al. (2002). Morphine glucuronide-to-morphine plasma ratios are unaffected by the UGT2B7, H268Y and UGT1A1*28 polymorphisms in cancer patients on chronic morphine therapy. *Eur J Clin Pharmacol, 58,* 353-356.

Ingelman-Sundberg, M. (2001). Genetic susceptibility to adverse effects of drugs and environmental toxicant: The role of the CYP family of enzymes. *Mutat Res, 482,* 11-19.

Katzung, B.G. (2003). *Basic & clinical pharmacology* (9th ed.). San Francisco, Calif: Lange Medical Books/McGraw-Hill.

Lugo, R.A., Satterfield, K.L., & Kern, S.E. (2006). Pharmacokinetics of methadone. *J Pain Palliat Care Pharmacother, 19,* 13-24.

Olson, J. (2003). *Clinical pharmacology made ridiculously simple* (2nd ed.). Miami, Fla: MedMaster.

Rollason, V. & Vogt, N. (2003). Reduction of polypharmacy in the elderly. *Drugs Aging, 20,* 817-832.

Schwartz, J.B. (2003). The influence of sex on pharmacokinetics. *Clin Pharmacokinet, 42,* 107-121.

Turnheim, K. (2003). When drug therapy gets old: Pharmacokinetics and pharmacodynamics in the elderly. *Exp Gerontol, 38,* 843-853.

Turnheim, K. (2004). Drug therapy in the elderly. *Exp Gerontol, 39,* 1731-1738.

Urso, R., Blardi. P., & Giorgi, G. (2002). A short introduction to pharmacokinetics. *Eur Rev Med Pharmacol Sci, 6,* 33-44.

U.S. Department of Health and Human Services Food and Drug Administration. (2006). *Electronic orange book.* Retrieved February 10, 2006, from www.fda.gov/cder/orange/default.htm.

Weinberg, D.S., Inturrisi, C.E., Reidenberg, B., et al. (1988). Sublingual absorption of selected opioid analgesics. *Clin Pharmacol Ther, 44,* 335-342.

CHAPTER 8

SLEEP

Catherine Vena

■

Sleep is an essential human need and an important component of human homeostasis. Despite an explosion of scientific discovery about sleep in the past 50 years, there is much to be discovered about the role of sleep in health and illness. However, research has shown that the lack of adequate sleep results in poor physical and mental function (Pilcher & Huffcutt, 1996). Because sleep has also been found to be important for immune, endocrine, and metabolic functions, insufficient or poorly timed sleep affects health and well-being (Akerstedt & Nilsson, 2003). Yet sleep problems are common in chronic illnesses such as cancer (Clark, Cunningham, McMillan, et al., 2004; Vena, Parker, Cunningham et al., 2004), cardiopulmonary disease (Gay, 2004; Parker & Dunbar, 2002), and neurological disorders such as Parkinson's disease (Rye, 2004) and Alzheimer's disease (Ancoli-Israel, Gehrman, Martin et al., 2003). Furthermore, sleep is frequently disturbed in populations characterized by chronic pain (Landis, Frey, Lentz et al., 2003) and is often associated with psychosocial distress such as anxiety, depression, or worry (Bixler, Vgontzas, Lin et al., 2002; Hall, Buysse, Nowell et al., 2000; Morin, Rodrigue, & Ivers, 2003). For the person experiencing a chronic or life-threatening illness, disturbed sleep has important implications for clinical outcomes. The sleep of family members, especially those who are caregivers for the chronically and terminally ill, is also at risk for being disrupted or inadequate due to either the patient's sleep problems or the burdens of caregiving, which places the family unit at risk for adverse outcomes (Carter, 2002, 2003). Therefore, it is important that advanced practice nurses (APNs) be proactive in assessing and promoting sleep in their palliative care practice. This chapter reviews normal sleep and sleep regulation, discusses factors that lead to disturbed sleep, and presents evidence-based interventions to promote sleep.

OVERVIEW OF NORMAL SLEEP

Despite the fact that a third of human existence is spent in the sleep state, there is little understanding of why sleep is needed or what mechanisms underlie its capacities for physical and mental restoration. As late as the early twentieth century, sleep was believed to be a passive, quiescent state intermediate between wakefulness and death. However, the discovery of rapid eye movement (REM) and the identification of the dramatic effects of sleep deprivation in the mid-twentieth century prompted an escalation in research concerning the physiology, neurobiology, and biobehavioral aspects of sleep (Akerstedt & Nilsson, 2003). It is now known that sleep is an active process characterized by a distinct architecture and rhythmicity. There are actually three discrete, functional states of the brain: waking, non-REM (NREM) sleep, and REM sleep. The cycling of these states is at two levels: the basic wake/sleep cycle and the within-sleep cycle of REM and NREM sleep. A complex array of behavioral, neuroendocrine, and central nervous system factors regulates these cycles. In optimal conditions, waking is consolidated during the day and sleeping is consolidated at night. In the presence of pathology or physical illness, it is possible to see intrusion of wakefulness into the sleeping period and, conversely, intrusion of sleep into the wake period.

Normal sleep consists of a sequence of various stages distinguished by electroencephalographic (EEG) activity, muscle tone, and eye movements (Silber, Krahn, & Morgenthaler, 2004). Sleep is initiated after an initial stage of drowsiness. The first stage, NREM sleep, is divided into stages 1 through 4, roughly corresponding to sleep depth. Each stage has its own "signature" of EEG activity. Stage 1 is characterized by mixed-frequency low-amplitude waves; stage 2 is characterized by K complexes and spindles; and stages 3 and 4 are characterized by progressively greater numbers of slow, high-amplitude waves. Stages 3 and 4 are also collectively termed slow-wave sleep (SWS) and are associated with the highest arousal threshold. REM sleep is characterized by EEG activity somewhat similar to stage 1 or wakefulness and by episodic bursts of eye movements and a loss of muscle tone. While often associated with dreaming, it is now known that dreaming can also occur during NREM sleep. Normal sleep architecture across the night consists of NREM alternating with REM sleep in approximately 90- to 120-minute cycles. A young adult will typically have four to six of these cycles as illustrated in Figure 8-1. Most SWS generally occurs during the first half of the night, while more REM sleep occurs during the second half. Stage 1 sleep represents 2% to 5% of total sleep; stage 2, 45% to 55%; and stages 3 and 4, about 13% to 23%. Typically, REM sleep accounts for 20% to 25% of total sleep (Carskadon & Dement, 2005). Brief arousals punctuate normal sleep, although only the longest of these are remembered. Arousals tend to increase in frequency as sleep quality deteriorates. Common terms used in conjunction with sleep are listed in Box 8-1.

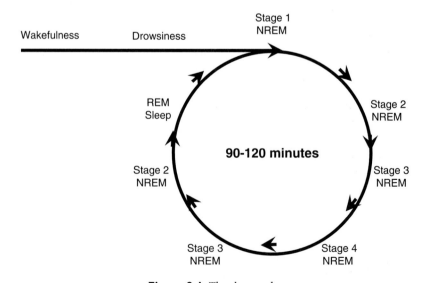

Figure 8-1 The sleep cycle.

Box 8-1   Sleep-Related Terms

Apnea Cessation of airflow at the nostrils and mouth lasting at least 10 seconds.

Arousal Abrupt change from sleep to wakefulness, from a "deeper" stage of non-REM sleep to a "lighter" stage.

Circadian rhythm Innate, daily fluctuation of behavioral and physiological functions, including sleeping and waking, generally tied to the 24-hour day-night cycle but sometimes to a different (e.g., 23- or 25-hour) periodicity when light/dark and other time cues are removed.

Excessive daytime sleepiness Difficulty in maintaining the alert, awake state.

Insomnia Sleep problems characterized by difficulty falling asleep, frequent awakenings during the night, or waking up earlier than desired that can result in getting up in the morning feeling nonrested and experiencing drowsiness during the day. Insomnia may be primary or secondary to other conditions.

K complex Sharp, negative, high-voltage EEG wave, followed by a slower, positive component. K complexes occur spontaneously during NREM sleep and define stage 2.

Light sleep Term used to describe non-REM sleep stage 1 and sometimes stage 2.

NREM sleep Non–rapid eye movement sleep; divided into four stages, 1 through 4. A stage of sleep in which brain activity and bodily functions slow down. NREM sleep accounts for the largest portion of the sleep cycle.

Periodic limb movement disorder Disorder characterized by periodic episodes of repetitive and highly stereotyped limb movements that occur during sleep.

Polysomnogram (PSG) Gold standard for objective measurement of sleep. PSG involves the continuous and simultaneous recording of physiological variables during sleep, i.e., EEG, EOG, EMG (the three basic stage scoring parameters), ECG, respiratory air flow, respiratory excursion, lower limb movement, and other electrophysiological variables.

REM density Function that expresses the frequency of eye movements per unit of time during REM sleep.

REM sleep Rapid eye movement sleep. REM sleep occurs in brief spurts of increased activity in the brain and body. REM is considered the dreaming stage of sleep. It is characterized by the darting of the eyes under the eyelids.

Restless legs syndrome (RLS) Disorder characterized by sensations in the legs that tend to occur when an individual is not moving and are usually worse in the evening. There is an almost irresistible urge to move the legs; the sensations are relieved by movement.

Sleep apnea syndrome Disorder characterized by repetitive episodes of reduced or absent respiratory airflow that occur during sleep and that are usually associated with a reduction in blood oxygen level. Symptoms include loud snoring and a gasping or snorting sound when the sleeping individual starts to breathe again. Although the individual may not be aware of having sleep apnea, the condition can disrupt the quality of sleep and result in daytime fatigue. The most common type, obstructive sleep apnea, occurs when the tongue or other soft tissue blocks the airway.

Sleep architecture NREM-REM sleep-stage and cycles.

Sleep debt Result of recurrent sleep deprivation that occurs over time when an individual does not experience a sufficient amount of the restorative daily sleep that is required to maintain a sense of feeling rested and refreshed.

Sleep deprivation Acute or chronic lack of sufficient sleep.

Data from Kryger, M.H., Roth, T., & Dement, W.C. (Eds.). (2005) *Principles and practice of sleep medicine* (4th ed.). Philadelphia: Elsevier Saunders; American Academy of Sleep Medicine (2005). *The international classification of sleep disorders: Diagnostic and coding manual, ICSD-2* (2nd ed.). Westchester, Ill: Author; and Silber, M.H., Krahn, L.E., & Morgenthaler, T.I. (2004). *Sleep medicine in clinical practice*, London: Taylor & Francis.

Continued

Box 8-1	Sleep-Related Terms—cont'd

Sleep diary (log) Daily, written record of an individual's sleep-wake pattern containing such information as time of retiring and arising, time in bed, estimated total sleep period, number and duration of sleep interruptions, quality of sleep, daytime naps, use of medications or caffeine beverages, nature of waking activities, and other data.

Sleep disorders Broad range of illnesses arising from many causes, including dysfunctional sleep mechanisms, abnormalities in physiological functions during sleep, abnormalities of the biological clock, and sleep disturbances that are induced by factors extrinsic to the sleep process.

Sleep efficiency (SE) Proportion of sleep in the episode filled by sleep; the ratio of TST to time in bed.

Sleep fragmentation Brief arousals occurring throughout the night, reducing the total amount of time spent in the deeper levels of sleep.

Sleep latency (SL) Time period measured from "lights out," or bedtime, to the beginning of sleep.

Sleep onset Transition from wake to sleep, normally into NREM stage 1.

Sleep pattern (24-hour sleep-wake pattern) Individual's clock hour schedule of bedtimes and rise times as well as nap behavior; may also include time and duration of sleep interruptions.

Slow-wave sleep (SWS) Common term for NREM stages 3 and 4 (also called delta or deep sleep).

Total sleep time (TST) Amount of actual sleep time in a sleep episode; the time is equal to the total sleep episode less the awake time.

Zeitgeber Environmental time cue that entrains biological rhythms to a specific periodicity. Known Zeitgebers are light, melatonin, and physical activity.

As humans age, the variabilities in sleep architecture and sleep-wake patterns increase. In general, relative to younger people, older people frequently have difficulty maintaining sleep and experience early morning awakenings, resulting in more time spent in bed relative to the amount of sleep. They also have more stage 1 sleep and less stage 2, 3, and 4 sleep. While total REM time decreases by a small percentage, the proportion of time spent in REM sleep to total sleep remains relatively unchanged into healthy old age (Bliwise, 2005). Objective changes in sleep architecture occur earlier and are more pronounced in men; however, women are more likely to voice subjective sleep complaints (Blazer, Hays, & Foley, 1995; Middelkoop, Smilde-van den Doel, Neven et al., 1996).

Normal aging plays a role in changes in sleep, but there is also evidence that psychosocial factors and medical illness may be significant contributors to disturbed sleep in the elderly. In a large survey, elders' sleep complaints were associated with respiratory symptoms, physical disability, depressive symptoms, and poor perceived health (Foley, Monjan, Brown et al., 1995). Other studies have demonstrated that in the absence of psychological, medical, and social factors that affect sleep, sleep problems in elders were much less frequent or even nonexistent (Bliwise, King, Harris et al., 1992; Ford & Kamerow, 1989; Gislason & Almqvist, 1987; Vitiello, Moe, & Prinz, 2002).

The Function of Sleep

A period of prolonged sleep loss is most likely to precipitate overwhelming sleepiness, which suggests that sleep is appetitive and fulfills essential needs. Despite the rapid increase in understanding of sleep physiology and pathology, the exact function of sleep remains unknown. Research has shown that REM and NREM sleep may serve specific biological functions. When individuals are restricted from entering REM sleep, they tend to spend longer periods in REM sleep during their next sleeping period. Furthermore, these REM periods are more intense and have more eye movements per minute than normal REM sleep. Similarly, individuals deprived of NREM sleep spend more time in NREM sleep during a recovery sleep period. EEGs measuring brain activity show that this "rebound" NREM sleep also differs from normal NREM sleep. This research suggests that the body needs adequate levels of both REM and NREM sleep and that the two kinds of sleep serve different biological purposes (Finelli, 2005).

While the exact function of sleep remains unclear, there are a number of theories. Some have suggested that sleep, especially NREM sleep, is necessary to reverse and/or restore biochemical and/or physiological processes through protein synthesis, cell division, and growth. Others have postulated that sleep serves to conserve energy through reduced metabolic rate and body temperature (Silber et al., 2004). There have also been numerous speculations on the functions of REM sleep, including brain restoration, consolidation of memory, and erasure of inappropriate memories (Siegel, 2001). Sleep also appears to be important for immune and endocrine function, metabolism, and thermoregulation (Krueger, Majde, & Obal, 2003; McGinty, Alam, Szymusiak et al., 2001; Steiger, 2003; Van Someren, 2000). None of these theories is supported unequivocally by current evidence. Most likely, sleep serves many functions.

Sleep Regulation

A basic understanding of the mechanisms that regulate sleep is necessary to appreciate how the sleep-wake cycle may be disrupted in palliative care patients. Two basic processes govern physiological sleepiness and wakefulness: process S and process C (Borbely, 1982). Process S is the homeostatic pressure to sleep that increases with the length of time an individual is awake and is eliminated by sleep. Process C, the circadian rhythm, is regulated by a clocklike mechanism in the brain (located in the suprachiasmatic nucleus). Process C represents the drive for wakefulness that is lowest in the early morning hours and highest at mid-day. The natural sleep-wake rhythm cycle is about 25 hours. However, cues from the environment (zeitgebers) entrain or "set" sleep's rhythm to a 24-hour schedule. As a result, humans depend on external cues such as exposure to light, regular meals, and social interactions to keep their diurnal cycle "on time."

Sleep propensity, sleep structure, and waking are regulated by a subtle and complex interaction of the two processes. Process C serves to maintain sleep as process S declines during the night and to maintain alertness as process S increases during the day (Borbely & Achermann, 2005). NREM sleep intensity is determined primarily by the homeostatic process (process S), and REM sleep by the circadian process (process C), while the ratio of REM to NREM sleep depends on both homeostatic and circadian factors. Factors that either interfere with or support these processes have the potential to significantly affect the timing, duration, and structure of sleep as well as daytime functioning.

EFFECTS OF IMPAIRED SLEEP

Impaired sleep may be the result of an inadequate amount of sleep or frequent disruption or fragmentation of sleep. The amount of sleep each person needs depends on many factors, including age. For most adults, 7 to 8 hours a night appears to be the best amount of sleep, although some people may need as few as 5 hours or as many as 10 hours of sleep each day (National Institute of Neurological Disorders and Stroke, 2005). The most common causes for inadequate amounts of sleep are self-imposed sleep restriction or lifestyle or work demands that require staying awake at night (Lee, Landis, Chasens et al., 2004). Caregivers are especially at risk for this type of sleep loss (Carter, 2002, 2003). Getting too little sleep creates a "sleep debt," which eventually demands repayment. Contrary to popular belief, humans do not adapt to getting less sleep than needed. Although individuals may become accustomed to a sleep-depriving schedule, adverse effects remain apparent. Sleep fragmentation can occur because of environmental conditions, but it is frequently the consequence of acute or chronic illness or primary sleep disorders. Both inadequate amounts of sleep and frequently interrupted sleep result in sleep loss, a condition with known adverse consequences. In addition to daytime sleepiness, sleep loss has been shown to produce impairment in cognitive function, including reduced attention, short-term memory, and problem-solving ability (Bonnet, 2005). Sleep fragmentation can also result in elevation of blood pressure, increases in urinary and serum catecholamines (an indicator of acute stress), arrhythmias, and progression of heart failure (Leung & Bradley, 2001; Sin, Logan, Fitzgerald et al., 2000). In addition, sleep loss has been shown to produce a catabolic state leading to negative nitrogen balance, alter immune function, increase oxygen consumption and carbon dioxide production, and disrupt thermoregulation (Bonnet, 2005). Thus, the lack of consolidated, restorative sleep places the palliative care patient and their caregivers at risk for adverse outcomes.

Factors Contributing to Disturbed Sleep in the Palliative Care Setting

Disturbed sleeping and waking are usually multifactoral. Some factors such as a history of primary sleep disorder and demographic or lifestyle factors predispose the patient to further problems with sleep when confronted with a chronic or life-threatening illness. Other factors, such as psychosocial, disease-related, and treatment-related factors, precipitate sleep-wake disturbance through further interference with sleep regulatory processes (process S and process C).

PRIMARY SLEEP DISORDERS

From population-based surveys, the National Sleep Foundation (NSF) estimates that at least 34% of Americans are at risk for primary sleep disorders such as insomnia, sleep apnea, and restless legs syndrome (NSF, 2005a). This means that tens of millions of Americans have undiagnosed and untreated sleep disorders. In addition, the average amount of sleep obtained by adults in this country is 6.9 hours per weeknight. Seventy-one percent of adults say they sleep less than 8 hours per night; 40% report sleeping less than 7 hours (NSF, 2005a). Thus, a significant number of patients seen in a palliative care practice may have a preexisting sleep disorder or chronic sleep deprivation, conditions that could worsen the effect of numerous precipitating factors associated with their disease process or treatments.

Demographic Factors

Researchers have identified increased reports of sleep problems in people who are older, female, single, and of lower socioeconomic status (Bliwise, 2005; Breslau, Roth, Rosenthal et al., 1997; Moore, Adler, Williams et al., 2002; Steptoe & Marmot, 2003). Of these factors, age appears to have the most significant impact on sleep. Elders have increased fragmentation of sleep, decreased amounts of deep sleep, and increased daytime napping that are linked to age-related changes that alter both homeostatic (process S) and circadian (process C) cycles, including (1) nocturia, (2) elevated autonomic activity that results in a greater susceptibility to arousal, and (3) decreased strength of circadian rhythms (Bliwise, 2005). Furthermore, primary sleep disorders such as sleep apnea (Young, Skatrud, & Peppard, 2004), periodic limb movements during sleep (Montplaisir, Allen, Walters et al., 2005), and insomnia are more prevalent in the elderly (Benca, Ancoli-Israel, & Moldofsky, 2004). While older men have more objective changes in sleep architecture, older women are more likely to complain of sleep difficulties (Rediehs, Reis, & Creason, 1990). Thus, elders in the palliative care setting may be at greater risk for disturbed sleep.

Lifestyle Factors

Lifestyle behaviors can influence quantity and quality of sleep (Lee-Chiong, 2002). Two factors that can interfere with both process S and process C are (1) the timing and duration of sleep periods and (2) conditions or agents that cause arousal in the sleep setting. Because the homeostatic drive for sleep is influenced by the amount of prior sleeping or waking, long naps taken during the daytime hours, especially late in the day, decrease the drive to sleep during the nocturnal sleep period (Monk, Buysse, Carrier et al., 2001). In addition, irregular bedtimes, staying longer in bed, and decreased daytime activity interfere with circadian activity-rest patterns (Lee-Chiong, 2002). Maintaining regular bed and rise times, as well as regular daily activity, enhances nocturnal sleep. Environmental factors and ingestion of common substances can interfere with process S by eliciting arousal. Room temperature, noise, and light level, as well as use of stimulants (such as caffeine in coffee and soft drinks and nicotine in tobacco products), can interfere with sleep onset or sleep continuity. Although alcohol ingestion is generally associated with sedation, falling blood alcohol levels produce sympathetic arousal so that sleep continuity after ingestion becomes a problem (Gillin, Drummond, Clark et al., 2005). These behaviors or conditions in combination can produce a profound effect on sleep.

Psychosocial Factors

Anxiety and depression are commonly encountered in palliative care practices. Researchers have found that anxiety related to a general stress burden is associated with numerous changes in sleep architecture, including a reduced amount of total sleep time, difficulty getting to sleep, reduced SWS, increased microarousals and stage 1 sleep, and reduced REM density (Hall et al., 2000; Kecklund & Akerstedt, 2004).

These findings suggest that anxiety can interfere with process S by causing increased physiological arousal. Disturbed sleep is also a key feature of depression. Sleep in persons diagnosed with major depression and dysthymia is characterized by changes in sleep architecture including decreased SWS, reduced REM latency, prolonged first REM period, and higher REM density (total eye movements/total REM time), as well as by sleep continuity disturbances and excessive daytime sleepiness (Benca, 2005). It has been hypothesized that these changes in sleep architecture may be due to deficiencies in process S (Borbely & Wirz-Justice, 1983) and changes in the circadian rhythm of body temperature (Avery, Wildschiodtz, Smallwood et al., 1986; Schultz & Lund, 1983). However, the role of depression and anxiety in sleep disturbance is not always clear. Increasing data indicate that sleep problems often precede clinical depression and anxiety (Breslau, Roth, Rosenthal et al., 1996; Ohayon & Roth, 2003).

Disease-Related Factors
Chronic Illness

Many persons with chronic illnesses, including cardiac diseases, lung diseases, renal failure, and cancer, report sleep problems (Parker, Bliwise, & Rye, 2000; Parker & Dunbar, 2002; Serber, Sears, Sotile et al., 2003; Silber et al., 2004; Vena et al., 2004). Common complaints among patients with these conditions include difficulty getting to sleep, frequent interruptions in sleep, daytime sleepiness, and fatigue. These complaints are likely the result of the disease process or treatments that have the potential to disturb sleep regulatory processes.

Pain

Disturbed sleep is a key complaint of patients experiencing both acute and chronic pain (Roehrs & Roth, 2005). Researchers have discovered that areas in the brain that process pain signals also regulate NREM sleep. This phenomenon may at least partially explain the interaction between pain and poor sleep (Basbaum & Jessell, 2000). Persons with pain have reduced amounts of SWS and often experience fragmented sleep related to the arousing property of pain (Lavigne, Zucconi, Castronovo et al., 2000). These findings suggest alterations in process S.

Sleep loss can also affect pain perception. Persons deprived of SWS or undergoing a cumulative sleep deficit (33% reduction in habitual amount) demonstrate a lowered pain threshold and increased somatic complaints (headache, sore joints) (Dinges, Pack, Williams et al., 1997; Lentz, Landis, Rothermel et al., 1999). Conversely, a good night of sleep may enhance mood and coping with pain. One group of investigators found that sleep quality was more likely to predict the following day's mood and physical symptoms than were mood and symptoms able to predict the following night's sleep quality (Totterdell, Reynolds, Parkinson et al., 1994).

Fatigue

Fatigue is a prevalent and disruptive symptom of many chronic illnesses, including heart failure, chronic lung disease, and cancer (Ancoli-Israel et al., 2003; Nordgren & Sorensen, 2003; Reishtein, 2005). There are many potential causes of fatigue in chronic illness, including preexisting physical conditioning, physical and psychological symptoms, and the consequences of treatments (Sharpe & Wilks, 2002). Several studies have demonstrated a link between fatigue and nocturnal sleep disturbance (Ancoli-Israel et al., 2003; Reishtein, 2005). Fatigue can lead to inactivity and daytime napping which interferes with process S. In turn, inactivity can also lead to a disruption in circadian activity/rest cycles (process C). Daytime sleepiness and "feeling drowsy" have also been identified as factors in the perceived level of fatigue (Ahsberg & Furst, 2001; Hwang, Chang, Rue et al., 2003). One study found that patients use the terms "lack of energy," "tiredness," and "fatigue" rather that "sleepiness" to describe their problem (Chervin, 2000). It may be that both patients and clinicians operationalize daytime sleepiness and fatigue in ways that contribute to confusing rather than distinguishing between the conditions (Pigeon, Sateia, & Ferguson, 2003).

Other Symptoms

Palliative care patients are likely to present with a number of other symptoms that interfere with sleep, including dyspnea, cough, nausea, gastrointestinal disturbances, and/or hot flashes (Albert, Davis, & Young, 2002; Blackler, Mooney, & Jones, 2004; Sachs, Shega, & Cox-Hayley, 2004; Walsh, Donnelly, & Rybicki, 2000). Although there is little research into the interaction of common nonpain symptoms and sleep, physical discomfort can delay onset of sleep or interrupt sleep (process S). The APN needs to carefully assess for the presence of these symptoms and their impact on sleep.

Treatment-Related Factors

It is becoming increasingly apparent that medical treatments have the potential to interfere with sleep regulatory processes and thus precipitate sleep loss. Sleep disturbances have been associated with hospitalization (Carvalhaes-Neto, Ramos, Suchecki et al., 2003; Redeker, 2000), surgery and anesthesia (Cronin, Kiefer, Davies et al., 2001; Redeker, Ruggiero, & Hedges, 2004; Rosenberg-Adamsen, Skarbye, Wildschiodtz et al., 1996), cancer therapies (Berger & Higginbotham, 2000; Capuron, Ravaud, & Dantzer, 2000; Miaskowski & Lee, 1999; Stein, Jacobsen, Hann et al., 2000), and hemodialysis (Parker et al., 2000). In addition, most palliative care patients received a number of medications to control the disease process or alleviate associated symptoms. A number of these may interfere with sleep or wakefulness. Impaired renal, hepatic, or neurological function in the chronically ill can further sensitize patients to adverse effects from their medications. It is beyond the scope of this chapter to provide a comprehensive review of the effect of medications on the sleep-wake cycle. However, the major types of drugs known to effect sleep and wakefulness are summarized in Table 8-1. It is common to think of the impact of analgesics, sedatives, and hypnotics on sleep and wakefulness. However, numerous other agents can have adverse effects on sleep regulation, particularly those with central nervous system effects (Schweitzer, 2005).

ASSESSMENT OF SLEEP

In light of the growing awareness of the potential for sleep loss and its adverse effects on the palliative care patient, it is important that the APN regularly assess for disturbed nocturnal sleep and daytime sleepiness. Although objective measures of sleep are available, an initial assessment relies on subjective information from the patient.

TABLE 8-1 ■ Drugs with Sleep-Impairing Properties

Category	Drug	Effect
Analgesics	Opioids	↓REM sleep ↓ Stage II ↓ Arousal
	Nonsteroidal antiinflammatory drugs (aspirin, ibuprofen, naproxen)	↑ Stage II ↓ SWS Altered thermoregulation
Antidepressants	Tricyclics (amitriptyline, doxepin, imipramine, trimipramine, desipramine, nortriptyline)	↓ REM, ↑ TST
	Selective serotonin reuptake inhibitors (fluoxetine, paroxetine, fluvoxamine)	↓ REM, ↓ TST
Antiemetics	Dopamine antagonists (phenothiazines, metoclopramide)	Drowsiness, sedation ↓ REM
	Anticholinergic agents (scopolamine)	Delayed REM onset ↓ REM sleep ↑ Stage II ↑ Body movement
	5-Hydroxytryptamine₃ (5-HT₃) antagonists (ondansetron, granisetron)	Drowsiness
Antihypertensives	β-Adrenergic receptor antagonists (propranolol, nadolol)	Insomnia, daytime sleepiness, nightmares, and vivid dreams
	α-Adrenergic agonists (clonidine, methyldopa)	Daytime sleepiness, insomnia, ↓ TST, ↓ SWS, REM changes
Anxiolytics	Benzodiazepines (alprazolam, diazepam, lorazepam)	↓ SWS/REM ↑ Stage II Shortened REM latency
Bronchodilators	Theophylline	↑ Arousals, ↓ TST
Corticosteroids	Prednisone, dexamethasone	Insomnia Bad dreams
Hypnotics	Benzodiazepines (flurazepam, triazolam, temazepam)	↓ SWS/REM (mild)
	Nonbenzodiazepines (zaleplon, zolpidem, zopiclone)	Minimal to no effects on SWS and REM ↓ Sleep latency

Data from Schweitzer, P.K. (2005). Drugs that disturb sleep and wakefulness. In M.H. Kryger, T. Roth, & W.C. Dement, (Eds.). *Principles and practice of sleep medicine* (4th ed.). Philadelphia: Elsevier Saunders; and Silber, M.H., Krahn, L.E., & Morgenthaler, T.I. (2004). *Sleep medicine in clinical practice*. London: Taylor & Francis.
REM, Rapid eye movement sleep; *SWS*, slow-wave sleep (stage 3-4 non-REM sleep); *TS*, total sleep time.

Several questionnaires have been designed to assess sleep quantity and quality, including the Pittsburgh Sleep Quality Index (PSQI) (Buysse, Reynolds, Monk et al., 1989), the St. Mary's Hospital Sleep Questionnaire (Ellis, John, Lancaster et al., 1981), the General Sleep Disturbance Scale (Lee, 1992), and the Sleep Questionnaire and Assessment of Wakefulness (SQAW) (Miles, 1982). The use of these questionnaires in primary care is difficult due to various factors, including length, complexity in scoring, and lack of defined cut-points in scores. Primary information is best obtained from a careful sleep-wake history. Collateral history from the patient's bed partner or caregiver can also provide vital information of which the patient may be unaware.

A sleep history should contain a subjective and behavioral account of a typical 24-hour day. Good sleep is characterized by the ability to fall asleep without difficulty (5 to 10 minutes), remain asleep throughout the night, awaken refreshed without the aid of an alarm clock, and remain alert and awake throughout the day. The BEARS system is a useful tool to organize taking a sleep history (see Table 8-2) (Owens, 2005). Another useful tool for assessing sleep patterns across time is the sleep diary or sleep log. Sleep diaries allow the APN to see night-to-night sleep patterns, sleep quality, and daily practices that affect sleep such as activity, naps, medications, and caffeine. Several sleep diaries are available online at the following Web sites.

TABLE 8-2 ■ BEARS Assessment System

Parameter	Objective	Initial Question	Follow-up Question
Bedtime	Find out what happens at sleep onset	Do you have difficulty falling asleep? Review: intake of alcohol, nicotine, chocolate, caffeine, medications	How long does it take you to fall asleep? What prevents you from falling asleep? How long have you had this problem?
Excessive daytime sleepiness	Determine the extent of daytime sleepiness	Do you find yourself falling asleep during the day when you don't want to?	How likely are you to fall asleep while reading, watching TV, during a conversation, while driving? Give Epworth Sleepiness Scale
Awakenings	Nightime: characterize the extent of awakenings	Are you having difficulty sleeping through the night?	What awakens you (pain, shortness of breath, etc)? How often and for how long are you awake? What keeps you from falling back asleep?
	Early morning: screen for mood disorder	Are you having any difficulty sleeping until the morning?	At what time do you usually awaken? What is your mood like in the morning?
Regularity and duration of sleep	Delineate sleep habits	What time do you usually go to bed and get up in the morning?	Do you feel that you usually get enough sleep?
Sleep disorders`	Screen for common sleep disorders	Have you or anyone else noticed that you snore loudly? Have you or anyone else noticed that your legs kick or twitch at night? Do you have an irresistible urge to move or other types of sensations in your arms or legs?	Have you or anyone else noticed that you stop breathing in your sleep? Does your bed partner go to another room of the house to sleep? Does this urge to move or sensation in your arms or legs become worse in the evening? Are these sensations relieved by moving or walking?

Data from the American Academy of Sleep Disorders: www.aasmnet.org/Resources.aspx?Resource_ID=5571; www.aasmnet.org/Resources.aspx?Resource_ID=5577; www.aasmnet.org/Resources.aspx?Resource_ID=1008.

- National Sleep Foundation (interactive diary): www.sleepfoundation.org/quiz/index.php?secid=&id=107#
- National Heart, Lung, and Blood Institute (NIH): www.nhlbi.nih.gov/health/public/sleep/starslp/teachers/sleep_diary.htm
- Shuteye.com (Sanofi Aventis): www.shuteye.com/solutions_patterns_diary.asp

Daytime sleepiness is also an important aspect of any sleep history. Often patients will not be cognizant of their level of sleepiness. As mentioned before, patients often characterize sleepiness as feeling "tired" or "fatigued." These complaints warrant a thorough investigation of nocturnal sleep and sleepiness. The Epworth Sleepiness Scale (ESS) (Johns, 1991) is widely used in practice to evaluate the level of daytime sleepiness in patients. The questionnaire contains eight items and measures the likelihood of falling asleep in hypothetical situations. Patients who score greater than 10 have excessive daytime sleepiness. The National Sleep Foundation (NSF) has also developed a Sleepiness Diary (NSF, 2005b). Like the sleep diary, this tool allows the APN to follow patterns of sleepiness across time.

Most sleep disorders are treatable. Many sleep problems can be solved with behavioral or brief pharmacological interventions. However, there are instances when a referral to a sleep specialist is in order for further evaluation. The decision to refer should be based on patient-family goals and the patient's place in the disease trajectory, which include:

- Sleep loss (insufficient sleep/fragmented sleep) not responsive to therapy and accompanied by daytime sleepiness
- Unexplained daytime sleepiness: ESS >10, falling asleep during the day without deliberate effort
- Symptoms of restless legs syndrome
- Symptoms of sleep apnea: loud snoring, awakening with gasping for breath, witnessed apneas during sleep
- Symptoms of periodic limb movement disorder: excessive limb movements or jerks during sleep (usually partner report)

INTERVENTIONS TO IMPROVE SLEEP IN PALLIATIVE CARE

Promoting Healthy Sleep Practices

Because disturbed sleep is due to multiple interacting factors, no single intervention is likely to produce desired outcomes. Given a basic understanding of the factors in palliative care patients that potentially alter sleep regulatory processes, the APN can implement patient-specific strategies to minimize disruption of sleep-wake cycles. It has been shown that poor sleep practices can complicate any disease or treatment factors that precipitate sleep-wake disturbances (Zarcone, 2000). Poor sleep habits tolerated in a healthy state may be less tolerable in the disease state. Therefore, APNs must consider evaluation of patient sleep habits and promotion of behaviors that enhance both process S and process C as first steps in any treatment plan. Sleep-promoting behaviors are listed in Table 8-3.

Treatment of Disturbing Symptoms

Controlling symptoms is a goal of palliative care and a means to improve quality of life. As discussed previously, a number of symptoms have been associated with sleep

TABLE 8-3 ■ Sleep Practices That Promote Sleep Homeostasis (Process S) and Circadian Rhythms (Process C)

	Promotes	
	Process S	Process C
Establish Routine Activity-Rest Patterns		
Get up and go to bed the same time every day.		X
Reduce time in bed to the average number of hours slept in the previous week.	X	X
Limit daytime sleep to brief naps (less than 1 hour) no later than 8 hours after waking.	X	
Engage in light exercise or increase activity in the morning or afternoon. Limit exercise 4 hours before bedtime.	X	X
Get at least 30 minutes exposure to sunlight or bright light within a half hour of arising.	X	X
Establish Dietary Habits that Promote Sleep		
Do not eat heavily for 3 hours before bedtime.	X	
A light bedtime snack is appropriate. Tryptophan content in dairy products and turkey may act as a natural sleep inducer.	X	
A hot drink may help to relax and warm you.	X	X
Make Sure Your Bed and Bedroom Are Pleasant and Relaxing		
Keep room dark. Avoid exposure to bright light if you have to get up at night.	X	X
If environmental noise is a problem, use earplugs or a "white noise" machine.	X	
Keep room well ventilated and temperature at a comfortable level.	X	
Make sure your mattress is comfortable and the pillow the correct height.	X	
Associate your bed with sleep. Try not to use the bed to watch television, listen to the radio, or read.	X	
Establish a Relaxing Bedtime Routine		
Avoid emotionally upsetting conversations or activities before bedtime.	X	
Make a list of pressing problems and simple solutions to be implemented the next day, then set your problems aside.	X	
Listen to relaxing music.	X	
Do relaxation exercises or meditate.	X	
Read something soothing until you are sleepy.	X	
Take a bath hot enough to raise your body temperature about 90 minutes before bedtime. Declining body temperature promotes sleepiness.	X	X
Avoid Stimulants at least 4 to 6 Hours before Bed		
Avoid caffeine: coffee, tea, cola, cocoa, chocolate.	X	
Check over-the-counter medications for caffeine content.	X	
Do not smoke after 7:00 P.M. or avoid smoking altogether.	X	
Use alcohol sparingly. Alcohol makes you sleepy, but it interrupts sleep in the second half of the sleep period.	X	

Data from Thorpy, M. (2004). Sleep hygiene. Retrieved October 23, 2004, from www.sleepfoundation.org/ask/sleephygiene.cfm; and Zarcone, V.P. (2000). Sleep hygiene. In M.H. Kryger, T. Roth, & W.C. Dement (Eds.). *Principles and practice of sleep medicine* (4th ed.). Philadelphia: Elsevier Saunders.

problems, including pain, dyspnea/cough, gastrointestinal disturbances (reflux, diarrhea, nausea/vomiting), and psychological manifestations (depression/anxiety). Research suggests that symptoms rarely occur in isolation but instead occur in groups or clusters (Dodd, Miaskowski, & Lee, 2004). Furthermore, it appears that the association between symptoms may be interactive (Parker, Kimble, Dunbar et al. 2005). In approaching symptoms that cluster together (e.g., sleep/pain/depression or sleep/dyspnea/anxiety), the APN should plan for behavioral and pharmacological interventions that address multiple symptoms.

Medications

When behavioral interventions alone do not resolve sleep-wake problems, the addition of medications may be warranted. The use of hypnotics in palliative care populations does not have evidence from rigorous randomized controlled trials (Hirst & Sloan, 2005); therefore, the choice of medications depends on the pharmacokinetics of the agent, goals of treatment, symptom presentation, and patient response. Commonly prescribed medications are listed in Table 8-4.

TABLE 8-4 ■ Hypnotic and Sedating Drugs

Medication	Dose	Half-life	Comments
Nonbenzodiazepine Hypnotics			
Zolpidem (Ambien)	5-10 mg	1.5-2.4 hours	Use caution in presence of liver failure and in the elderly. May cause rebound insomnia if withdrawn abruptly. May cause rebound morning anxiety. Eszopiclone has been shown effective and safe for long-term use.
Zaleplon (Sonata)	5-10 mg	1 hour	
Eszopiclone (Lunesta)	1-3 mg	6 hours	
Benzodiazepine Hypnotics			
Tamezepam (Restoril)	15-30 mg	8-20 hours	May develop dependency. Caution in patients with liver failure. Longer-acting medications associated with daytime sleepiness and impaired performance. Avoid rapid withdrawal. Use with caution in the elderly.
Estazolam (ProSom)	1-2 mg	8-24 hours	
Triazolam (Halcion)	0.125-0.25 mg	2-6 hours	
Melatonin Receptor Agonist			
Remelteon (Rozerem)	8 mg	0.5-1.5 hours	Contraindicated in severe liver failure. Do not take after a high-fat meal. For use with sleep-onset insomnia.
Antidepressants			
Tricyclic			
Amitriptyline (Elavil)	25-50 mg (Maximum 150)	10-50 hours	Cautious use with elders due to anticholinergic effects. May be used as adjunct for neuropathic pain. Very sedating. Not FDA approved for primary insomnia.
Selective Serotonin Reuptake Inhibitors			
Trazodone (Desyrel)	25-100 mg	5-9 hours	Not FDA approved for insomnia. Doses usually used for insomnia are below recommended doses for depression. Not considered best antidepressant due to excessive daytime sedation at therapeutic doses.

Continued

TABLE 8-4 ■ Hypnotic and Sedating Drugs—cont'd

Medication	Dose	Half-life	Comments
Antidepressants—cont'd			
Other			
Mirtazapine (Remeron)	15-45 mg	20-40 hours	Not FDA approved for insomnia. May be useful for sleep with coexisting mood disorder due to sedating properties. Increases appetite. Weight gain common.
Antihistamines			
Diphenhydramine (Benadryl)	25-50 mg	3-12 hours	Not much data to support use for sleep. May cause morning sedation. Should only be used short term. Use with great caution in elders. Has been shown to cause cognitive impairment and delirium.
Doxylamine (Unisom)	12.5-25 mg	9 hours	Potent antihistamine with strong anticholinergic effects. Use with caution in elders.

Data from Roth, T., Stubbs, C., & Walsh, J.K. (2005). Ramelteon (TAK-375), a selective MT1/MT2-receptor agonist, reduces latency to persistent sleep in a model of transient insomnia related to a novel sleep environment, *Sleep, 28*, 303-307; Silber, M.H., Krahn, L.E., & Morgenthaler, T.I. (2004). *Sleep medicine in clinical practice*, London: Taylor & Francis; and Walsh, J.K., Roehrs, T., & Roth, T. (2005). Pharmacologic treatment of primary insomnia. In M.H. Kryger, T. Roth, & W.C. Dement, (Eds.). *Principles and practice of sleep medicine* (4th ed.). Philadelphia: Elsevier Saunders.

A careful evaluation of each patient's medication regimen is also warranted. Many medications have arousing properties that will interfere with nocturnal sleep. These medications should be avoided in the evening. Examples include steroids, arousing selective serotonin reuptake inhibitors (fluoxetine, paroxetine, sertraline), buproprion, and diuretics.

CONCLUSION

Palliative care patients are susceptible to severe disturbances in sleep that have the potential to impair tissue repair, immune function, endocrine function, and metabolism—conditions that affect overall morbidity and mortality. Some of the factors that underlie sleep disturbances include predisposing factors, such as a history of a primary sleep disorder, demographic factors, and lifestyle factors, and precipitating factors, such as psychosocial, disease-related, treatment-related, and environmental conditions. These factors have the potential to disrupt sleep regulatory mechanisms. APNs can promote sleep by recognizing which factors may be operable in individual patients and implementing strategies to minimize disruption in sleep and promote daytime alertness.

Box 8-2   Additional Resources

American Academy of Sleep Medicine
- Education site: www.sleepeducation.com
- Education for health professionals: www.aasmnet.org/MedSleep_Resources.aspx (look under specific authors)

National Sleep Foundation
- www.sleepfoundation.org

REFERENCES

Ahsberg, E. & Furst, C.J. (2001). Dimensions of fatigue during radiotherapy. *Acta Oncol, 40*, 37-43.

Akerstedt, T. & Nilsson, P.M. (2003). Sleep as restitution: An introduction. *J Intern Med, 254*, 6-12.

Albert, N.M., Davis, M., & Young, J. (2002). Improving the care of patients dying of heart failure. *Cleve Clin J Med, 69*, 321-328.

Ancoli-Israel, S., Gehrman, P., Martin, J.L., et al. (2003). Increased light exposure consolidates sleep and strengthens circadian rhythms in severe Alzheimer's disease patients. *Behav Sleep Med, 1*, 22-36.

Avery, D.H., Wildschiodtz, G., Smallwood, R.G., et al. (1986). REM latency and core temperature relationships in primary depression. *Acta Psychiatr Scand, 74*, 269-280.

Basbaum, A.I. & Jessell, T.M. (2000). The perception of pain. In E.R. Kandel, J.H. Schwartz, & T.M. Jessell (Eds.). *Principles of neuroscience* (4th ed., pp. 472-491). New York: McGraw-Hill.

Benca, R.M. (2005). Mood disorders. In M.H. Kryger, T. Roth, & W.C. Dement (Eds.). *Principles and practice of sleep medicine* (3rd ed., pp. 1311-1326). Philadelphia: Elsevier Saunders.

Benca, R.M., Ancoli-Israel, S., & Moldofsky, H. (2004). Special considerations in insomnia diagnosis and management: Depressed, elderly, and chronic pain populations. *J Clin Psychiatry, 65 (Suppl 8)*, 26-35.

Berger, A.M. & Higginbotham, P. (2000). Correlates of fatigue during and following adjuvant breast cancer chemotherapy: A pilot study. *Oncol Nurs For, 27*, 1443-1448.

Bixler, E.O., Vgontzas, A.N., Lin, H.M., et al. (2002). Insomnia in central Pennsylvania. *J Psychosom Res, 53*, 589-592.

Blackler, L., Mooney, C., & Jones, C. (2004). Palliative care in the management of chronic obstructive pulmonary disease. *Br J Nurs, 13*, 518-521.

Blazer, D.G., Hays, J.C., & Foley, D.J. (1995). Sleep complaints in older adults: A racial comparison. *The Journals of Gerontology. Series A, Biol Sci Med Sci, 50*, M280-M284.

Bliwise, D.L. (2005). Normal aging. In M.H. Kryger, T. Roth, & W.C. Dement (Eds.). *Principles and practice of sleep medicine* (4th ed., pp. 24-38). Philadelphia: Elsevier Saunders.

Bliwise, D.L., King, A.C., Harris, R.B., et al. (1992). Prevalence of self-reported sleep in a healthy population aged 50-65. *Soc Sci Med, 34*, 49-55.

Bonnet, M.H. (2005). Acute sleep deprivation. In M.H. Kryger, T. Roth, & W.C. Dement (Eds.). *Principles and practice of sleep medicine* (4th ed., pp. 51-66). Philadelphia: Elsevier Saunders.

Borbely, A.A. (1982). A two-process model of sleep regulation. *Hum Neurobiol, 1*, 195-204.

Borbely, A.A. & Achermann, P. (2005). Sleep homeostasis and models of sleep regulation. In M.H. Kryger, T. Roth, & W.C. Dement (Eds.). *Principles and practice of sleep medicine* (4th ed., pp. 405-417). Philadelphia: Elsevier Saunders.

Borbely, A.A. & Wirz-Justice, A. (1983). Sleep, sleep deprivation and depression: A hypothesis derived from a model of sleep regulation. *Hum Neurobiol, 1*, 205-210.

Breslau, N., Roth, T., Rosenthal, L., et al. (1996). Sleep disturbance and psychiatric disorders: A longitudinal epidemiological study of young adults. *Biol Psychiatry, 39*, 411-418.

Breslau, N., Roth, T., Rosenthal, L., et al. (1997). Daytime sleepiness: An epidemiological study of young adults. *Am J Pub Health, 87*, 1649-1653.

Buysse, D.J., Reynolds, C.F., III., Monk, T.H., et al. The Pittsburgh Sleep Quality Index: A new instruments for psychiatric practice and research. *Psychiatry Res, 28*, 193-213.

Capuron, L., Ravaud, A., & Dantzer, R. (2000). Early depressive symptoms in cancer patients receiving interleukin 2 and/or interferon alfa-2b therapy. *J Clin Oncol, 18*, 2143-2151.

Carskadon, M.A. & Dement, W.C. (2005). Normal human sleep: An overview. In M.H. Kryger, T. Roth, & W.C. Dement (Eds.). *Principles and practice of sleep medicine* (4th ed., pp. 13-23). Philadelphia: Elsevier Saunders.

Carter, P.A. (2002). Caregivers' descriptions of sleep changes and depressive symptoms. *Oncol Nurs For Online, 29*, 1277-1283.

Carter, P.A. (2003). Family caregivers' sleep loss and depression over time. *Cancer Nurs, 26*, 253-259.

Carvalhaes-Neto, N., Ramos, L.R., Suchecki, D., et al. (2003). The effect of hospitalization on the sleep pattern and on cortisol secretion of healthy elderly. *Exp Aging Res, 29*, 425-436.

Chervin, R.D. (2000). Sleepiness, fatigue, tiredness, and lack of energy in obstructive sleep apnea. *Chest, 118*, 372-379.

Clark, J., Cunningham, M., McMillan, S.C., et al. (2004). Sleep-wake disturbances in people with cancer. Part II: Evaluating the evidence for clinical decision making. *Oncol Nurs For, 31,* 747-771.

Cronin, A.J., Keifer, J.C., Davies, M.F., et al. (2001). Postoperative sleep disturbance: Influences of opioids and pain in humans. *Sleep, 24,* 39-44.

Dinges, D.F., Pack, F., Williams, K., et al. (1997). Cumulative sleepiness, mood disturbance, and psychomotor vigilance performance decrements during a week of sleep restricted to 4-5 hours per night. *Sleep, 20,* 267-267.

Dodd, M.J., Miaskowski, C., & Lee, K.A. (2004). Occurrence of symptom clusters. *J Nat Cancer Inst Monogr, 32,* 76-78.

Ellis, B.W., Johns, M.W., Lancaster, R., et al. (1981). The St. Mary's Hospital Sleep Questionnaire: A study of reliability. *Sleep, 4,* 93-97.

Finelli, L.A. (2005). Sleep deprivation: Cortical and EEG changes. In C.A. Kushida (Ed.). *Sleep deprivation: Basic science, physiology, and behavior* (pp. 223-264). New York: Marcel Dekker.

Foley, D.J., Monjan, A.A., Brown, S.L., et al. (1995). Sleep complaints among elderly persons: An epidemiologic study of three communities. *Sleep, 18,* 425-432.

Ford, D.E. & Kamerow, D.B. (1989). Epidemiologic study of sleep disturbance and psychiatric disorders: An opportunity for prevention? *JAMA, 262,* 1479-1484.

Gay, P.C. (2004). Chronic obstructive pulmonary disease and sleep. *Respira Care, 49,* 39-51.

Gillin, J.C., Drummond, S.P.A., Clark, C.P., et al. (2005). Medication and substance abuse. In M.H. Kryger, T. Roth, & W.C. Dement (Eds.). *Principles and practice of sleep medicine* (4th ed., pp. 1345-1358). Philadelphia: Elsevier Saunders.

Gislason, T. & Almqvist, M. (1987). Somatic diseases and sleep complaints. *Acta Med Scand, 221,* 475-481.

Hall, M., Buysse, D.J., Nowell, P.D., et al. (2000). Symptoms of stress and depression as correlates of sleep in primary insomnia. *Psychosom Med, 62,* 227-230.

Hirst, A. & Sloan, R. (2005). Benzodiazepines and related drugs for insomnia in palliative care. *Cochrane Database System Review, 3.*

Hwang, S.S., Chang, V.T., Rue, M., et al. (2003). Multidimensional independent predictors of cancer-related fatigue. *J Pain Symptom Manage, 26,* 604-614.

Johns, M.W. (1991). A new method for measuring daytime sleepiness: The Epworth Sleepiness Scale. *Sleep, 14,* 540-545.

Kecklund, G. & Akerstedt, T. (2004). Apprehension of the subsequent working day is associated with a low amount of slow wave sleep. *Biol Psychiatry, 66,* 169-176.

Krueger, J.M., Majde, J.A., & Obal, F. (2003). Sleep in host defense. *Brain Behav Immun, 17 (Suppl 1),* S41-S47.

Kryger, M.H., Roth, T., & Dement, W.C. (Eds.). (2005). *Principles and practice of sleep medicine* (4th ed.). Philadelphia: Elsevier Saunders.

Landis, C.A., Frey, C.A., Lentz, M.J., et al. (2003). Self-reported sleep quality and fatigue correlates with actigraphy in midlife women with fibromyalgia. *Nurs Res, 52,* 140-147.

Lavigne, G., Zucconi, M., Castronovo, C., et al. (2000). Sleep arousal response to experimental thermal stimulation during sleep in human subjects free of pain and sleep problems. *Pain, 84,* 283-290.

Lee, K.A. (1992). Self-reported sleep disturbances in employed women. *Sleep, 15,* 493-498.

Lee, K.A., Landis, C., Chasens, E.R., et al. (2004). Sleep and chronobiology: Recommendations for nursing education. *Nurs Outlook, 52,* 126-133.

Lee-Chiong, T.L. (2002). Manifestation and classification of sleep disorders. In T.L. Lee-Chiong, M.J. Sateia, & M.A. Carskadon (Eds.). *Sleep medicine* (pp. 125-142). Philadelphia: Hanley & Belfus.

Lentz, M.J., Landis, C.A., Rothermel, J., et al. (1999). Effects of selective slow wave sleep disruption on musculoskeletal pain and fatigue in middle aged women. *J Rheumatol, 26,* 1586-1592.

Leung, R.S. & Bradley, T.D. (2001). Sleep apnea and cardiovascular disease. *Am J Respir Crit Care Med, 164,* 2147-2165.

McGinty, D., Alam, M.N., Szymusiak, R., et al. (2001). Hypothalamic sleep-promoting mechanisms: Coupling to thermoregulation. *Arch Ital Biol, 139,* 63-75.

Miaskowski, C. & Lee, K.A. (1999). Pain, fatigue, and sleep disturbances in oncology outpatients receiving radiation therapy for bone metastasis: A pilot study. *J Pain Symptom Manage, 17,* 320-332.

Middelkoop, H.A., Smilde-van den Doel, D.A., Neven, A.K., et al. (1996). Subjective sleep characteristics of 1,485 males and females aged 50-93: Effects of sex and age, and factors related to self-evaluated quality of sleep. *J Gerontol 51*, M108-M115.

Miles, L. (1982). Sleep Questionnaire and Assessment of Wakefulness (SQAW). In C. Guilleminault (Ed.). *Sleeping and waking disorders: Indications and techniques* (pp. 384-413). Menlo Park, Calif: Addison-Wesley.

Monk, T.H., Buysse, D.J., Carrier, J., et al. (2001). Effects of afternoon "siesta" naps on sleep, alertness, performance, and circadian rhythms in the elderly. *Sleep, 24*, 680-687.

Montplaisir, J., Allen, R.P., Walters, A.S., et al. (2005). Restless legs syndrome and periodic limb movement disorder. In M.H. Kryger, T. Roth, & W.C. Dement (Eds.). *Principles and practice of sleep medicine* (4th ed., pp. 839-852). Philadelphia: Elsevier Saunders.

Moore, P.J., Adler, N.E., Williams, D.R., et al. (2002). Socioeconomic status and health: The role of sleep. *Psychosom Med, 64*, 337-344.

Morin, C.M., Rodrigue, S., & Ivers, H. (2003). Role of stress, arousal, and coping skills in primary insomnia. *Psychosom Med, 65*, 259-267.

National Institute of Neurological Disorders and Stroke (2005). *Brain basics: Understanding sleep.* Retrieved May 20, 2006, from www.ninds.nih.gov/disorders/brain_basics/understanding_sleep.htm.

National Sleep Foundation (2005a). *Sleep in America.* Retrieved May 20, 2006, from www.sleepfoundation.org/hottopics/index.php?secid=16&id=245.

National Sleep Foundation (2005b). *Sleepiness diary.* Retrieved May 20, 2006, from www.sleepfoundation.org/quiz/index.php?secid=&id=110.

Nordgren, L. & Sorensen, S. (2003). Symptoms experienced in the last six months of life in patients with end-stage heart failure. *Eur J Cardiovasc Nurs, 2*, 213-217.

Ohayon, M.M. & Roth, T. (2003). Place of chronic insomnia in the course of depressive and anxiety disorders. *J Psychiatr Res, 37*, 9-15.

Owens, J. (2005). *Taking a sleep history.* Retrieved May 20, 2006, from www.aasmnet.org/Resources.aspx?Resource_ID=1008.

Parker, K.P. Bliwise, D.L., & Rye, D.B. (2000). Hemodialysis disrupts basic sleep regulatory mechanisms: Building hypotheses. *Nurs Res, 49*, 327-332.

Parker, K.P. & Dunbar, S.B. (2002). Sleep and heart failure. *J Cardiovasc Nurs, 17*, 30-41.

Parker, K.P., Kimble, L.P., Dunbar, S.B., et al. (2005). Symptom interactions as mechanisms underlying symptom pairs and clusters. *J Nurs Schol, 37*, 209-215.

Pigeon, W.R., Sateia, M.J., & Ferguson, R.J. (2003). Distinguishing between excessive daytime sleepiness and fatigue: Toward improved detection and treatment. *J Psychosom Res, 54*, 61-69.

Pilcher, J.J. & Huffcutt, A.I. (1996). Effects of sleep deprivation on performance: A meta-analysis. *Sleep, 19*, 318-326.

Redeker, N.S. (2000). Sleep in acute care settings: An integrative review. *J Nurs Schol, 32*, 31-38.

Redeker, N.S., Ruggiero, J., & Hedges, C. (2004). Patterns and predictors of sleep pattern disturbance after cardiac surgery. *Res Nurs Health, 27*, 217-224.

Rediehs, M.H., Reis, J.S., & Creason, N.S. (1990). Sleep in old age: Focus on gender differences. *Sleep, 13*, 10-24.

Reishtein, J.L. (2005). Relationship between symptoms and functional performance in COPD. *Res Nurs Health, 28*, 39-47.

Roehrs, T. & Roth, T. (2005). Sleep and pain: Interaction of two vital functions. *Semin Neurol, 25*, 106-116.

Rosenberg-Adamsen, S., Skarbye, M., Wildschiodtz, G., et al. (1996). Sleep after laparoscopic cholecystectomy. *Br J Anaesth, 77*, 572-575.

Rye, D.B. (2004). The Two Faces of Eve: Dopamine's modulation of wakefulness and sleep. *Neurology, 63 (8 Suppl 3)*, S2-S7.

Sachs, G.A., Shega, J.W., & Cox-Hayley, D. (2004). Barriers to excellent end-of-life care for patients with dementia. *J Gen Internal Med, 19*, 1057-1063.

Schultz, H. & Lund, R. (1983). Sleep onset REM episodes are associated with circadian parameters of body temperature. A study in depressed patients and normal controls. *Biol Psychiatry, 18*, 1411-1426.

Schweitzer, P.K. (2005). Drugs that disturb sleep and wakefulness. In M.H. Kryger, T. Roth & W.C. Dement (Eds.). *Principles and practice of sleep medicine* (4th ed., pp. 499-518). Philadelphia: Elsevier Saunders.

Serber, E.R., Sears, S.F., Sotile, R.O., et al. (2003). Sleep quality among patients treated with implantable atrial defibrillation therapy: Effect of nocturnal shock delivery and psychological distress. *J Cardiovasc Electrophysiol, 14,* 960-964.

Sharpe, M. & Wilks, D. (2002). Fatigue. *Br Med J, 325,* 480-483.

Siegel, J.M. (2001). The REM sleep-memory consolidation hypothesis. *Science, 294,* 1058-1063.

Silber, M.H., Krahn, L.E., & Morgenthaler, T.I. (2004). *Sleep medicine in clin practice.* London: Taylor & Francis.

Sin, D.D., Logan, A.G., Fitzgerald, F.S., et al. (2000). Effects of continuous positive airway pressure on cardiovascular outcomes in heart failure patients with and without Cheyne-Stokes respiration. *Circulation, 102,* 61-66.

Steiger, A. (2003). Sleep and endocrinology. *J Intern Med, 254,* 13-22.

Stein, K.D., Jacobsen, P.B., Hann, D.M., et al. (2000). Impact of hot flashes on quality of life among postmenopausal women being treated for breast cancer. *J Pain Symptom Manage, 19,* 436-445.

Steptoe, A. & Marmot, M. (2003). Burden of psychosocial adversity and vulnerability in middle age: Associations with biobehavioral risk factors and quality of life. *Psychosom Med, 65,* 1029-1037.

Totterdell, P., Reynolds, S., Parkinson, B., et al. (1994). Associations of sleep with everyday mood, minor symptoms and social interaction experience. *Sleep, 17,* 466-475.

Van Someren, E.J. (2000). More than a marker: Interaction between the circadian regulation of temperature and sleep, age-related changes, and treatment possibilities. *Chronobiol Internat, 17,* 313-354.

Vena, C., Parker, K.P., Cunningham, M., et al. (2004). Sleep-wake disturbances in people with cancer. Part I: An overview of sleep, sleep regulation, and effects of disease and treatment. *Oncol Nurs For, 31,* 735-746.

Vitiello, M.V., Moe, K.E., & Prinz, P.N. (2002). Sleep complaints cosegregate with illness in older adults: Clinical research informed by and informing epidemiological studies of sleep. *J Psychosom Res, 53,* 555-559.

Walsh, D., Donnelly, S., & Rybicki, L. (2000). The symptoms of advanced cancer: Relationship to age, gender, and performance status in 1,000 patients. *Support Care Cancer, 8,* 175-179.

Young, T., Skatrud, J., & Peppard, P.E. (2004). Risk factors for obstructive sleep apnea in adults. *JAMA, 291,* 2013-2016.

Zarcone, V.P. (2000). Sleep hygiene. In M.H. Kryger, T. Roth, & W.C. Dement (Eds.). *Principles and practice of sleep medicine,* (3rd ed., pp. 657-661). Philadelphia: Saunders.

CHAPTER 9

NUTRITION

Suzanne W. Dixon

■

The issue of nutrition support in the palliative care environment is controversial. Between the extremes of solely appetite-driven dietary intake and feeding aggressively with enteral or parenteral nutrition until death lies the gray area of if, when, and how much to feed individuals with known terminal disease. Further complicating this issue are discrepant perceptions of the patient, family, and the clinician, as well as the cultural context in which death occurs. Many families equate feeding and nourishment with love (Poole & Froggatt, 2002), leading to a desire to aggressively feed the patient, even if this is not likely to improve comfort or length of life. For other families, past negative experiences with aggressive nutrition interventions lead to a rejection of nutrition support under all circumstances (Back & Arnold, 2005). And a study of advanced cancer patients in Europe has demonstrated that cultural values likely affect the decision to aggressively implement nutrition support (McKinlay, 2004).

The role of the clinician is to help patients and families navigate through this difficult and emotionally fraught time, while respecting patient autonomy, desires, and needs. The clinician is in the unique position to help involved individuals weigh the risks and benefits of various nutrition interventions and to determine whether aggressive intervention is likely to improve comfort, pain, and length of life in a meaningful way (Fine, 2006; Fuhrman & Herrmann, 2006).

DEFINITIONS

It is vitally important for the clinician to understand the difference between *anorexia* and *cachexia*. These terms often are used interchangeably, but they are not the same. Anorexia is a lack of appetite. Cachexia is the term used to describe the disordered metabolism characteristic of certain diseases and/or conditions including, but not limited to, cancer, sepsis, chronic infections, HIV/AIDS, congestive heart failure, chronic obstructive pulmonary disease, and other conditions resulting in systemic inflammation (Delano & Moldawer, 2006). Anorexia is a feature of cachexia, but anorexia does not cause cachexia. Cachexia and subsequent anorexia can lead to weight loss, loss of muscle mass, loss of functional status, and decline in length and quality of life for patients with advanced illnesses.

PATHOPHYSIOLOGY

The weight loss associated with simple anorexia can be ameliorated with appropriate energy and protein, because this condition is not characterized by the metabolic aberrations that underlie cachexia. The loss of weight, muscle mass, and functional status characteristic of cachexia cannot be addressed with calories and protein alone. If the underlying metabolic derangement of cachexia is not addressed, nutrition support is unlikely to halt weight loss, although it may improve quality of life. In this circumstance, nutrition intervention risks, such as increased discomfort and infection, and benefits, including improved quality of life, must be carefully considered.

The cause of cachexia is not completely understood, but it is thought to result from the overproduction of proinflammatory (procachectic) mediators called cytokines and interferons. Tumor necrosis factor, interleukins 1 and 6, interferon γ, and proteolysis-inducing factor are believed to be among the most important mediators in the cachexia response (Argiles, Busquets, & Lopez-Soriano, 2005; Deans, Wigmore, Gilmour et al., 2006; DeJong, Busquets, Moses et al., 2005; Delano & Moldawer, 2006; Tisdale, 2005). Current research is focusing on additional novel molecules and pathways that may play a role in the development and progression of cachexia, including ghrelin, leptin, myostatin, and the ubiquitin-proteasome pathway (Akashi, Springer, & Anker, 2005; Filippatos, Anker, & Kremastinos, 2005; Jespersen, Kjaer, & Schjerling, 2006; Wolf, Sadetzki, Kanety et al., 2006).

The presence of these mediators can result in anorexia, hypermetabolism, and alterations in normal metabolic pathways. In simple starvation, the healthy body readily adapts to a calorie deficit by decreasing metabolic rate and shifting to fatty acids as a primary energy source, thereby preserving lean body mass. In cachexia, the body fails to make this adaptation, which can lead to disproportionate wasting of lean body mass and loss of strength and functional status. This can lead to a decline in quality of life, comfort, and functionality of the patient who is terminally ill (Anker, Steinborn, & Strassburg, 2004; Cox & McCallum, 2000; Muscaritoli, Bossola, Aversa et al., 2006; Strasser & Bruera, 2002; Van Cutsem & Arends, 2005).

MANIFESTATIONS OF CACHEXIA

The primary manifestations of cachexia include, but are not limited to, anemia, anorexia, dehydration, early satiety, electrolyte imbalances, fatigue, loss of lean body mass, malaise, micronutrient deficiency, taste alterations, weakness, and weight loss. In the palliative care setting, the goal of nutrition intervention for cachexia is to address as many of these issues as possible to improve the quality of life and functionality without increasing discomfort, pain, fluid retention, or other symptoms.

Metabolic Abnormalities of Cachexia

Ideally, addressing the underlying metabolic abnormalities of cachexia is the first step to improved quality of life, functionality, and symptomatology in the palliative care setting. Unfortunately, pharmacologic interventions for cachexia have had limited success and are only appropriate in carefully selected patients (Strasser & Bruera, 2002; Wilcock, 2006).

The use of omega-3 fatty acids is one intervention designed to ameliorate the underlying metabolic aberrations of cachexia (Elia, Van Bokhorst-de van der Schueren, Garvey et al., 2006). Evidence suggests that the metabolic alterations that contribute to cancer cachexia can be normalized by increased intake of eicosapentaenoic acid (EPA), one type of omega-3 fatty acids (Barber, 2002; Barber & Fearon, 2001; Barber, Fearon, Tisdale et al., 2001; Barber, McMillan, Preston et al., 2000; Barber, Ross, Voss et al., 1999;

Burns, Halabi, Claman et al., 1999; Harman, 2002; Jho, Babcock, Helton et al., 2003; Moses, Slater, Preston et al., 2004; Wigmore, Barber, Ross et al., 2000). Research on the benefits of EPA for addressing cachexia has been conducted predominantly in cancer populations. However, given that common pathophysiologic mechanisms appear to underlie cachexia that occurs in various disease states, it is reasonable to assume that administration of omega-3 fatty acids is a useful approach in all of these cases (Coletti, Moresi, Adamo et al., 2005; Hehlgans & Pfeffer, 2005; Witte & Clark, 2002).

Research has indicated that amounts up to 18 g/day of EPA are well tolerated (Barber & Fearon, 2001). The most common dose-limiting symptom is diarrhea (Barber & Fearon, 2001). It is important to note, however, that *a dose of 2.2 g of EPA per day* is believed to be effective and that this lower dose is associated with minimal risk of side effects (Fearon, Von Meyenfeldt, Moses et al., 2003; Moses et al., 2004).

Patient education is a key component of appropriate use of EPA. Three double-blind, placebo-controlled trials failed to find a benefit from an EPA-enhanced liquid nutritional supplement in cachectic cancer patients. However, in *not one of these trials was the therapeutic minimum dose reached* of 2.2 g of EPA per day (Bruera, Strasser, Palmer et al., 2003; Fearon et al., 2003; Jatoi, Rowland, Loprinzi et al., 2004). Furthermore, post-hoc analyses indicated a strong correlation between higher EPA intakes and significantly improved outcomes, including halt in weight loss, improved quality of life, and reductions in inflammatory biomarkers. These trials highlight the importance of educating patients on the therapeutic nature of an EPA-containing supplement so that this is not treated as simply "another supplement to try."

EPA can be incorporated into the diet through specialized oral/enteral formulas such as RESOURCE Support (Novartis Medical Support) and ProSure (Ross/Abbott Laboratories) or EPA-containing fish oil supplements. Fish oil supplements are available in gelatin capsule and deodorized liquid form. For typical gelatin capsule supplements, approximately 8 to 10 capsules per day are required to reach 2.2 g of EPA. Many patients have difficulty swallowing pills, and for this group, the deodorized liquid form of fish oil may be a better option (The Very Finest Fish Oil [Carlson Laboratories] is an example of a liquid product that is well tolerated by many patients). Generally, it has been recognized that food sources of EPA do not provide a dose that is sufficient to halt cachexia.

MANAGEMENT OF NUTRITION IMPACT SYMPTOMS

The nature of appropriate nutrition intervention should be guided by the setting in which it occurs. Suggested interventions that can be used by the clinician when educating the patient and family in the palliative and end-of-life care settings include the following.

Palliative Care Setting

The caregiver must treat and manage the symptoms that may affect nutritional intake and interfere with the patient's desire to eat, including constipation; bloating; diarrhea; feelings of fullness, early satiety, and poor appetite; altered sense of taste and smell; dry mouth and/or thick saliva; sore mouth and/or throat; nausea and/or vomiting; and pain.

Patient and Family Education
Constipation

While many health care professionals dismiss constipation as a relatively trivial problem, resulting in a lack of attention to the subject, constipation is experienced by more than 50% of cancer patients (Smith, 2001), a group that comprises a significant proportion of the palliative care population. Constipation causes physical and emotional distress in patients who experience it, and the frequent use of pain management medications makes constipation common in the palliative care population (Staats, Markowitz, & Schein, 2004). Unfortunately, the need to treat constipation often is due to a failure to prevent it (Smith, 2001).

In addition to *preventive* constipation management medication protocols, which should be initiated *prior* to onset of constipation, nutrition intervention can be beneficial. While some literature suggests that constipation is not strongly related to dietary factors (Muller-Lissner, Kamm, Scarpignato, & Wald, 2005), numerous studies and reports indicate that nutrition can and should be an important part of constipation management (Geriatrics, 2005; Khaja, Thakur, Bharathan et al., 2005; Wilson, 2005; Wisten & Messner, 2005). It is important for the APN to encourage ongoing communication between the patient and family and their health care team about medication options that are useful for constipation management. Nutrition approaches work best in combination with medication. Suggested nutrition interventions for constipation include the following (American Cancer Society, 2006a; Dobbin & Hartmuller, 2000):

- Eat at regular times each day.
- Drink 8 to 10 cups of noncaffeinated fluid each day. If additional calories are needed to meet nutritional needs, focus on calorie-containing beverages including 100% fruit juices, milk, soy milk, rice milk, and any other tolerated beverages.
- Include water, prune juice (2 to 4 ounces to assess tolerance), warm juices, and teas as a portion of fluid intake. Drink two cups of warm liquid (can include coffee) with breakfast every day.
- Include foods high in *insoluble* fiber, **only if tolerated**. This includes *whole-grain* breads containing a minimum of 4 g of fiber per slice; cereals containing a minimum of 6 to 8 g of fiber per serving; whole-grain pastas; raw and cooked vegetables including skins and peels, such as apples, carrots, and green leafy vegetables; popcorn; and beans, such as navy beans, kidney beans, black beans, and lentils. If gas, bloating, and/or abdominal distention is present, **do not** increase insoluble fiber in the diet. Do not increase insoluble fiber if a low-residue diet has been prescribed.
- Eat a good breakfast that includes a hot drink and high-fiber foods, such as bran cereals, oatmeal, or Cream of Wheat (Kraft Foods).
- If additional calories are needed to meet nutritional needs, try a *fiber-containing*, high-calorie, high-protein, liquid supplement (e.g., Ensure Plus with Fiber [Ross/Abbott Laboratories]).
- Try adding in a fiber supplement such as Benefiber (Novartis Consumer Health) or Metamucil (Procter & Gamble). Benefiber may be better tolerated. Be sure patient consumes adequate fluids with fiber supplements.

- Try mixing three parts wheat bran, two parts applesauce, and one part prune juice and eating three times per day or as needed to help promote bowel movements. This mixture can be spread on whole-grain toast.
- Try dried fruit such as apricots, figs, or raisins. If gas, bloating, and/or abdominal distention is present, **do not** increase insoluble fiber in the diet. Do not increase insoluble fiber if a low-residue diet has been prescribed.

Bloating*

The APN should encourage ongoing communication between the patient and family and their health care team about medication options for decreasing gas production. Nutrition approaches work best in combination with medication.

- Limit foods and drinks that cause gas, including carbonated beverages, broccoli, cabbage, cauliflower, cucumbers, peppers, beans, peas, onions, and garlic. A food and symptom diary can help identify other, individual triggers of gas and bloating from particular ingested foods.
- Lessen the amount of air swallowed by eating slowly and avoiding excessive talking while chewing and swallowing.
- Do not use straws to drink liquids.
- Avoid chewing gum.

Diarrhea†

- Encourage ongoing communication between the patient and family and their health care team about medication options for managing diarrhea. Nutrition approaches work best in combination with medication.
- Increase intake of foods high in *soluble* fiber, including oatmeal, white rice, bananas, white toast, applesauce, and canned fruits without the skins, such as peaches and pears.
- Drink 6 to 8 cups of fluids each day to replace losses. Include nonwater beverages, such as Gatorade (Stokely-Van Camp, Inc.) or Pedialyte (Abbott Laboratories), to help replace lost electrolytes. Do not rehydrate solely with water; this can contribute to electrolyte abnormalities.
- Drink fluids at room temperature. Avoid very hot and very cold drinks.
- With each loose bowel movement, drink 1 additional cup of electrolyte-containing fluid, such as Gatorade or Pedialyte.
- Try nonacidic juices, such as apple juice, apricot nectar, peach nectar, or pear nectar.
- *Sip* broth and sports drinks to replace electrolyte losses.
- Eat very small, frequent meals. Encourage a "bite-at-a-time" approach to eating.
- Drink fluids between meals rather than with meals (e.g., separate liquids from solids).
- Lie down immediately after eating.
- Snack on salty, bland foods, such as crackers and pretzels, to replace lost sodium.
- Consider powdered glutamine (amino acid) supplement, mixed with liquid, at a dose of 10 g, three times daily (research-supported brands of glutamine include

*Cox & McCallum, 2000; and Dobbin & Hartmuller, 2000.
†American Cancer Society, 2006b; Can, Besirbellioglu, Avci, et al., 2006; Chermesh & Eliakim, 2006; Coeffier, Hecketsweiler, Hecketsweiler et al., 2005; Cox & McCallum, 2000; Dobbin & Hartmuller, 2000; Heiser et al., 2004; Novak & Katz, 2006; Rushdi, Pichard, & Khater, 2004; Savarese, Savy, Vahdat et al., 2003; and Savarese, Al-Zoubi, & Boucher, 2000.

RESOURCE GlutaSolve [Novartis Medical Nutrition] and Sympt-X [Cambridge Nutraceuticals/Baxter Pharmaceuticals]). Glutamine may be contraindicated if renal and/or hepatic function is impaired.

- Try probiotic supplements that contain a broad spectrum of probiotic flora including *Lactobacillus acidophilus, Lactobacillus casei, Lactobacillus reuteri, Lactobacillus rhamnosus, Bifidobacterium bifidum, Bifidobacterium longum,* and/or *Streptococcus thermophilus.*
- Avoid foods high in *insoluble* fiber, such as fresh fruit with the peel (the flesh of the fruit is okay), raw vegetables (well-cooked vegetables are okay), whole-grain breads and cereals, beans, peas, and popcorn.
- Limit fatty and greasy foods.
- Limit or eliminate dairy products (except yogurt) if helpful. Include yogurt to replace normal and healthy gut flora.
- Consider utilizing a rice congee that is made of 1 cup long-cooking rice combined with 6 cups water and 1 tablespoon of salt; cook according to package directions (typically about 40 minutes). Eat and drink this soupy mixture.

Feelings of Fullness, Early Satiety, and Poor Appetite*

- Incorporate a minimum of 2.2 g of EPA into the diet to halt cachexia, which may be contributing to poor appetite. EPA can be incorporated into the diet through specialized oral/enteral formulas such as RESOURCE Support (Novartis Medical Support) and ProSure (Ross/Abbott Laboratories) or EPA-containing fish oil supplements. Fish oil supplements are available in gelatin capsule and deodorized liquid form. Patients and families must be educated to reach therapeutic dose (at least 2.2 g of EPA per day) to maximize possibility of benefit.
- Assess zinc status and supplement as indicated.
- Avoid intake of noncaloric beverages such as water and tea in large quantities.
- Eat very small, frequent meals. Encourage a "bite-at-a-time" approach to eating.
- Focus on eating one to two bites every 20 minutes throughout the day.
- Make eating more enjoyable by setting an attractive table, playing favorite music, or watching television.
- Eating is a social activity. If patient is unable to eat at the table, have family join patient where he or she is able to eat. Prevent patient from eating alone, if at all possible.
- Keep snacks handy to eat immediately (hunger may last only a few minutes), such as granola bars; nuts; pudding cups; chips; crackers; pretzels; single serving sizes of tuna, chicken, or fruit; dried fruit; and/or trail mix.
- Eat favorite foods at any time of the day; for example, if breakfast foods are appealing, eat them for dinner. No foods are off-limits.
- Eat every hour at a minimum—do not wait until hungry. Relying on appetite is not a good guide when introducing appropriate nutrition.
- Treat food like medicine—set times to eat, such as every 30 minutes to 1 hour and encourage at least one or two bites of any food during "medication" times (quantity and type of food are less important; frequency of eating is more important).

---

*American Cancer Society, 2006e; Elia et al., 2006; and Polisena, 2000.

- Drink high-calorie, high-protein drinks such as shakes and liquid nutritional supplements.
- Consider fortified juice-based supplements such as Enlive! (Ross/Abbott Laboratories) if taste fatigue of other "creamy" textured supplements is a problem.
- Encourage fluids between meals, rather than with meals (e.g., separate liquids from solids). Liquids can cause stomach distension and worsen feelings of fullness, making intake of calorie-rich solids problematic.

Altered Sense of Taste and Smell*

- Encourage ongoing communication between the patient and family and their health care team about specific conditions that can create unpleasant mouth taste. For example, infections such as thrush and zinc deficiency can alter sense of taste and smell. These problems can be treated with medication and/or nutritional supplementation. Nutrition approaches work best when combined with medication.
- If indicated, use a zinc supplement of 220 mg of zinc sulfate two times per day. Use supplement for up to 3 months. Short-term zinc supplementation may help with altered sense of taste, but long-term zinc supplementation may contribute to impaired immune status, micronutrient malabsorption, and other health problems.
- Provide education on fastidious mouth care to prevent secondary bacterial infections.
- Avoid food smells.
- Consider foods that have minimal odors and short cooking time, such as scrambled eggs, plain pasta, yogurt, pudding, oatmeal, and Cream of Wheat.
- Season foods with tart flavors such as lemon, citrus, vinegar, and pickled items *(avoid if sore mouth or throat is present)*.
- Flavor foods with spices not normally used, such as basil, oregano, rosemary, tarragon, mustard, catsup, or mint.
- Marinate and cook meats in sweet juices, fruits, dressings, or wine, such as sweet and sour pork, chicken with honey glaze, or beef with Italian dressing.
- Rinse mouth with tea, ginger ale, saltwater, or baking soda and water to clear taste buds prior to eating.
- Suck on lemon drops or mints or chew gum *(avoid if sore mouth or throat is present*; avoid sugarless gums and candies if diarrhea is present).
- Encourage patient to experiment often. Very unusual flavors, such as a pickle juice milk shake, may be acceptable to a patient with altered sense of taste and smell.

Dry Mouth and Thick Saliva†

- Encourage ongoing communication between the patient and family and the health care team about what is creating a dry mouth and/or thick saliva. Medication options may be available to alleviate severe xerostomia. Nutrition approaches work well in combination with medications.

---

*American Cancer Society, 2006h; Cox & McCallum, 2000; Dobbin & Hartmuller, 2000; Heckmann et al., 2005; Polisena, 2000; Ripamonti et al., 1998; and Shay & Mangian, 2000.
†American Cancer Society, 2006c, 2006d; American Institute for Cancer Research, 2006; Cox & McCallum, 2000; Dobbin & Hartmuller, 2000; and Guggenheimer & Moore, 2003.

- Encourage adequate mouth care to prevent secondary bacterial infections.
- Drink 8 to 12 cups of liquid a day and take a water bottle when leaving the house (adequate and even extra fluids can help loosen mucus). Use nonacidic juices and other high-calorie liquids to increase calorie intake if weight loss is a problem.
- Consider 100% papaya juices or eating papayas, which contain an enzyme (papain) that can help to break up thick saliva.
- Introduce 100% pineapple juice or pineapple, which can help to thin mucus (avoid if sore mouth or throat is present).
- Use a straw to drink liquids to bypass mouth sores (avoid if bloating and gas are present).
- Eat soft foods at room temperature or cold. Try blenderized fruits and vegetables, soft-cooked chicken and fish, well-thinned cereals, Popsicles, and shakes/smoothies made with juices and fruit; if dairy foods increase mucus production, try making a smoothie with a nondairy alternative such as soy or rice milk).
- Try limiting intake of dairy products, which may promote mucus secretions; use a nondairy alternative such as soy or rice milk.
- Suck on lemon drops (avoid if sore mouth or throat is present) or frozen grapes or ice chips (do not chew ice, as this can damage teeth).
- Try mixing 1 cup of peach or papaya nectar with 1/2 cup of club soda and drink (avoid if sore mouth or throat is present).
- Avoid commercial mouthwashes; these contain alcohol, which is drying.
- Try alcohol-free mouthwashes and gums, such as Biotene (Laclede).
- Avoid alcoholic beverages, caffeinated beverages, chocolate, and tobacco products. These are drying to the mouth.
- Use a cool mist humidifier to moisten room air (keep clean to avoid spreading bacteria, fungi, or mold).

Sore Mouth and Throat*

- Encourage ongoing communication between the patient and family and their health care team about medication options for managing mouth and throat pain. Nutrition approaches work best in combination with medication.
- Encourage fastidious mouth care to prevent secondary bacterial infections.
- Eat soft, bland foods, such as creamed soups, cooked cereals, macaroni and cheese, yogurt, pudding, mashed potatoes, eggs, custards, casseroles, cheese cake, and milk shakes or smoothies.
- Drink through a straw to bypass mouth sores (avoid if bloating is present).
- Eat high-protein, high-calorie foods to promote healing.
- Consider a powdered glutamine (amino acid) supplement, dissolved into warm water, at a dose of 10 g, three times daily (research-supported brands of glutamine include RESOURCE GlutaSolve [Novartis Medical Nutrition] and Sympt-X [Cambridge Nutraceuticals/Baxter Pharmaceuticals]). Swish and swallow the glutamine mixture for best results. Glutamine may be contraindicated if renal and/or hepatic function is impaired.

---

*American Cancer Society, 2006f, 2006g; American Institute for Cancer Research, 2006; Anderson, Schroeder, & Skubitz, 1998; Anonymous, 2005; and Peterson, 2006.

- Blend or moisten foods with yogurt; pudding; soft cereals such as oatmeal, Cream of Wheat, and Malt-O-Meal (Malt-O-Meal Company); warm water; nonacidic juices; milk; soy milk; rice milk; gravy; butter; cream; or sauces.
- Soften foods such as bread by soaking in milk.
- Stick to nonacidic juices such as apple juice; peach, pear, or apricot nectars; and grape juice *(do not use grape juice if diarrhea is present)*.
- Avoid tart, acidic, or salty beverages and foods such as citrus, pickled items, and tomato-based foods.
- Avoid alcohol, caffeine, and tobacco.

Nausea and Vomiting*

- Incorporate a minimum of 2.2 g of EPA into the diet to halt cachexia, which may be contributing to poor appetite. EPA can be incorporated into the diet through specialized oral/enteral formulas such as RESOURCE Support (Novartis Medical Support) and ProSure (Ross/Abbott Laboratories) or EPA-containing fish oil supplements. Fish oil supplements are available in gelatin capsule and deodorized liquid form. Patients and families must be educated to reach therapeutic dose ($\geq$2.2 g of EPA per day) to maximize possibility of benefit.
- Encourage ongoing communication between patient and family and the health care team about medication options to manage nausea and vomiting. Encourage the use of medications as prescribed, even if not feeling nauseous. Educate that it is *easier to prevent nausea and vomiting* than it is to treat it. Nutrition approaches are ineffective if intractable, untreated nausea and vomiting are present.
- Eat small frequent meals and snacks to avoid an empty stomach, which may worsen nausea.
- Eat bland foods such as oatmeal, pasta, rice, plain pancakes, and potatoes.
- Try warm salty foods and liquids, such as soups or broths, and cooked hot cereals such as oatmeal or Cream of Wheat.
- Try dry salty foods, such as crackers, toast, dry cereal, or breadsticks, every 1 to 2 hours.
- Avoid offensive food smells.
- Have someone other than the patient prepare his or her food.
- Consider foods that have minimal odors and short cooking time, such as scrambled eggs, plain pasta, yogurt, pudding, shakes and smoothies, oatmeal, Cream of Wheat, plain baked chicken, or instant mashed potatoes.
- Avoid eating in a room that is uncomfortably warm or has poor ventilation.
- Rinse out mouth before and after meals.
- Sip warm, flat ginger ale.
- Sip ginger tea, chamomile tea, or peppermint tea *(avoid peppermint tea and other peppermint-flavored foods if reflux is present)*.
- Position in a sitting position when eating.
- Do not lay down after eating for at least 1 hour.
- Consider limiting dairy products if helpful.
- Avoid overly sweet, fatty, fried, or rich foods such as desserts and French fries.

---

*Bruera et al., 2003; Fearon et al., 2003; Harman, 2002; Jho et al., 2003; Moses et al., 2004; and Polisena, 2000.

Pain

- Provide appropriate analgesics. Unmanaged, intense pain can contributes to lack of appetite and inability to eat. In the presence of unmanaged pain, eating is of little importance.
- Encourage ongoing communication between the patient and family and the health care team to ensure optimal pain management. Educate that there are many options for pain management and that different medications can be tried.

Enteral Nutrition Support

Enteral nutrition is an aggressive intervention but is appropriate to support the patient if it will improve quality and/or length of life in a meaningful way (Cox, 2006; Dormann, 2004; Hopkins, 2004; Lundholm, Daneryd, Bosaeus et al., 2004). Enteral nutrition should be given only when the patient wants it, is motivated to learn and follow the instructions on tube feeding, and has a functioning gut.

Enteral nutrition is *not necessarily contraindicated* by conditions such as intractable nausea and vomiting, obstruction, or gastroparesis. It may be possible to bypass these issues/areas with a jejunal feeding tube instead of a gastric feeding tube. Indications include patients who fail to meet a minimum of 50% of required nutrient needs orally for 5 days or longer or who have protein-energy malnutrition and severe dysphagia. Contraindications for this intervention include intestinal obstruction distal to the feeding site; ileus; unmanageable hypomotility of the intestine; severe, intractable diarrhea that is unresponsive to treatment including resolution of underlying infection, antidiarrheal medications, and diet modifications; high output enterocutaneous fistulas; and acute pancreatitis.

Enteral nutrition is contraindicated if the prognosis does not warrant aggressive nutritional support. This is an individual decision that must be discussed with the patient and family and managed on a case-by-case basis. Issues to consider include patient desires and needs, mores and values, cultural context, and sociofamilial issues.

Research has indicated that enteral feeding is used more often in for-profit settings and when state-stipulated weight loss and dehydration regulations are present (Cox, 2006). This finding is important because in certain disease states, such as dementia, tube feeding is not proven to reduce rates of aspiration pneumonia, pressure sores, or infections. Furthermore, tube feeding does not prolong survival, improve function, or provide palliation in this population (Finucaine, Christmas, & Travis, 1999; Li, 2002). All of these issues must be considered and discussed honestly with the patient and the family to allow for an informed choice regarding enteral nutrition.

Initiating enteral nutrition includes the following steps:

- Consult a registered dietitian (RD) to determine nutrient needs and to select formula (e.g., high protein, fiber containing, elemental, etc.) and administration method (pump, gravity feeding, or bolus feeding).
- Troubleshoot common, simple enteral feeding problems (Table 9-1).
- Address micronutrient deficiencies: If patient is not close to death, the use of vitamin and mineral supplements, such as an iron supplement for iron deficiency

TABLE 9-1 ■ Troubleshooting for Simple Enteral Feeding Problems*

Problem	Possible Causes	Solutions
Feeding Tube Clog *Note: DO NOT try to clear blockage by inserting an object into the tube as this could injure the stomach lining or damage the tube. DO NOT use cranberry juice, other juices, meat tenderizer, soda, colas, or any other carbonated beverage to attempt to unclog tube. These products cause the protein in tube feeding formulas to coagulate, form clogs, and worsen existing clogs.*	Inadequate flushing before or after administering feedings and/or medications. Attempting to place anything other than enteral feeding formula, water, or crushed and dissolved medications through the tube.	Attempt to flush tube with a syringe filled with 30 ml of warm water. If unsuccessful, fill syringe with water again and move plunger back and forth gently several times until tube clears. Avoid excessive force when trying to unclog a feeding tube. Use a product designed to dissolve enteral feeding clogs, such as Viokase or a similar product. If unsuccessful, call your home care nurse, physician, or registered dietitian.
Leakage Around the Tube	Improper positioning, such as laying flat during feeding. Feeding too rapidly. A blocked tube. The tube is out of position.	Sit at least 45 degrees upright during feeding and for at least 1 hour after feeding. Slow the feeding rate by $1/4$ to $1/2$. If it appears that the tube is clogged, use instructions above to unclog tube. To check for the tube being out of position, measure the length of the tube or locate the mark on tube. If the tube is longer than it should be compared to when it was first placed or if the mark is further out that just flush with your skin, contact your health care provider immediately—the tube may need to be replaced.
Diarrhea	Feeding too rapidly. Using a formula with an osmolality that is too high. Using a formula without any fiber. Maldigestion/malabsorption	Slow the feeding rate by $1/4$ to $1/2$ the previous feeding rate. Switch to an isotonic formula. Flavored, oral liquid products such as Ensure or Boost are not designed for tube feeding and can cause diarrhea, especially if the tube is placed in the jejunum rather than the stomach. Change all or some of the feeding formula to a fiber containing formula. Use an elemental formula or a formula that contains medium-chain triglycerides as the fat source to address malabsorption.

*Contact a registered dietitian or physician if these measures fail to correct the problem.

anemia (microcytic), or vitamin B_{12} and folic acid supplements (for macrocytic/megaloblastic anemia), may be beneficial. However, the benefit of micronutrient supplementation must be weighed against potential discomfort it may cause. For example, iron supplementation can exacerbate constipation and may contribute to nausea. It may be more beneficial to discontinue vitamin and mineral supplements that contribute to gastrointestinal stress, nausea, constipation, or diarrhea if these conditions diminish quality of life to a significant degree. This issue must be discussed with the patient, family, and other caregivers. The risks and benefits of supplementation should be decided on a case-by-case basis.

Parenteral Nutritional Support*

In *select* cases, the use of parenteral nutrition may be warranted. If the prognosis is more than 3 months to live and no other route of administration is available, parenteral nutrition may provide some benefit to the patient who is receiving palliative care. A study by the Japan Palliative Oncology Study Group indicated that artificial hydration can alleviate dehydration signs but may worsen peripheral edema, ascites, and pleural effusions (Morita, Hyodo, Yoshimi et al., 2005). Potential benefits of artificial hydration therapy and parenteral nutrition must be balanced against the risk of worsening fluid retention. This is an excellent example of how the physical costs and benefits of an aggressive supportive intervention must be weighed to allow for informed choice by the patient and family.

Parenteral nutrition may be inappropriate for the following reasons:
- It does not add quality or length of life.
- The risks, including infection, hepatic and renal complications, and fluid management, often outweigh the benefits.
- It is costly.
- It is invasive.
- It requires frequent blood work (no less than weekly) and intensive management by a nutrition support RD or pharmacist.
- It can contribute to and/or exacerbate other complications including ascites, edema, and hepatic and renal dysfunction.

The *most important role* for the palliative care clinician is to educate the patient and family on the risks and benefits of parenteral nutrition on a case-by-case basis. The request for parenteral nutrition from a family may be driven by a desire to provide nourishment and support. Providing the patient and family with an understanding of the potential complications and discomfort of parenteral nutrition will allow the patient and the family to make an informed choice.

Pharmacologic Support

Table 9-2 identifies the basic pharmacologic approaches for managing select nutrition-impact symptoms that commonly occur in patients in the palliative care environment.

---

*Bruera et al., 2005; Mirhosseini, Fainsinger, & Baracos, 2005; Morita et al., 2005; Orrevall, Tishelman, & Permert, 2005; Orrevall et al., 2004; and Plonk & Arnold, 2005.

TABLE 9-2 ■ Pharmacologic Options to Consider for Nutrition Impact Symptoms

Symptom	Pharmacologic Options
Sore mouth and mucositis	Equal parts Benadryl (diphenhydramine), viscous lidocaine, and Maalox (aluminum hydroxide/magnesium hydroxide) or Mylanta (aluminum hydroxide/magnesium hydroxide/simethicone)
	Equal parts Nystatin, Maalox, Benadryl, and viscous lidocaine
Thick saliva and dry mouth	Guaifenesin (expectorant)
	Saliva stimulators: Salagen tablets (pilocarpine hydrochloride)
	Saliva replacers: Xero-Lube (sodium fluoride), Salivart (carboxymethylcellulose sodium), Moi-Stir (carboxymethylcellulose sodium), Salix (carboxymethylcellulose sodium), Optimoist (hydroxyethyl cellulose)
	Mouth moisturizers
Lack of appetite	Megestrol acetate (Megace)
	Dexamethasone (Decadron)
	Dronabinol (Marinol)
	Cyproheptadine (antihistamine)
	Fluoxymesterone (androgenic)
	Selective serotonin reuptake inhibitors
	Ritalin
Constipation	Over-the-counter constipation medications used in combination as directed by nursing staff and medical care team to relieve constipation; prevention is key.
Nausea and vomiting	First-line antiemetics: dopamine antagonists, serotonin receptor antagonists, corticosteroids, dopamine antagonists, butyrophenones, phenothiazines, benzodiazepines, antihistamines
	Marinol
	Erythromycin
	Metoclopramide (Reglan)

A number of agents have been used to promote and stimulate appetite in the nutritionally challenged patient. In severe cases of advanced cachexia, anabolic agents also may be indicated. Appetite-stimulating medications include the following:

■ Cyproheptadine hydrochloride (Periactin)—slight increase in appetite and intake with use of this agent; may not prevent persistent weight loss but may improve quality of life due to improved appetite (Mattox, 2005)
■ Cannabinoids (dronabinol [Marinol])—5 to 10 mg orally twice daily—increased appetite, decreased nausea, trend toward stabilized weight; may be particularly beneficial for anorectic patients at end-of-life (Morley, 2002; Walsh, Nelson, & Mahmoud, 2003)
■ Corticosteroids—decreased nausea, increased sense of well-being, and increased appetite have been documented, but beneficial effects are time-limited and should be weighed against long-term adverse effects that may include Cushing's syndrome, proximal myopathy, immunosuppression, steroid-induced diabetes, and exacerbation of delirium (Tisdale, 2006)
■ Megestrol acetate (Megace)—800 mg/day orally—a number of studies demonstrate beneficial effects on appetite and weight gain at 800 mg/day dosage; more

effective in men when given with testosterone; may be more effective than dronabinol in advanced cancer patients; possible side effects include edema, thrombosis, and vaginal bleeding; *should not be used in bed-bound patients* due to risk of deep vein thrombosis (Jatoi, Windschitl, Loprinzi et al., 2002; Morley, 2002; Pascual Lopez, Rogue i Figuls, Urrutia Cuchi et al., 2004).

End-of-Life Care Setting

Patient and family education on the dying process and on "what to expect" as death approaches is one of the most important roles of the clinician in the palliative care setting (American Medical Association, 2001; Beider, 2005; McKinlay, 2004). It is important to inform the patient and family on the following aspects of death and dying:

1. A decrease in food and fluid intake is a normal part of the "physiology" of dying.
2. In the last weeks to days of life, there is a marked decline in upper and lower gastrointestinal functioning, as well as a decrease in the senses of taste and smell. Education of family members and caregivers at this stage is *very* important.
3. The physical sensations of "starving" are not present at end-of-life. The patient feels little discomfort from decreasing nutritional status. Hunger is nonexistent. Forcing the issue of food is counterproductive and can result in resentment and a decreased quality of life.
4. Maintenance of strength and nutritional status at this time is unrealistic. Caregivers should be encouraged to show love and support in ways that do not involve the preparation or provision of food.
5. Dehydration is a normal part of the end-stage of the dying process. Often, the only discomfort associated with dehydration is a dry mouth. This can be alleviated with sips of water, ice chips, or moistened swabs.
6. Artificial hydration should be evaluated and used appropriately.
7. If artificial hydration or nutrition support is already in place, decreasing the amount of the infusion to 500 to 600 ml/day may help to avoid discomfort from increased urinary output, gastrointestinal and pharyngeal secretions, and pulmonary edema. Stopping hydration altogether is an option if desired by the patient and family.
8. According to the American Medical Association Code of Ethics, human dignity is the primary obligation if it conflicts with prolonging life. All competent patients have the right to accept or reject any form of medical treatment, including artificial hydration and nutrition. If an advance directive is in place, this should specify patient desires with regard to supportive interventions, including fluids and artificial nutrition, at end-of-life.
9. If a patient expresses a desire to undertake voluntary cessation of eating and drinking, the following issues must be considered and addressed:
   a. Patient characteristics: Persistent, unrelenting, otherwise unrelievable symptoms that are deemed unacceptable to patient and family, including, but not limited to, pain, seizures, weakness, and extreme fatigue
   b. Patient informed consent
      (1) Patient must be fully competent.

(2) Patient must be fully informed of all treatment and symptom management options.

(3) Patient must be evaluated by a mental health professional to rule out treatable depression or other mental health conditions; a second opinion is strongly recommended.

(4) A written informed consent is in place.

c. Terminal prognosis: typically days to weeks

d. Palliative care: Must be available, in place, and unable to adequately relieve suffering.

e. Family participation: Clinicians should strongly encourage frank discussion. Consensus should be reached, if possible, among patient, immediate family members, and caregivers.

f. Patient incompetence: Food and fluids (oral) must not be denied from incompetent patients who are willing and able to eat.

g. Second opinions: Must be obtained from experts in underlying disease, mental health, pain management, and palliative care.

10. If all of these issues are addressed and managed, voluntary refusal of food and fluids may be an appropriate option. Artificial nutrition and hydration is considered a life-sustaining medical therapy similar to medications, surgery, dialysis, mechanical ventilation, or other medical interventions. Decisions regarding this issue should be handled under the same ethical and legal standards as other medical interventions. If the benefits of an intervention outweigh the costs, it is justified. If it is not beneficial or if, for this patient, the costs are higher than the benefits, it is not justified. Discontinuation of nutrition and hydration generally is *not* considered justified in the following situations.

a. The patient will die of malnutrition before he or she would succumb to the disease process. Example: Patient with severe dysphasia secondary to head and neck cancer, in whom the primary diagnosis will not result in death before malnutrition, if nutrition support and hydration are not provided.

b. There are untreated mental health issues such as depression.

c. The patient has a strong desire to "get affairs in order" such as writing a will or attending a specific family event.

d. A new acute, but treatable, diagnosis arises.

PATIENT OUTCOMES

The goal of palliative nutrition care should include the following outcomes:

■ Anemia, anorexia, dehydration, early satiety, electrolyte imbalances, fatigue, loss of lean body mass, malaise, micronutrient deficiency, taste alterations, weakness, and weight loss are corrected when feasible.

■ When maintenance of nutritional and hydration status are no longer reasonable goals, patient's discomfort is addressed, such as providing ice chips for a dry mouth.

■ When maintenance of nutritional status and strength are no longer reasonable goals, patient's desires are addressed, such as providing whatever food and nutrition

the patient wants (e.g., provision of favorite foods even if doing so does not improve nutritional status or meet nutritional needs).
- Patient maintains control over his or her intake.

PROFESSIONAL COMPETENCIES

- Assess and evaluate early manifestations of cachexia/anorexia and dehydration in order to ensure timely and beneficial interventions.
- Initiate interventions used to increase appetite and dietary intake, and calories, when feasible.
- Identify the risks and benefits of artificial nutrition and hydration and include the evaluation of the invasive nature of such interventions.
- Evaluate the effectiveness of interventions and modify the treatment plan to optimize patient comfort and dignity.

MEASUREMENT INSTRUMENTS

- Twenty-four–hour food recall
- Comprehensive diet history
- Nutrition needs assessment (calorie and fluid needs for maintenance of nutrition and hydration status)
- Laboratory measures, if available, including comprehensive metabolic panel and measures of micronutrient status

REFERENCES

Akashi, Y.J., Springer, J., & Anker, S.D. (2005) Cachexia in chronic heart failure: prognostic implications and novel therapeutic approaches. *Curr Heart Fail Rep, 2,* 198-203.

American Cancer Society. (2006a). *Constipation.* Retrieved March 5, 2006, from www.cancer.org/docroot/MBC/content/MBC_2_3X_Constipation.asp?sitearea=MBC.

American Cancer Society. (2006b). *Diarrhea.* Retrieved March 6, 2006, from www.cancer.org/docroot/MBC/content/MBC_2_3X_Diarrhea.asp?sitearea=MBC.

American Cancer Society. (2006c). *Dry mouth or thick saliva.* Retrieved March 8, 2006, from www.cancer.org/docroot/MBC/content/MBC_6_2X_Dry_Mouth_or_Thick_Saliva.asp?sitearea=MBC.

American Cancer Society. (2006d). *Dry mouth.* Retrieved March 6, 2006, from www.cancer.org/docroot/MBC/content/MBC_2_3x_Dry_Mouth.asp.

American Cancer Society. (2006e). *Poor appetite.* Retrieved March 6, 2006, from www.cancer.org/docroot/MBC/content/MBC_2_3X_Appetite.asp?sitearea=MBC.

American Cancer Society. (2006f). *Sore or irritated mouth or throat.* Retrieved March 2, 2006, from www.cancer.org/docroot/MBC/content/MBC_6_2x_Sore_or_Irritated_Mouth_or_Throat.asp?sitearea=MBC.

American Cancer Society. (2006g). *What about sore mouth, gums, and throat problems?* Retrieved March 1, 2006, from www.cancer.org/docroot/MBC/content/MBC_2_2X_What_About_Sore_Mouth_Gums_and_Throat_Problems.asp?sitearea=MBC.

American Cancer Society. (2006h). *When things aren't tasting right.* Retrieved March 3, 2006, from www.cancer.org/docroot/MBC/content/MBC_6_2X_When_Things_Arent_Tasting_Right.asp?sitearea=MBC.

American Institute for Cancer Research. (2006). *Nutrition of the cancer patient.* Retrieved February 19, 2006, from https://aicr.donortrust.com/bookform.asp?item=booklets.

American Medical Association. (2001). *End-of-life care*. Retrieved February 24, 2006, from www.ama-assn.org/ama/pub/category/14730.html.

Anderson, P.M., Schroeder, G., & Skubitz, K.M. (1998). Oral glutamine reduces the duration and severity of stomatitis after cytotoxic cancer chemotherapy. *Cancer, 83*, 1433-1439.

Anker, S.D., Steinborn, W., & Strassburg, S. (2004). Cardiac cachexia. *Ann Med, 36*, 518-529.

Anonymous. (2005). Experimental L-glutamine agent shown effective in oral mucositis. *J Support Oncol, 3*, 414.

Argiles, J.M., Busquets, S., & Lopez-Soriano, F.J. (2005). The pivotal role of cytokines in muscle wasting during cancer. *Int J Biochem Cell Biol, 37*, 1609-1619.

Back, A.L. & Arnold, R.M. (2005). Dealing with conflict in caring for the seriously ill: "It was just out of the question." *JAMA, 293*, 1374-1381.

Barber, M.D. (2002). Cancer cachexia and its treatment with fish-oil-enriched nutritional supplementation. *Nutrition, 17*, 751-755.

Barber, M.D. & Fearon, K.C. (2001). Tolerance and incorporation of a high-dose eicosapentaenoic acid diester emulsion by patients with pancreatic cancer cachexia. *Lipids, 36*, 347-351.

Barber, M.D., Fearon, K.C., Tisdale, M.J., et al. (2001). Effect of a fish oil-enriched nutritional supplement on metabolic mediators in patients with pancreatic cancer cachexia. *Nutr Cancer, 40*, 118-124.

Barber, M.D., McMillan, D.C., Preston, T., et al. (2000). Metabolic response to feeding in weight-losing pancreatic cancer patients and its modulation by a fish-oil-enriched nutritional supplement. *Clin Sci, 98*, 389-399.

Barber, M.D., Ross, J.A., Voss, A.C., et al. (1999). The effect of an oral nutritional supplement enriched with fish oil on weight-loss in patients with pancreatic cancer. *Br J Cancer, 81*, 80-86.

Beider, S. (2005). An ethical argument for integrated palliative care. *Evid Based Complement Alternat Med, 2*, 227-231.

Bruera, E., Sala, R., Rico, M.A., et al. (2005). Effects of parenteral hydration in terminally ill cancer patients: A preliminary study. *J Clin Oncol, 23*, 2366-2371.

Bruera, E., Strasser, F., Palmer, J.L., et al.(2003) Effect of fish oil on appetite and other symptoms in patients with advanced cancer and anorexia/cachexia: a double-blind, placebo-controlled study. *J Clin Oncol, 21*, 129-134.

Burns, C.P., Halabi, S., Claman, G.H., et al. (1999). Phase I clinical study of fish oil fatty acid capsules for patients with cancer cachexia: Cancer and Leukemia Group B Study 9473. *Clin Cancer Res, 5*, 3942-3947.

Can, M., Besirbellioglu, B.A., Avci, I.Y., et al. (2006). Prophylactic *Saccharomyces boulardii* in the prevention of antibiotic-associated diarrhea: A prospective study. *Med Sci Monitor, 12*, PI19-PI22.

Chermesh, I. & Eliakim, R. (2006). Probiotics and the gastrointestinal tract: where are we in 2005? *World J Gastroenterol, 12*, 853-857.

Coeffier, M., Hecketsweiler, B., Hecketsweiler, P., et al. (2005). Effect of glutamine on water and sodium absorption in human jejunum at baseline and during PGE1-induced secretion. *J Appl Physiol, 98*, 2163-2168.

Coletti, D., Moresi, V., Adamo, S., et al. (2005). Tumor necrosis factor-alpha gene transfer induces cachexia and inhibits muscle regeneration. *Genesis, 43*, 120-128.

Cox, A. (2006). End-of-life nutrition and hydration—Issues and ethics. *Today's Dietitian, 7*, 35.

Cox, A. & McCallum, P.D. (2000). Medical nutrition therapy in palliative care. In P.D. McCallum & C.G. Polisena (Eds.). *The Clinical Guide to Oncology Nutrition* (pp. 143-149). Chicago: The American Dietetic Association.

Deans, D.A., Wigmore, S.J., Gilmour, H., et al. (2006). Expression of the proteolysis-inducing factor core peptide mRNA is upregulated in both tumour and adjacent normal tissue in gastro-oesophageal malignancy. *Br J Cancer, 94*, 731-736.

DeJong, C.H., Busquets, S., Moses, A.G., et al.(2005). Systemic inflammation correlates with increased expression of skeletal muscle ubiquitin but not uncoupling proteins in cancer cachexia. *Oncol Rep, 14*, 257-263.

Delano, M.J. & Moldawer, L.L. (2006). The origins of cachexia in acute and chronic inflammatory diseases. *Nutr Clin Pract, 21*, 68-81.

Dobbin, M. & Hartmuller, V.W. (2000). Suggested management of nutrition-related symptoms. In P.D. McCallum & C.G. Polisena (Eds.). *The clin guide to oncol nutrition* (pp. 164-167). Chicago: The American Dietetic Association.

Dormann, A.J. (2004). Endoscopic palliation and nutritional support in advanced gastric cancer. *Digest Dis, 22,* 351-359.

Elia, M., Van Bokhorst-de van der Schueren, M.A., Garvey, J., et al. (2006). Enteral (oral or tube administration) nutritional support and eicosapentaenoic acid in patients with cancer: A systematic review. *Int J Oncol, 28,* 5-23.

Fearon, K.C., Von Meyenfeldt, M.F., Moses, A.G., et al. (2003) Effect of a protein and energy dense N-3 fatty acid enriched oral supplement on loss of weight and lean tissue in cancer cachexia: A randomised double blind trial. *Gut, 52,* 1479-1486.

Filippatos, G.S., Anker, S.D., & Kremastinos, D.T. (2005). Pathophysiology of peripheral muscle wasting in cardiac cachexia. *Curr Opin Clin Nutr Metabol Care, 8,* 249-254.

Fine, R.L. (2006). Ethical issues in artificial nutrition and hydration. *Nutr Clin Pract, 21,*118-125.

Finucaine, T., Christmas, C., & Travis, K. (1999). Tube feeding in patients with advanced dementia. *JAMA, 282,* 1365-1381.

Fuhrman, M.P. & Herrmann, V.M. (2006). Bridging the continuum: Nutrition support in palliative and hospice care. *Nutr Clin Pract, 21,* 134-141.

Geriatrics. (2005). Patient handout. Does constipation ruin your day? What you eat, drink, and do can make a difference. *Geriatrics, 60,* 19.

Guggenheimer, J. & Moore, P.A. (2003). Xerostomia: Etiology, recognition and treatment. *J Am Dent Assoc, 134,* 61-69.

Harman, W.E. (2002). Omega-3 fatty acids to augment cancer therapy. *J Nutr, 132,* 3508S-3512S.

Heckmann, S.M., Hujoel, P., Habiger, S., et al. (2005) Zinc gluconate in the treatment of dysgeusia— A randomized clinical trial. *J Dent Res, 84,* 35-38.

Hehlgans, T. & Pfeffer, K. (2005). The intriguing biology of the tumour necrosis factor/tumour necrosis factor receptor superfamily: Players, rules and the games. *Immunology, 115,* 1-20.

Heiser, C.R., Ernst, J.A., Barrett, J. et al. (2004). Probiotics, soluble fiber, and L-glutamine (GLN) reduce nelfinavir (NFV)- or lopinavir/ritonavir (LPV/r)-related diarrhea. *J Int Assoc Phys AIDS Care (Chic), 3,* 121-129.

Hopkins, K. (2004). Food for life, love and hope: An exemplar of the philosophy of palliative care in action. *Proc Nutr Soc, 63,* 427-429.

Jatoi, A., Rowland, K., Loprinzi, C.L., et al.; North Central Cancer Treatment Group. (2004). An eicosapentaenoic acid supplement versus megestrol acetate versus both for patients with cancer-associated wasting: A North Central Cancer Treatment Group and National Cancer Institute of Canada collaborative effort. *J Clin Oncol, 22,* 2469-2476.

Jatoi, A., Windschitl, H.E., Loprinzi, C.L., et al. (2002). Dronabinol versus megestrol acetate versus combination therapy for cancer-associated anorexia: A North Central Cancer Treatment Group study. *J Clin Oncol, 20,* 567-573.

Jespersen, J., Kjaer, M., & Schjerling, P. (2006). The possible role of myostatin in skeletal muscle atrophy and cachexia. *Scand J Med Sci Sports, 16,* 74-82.

Jho, D., Babcock, T.A., Helton, W.S., et al. (2003). Omega-3 fatty acids: Implications for the treatment of tumor-associated inflammation. *Am Surg, 69,* 32-36.

Khaja, M., Thakur, C.S., Bharathan, T., et al. (2005). 'Fiber 7' supplement as an alternative to laxatives in a nursing home. *Gerodontology, 22,* 106-108.

Li, I. (2002). Feeding tubes in patients with severe dementia. *American Family Physician, 65,* 1605-1610.

Lundholm, K., Daneryd, P., Bosaeus, I., et al. (2004). Palliative nutritional intervention in addition to cyclooxygenase and erythropoietin treatment for patients with malignant disease: Effects on survival, metabolism, and function. *Cancer, 100,* 1967-1977.

Mattox, T.W. (2005). Treatment of unintentional weight loss in patients with cancer. *Nutr Clin Prac, 20,* 400-410.

McKinlay, A.W. (2004). Nutritional support in patients with advanced cancer: Permission to fall out? *Proc Nutr Soc, 63,* 431-435.

Mirhosseini, N., Fainsinger, R.L., & Baracos, V. (2005). Parenteral nutrition in advanced cancer: indications and clinical practice guidelines. *J Palliat Med, 8,* 914-918.

Morita, T., Hyodo, I., Yoshimi, T., et al.; Japan Palliative Oncology Study Group. (2005). Association between hydration volume and symptoms in terminally ill cancer patients with abdominal malignancies. *Ann Oncol, 16,* 640-647.

Morley, J.E. (2002). Orexigenic and anabolic agents. *Clin Geriatr Med, 18,* 853-866.

Moses, A.W., Slater, C., Preston, T., et al. (2004). Reduced total energy expenditure and physical activity in cachectic patients with pancreatic cancer can be modulated by an energy and protein dense oral supplement enriched with n-3 fatty acids. *Br J Cancer, 90,* 996-1002.

Muller-Lissner, S.A., Kamm, M.A., Scarpignato, C., et al. (2005). Myths and misconceptions about chronic constipation. *Am J Gastroenterol, 100,* 232-242.

Muscaritoli, M., Bossola, M., Aversa, Z., et al. (2006). Prevention and treatment of cancer cachexia: New insights into an old problem. *Eur J Cancer, 42,* 31-41.

Novak, J. & Katz, J.A. (2006). Probiotics and prebiotics for gastrointestinal infections. *Curr Infect Dis Rep 8,* 103-109.

Orrevall, Y., Tishelman, C., Herrington, M.K., et al. (2004). The path from oral nutrition to home parenteral nutrition: A qualitative interview study of the experiences of advanced cancer patients and their families. *Clin Nutr, 23,* 1280-1287.

Orrevall, Y., Tishelman, C., & Permert, J. (2005). Home parenteral nutrition: A qualitative interview study of the experiences of advanced cancer patients and their families. *Clin Nutr, 24,* 961-970.

Pascual Lopez, A., Roque i Figuls, M., Urrutia Cuchi, G., et al. (2004). Systematic review of megestrol acetate in the treatment of anorexia-cachexia syndrome. *J Pain Symptom Manage, 27,* 360-369.

Peterson, D.E. (2006). New strategies for management of oral mucositis in cancer patients. *J Support Oncol, 4,* 9-13.

Plonk, W.M. & Arnold, R.M. (2005). Terminal care: The last weeks of life. *J Palliat Med, 8,* 1042-1054.

Polisena, C.G. (2000). Nutrition concerns with the radiation oncology patient. In P.D. McCallum & C.G. Polisena (Eds.). *The clinical guide to oncology nutrition* (pp. 70-78). Chicago: American Dietetic Association.

Poole, K. & Froggatt, K. (2002). Loss of weight and loss of appetite in advanced cancer: A problem for the patient, the carer, or the health professional? *Palliat Med, 16,* 499-506.

Ripamonti, C., Zecca, E., Brunelli, C., et al. (1998). A randomized, controlled clinical trial to evaluate the effects of zinc sulfate on cancer patients with taste alterations caused by head and neck irradiation. *Cancer, 82,* 1938-1945.

Rushdi, T.A., Pichard, C., & Khater, Y.H. (2004). Control of diarrhea by fiber-enriched diet in ICU patients on enteral nutrition: A prospective randomized controlled trial. *Clin Nutr, 23,* 1344-1352.

Savarese, D., Al-Zoubi, A., & Boucher, J. (2000). Glutamine for irinotecan diarrhea. *J Clin Oncol, 18,* 450-451.

Savarese, D.M., Savy, G., Vahdat, L., et al. (2003). Prevention of chemotherapy and radiation toxicity with glutamine. *Cancer Treat Rev, 29,* 501-513.

Shay, N.F. & Mangian, H.F. (2000). Neurobiology of zinc-influenced eating behavior. *J Nutr, 130,* 1493S-1499S.

Smith, S. (2001). Evidence-based management of constipation in the oncology patient. *Eur J Oncol Nurs, 5,* 18-25.

Staats, P.S., Markowitz, J., & Schein, J. (2004). Incidence of constipation associated with long-acting opioid therapy: A comparative study. *South Med J, 97,* 129-134.

Strasser, F. & Bruera, E.D. (2002). Update on anorexia and cachexia. *Hematol Oncol Clin North Am, 16,* 589-617.

Tisdale, M.J. (2005). Molecular pathways leading to cancer cachexia. *Physiology, 20,* 340-348.

Tisdale, M.J. (2006). Clinical anticachexia treatments. *Nutr Clin Prac, 21,* 168-174.

Van Cutsem, E. & Arends, J. (2005). The causes and consequences of cancer-associated malnutrition. *Eur J Oncol Nurs, 9,* S51-S63.

Walsh, D., Nelson, K.A., & Mahmoud, F.A. (2003). Established and potential therapeutic applications of cannabinoids in oncology. *Support Care Cancer, 11,* 137-143.

Wigmore, S.J., Barber, M.D., Ross, J.A., et al. (2000). Effect of oral eicosapentaenoic acid on weight loss in patients with pancreatic cancer. *Nutr Cancer, 36,* 177-184.

Wilcock, A. (2006). Anorexia: A taste of things to come? *Palliat Med, 20,* 43-45.

Wilson, L.A. (2005). Understanding bowel problems in older people: Part 2. *Nurs Older People, 17,* 24-29.

Wisten, A. & Messner, T. (2005). Fruit and fibre (Pajala porridge) in the prevention of constipation. *Scand J Caring Sci, 19,* 71-76.

Witte, K.K. & Clark, A.L. (2002). Nutritional abnormalities contributing to cachexia in chronic illness. *Int J Cardiol, 85,* 23-31.

Wolf, I., Sadetzki, S., Kanety, H., et al. (2006). Adiponectin, ghrelin, and leptin in cancer cachexia in breast and colon cancer patients. *Cancer, 106,* 966-973.

UNIT III

ADVANCED DISEASE MANAGEMENT

CHAPTER 10

CARDIOVASCULAR DISEASE

Carol L. Scot and Kim Anne Pickett

■

OVERVIEW

The cardiovascular (CV) system includes the heart and the blood vessels. These vessels include the arteries, veins, and capillaries that feed the tissues throughout the body. Cardiovascular disease (CVD) accounted for 38% of the approximately 2,400,000 deaths in the United States in 2002 (American Heart Association [AHA], 2005). Of the approximately 912,000 deaths from CVD in 2002, 53% were due primarily to coronary artery disease (CAD) and 18% were due to stroke. In addition, CVD is a contributing factor in another 500,000 deaths, meaning that in 2002 CVD mortality was nearly 60% of total mortality in the United States (AHA, 2005).

CVD is caused or worsened by comorbidities such as diabetes, high blood pressure, hyperlipidemia, kidney disease, and/or connective tissue disease. Patients with multiple medical problems present the palliative care clinician with challenges in balancing the risks and benefits of treatments.

ETIOLOGY AND PATHOPHYSIOLOGY

Atherothrombotic Disease

Arteriosclerosis is a generic term for thickened and stiffened arteries. Atherosclerosis is the term used to describe the thickened and hardened lipid-rich lesions (plaques) of the larger muscular and elastic arteries (Fuster, 2004). Atherothrombotic CVD is a diffuse condition involving areas of thrombotic change in vessels of the heart (coronary arteries), brain (carotid, vertebral, cerebral arteries), aorta, and peripheral arteries (Fuster, 2004). Thrombosis, which most often results from the rupture of an unstable atherosclerotic plaque, is generally one of the most significant manifestations of atherosclerotic disease.

Hyperlipidemia, hypertension, smoking, diabetes, a high-fat diet, obesity, physical inactivity, and genetic factors all contribute to the vasoconstriction and increased blood levels of low-density lipoprotein, which promote damage and the formation of plaque within the arteries, leading to the development of atherosclerosis (Fuster, 2004).

Lipid-rich plaques form on the inner surface of arteries, especially in the areas of disturbed blood flow around bends and near bifurcations. The plaque formation itself further disrupts blood flow. If the plaque ruptures, a thrombus forms and platelets are deposited around the thrombus, which partially or completely occludes the artery. In the coronary arteries, a partial occlusion decreases blood flow to the myocardium;

the resultant decreased oxygenation can create angina. Complete occlusion causes a myocardial infarction (MI). Similar occlusions can occur within the brain, with partial occlusions causing transient ischemic attacks and complete occlusions often causing ischemic strokes. When patients present with clinical evidence of vascular occlusion, approximately 3% to 8% have symptomatic disease in all three main arterial districts (systemic, cardiac, brain) and 23% to 32% have disease in two arterial districts (Fuster, 2004).

Coronary Artery Disease

CAD results from the narrowing of the coronary arteries due to atherosclerosis. CAD is the primary cause of angina—the crushing, breathtaking pain related to ischemia of the myocardium. Anginal pain is most commonly located over the left precordium, but pain beginning at the sternum and radiating to the neck, shoulder, arms, or jaw is not uncommon. The pain builds up in less than a minute and usually subsides in 5 to 15 minutes, or more quickly if the patient uses nitroglycerin (Hunt, Abraham, Chin et al., 2005).

Angina may be due to a fixed coronary obstruction, a superimposed thrombus, or vasospasm. Stable angina occurs predictably, precipitated by the same factors each time it occurs, usually as the result of increased physical activity. Stable angina is usually due to a fixed coronary artery lesion (Hunt et al., 2005). With walk-through angina, the discomfort lessens with continued activity. Nocturnal angina occurs with recumbency, either soon after lying down or hours later. Postprandial angina develops during or after meals because of increased oxygen demand of the muscles of mastication and the activity of the digestive system.

Unstable angina is the initial presentation of angina, or a worsening of stable angina, in either frequency or intensity. Unless a patient is already designated as comfort care only, unstable angina should be considered a medical emergency, which requires an immediate cardiac evaluation. Patients with heart failure (HF) may still experience angina and be at risk for an MI (Theroux, 2004).

Cardiomyopathies

Disease of the heart muscle itself, or cardiomyopathy, is a term used to designate disorders originating within the myocardium. The heart muscle may be damaged by ischemia from CAD. The response of the heart to ischemic injury triggers a cascade of neurohormonal changes that, over time, remodel the heart in ways that are immediately beneficial but eventually harmful. The ischemic ventricle thickens and enlarges to be able to generate more force, but ultimately this cardiomegaly causes more problems (Stevenson, 2004).

All other forms of heart muscle disease are grouped together as nonischemic cardiomyopathy. Nonischemic cardiomyopathies account for about 5% to 10% of the 5 million patients in the United States diagnosed with HF (Stevenson, 2004).

Causes of nonischemic cardiomyopathy include (1) the storage diseases (diseases in which abnormal substances, or an overabundance of a usually benign substance, are deposited in normal body tissues, like the heart muscle) such as Gaucher disease, hemochromatosis, and amyloidosis; (2) systemic conditions, including hypertension, diabetes, hyperthyroidism, and hypocalcemia; (3) exposure to cardiac toxins, such as alcohol, cocaine, methamphetamine, anthracycline, or trastuzumab; and (4) myocarditis, which is infectious or noninfectious inflammation of the heart muscle (Hunt, et al., 2005; Stevenson, 2004).

Most patients with nonischemic cardiomyopathy have none of these causes. Their diagnosis is the diagnosis of exclusion—dilated idiopathic cardiomyopathy. Thirty percent of these patients are thought to have an inherited form of nonischemic cardiomyopathy (Mestroni, 2003).

Congenital Heart and Valvular Heart Disease

By definition, a newborn with a malformed heart or great vessels is immediately in ACC/AHA guidelines stage B (structural heart abnormalities) or stage C or D if the malformation causes HF (Table 10-1).

Many congenital heart conditions can be surgically corrected or palliated, allowing survival into adulthood, with HF always a possibility or a reality. Approximately 32,000 infants are diagnosed with congenital heart disease each year in the United States. An estimated 20% die in the first year of life; this is a substantial decrease from the 40% who were reported to have died in the first year of life in the late 1960s. Approximately 80% of the first-year survivors live to reach adulthood. The estimated prevalence of adults with congenital heart disease in the United States is 800,000 (Marelli, 2004).

Minor congenital abnormalities can go undetected and produce little or no symptoms through youth and midlife yet become significant in the elderly—notably, atrial septal defect, mitral regurgitation, and bifid aortic valve. Two percent of the general adult population have the congenital anomaly of a bifid aortic valve. A person with this condition may live and die without ever knowing it. Many, however, become symptomatic as they age, because the abnormal valve is subject to stenosis. Half of all operations for aortic stenosis in adults are due to a bifid aortic valve (Marelli, 2004).

TABLE 10-1 ■ The New York Heart Association Functional Classification of Heart Failure

	Functional Class		Stage of Heart Failure
I	No limitation of physical activity. Ordinary physical activity does not cause undue fatigue, palpitation, or dyspnea.	A	At high risk for developing heart failure (pre–heart failure)
II	Symptoms with ordinary exertion.	B	Structural heart disease and systolic left ventricular dysfunction but asymptomatic
III	Marked limitation of physical activity. Symptoms with less than ordinary exertion.	C	Systolic dysfunction; currently has symptoms or has history of prior symptoms
IV	Unable to carry out any physical activity without discomfort. Symptoms of cardiac insufficiency at rest.	D	End-stage/advanced systolic dysfunction

Data from New York Heart Association. (1994). *1994 Revisions to classification of functional capacity and objective assessment of patients with diseases of the heart.* Retrieved May 29, 2006, from www.americanheart.org/ presenter.jhtml?identifier=1712; and American College of Cardiology/American Heart Association. (2005). *Guideline update for the diagnosis and management of chronic heart failure in the adult.* Retrieved May 29, 2006, from www.acc.org/clinical/guidelines/failure/index.pdf.

Valvular heart disease can also be acquired. The mitral valve can be damaged by an MI and then require replacement.

Rheumatic heart disease, both the acute myocardial inflammation and the valvular damage, has been reduced by the use of penicillin for group A streptococcal upper respiratory infections. However, other infective agents can cause endocarditis.

Chronic Heart Failure

Patients living with the limitations associated with advanced cardiac disease have experienced a progressive course that typically has taken them through multiple diagnostics, emergent care situations, and routine medical evaluation over several years. Chronic HF is due to many causes: CAD, nonischemic cardiomyopathy, valvular heart disease, malignancy and its associated treatments, or other toxins. HF is the final common pathway when the intricately timed electromuscular pump of the heart can no longer perform its life-sustaining functions, despite the technological advancements currently available. Because palliative care is often focused on HF, the remainder of this chapter discusses HF, its incidence, and its management.

DEFINITION AND INCIDENCE

Heart failure is a broad term for a clinical syndrome characterized by the inability of the heart to maintain an adequate cardiac output to sustain the demands of the tissues. HF can result from left or right ventricular dysfunction and is usually characterized by symptoms such as fatigue and dyspnea and signs such as fluid volume overload (Albert, 2005).

The syndrome of HF historically has been considered to be synonymous with diminished contractility of the left ventricle (LV), resulting in a reduced left ventricular ejection fraction (LVEF). This is commonly known as systolic HF (Hunt et al., 2005). However, it is currently understood that HF also exists in many patients who have a normal or near-normal ejection fraction. Diastolic failure, in which increased resistance to ventricular filling during diastole is noted, is present with a preserved LVEF of 40% or more (Albert, 2005). The current incidence of diastolic failure is believed to be approximately 50% of all patients diagnosed with HF (McEntegart & Gray, 2004).

Some causes of diastolic HF (HF with a normal LVEF) are hypertensive heart disease, chronic pulmonary disease, valvular disease, restrictive (infiltrative) cardiomyopathies (amyloidosis, sarcoidosis, hemochromatosis), pericardial constriction, pulmonary hypertension, and obesity. HF that is associated with a normal LVEF is prevalent among elderly women, most of whom have concomitant diseases such as hypertension, diabetes mellitus, CAD, and/or atrial fibrillation. In the aging population coupled with the prevalence of diabetes, advanced practice nurses (APNs) should expect to see more patients in this category (Hunt et al., 2005).

Decreased cardiac output and high ventricular filling pressures are the two basic disorders in HF (Albert, 2005). Typically, the "congestive" manifestations include signs and symptoms such as orthopnea, paroxysmal nocturnal dyspnea, edema, ascites, and jugular venous distention, although it is important to note that not every patient with HF may present with congestive features. For that reason, the preferred term is *chronic heart failure* or *heart failure*.

As the incidence of survival in acute heart disease has increased, the number of people living with chronic heart disease has risen. HF has been diagnosed in approximately 5 million persons in the United States, with over 550,000 new diagnoses each year. HF was the primary and secondary diagnosis in 3.6 million hospitalizations in 1999 (Koelling, Chen, Lubwama et al., 2004). HF was the primary cause of death for 53,000 patients in 2001 and approximately 55,000 in the 2002 (Hunt et al., 2005).

PATHOPHYSIOLOGY OF HEART FAILURE

Over the years, theories regarding the pathophysiologic processes of HF progressed from an initial belief that viewed HF as a low cardiac output state that was treated with inotropic therapy to the most recent model that describes neurohormonal activation and inflammatory response (Davis, Albert, & Young, 2005). HF may be classified as systolic (LVEF less than 40%) or diastolic (decreased ventricular compliance with a normal LVEF).

To understand current recommended treatment, health care providers should be familiar with the pathophysiology of HF. Although the process is complex, there are three general processes that occur in response to stress or injury of the myocardium: neuroendocrine activation, ventricular remodeling, and immune system upregulation (Albert, Eastwood, & Edwards, 2004). When the injured myocardium is unable to contract with sufficient force to maintain adequate organ perfusion, these three processes are activated to increase cardiac output. However, these compensatory mechanisms become counterproductive over time and lead to ventricular remodeling. Ventricular remodeling, in which myocytes elongate and form a spherical shape, further activates neurohormones and cytokines to adversely affect cardiac structure and function. This contributes to stress on the myocardium and contributes to morbidity and mortality (Albert, 2005). One of the primary goals in treatment of HF is to reverse ventricular remodeling, irregardless of whether the patient is in acute or chronic HF (Albert et al., 2004).

STAGING

For decades, the New York Heart Association (NYHA) functional classification of HF patients has been useful in helping researchers and clinicians compare the severity of HF between groups of patients or to compare a single patient's physical function throughout the course of disease (see Table 10-1). Patients often move back and forth between levels of clinical functioning. For example, an impaired patient functioning in class IV (completely incapacitated, with symptoms at rest) as a result of exacerbating factors that include a recent MI, anemia, thyroid disease, or not adhering to prescribed medications could return to class III (less than ordinary physical exertion causes symptoms) after rehabilitation.

The ACC/AHA Task Force on Heart Failure Practice Guidelines has published guidelines for the diagnosis and management of chronic HF. These guidelines were first published in 1995 and revised in 2001 and 2005. The primary emphasis has been to develop a staging system that could reliably and objectively identify patients during the course of disease and link treatments based upon each stage of illness

(Hunt et al., 2005). This staging system is intended to complement, but not replace, the NYHA functional classification.

DIAGNOSIS

The chest radiograph, when considered with the clinical assessment of the patient and the 12-lead electrocardiogram (ECG), can have a high predictive value for HF. The chest radiograph may show cardiomegaly and pulmonary venous congestion. The ECG may reveal left ventricular hypertrophy, changes suggestive of ischemic heart disease, or an arrhythmia such as atrial fibrillation. However, neither chest radiography nor the 12-lead electrocardiogram provides sensitive information regarding the degree of HF or its etiology (McEntegart & Gray, 2004).

The most widely used and most preferred test to confirm HF is a two-dimensional echocardiogram with Doppler flow studies. This test can confirm the diagnosis of HF (systolic or diastolic) and reveal measurements such as wall motion abnormalities, LVEF, and chamber size, thus helping to determine etiology and guide further management (Davis et al., 2005).

Brain natriuretic peptide (BNP) is a neurohormone released by the cardiac ventricles in response to fluid overload and volume expansion in the failing heart. BNP elevations are seen in both systolic and diastolic failure, although the BNP does not aid in distinguishing systolic from diastolic failure (Davis et al., 2005; Wu & Yu, 2005). Although BNP blood levels are sometimes used to support a diagnosis of HF, further studies are needed regarding the use of BNP levels in guiding therapy. It is important to note that, as with any other laboratory data, the clinical presentation of the patient must also be considered (McEntegart & Gray, 2004).

HISTORY AND PHYSICAL EXAMINATION

History

Patients who are diagnosed with HF and who are in need of palliative care have typically undergone repeated invasive and noninvasive diagnostic testing that may include electrocardiograms, chest and other radiographs, blood and urine tests, echocardiograms, radionucleotide testing, magnetic resonance imagining, and angiography. Some patients may have undergone an endomyocardial biopsy, ablation of malfunctioning electrical nodes or pathways, coronary artery bypass grafting (sometimes repeatedly), pacemaker and defibrillator implantation, or heart transplantation. The records of these tests and procedures, as well as records from hospital admissions and from other clinicians the patient has seen or is seeing, form an important part of the patient's medical history.

The typical medical interview with all its subparts, including chief complaint, history of present illness, past medical history, past surgical history, allergies, medications, family history, social history, and review of systems, is an important factor for the APN to evaluate. Past medical records can and should provide much of this information to the APN.

When the APN knows the patient's previous medical history, the "history" becomes a present-day evaluation, focusing on current symptoms and functioning.

Specific questions about sleep, self-care, household chores, ability to do what he or she would like to do, and pain, palpitations, breathlessness, cough, poor appetite, nausea, weight loss, anxiety, depression, confusion, dizziness on arising, fainting, or falls can help the APN in developing a picture of the patient's self-assessment of his or her sense of well-being and functioning.

Physical Examination

After taking the medical history, including all current concerns, the APN performs the physical examination, focusing on the signs associated with any specific symptoms the patient has mentioned. The physical examination includes an overall examination of the patient as well as the following.

Vascular Assessment

During auscultation of a normal heart, two heart sounds are produced, which represent the mitral and tricuspid valves closing (S1) and the aortic and pulmonary valves closing (S2). The APN evaluating a patient with HF should also be mindful of the third heart sound (S3). When present, the S3 sound, or ventricular gallop, is a low-pitched sound noted after the S1 and S2 sounds during cardiac auscultation and is associated with increased filling pressures of the cardiac ventricles (McEntegart & Gray, 2004). An S3 sound is usually abnormal in adults over the age of 40. It is often one of the first clinical signs of HF and is best heard with the bell of the stethoscope when the patient is in the left lateral position (McEntegart & Gray, 2004).

Jugular venous pressure (JVP), as measured from the sternal angle, is a clinical measure of central venous pressure. Although determination of JVP can be a difficult skill to master, it is one of the most significant physical indicators of fluid volume overload in patients with HF. Deoxygenated blood from the internal jugular vein drains via the superior vena cava into the right atrium; therefore, patients with fluid overload and elevated right atrial pressure generally present with elevated JVP (McEntegart & Gray, 2004).

JVP is usually assessed on the right side of the neck, with the patient sitting at a 45-degree angle. The patient's head should be tilted slightly backward and toward the left, away from the examiner. The examiner checks for engorgement of the internal jugular vein, which runs between the two heads of the sternocleidomastoid muscle toward the angle of the patient's jaw. JVP has a good positive predictive value, which means that if it is elevated, the patient most likely has HF, but unfortunately, it is not elevated in many HF patients (McEntegart & Gray, 2004).

Pulse and blood pressure, which are general indicators of the patient's hemodynamic stability, should be evaluated. Apical and radial pulses should be assessed, and orthostatic blood pressures should be obtained in a patient reporting symptoms of orthostatic hypotension.

The rate and rhythm of the pulse are important components of the physical examination. The patient with HF often presents with bradycardia (heart rate less than 60 bpm), most commonly due to β-blocker therapy. If the patient is bradycardic in the absence of β-blocker therapy, further investigation is warranted to rule out the possibility of other conditions such as heart block (McEntegart & Gray, 2004).

Resting tachycardia and/or a marked tachycardia with minimum exertion should be noted as well. Tachycardia, although part of the heart's normal response to increased sympathetic activity, may develop in severe HF but may also be suppressed with β-blocker therapy. Tachycardia can also be a sign of decompensating HF; other indicators, as well as the patient's clinical presentation, should be considered to obtain the entire clinical picture (McEntegart & Gray, 2004).

Atrial fibrillation is the most common arrhythmia in HF patients. The pulse is typically irregularly irregular (McEntegart & Gray, 2004). According to Wu and Yu (2005), patients with diastolic HF tolerate tachycardia especially poorly, and if atrial fibrillation is present in this population, β-blocker or calcium channel blocker therapy should be considered.

Respiratory Assessment

The respiratory assessment includes auscultation of lung sounds, respiratory rate, any use of accessory muscles, and whether the patient appears dyspneic at rest or on exertion. The most common abnormal respiratory sounds noted in HF are crackles or rales, which are caused by opening of the alveoli when there is fluid within them (McEntegart & Gray, 2004). However, the absence of pulmonary rales is not necessarily a clinically significant finding, as rales are absent in 80% of HF patients due to compensatory mechanisms that increase pulmonary lymphatic flow (Davis et al., 2005).

Edema

Edema in HF is initiated by the fall in cardiac output, leading to activation of the sympathetic nervous and renin-angiotensin-aldosterone systems. One of the primary effects of renin-angiotensin-aldosterone system activation is sodium retention; as a result, increased venous pressure is distributed to smaller vessels, leading to fluid in the soft tissues and producing edema (McEntegart & Gray, 2004).

The presence of edema is not an early sign of fluid volume overload; it is estimated that a patient can gain up to 10 pounds before edema is clinically detected. Obtaining regular weights, in conjunction with monitoring other symptoms and signs, is an important component of assessing fluid volume status (McEntegart & Gray, 2004).

Fluid can also accumulate as ascites; the accumulation of fluid may develop over time and be manifested as slowly increasing abdominal girth. Although typically associated with right ventricular HF, patients may also present when the etiology is LV failure as well. The presence of ascites can be confirmed with eliciting the sign of shifting dullness (McEntegart & Gray, 2004).

ASSOCIATED SIGNS AND SYMPTOMS

In discussing the signs and symptoms of disease, it is important to remember their distinction. A *sign* can be seen, measured, and/or described by an observer. A *symptom* can be described only by the patient who experiences it.

Congruent signs and symptoms are powerful indicators of disease, helping the APN make a confident diagnosis. Reconciling incongruent signs and symptoms is part of the art of nursing.

Key symptoms of HF include localized signs and symptoms (such as dyspnea, pain, orthopnea, paroxysmal nocturnal dyspnea, ascites, and edema) and generalized symptoms (fatigue, anorexia, cachexia, and weight loss) (Davis et al., 2005).

Fluid Retention

The hallmark sign of HF is fluid retention. When the ventricle operates under abnormal diastolic conditions (cannot fill adequately) or abnormal systolic conditions (inadequate ejection fraction), a back pressure develops that increases venous pressure and forces transudation of fluid into the tissues. Dysfunction of the left ventricle causes back pressure into the pulmonary system and pulmonary congestion. Dysfunction of the right ventricle (often due to the dysfunction of the left ventricle) causes back pressure into the systemic system, which results in peripheral edema.

These signs of fluid retention—edema and pulmonary congestion—are a focus of the physical examination in the HF patient.

Pulmonary Fluid Retention

Pulmonary congestion first occurs in the interstitial lung spaces—the walls of alveoli and bronchioles. Eventually, small amounts of the fluid enter the alveolar sac and present as rales and rhonchi, often accompanied by labored breathing.

Pleural effusions are due to transudation of fluid into the potential space between the serosal surfaces of the lung (visceral pleura) and inner thoracic wall (parietal pleura). They can be identified by chest dullness to percussion and fluid seen in the pleural space on chest radiograph.

Acute pulmonary edema occurs when fluid fills not only the interstitial lung spaces but also the alveoli. In pulmonary edema, the lung sounds may resemble asthma, with wheezing and even musical sounds. The patient may be struggling to breathe, cyanotic, and coughing, with frothy, occasionally blood-tinged, sputum.

Systemic Fluid Retention

Right ventricle failure can precipitate hepatic congestion. External pressure applied to the right upper quadrant can produce hepatojugular reflux (or abdominal-jugular reflux), a pressure wave, and engorgement in the jugular vein can be observed. As the liver becomes more congested, it may become large and tender. Eventually, the liver capsule becomes thicker and no longer tender.

In peripheral tissues, edema develops mostly in dependent areas, due to gravity. The swelling of the abdomen, scrotum, and lower extremities in ambulatory patients worsens during the daytime and improves at night, with recumbent positioning. HF patients may present with leg or abdominal swelling as their only, or major, complaint. Edema in bed-bound patients can be more subtle, affecting the entire dependent areas of the back and limbs.

Significant fluid retention in the peritoneal space (ascites) can be determined by a careful abdominal examination that elicits shifting and/or horseshoe dullness.

Fluid retention of the internal organs themselves, such as in the walls of the stomach and bowel, cannot be assessed in the physical examination. This fluid retention can sometimes be seen on abdominal radiographs but is more accurately viewed on abdominal computed tomography scans. More often, it will be inferred from symptoms of anorexia, nausea, vomiting, or diffuse abdominal pain.

Symptoms

Although the signs of fluid retention are fairly specific to HF, the symptoms are less specific. The cardinal symptoms of fatigue, dyspnea, and exercise intolerance can be present in many other conditions such as malignancy, pulmonary disease, and aging, all of which may occur alone, or as comorbidities in any combination.

Fatigue

Fatigue has been identified by patients as one of the most problematic symptoms in the palliative care setting as it limits valued life-affirming activities they were previously able to perform. Manifestations of fatigue can include inability to maintain routines, impaired ability to concentrate, disinterest in surroundings, decreased libido, lethargy, and listlessness.

Dyspnea

Dyspnea is the subjective sensation of difficulty in breathing, breathlessness, or shortness of breath. At first, it may be experienced only on exertion. As HF worsens, the patient may develop orthopnea, which is dyspnea that develops or worsens when the patient is in a recumbent position. Nocturnal dyspnea may occur in the recumbent position or while partially elevated. A patient may be able to fall asleep but have pulmonary fluid retention that worsens as he or she sleeps. The patient wakens with paroxysmal nocturnal dyspnea, which is severe breathlessness that interrupts sleep, and this may require the patient to sit up or stand up and move around until the dyspnea lessens. Paroxysmal nocturnal dyspnea may be due to the increased blood return from dependent edema that occurs in the recumbent position.

Dyspnea usually occurs first on exertion and progresses to dyspnea at rest (Pina, Apstein, Balady et al., 2003). Both dyspnea and fatigue can limit exercise tolerance and further promote fluid retention and eventual pulmonary congestion and peripheral edema (Hunt et al., 2005).

Exercise Intolerance

Decreased exercise capability is the logical concomitant to fatigue and dyspnea and can be the symptom that first brings a patient to medical care. A person may not recognize dyspnea or fatigue if it comes on slowly but may become sharply aware of his or her inability to accomplish physically what had been usual before.

Lack of oxygen to muscle tissue forces the muscle to use glucose for energy instead of oxygen, and the muscle develops lactic acid. Lactic acidosis and loss of muscle mass may contribute to exercise intolerance, as well as to generalized pain.

Exercise intolerance is one of the ambiguous manifestations of disease that may be either a symptom only described by the patient or a sign that can be measured. A suggested evaluation to measure exercise tolerance (and therefore record it as a sign) is the 6-minute walk. This diagnostic tool assesses the distance a patient can walk in 6 minutes. Because exercise can be limited by other conditions—pulmonary disease, arthritis, and generalized deconditioning—it may not be a usable tool for all HF patients (McGavigan & Dunn, 2004).

Gastrointestinal Symptoms and Cardiac Cachexia

The role of HF in producing nonspecific gastrointestinal (GI) symptoms such as anorexia, early satiety, nausea, diffuse abdominal discomfort, malabsorption, and a rare form of protein-losing enteropathy is often overlooked, which can lead to extensive diagnostic testing or unnecessary discontinuation of medications.

When the patient experiences unintended weight loss and loss of muscle mass, he or she has developed the syndrome of cardiac cachexia. Cardiac cachexia occurs in up to 50% of patients (McGavigan & Dunn, 2004). The cause of cardiac cachexia is unclear but may be the result of several factors, including elevated levels of proinflammatory cytokines (e.g., tumor necrosis factor [TNF]), elevated metabolic rates, loss of appetite, and malabsorption. Cardiac cachexia is associated with a poor prognosis (Davis et al., 2005).

INTERVENTIONS

Early recognition of changes in baseline clinical status of the HF patient is crucial to minimize the incidence of acute exacerbations. Recent studies have indicated a correlation between fluid volume overload/sodium retention and rehospitalization in the end-stage HF patient (Albert, 2005; Tsuyuki, McCelvie, Arnold et al., 2001). Therefore, it is extremely important for the APN to discuss a plan of care and lifestyle recommendations with the patient and family. By incorporating lifestyle changes focused on prevention of fluid volume overload such as weighing daily and reporting early weight gains, limiting dietary sodium, and limiting fluids when indicated, the APN and patient can recognize status changes early and intervene.

Lifestyle recommendations for patients with HF often include limiting dietary sodium, obtaining regular physical exercise, weight control, cessation of smoking, and avoidance of alcohol and recreational drugs. Nursing interventions for patients with dyspnea, such as using a fan or repositioning the patient, are also helpful. Medical treatments address controlling symptoms, blood pressure, and diabetes. Medical management is discussed next.

MANAGEMENT OF CHRONIC HEART FAILURE

The ACC/AHA Guidelines for the Diagnosis and Management of Chronic Heart Failure in the Adult have been and will be referenced frequently throughout this discussion. This lengthy document, based on 694 current clinical references, gives authoritative recommendations for the medical care of HF patients, from those who are at risk for the disease to those dying of it. The recommendations are aimed at preserving cardiac function and decreasing ischemic burden.

Interventions given in the ACC/AHA guidelines are organized according to the patient's NYHA functional classification and ACC/AHA stage, as detailed in Table 10-1. In the ACC/AHA staging system, patients in stage A are classified "at risk" for HF, while patients in stage B are classified as having HF but being asymptomatic. Palliative care patients fall into stage C (systolic dysfunction; currently has symptoms) or stage D (end-stage/advanced systolic dysfunction).

Although historically patients with HF with diastolic dysfunction were believed to require separate treatment, researchers such as Wu and Yu (2005) are gathering data that indicate that treatment for both of these diseases are similar. However, Wu and Yu point out that patients with diastolic dysfunction do not tolerate tachycardia as well as might patients with systolic dysfunction.

Patients in stage C have structural heart disease and prior or current symptoms of HF. For them, the same lifestyle recommendations apply as for stage A and B patients (smoking cessation, exercise, and the control of weight, hypertension, and blood lipid levels), with the additional recommendation for dietary salt restriction, usually "no added salt" or 2 g or less of sodium per day. Medications added are diuretics for fluid retention, angiotensin-converting enzyme inhibitors (ACEIs), or β-blockers; other possible medications are aldosterone antagonists, adrenergic receptor blockers (ARBs), digitalis, hydralazine, and nitrates (Hunt et al., 2005).

Not all medications in each group are recommended for use at stage C. The only β-blockers recommended are bisoprolol, carvedilol, and metoprolol succinate. All ACEIs may be used except benazepril, moexipril, and perindopril. Of the ARBs, only candesartan and valsartan are recommended (Hunt et al., 2005).

A patient in stage C can have a widely varying clinical status, from relatively symptom free to being hospitalized. The syndrome may be completely controlled for long periods of time, with only minor episodes of increased symptoms. Over time, or suddenly, the disease may worsen and require increased interventions. Biventricular pacing devices and implantable cardioverter-defibrillators (ICDs) may be recommended and may provide marked improvement in the patient's quality of life, enabling him or her to enter another period of improved functioning.

For patients whose disease has progressed to stage D, or end-stage HF, the symptoms are no longer mild or intermittent but are refractory. Despite maximal medical therapy, these patients are disabled, with symptoms at rest. There are no overall recommendations made for medication in stage D. At this stage, either experimental or only comfort medications will be used (Hunt et al., 2005).

Patients in stages C and D should be encouraged to avoid aspirin and nonsteroidal antiinflammatory drugs, which block ACEI activity, worsen renal function, and increase retention of sodium and fluid in HF (Masoudi, Wang, Inzucchi et al., 2003).

Congestion is one of the most problematic symptoms with end-stage HF. Most patients are on loop diuretics, usually furosemide (Lasix). However, bioavailability in furosemide varies (it is believed to be approximately 50%, although the range is 10% to 90%), and if the patient is experiencing "diuretic resistance," it may be helpful to switch to another loop diuretic, such as bumetanide (Bumex) or torsemide (Demadex) (Taylor, 2003).

DEVICE THERAPY

Electrophysiologic devices that are commonly used are cardiac resynchronization therapy, biventricular pacing (pacemakers), and ICDs for cardioversion and defibrillation as needed. These devices are targeted for patients with structural heart disease and HF. Patients with device therapy tend to experience improved quality of life, increased exercise tolerance, and improved mortality (Davis et al., 2005).

Ventricular arrhythmias (particularly ventricular fibrillation and ventricular tachy-cardia) are common in patients with reduced LVEF, and drug therapy alone may not always be effective in arrhythmia prevention (Taylor, 2003). The ICD provides moni-toring and treatment for cardiac arrhythmias and, when appropriate, delivers an elec-tric shock for recognizably lethal rhythms such as ventricular flutter or fibrillation. These shocks are strong enough to be uncomfortable for the patient; many patients experience the sensation of "being kicked in the chest."

It is important to make a distinction between pacemakers and ICDs when provid-ing the palliative care or hospice patient with information. Although both devices can be deactivated in a painless and noninvasive manner, the deactivation of a pacemaker may be likely to induce symptomatic bradycardia and perhaps a poorer quality of death, whereas deactivating an ICD is unlikely to decrease quality of life (except that a fatal arrhythmia would not be corrected) and will prevent the distress of shocks (Ballentine, 2005).

The ACC/AHA guidelines recommend discussion of the option of inactivating ICDs for patients with HF at end-of-life (Hunt et al., 2005), but each patient must be afforded the opportunity to make a well-informed decision based on his or her goals.

Palliative Care

The ACC/AHA guidelines, while medically comprehensive, do not address key corner-stones of palliative care.

Medications that prolong survival have also been shown to reduce symptoms and improve a patient's perceived quality of life and are important in palliative therapy. A predicament often occurs when an end-of-life patient, even one who actively sought palliative or hospice care, is offered a surgical, diagnostic, or interventional procedure toward the end of his or her life. This presents a quandary for the patient and physi-cian. Many patients (and physicians) are conditioned to think that mechanical treat-ments, such as procedures, tend to be effective, whereas medical therapy is simply "palliative" and will not be as effective (Taylor, 2003).

Hauptman and Havranek (2005) explored the palliative and HF care models and believe that palliative care can and should be integrated with traditional HF care. The authors also suggest that the dual nature should be considered a normal approach to treat-ment in HF. In this model, hospice care is a form of palliative care in which the patient has opted not to receive life-prolonging treatment (Hauptman & Havranek, 2005).

When discussing palliative care options with the HF patient, the APN identifies the patient's goals and expectations of care. These discussions between clinician and patient provide an opportunity to evaluate care options and to develop a plan of care in the face of a poor prognosis. The two must explore the patient's current problems, plans, hopes, fears, and values. An APN who is planning the care and management of the patient living with and dying from advanced cardiac disease needs a clear under-standing not only of the best recommendations for the patient's medical care but also of what the patient and his or her family expect and want in terms of care manage-ment. As the physician William Osler said, "It is much more important to know what sort of patient has the disease than to know what sort of disease the patient has."

One study has shown that HF patients are less informed about the course of HF and its prognosis, and less involved in clinical decisions, than are cancer patients

(Murray, Boyd, Kendall et al., 2002). This may be due to several factors. Patients, and often clinicians, may not consider HF a terminal disease like cancer, even though the mortality rate of HF is worse than that of many cancers. The unpredictable course and nontraditional trajectory of HF compared with the often-steady decline in cancer is another factor.

Many patients are also dealing with comorbidities such as diabetes, depression, arthritis, pulmonary disease, thyroid disease, cancer, or a combination of these. Only the patient can say which condition bothers and worries him or her the most. Together, the patient and the APN can decide what treatments can be used to benefit one condition without negatively affecting another. A patient with severe arthritis may fear giving up nonsteroidal antiinflammatory drugs to benefit his heart disease but may find the arthritic pain can be controlled with acetaminophen and the less-potent opioids.

The goal of the APN is to educate the patient about his or her disease and to involve him or her in clinical decisions. As the APN and the patient plan care, the APN probes for what sort of patient has the disease.

Is this patient a person in midlife with projects, plans, and responsibilities that make her say she has to keep functional, has to stay alive and active, and will do anything to accomplish it? Is he a crusty fellow who is never going to take diuretics on a day he is leaving home or give up his cigars or salty food? Is the patient someone who is tired of going to the hospital but is willing to do so if it occurs only once or twice a year? Perhaps this is that same patient a year later, when she has had almost continuous exacerbations and hospitalizations and is now in stage D HF with intractable symptoms. She has had a biventricular pacer and an ICD but is reaching the end-of-life despite it.

The same patient may still even voice a preference to not have her ICD deactivated yet, on the chance that the ventricular fibrillation she experiences is reversible (e.g., in cases of hypokalemia). If the patient does wish to have the ICD deactivated and is competent, there is ethical justification for that decision as well (Ballentine, 2005). Members of the health care team have an obligation to respect the patient's goals and to encourage autonomy whenever appropriate.

Every patient, no matter where he or she is on the trajectory of HF and choice of care, needs to have an advanced directive completed. (Please refer to Chapter 4, with its discussion of the importance of advance directives.)

The patient, with the APN's support, will choose principally "live longer" or principally "feel better" care. Live-longer care emphasizes treatment to preserve cardiac function and decrease the ischemic burden, even if the treatments have risk or unpleasant side effects. Even in this mode, few cardiac diagnostic tests (beyond the physical examination) need to be repeated. Once the nature and cause of the pathophysiology leading to the development of HF have been identified, clinicians should focus on the clinical assessment and management of the patient (Hunt et al., 2005).

Diagnostic testing will be used mostly to monitor effects of medications. Blood counts, digoxin level, Coumadin (warfarin) effects (prothrombin time or international normalized ratio), and effects of diuretics on electrolytes, blood urea nitrogen, and creatinine may all need to be followed.

Many patients entering palliative care or hospice care are told by clinicians that there is nothing more that can be done. A more helpful approach may be to emphasize to the patient that the clinician is still able to help, in terms of providing pain control, comfort, and emotional support.

End-of-Life Care

For some patients and their families, the change from care emphasizing "live longer" to care emphasizing comfort and the best short-term functioning may be confusing, and the particulars will need to be discussed more than once. Everyone involved—the patient, all the people who matter to the patient, and the medical personnel—need to know the current game plan.

Is the patient truly done with acute hospitalizations, intensive investigation of any changes, and life support? Or would he or she, or some family member, still choose such measures or insist on them? If there is dissension in the group, can it be resolved in advance of an emergent situation?

Once these decisions are made, attention turns to management of the patient with the terminally failing heart. If the patient is still able to take oral medications, the medications will all be reviewed. Each medication must be evaluated in terms of whether it is being used for comfort, cure, or prevention.

Most of the medications used for advanced HF contribute to the patient's comfort by reducing symptoms and should be continued as long as possible.

ACEIs, β-blockers, and aldosterone inhibitors slow ventricular remodeling and improve symptoms (Davis et al., 2005) and should be continued. Diuretics, nitrates, and digoxin do not alter the course of HF by altering the neurohormonal response. However, they will also relieve symptoms and should be continued as well (Davis et al., 2005).

Opioids (e.g., morphine) should be continued if the patient is in pain or dyspneic. Opioids dilate pulmonary vasculature and help alleviate the dyspnea related to congestive HF (Abernethy, Currow, Frith et al., 2003; Davis et al., 2005). Intravenous inotropic agents, in some instances, may be indicated in palliative care as well (Davis et al., 2005).

HF cannot be cured, but other concurrent conditions may be. If the patient has a painful urinary tract, sinus, or lung infection, an antibiotic may be curative and also contribute to comfort. Depression and pain are also important symptoms in HF (Davis et al., 2005) and should be treated as well. Many patients report feeling better when thyroid conditions remain treated, and palliative care and end-of-life patients should be offered the same consideration.

When all of the patient's distressing symptoms are controlled, dying often appears to be an ongoing lessening of energy. The patient goes from having enough energy to stand and walk, to needing assistance with standing, to being unable to sit up, to being unable to turn in bed. Finally, the heart no longer beats and the lungs do not breathe.

During this time, the patient needs total care. He or she needs medication and food administered; repositioning to prevent the development of pressure ulcers; toileting; bathing; and, while conscious, amusement—and always company.

For a person who can no longer swallow and who has no established venous access, other routes to deliver medication are needed. The rectal, transdermal, subcutaneous, sublingual, and inhalation (aerosols) routes can all be effective. Many medications are available in rectal suppository form, and many oral medications can be given rectally with good effect, including slow-release morphine and diuretics.

A subcutaneous infusion of highly concentrated morphine, hydromorphone, lorazepam, or midazolam through a small needle works as effectively as an intravenous infusion, with much less fluid burden.

CONCLUSION

Because CVD is so prevalent, an APN can expect to see many such patients and can be a positive influence for each of them. APNs have a crucial role in collaborating with physicians and other members of the health care team to provide physical, psychosocial, and spiritual care for the cardiovascular patient.

REFERENCES

Abernethy, A.P., Currow, D.C., Frith, P., et al. (2003). Randomised, double blind, placebo controlled crossover trial of sustained release morphine for the management of refractory dyspnoea. *Br Med J, 327,* 523-528.

Albert, N.M. (2005). Cardiovascular. In K. Kuebler, M. Davis, & C. Moore (Eds.). *Palliative practice: An interdisciplinary approach.* St. Louis: Mosby.

Albert, N.M., Eastwood, C.A., & Edwards, M.L. (2004). Evidence-based practice for acute decompensated heart failure. *Crit Care Nurse, 24,* 14-29.

American College of Cardiology/American Heart Association. (2005). *Guideline update for the management of patients with chronic stable angina.* Retrieved March 11, 2006, from http://content.onlinejacc.org/cgi/reprint/46/6/e1.

American Heart Association. (2005). *Heart disease and stroke statistics: 2005 Update.* Dallas: Author.

Ballentine, J. (2005). Pacemaker and defibrillator deactivation in competent hospice patients: An ethical consideration. *Am J Hospice Palliat Med, 22,* 14-19.

Davis, M.P., Albert, N.M., & Young, J.B. (2005). Palliation of heart failure. *Am J Hospice Palliat Med, 22,* 211-222.

Fuster, V. (2004). Atherosclerosis, thrombosis, and vascular biology. In L. Goldman & D. Ausiello (Eds.). *Cecil textbook of medicine* (22nd ed., pp. 327-336). Philadelphia: Saunders.

Hauptman, P.J. & Havranek, E.P. (2005). Integrating palliative care into heart failure care. *Arch Int Med, 165,* 374-378.

Hunt S., Abraham, W., Chin, M., et al. (2005). ACC/AHA 2005 Guideline update for the diagnosis and management of chronic heart failure in the adult: A report of the American College of Cardiology/American Heart Association Task Force on Practice Guidelines, American College of Cardiology web site. Available at www.acc.org/clinical/guidelines/failure/index.pdf.

Koelling, T.M., Chen, R.S., Lubwama, R.N., et al. (2004) The expanding national burden of heart failure in the United States: The influence of heart failure in women. *Am Heart J, 147,* 74-78.

Marelli, A.J. (2004). Congenital heart disease in adults. In L. Goldman & D. Ausiello (Eds.). *Cecil textbook of medicine* (22nd ed., pp. 371-389). Philadelphia: Saunders.

Masoudi, F., Wang, Y., Inzucchi, S., et al. (2003). Melformin and thiazolidine dione use in Medicare patients with heart failure. *JAMA, 290(1),* 81-85.

McEntegart, M. & Gray, E. (2004). Assessing the patient with heart failure. In S. Stewart & L. Blue (Eds.). *Improving outcomes in chronic heart failure: Specialist nurse intervention from research to practice* (2nd ed.). London: BMJ Publishing.

McGavigan, A.D. & Dunn, F.G. (2004). Palliative medicine for patients with end-stage heart disease. In D. Doyle, G. Hanks, N.I. Cherny, & K. Calman (Eds.). *Oxford textbook of palliative medicine* (3rd ed., pp 917-922). Oxford: Oxford University Press.

Mestroni, L (2003). Genomic medicine and atrial fibrillation. *J Am Coll Cardiol, 41,* 2193-2196.

Murray, S.A., Boyd, K., Kendall, M., et al. (2002). Dying of lung cancer or cardiac failure: Prospective qualitative interview study of patients and their careers in the community. *Br Med J, 325,* 929-932.

Pina, I.L., Apstein, C.S., Balady, G.J., et al.; American Heart Association Committee on Exercise, Rehabilitation, and Prevention. (2003). Exercise and heart failure: A statement from the

American Heart Association Committee on Exercise, Rehabilitation, and Prevention. *Circulation, 107,* 1210-1225.

Stevenson, L.W. (2004). Diseases of the myocardium. In L. Goldman & D. Ausiello (Eds.). *Cecil textbook of medicine* (22nd ed., pp. 441-453) Philadelphia: Saunders.

Taylor, G. (2003). Heart disease. In G. Taylor & J. Kurent, J. (Eds.). *A clinician's guide to palliative care.* Malden, Mass: Lippincott, Williams & Wilkins.

Theroux, P. (2004). Angina pectoris. In L. Goldman & D. Ausiello (Eds.). *Cecil textbook of medicine* (22nd ed.). Philadelphia: Saunders.

Tsuyuki, R.T., McCelvie, R.S., Arnold, M.O., et al. (2001). Acute precipitants of congestive heart failure exacerbations. *Arch Intern Med, 161,* 2337-2342.

Wu, E.B. & Yu, C.M. (2005). Management of diastolic heart failure—A practical review of pathophysiology and treatment trial data. *Int J Clin Pract, 59,* 1239-1246.

CHAPTER 11

PULMONARY DISEASE

Kim K. Kuebler and Rhalene Gabuat Patajo

■

The increased prevalence of nonmalignant pulmonary disease is often underestimated because chronic obstructive pulmonary disease (COPD) is often underdiagnosed and poorly defined (Global Initiative for Chronic Obstructive Lung Disease [GOLD], 2005; Voelkel & Agusti, 2004). COPD is a major cause of morbidity and mortality throughout the world and is the fourth leading cause of death in the United States. In 2000, COPD was listed as the underlying cause of death for almost 119,000 American adults, which is a 67% increase compared with 52,000 deaths in 1980 (Centers for Disease Control and Prevention [CDC], 2002). By 2020, COPD is predicted to become the third leading cause of death in the United States and worldwide (GOLD, 2005; National Heart, Lung, and Blood Institute [NHLBI], 2001).

The increase in age-adjusted mortality rates for COPD between 1965 and 1998 distinguishes it from other diseases such as coronary heart disease or stroke, which have demonstrated a decrease in mortality rates over the same period of time (Anderson, 2002; Minino, Arias, Kochanek et al., 2002). COPD is the only leading cause of death in the United States for which the death rate is increasing (Doherty, 2005). The World Health Organization (WHO) estimates that 2.5 million deaths worldwide were the result of COPD in 2001 (WHO, 2003). In 2002 in the United States, the annual direct costs for COPD were more than $32 billion (Hilleman, Dewan, Malesker et al., 2000; NHLBI, 2002). Because of the morbidity and mortality associated with COPD, the economic implications of COPD in the United States are significant.

Of the estimated 24 million cases in the United States, less than 50% of these patients are given an accurate diagnosis of COPD (Mannino, Homa, Akinbami et al., 2002). The lack of proper diagnosis is fueled in part by clinical misconceptions of the demographics of this disease (Dransfield & Bailey, 2005). For the first time in history, the number of deaths in the United States from COPD was higher among women than among men in 2000, and the COPD death rate for women tripled from between 1980 and 2000 (CDC, 2002). In addition, the majority of COPD cases occur in patients younger than 65 years; in 2000, only 30% of reported cases occurred in older age groups. This evidence challenges the traditional assumption that COPD is a disease of the elderly male patient (CDC, 2003).

Pulmonary function and exercise abilities differ between geriatric and younger populations (Chan & Welsh, 1998). The elderly are susceptible to an increased risk of pulmonary disease over time, and the presentation of these diseases will differ in the middle-aged adult and the elderly (Chan & Welsh, 1998). The elderly patient will have less respiratory reserve to blunt a hypoxic or hypercarbic drive or to perceive the experience of dyspnea (Chan & Welsh, 1998). The burden of COPD in an increasingly aging society is likely only to increase, and so the importance of integrating palliative management for the myriad accompanying symptoms is critical.

DEFINITION

The current and widely accepted definition of COPD was proposed by WHO and NHLBI through an initiative identified as GOLD (2005). This collaborative project identified new guidelines for the diagnosis and treatment of COPD (Bramen & Peters, 2005). Prior to the GOLD guidelines, COPD was defined as a disease process caused by chronic bronchitis and emphysema. This definition has been replaced by new information suggesting that COPD is a result of airflow limitation—a reaction to the abnormal inflammatory response in the lungs from prolonged exposure to noxious gases. The American Thoracic Society (ATS) and the European Respiratory Society (ERS) offer a joint definition of COPD identical to the GOLD guidelines, describing COPD as "a preventable and treatable disease state characterized by airflow limitation that is not fully reversible" (ATS, 2004). "Airflow limitation is usually progressive and is associated with an abnormal inflammatory response of the lungs to noxious particles of gases primarily caused by cigarette smoking" (ATS, 2004). Although the new GOLD definition for COPD no longer identifies this disease as an irreversible process, both guidelines recommend the use of staging criteria to prognosticate COPD, ranging from "at risk" to "very severe" disease (ATS, 2004; GOLD, 2005). However, COPD is considered a progressive disease, and the goal of care is often to reduce the progression of disability and symptoms.

COPD encompasses both chronic bronchitis and emphysema. Chronic bronchitis occurs in most patients with COPD in the earlier phases of the disease, whereas emphysema is less common and often presents much later in the course of disease, accompanied by significant symptom burden (cachexia, dyspnea, fatigue, etc.). Chronic bronchitis is defined by the ATS/ERS guidelines as "chronic productive cough, lasting for three months over two successive years in a patient in whom other causes of productive cough have been excluded" (ATS, 2004). Emphysema is further defined as "permanent enlargement of the airspaces distal to the terminal bronchioles, accompanied by destruction of the walls of the alveoli without obvious fibrosis" (ATS, 2004).

THE COPD PATIENT

Many clinicians hold stereotypical views on the "typical" COPD patient as being elderly and male. The validity of this traditional approach to COPD was analyzed through a retrospective study of more than 2100 COPD patients managed by the National Jewish Medical and Research Center (Tinkelman & Corsello, 2003). This study was designed to evaluate the socioeconomic, demographic, and resource utilization of current COPD patients. The investigators concluded that COPD patients are younger than previously identified and are typically described by the following characteristics:

- Continues to smoke cigarettes despite having moderate to severe disease
- Just as likely to be female (52.7%) as male (47.3%)
- Older than 40 years
- Just as likely to be employed as unemployed

- Just as likely to be younger than 65 years (49.7%) as to be older than 65 years (50.3%)
- Is not diagnosed in the early stages of disease
- Has increased use of health care services compared to same-age individuals in the general population (Doherty, 2005; Tinkelman & Corsello, 2003)

The diagnosis of COPD has been historically assigned to patients who have emphysema, chronic bronchitis, or a mixture of the two. Many patients will complain of having increased dyspnea over several years and are positive for chronic cough, poor exercise tolerance, and evidence of airway obstruction such as overinflated lungs and poor gas exchange (West, 2003). Appropriate diagnosis, therefore, is absolutely essential when effectively managing a specific pulmonary disease.

ETIOLOGY AND PATHOPHYSIOLOGY

The classic epidemiologic studies of Fletcher and Peto (1977) revealed that death and disability from COPD were related to an accelerated decline in lung function over time, with a loss of more than 50 mL per year in the forced expiratory volume over 1 second (FEV_1) compared with a normal loss of approximately 20 mL per year. A reduction in FEV_1 in the face of progressive disease over time contributes to increased dyspnea on exertion and slowly advances to respiratory failure (Barnes, 2004).

There is considerable debate regarding the reasons for the accelerated loss of FEV_1 and its relation to the pathogenesis of COPD. However, there are four major mechanisms that have been implicated (Barnes, 2004):

1. Loss of elasticity and the destruction of the alveolar attachments of airways during expiration
2. Increased cholinergic bronchomotor tone in the airways via release of acetylcholine by way of the parasympathetic nervous system
3. Narrowing of small airways as a result of inflammation and scarring
4. Mucus blocking of small airways

All four of these mechanisms can interact with one another and are often induced from cigarette smoking and the inhalation of noxious particles. Narrowing of the small airways results in hyperinflation of the lungs and air trapping contributing to dyspnea and cough (Barnes, 2004). The structural changes that occur in the aging lung and chest wall produce predictable alterations in pulmonary function tests. The elderly patient will tend to have a decrease in his or her vital capacity, which is a direct result of the following (Chan & Welsh, 1998):

- Increased chest wall stiffness (muscle atrophy, weakness, arthritis, etc.)
- Loss of elastic recoil of the lung and supportive connective tissue
- Decreased respiratory force generated by respiratory muscles

Obstructive and Restrictive Airway Disease

The differentiations in obstructive and restrictive airway diseases are often blurred and may give rise to the difficulties in definition, diagnosis, and management of specific diseases (i.e., asthma, COPD, bronchitis, emphysema, and malignancies). Obstructive airway disease is an increased resistance to airflow and can be caused by conditions that occur inside the pulmonary lumen, within the wall of the airway, and/or in the peribronchial region (West, 2003). Airway lumen, for example, may be blocked by excessive secretions often found in patients with chronic bronchitis. Other examples of airway lumen blockage include a partially occluded lumen from pulmonary edema, aspiration of a foreign object, or any substance that creates a partial or complete blockage within the airway lumen (West, 2003).

Disease that affects the internal wall of the airway includes the contraction of the bronchial smooth muscle that occurs in asthma as a result of the inflammatory process of the airway epithelium. Hypertrophy of the mucus glands that accompanies chronic bronchitis can also interfere with airway obstruction within the lumen (West, 2003). Prolonged exposure to noxious gas contributes to the destruction of the lung parenchyma, which causes a loss of the radial traction of the connective tissues within the lung and consequent airway narrowing (West, 2003).

Cigarette smoke accounts for more than 90% of cases of COPD in developed countries; however, COPD occurs in only a minority of smokers (10% to 20%), indicating individual variations in susceptibility to this disease (Barnes, 2004). Research in this area is ongoing and includes evaluation of patient-specific phenotype, pathologic mediators of disease, involved cellular mechanisms, and newly identified environmental factors.

Emphysema

Emphysema is characterized by an enlargement of the air spaces (alveoli) distal to the terminal bronchiole with associated airway lumen destruction (West, 2003). The associated loss of elasticity and the destruction of the alveolar attachments in the lung promote narrow airways and air trapping (hyperinflation) (Barnes, 2004). Cigarette smoke may stimulate the neutrophil to release excessive amounts of the enzyme lysosomal elastase. This results in the destruction of elastin, an important structural protein in the lung (West, 2003). Neutrophil elastase also binds to type IV collagen, an important molecule that influences the strength of the pulmonary capillary and the integrity of the alveolar wall (West, 2003).

Chronic Bronchitis

This disease is associated with an excessive production of mucus secretions within the bronchial tree. Hypertrophy of the mucus glands in the large airway and chronic inflammation of the airway contribute to airway narrowing—a result of lumen thickening, inflammation, and scarring in the small airways (West, 2003). In chronic bronchitis, excessive amounts of mucus are found in the airways, and thickened mucus may occlude some small bronchi (West, 2003). Small airways are narrowed and show inflammatory changes that include cellular infiltration and airway edema. Granulation tissue and peribronchial fibrosis occur over time (West, 2003).

Asthma

Asthma is an inflammatory response of the airways to various stimuli (antigens) that potentiate airway narrowing. The airways of an asthmatic patient respond to stimuli by hypertrophied smooth muscle that contracts and produces bronchoconstriction. The bronchial airway contains hypertrophy of the mucus glands and edema of the bronchial wall with an increased integration of eosinophils and lymphocytes (West, 2003).

Restrictive Disease

Restrictive diseases are those in which the expansion of the lung is restricted because of alterations in the lung parenchyma or because of disease of the pleura, chest wall, or neuromuscular apparatus. They are characterized by a reduced vital capacity and a small resting lung volume, but the airway resistance is not increased. It is important to note that restrictive and obstructive conditions can be present concurrently.

- **Diffuse interstitial pulmonary fibrosis** Thickening of the interstitium of the alveolar wall may be caused by an immunologic reaction. The patient presents with dyspnea, rapid and shallow breathing, and an irritating, unproductive cough.
- **Sarcoidosis** Granulomatous tissue is present in several organs (lymph nodes, lungs, skin, eyes, liver, spleen, etc.). Fibrotic changes in the alveolar walls are seen, and pulmonary fibrosis and cor pulmonale may develop.
- **Hypersensitivity pneumonitis** This occurs with exposure to inhaled organic dusts. Fibrotic changes occur in advanced cases, and the patient is frequently dyspneic.
- **Interstitial disease caused by drugs, poisons, radiation** Busulfan, nitrofurantoin, amiodarone, bleomycin, antineoplastic drugs, and oxygen may cause an acute pulmonary reaction, which can proceed to interstitial fibrosis. Therapeutic radiation causes acute pneumonitis followed by fibrosis.
- **Collagen disease** Interstitial fibrosis may be found in patients with generalized scleroderma, systemic lupus erythematosus, or rheumatoid arthritis.
- **Lymphangitis carcinomatosa** Spread of carcinoma tissue through pulmonary lymphatics leads to prominent dyspnea.
- **Pneumothorax** This occurs in a variety of conditions, including rupture of a bulla in COPD, rupture of a cyst in advanced fibrotic disease, or during mechanical ventilation with high airway pressures, and often precipitates breathlessness/dyspnea.
- **Pleural effusion** Fluid in the pleural space frequently accompanies serious disease, and the patient often reports dyspnea if the effusion is large.
- **Scoliosis** Bone deformities can cause an increased work of breathing.
- **Ankylosing spondylitis** Gradual immobility of the vertebral joints and fixation of the ribs result in reduced movement of the chest wall.
- **Neuromuscular disorders** Poliomyelitis, Guillain-Barré syndrome, amyotrophic lateral sclerosis, myasthenia gravis, and muscular dystrophies affect the muscles or nerves of respiration (West, 2003).

HISTORY AND PHYSICAL EXAMINATION

History

Diagnosing and managing advanced pulmonary disease require a history of exposure to risk factors that contribute to airflow limitation with or without symptoms (GOLD, 2005). COPD, however, should be considered in any patient who has had cough, sputum production, or dyspnea and who smokes or is exposed to noxious gases (Table 11-1).

TABLE 11-1 ■ COPD Patient History Taking

	Signs and Symptoms
Chronic cough	Intermittent or every other day
	Occurs throughout the day
	Rarely occurs only during nocturnal hours
Chronic sputum production	Any pattern of chronic sputum production
Dyspnea	Progressive (worsens over time)
	Persistent, daily
	Patient complains of an increased effort to breathe
	Unable to exercise
	Worse during respiratory infections
Risk factors	Tobacco smoke
	Occupational dusts and chemicals
	Smoke from home cooking, heating fuels

From Global Initiative for Chronic Obstructive Lung Disease (GOLD). (2005). *Global strategy for the diagnosis, management, and prevention of chronic obstructive pulmonary disease.* Bethesda: U.S. Department of Health and Human Services, Public Health Services, National Institutes of Health, National Heart, Lung and Blood Institute.

Patient history should include an evaluation of clinical symptoms; these symptoms are often present and ignored for many years before the development of airflow limitation. However, for a patient with a new diagnosis of COPD, a detailed medical history should also include:

- Past medical history of asthma, allergies, sinusitis, frequent respiratory infections in childhood, nasal polyps, and/or other respiratory difficulties in the adult patient
- Family history of COPD, α-1 deficiency, or other chronic respiratory diseases
- Pattern of symptom development that would include age of onset, dyspnea in colder temperatures, with physical exertion, aggravating/relieving factors, and so on
- History of respiratory exacerbations and/or frequent hospitalizations
- Concomitant comorbidities such as respiratory infections, ischemic heart disease, hypertension, congestive heart failure, or asthma (Kesten, 2001)
- Review of current medications (β-blockers are contraindicated in COPD patients)
- Patient-perceived quality of life
- Whether social and family support are available
- Reduction of risk factors (GOLD, 2005)

As patients develop moderate to severe COPD (FEV_1 less than 50%), they often present with

- Sleep apnea or nocturnal O_2 desaturation
- Pulmonary hypertension with exertion (exercise)
- Hypercarbia
- Weight loss, muscle wasting (cachexia)
- Increased incidence of depression
- Pulmonary hyperinflation (on chest radiograph) (Voelkel & Agusti, 2004)

Physical Examination

Objective evaluation of the COPD patient may vary from patient to patient, but common findings often include the following (GOLD, 2005):

- Central cyanosis or a bluish, pale discoloration of the mucous membranes
- Chest wall structural abnormalities that resemble a "barrel-shaped" chest, horizontal ribs, and/or protruding abdomen
- Reduction in cardiac dullness, difficulty in auscultation heart apex beat, due to pulmonary hyperinflation (best auscultated over the xiphoid area)
- Resting shallow respiratory rate of 20 breaths per minute, reduced breath sounds
- Prolonged expiratory effort, pursed lip breathing, and use of accessory muscles to breathe

DIAGNOSTICS

It is important to efficiently decide and administer diagnostics that will not add further symptom burden to the pulmonary patient, bearing in mind that a major differential diagnosis for COPD is asthma. In patients with chronic asthma, a clear distinction from COPD is not possible by using current imaging and physiological diagnostics (GOLD, 2005). It is assumed that both COPD and asthma coexist in this patient population. Other differential diagnoses are easier to differentiate from COPD (GOLD, 2005).

Because COPD is a progressive disease, the monitoring of pulmonary function through spirometry is ideal when evaluating worsening of disease. Evaluating arterial blood gas measurement is recommended for patients with a FEV_1 less than 40% predicted or if respiratory failure or right-side heart failure is present. This should be considered only in the patient who is seeking aggressive interventions and not in the patient seeking only symptom management. Chest radiographs and spirometry may be the only diagnostic measurements needed in the palliative care setting to discern changes in pulmonary function. A complete blood cell count with differential can also identify dyspnea that is related to anemia. It is important to note that polycythemia (hematocrit greater than 55%) can develop in the presence of atrial hypoxemia and in patients who currently smoke (GOLD, 2005).

PHARMACOLOGIC INTERVENTIONS

Several guidelines have been established to help clinicians treat patients with COPD. As previously mentioned, major treatment guidelines have been endorsed by organizations such as GOLD and ATS/ERS. According to these organizations, the goals of COPD treatment should include the following (ATS, 2004; GOLD, 2005):

- Prevent disease progression
- Relieve symptoms of dyspnea and improve airflow limitation and lung function
- Improve exercise tolerance
- Improve quality of life
- Prevent and/or treat complications
- Prevent and/or treat exacerbations
- Reduce mortality

Currently, there is no treatment modality available to stop the progression of this irreversible disease. Because smoking is the leading cause of approximately 90% of all cases of COPD, smoking cessation is recommended to slow down disease progression (Decramer, 2005). Long-term oxygen therapy, used properly, has been shown to decrease mortality. However, because no treatment actually stops disease progression, the major focus in COPD treatment is to treat the symptoms and complications associated with the disease, to improve health status, and to improve exercise tolerance (GOLD, 2005).

There are several classes of drugs that are used to treat COPD: anticholinergics, β-agonists, steroids, theophylline, and others. Treatments are also available that combine different drug classes into one convenient form. The major COPD guidelines have recommended specific uses for each of the classes based on the patient's disease severity, as measured by airflow limitation (FEV_1).

Inhaled medications are preferred for COPD, to deliver the drug directly to the site of action and to minimize the systemic side effects. This is particularly important in elderly patients who may have comorbid conditions. However, it is ultimately patient factors such as tolerability, convenience, proper inhaler technique, and cost that drive the choice of medications (Dolovich, Ahrens, Hess et al., 2005).

Anticholinergics

Because cholinergic activity is an important and distinctive feature in COPD, anticholinergics are recommended as first-line treatment in national and international COPD guidelines (GOLD, 2005; ATS, 2004). Anticholinergics decrease bronchoconstriction, decrease mucus secretion, and decrease bronchial vasodilation, thereby decreasing the symptoms of dyspnea and cough.

For several decades, only short-acting anticholinergics have been available, with ipratropium being the agent most commonly used. Tiotropium became the first long-acting anticholinergic agent approved for once-daily administration. All anticholinergics affect the muscarinic receptors in the airways. Tiotropium, however, has specific selectivity for the M_1 and M_3 receptors, providing long duration of action. Tiotropium has shown to improve lung function, improve dyspnea, reduce COPD exacerbations and related hospitalizations, and improve health-related quality of life (Barr, Bourbeau, Camargo et al., 2005).

Anticholinergics are available in metered-dose inhalers, dry powder inhalers, and nebulized forms. Short-acting anticholinergics can be given as needed for symptom relief or on a regular basis to prevent exacerbations, whereas long-acting anticholinergics are used as maintenance therapy to prevent exacerbations.

With anticholinergics, the most common side effect is dry mouth. This may be particularly pronounced in the elderly COPD patient, although this side effect decreases over time, allowing the patient to maintain therapy without the need for withdrawal (Tashkin & Cooper, 2004).

β-Agonists

As bronchodilators, β-agonists are also recommended as first-line treatment for COPD. β-Agonists cause bronchodilation indirectly by blocking the adrenergic receptors found on airway smooth muscle. β-Agonists improve lung function, decrease symptoms, improve exercise-induced dyspnea, decrease exacerbations, and increase health-related quality of life (Sin, McAlister, Man et al., 2003).

Short-acting and long-acting β-agonists are available in metered-dose inhalers, dry-powder inhalers, solutions for nebulization, and other combinations. For patients with intermittent episodes of dyspnea or COPD exacerbations, short-acting β-agonists may be used. Long-acting β-agonists may be used as an option for convenient maintenance therapy.

Tremor and tachycardia are a class effect of β-agonist use and are unlikely to be problematic unless the patient has preexisting heart conditions (Tashkin, 2005). Tremors can be most troublesome in older patients and may limit the dose that is tolerated (GOLD, 2005).

Corticosteroids

The exact mechanism is unknown, but corticosteroids work by affecting the inflammation cascade in COPD, although the inflammation in COPD is not completely suppressed by corticosteroids. This may be due to the fact that corticosteroids prolong the survival of neutrophils rather than suppress the neutrophilic inflammation in COPD (Barnes, 2000).

There are several forms of treatment with corticosteroids: oral, nebulized, and inhaled. Due to the side effect profile of oral corticosteroids, clinicians are encouraged to use the least amount for the shortest period of time (approximately 2 weeks) and then to transition to an inhaled corticosteroid for maintenance treatment if the patient is classified as severe or for very severely affected patients who experience frequent exacerbations (GOLD, 2005).

Oral corticosteroids have demonstrated a beneficial effect in treating acute exacerbations of COPD, improving clinical outcome and reducing the length of hospitalization. The reasons for this discrepancy between the responses to corticosteroids in acute and chronic COPD may be related to differences in the inflammatory response (e.g., increased numbers of eosinophils) or airway edema in exacerbations (Barnes, 2000).

According to COPD guidelines, inhaled corticosteroids should be reserved for the more severe patients in late-stage COPD (GOLD, 2005). The benefit of inhaled corticosteroids has not been established with regard to FEV_1 or hyperinflation. There is, however, a benefit seen in reducing exacerbations, thus acknowledging its place in treating more severe patients who experience an increased number of exacerbations.

When using corticosteroids, caution is warranted with regard to adverse effects. The most common adverse effects include oral thrush (with inhaled formulations), dysphonia (with inhaled formulations), and skin bruising (Man & Sin, 2005). In general, use of inhaled corticosteroids appears to be relatively safe compared with prolonged courses of oral corticosteroids, especially patients with more severe COPD who may find that the benefits outweigh the side effect risks (Calverley, 2005).

Theophylline

Even with the availability of new and more tolerable medications for COPD, theophylline is still widely used. Although the exact mechanism is unknown, theophylline improves lung function and ventilatory capacity by causing dilatation of the small airways and improves arterial blood gas tensions with effects on respiratory muscles (Ram, 2005).

The role for theophylline is established in asthma but is not fully defined in COPD, as only very small studies have been done. It is generally reserved as a last resort, according to guideline recommendations for theophylline and other xanthine derivatives (GOLD, 2005). It may benefit patients who remain symptomatic after the failure of first-line therapy.

Due to a very narrow therapeutic index, close laboratory monitoring is needed with theophylline therapy. Theophylline is associated with dose-related adverse effects, including nausea, vomiting, seizures, and arrhythmias. If a patient must be treated with theophylline, benefits must outweigh the risks of side effects and possible drug interactions (Rennard, 2004).

Opioids

Opioids are commonly used to treat dyspnea and pain in patients with advanced lung disease. As COPD progresses to more severe COPD, dyspnea may often be debilitating and opioids have been used to suppress the sensation of dyspnea in the patient with chronic, stable COPD. The possible mechanisms of action of opioids include reduction in the central perception of dyspnea (similar to the reduction in the central perception of pain), reduction in anxiety associated with dyspnea, reduction in sensitivity to hypercapnia, reduction in oxygen consumption, and improved cardiovascular function (Jennings, Davies, Higgins, et al., 2002).

Oral, parenteral, and nebulized opioids have been used to treat dyspnea and pain. However, available data support only the use of oral and parenteral formulations due to potential respiratory depression and worsening hypercapnia. Nebulized opioids should be discouraged, as current data do not support their use (Foral, Malesker, Huerta et al., 2004; GOLD, 2005).

Anxiolytics

The role of anxiety in dyspnea remains unclear. Many patients report anxiety concurrent with the feeling of breathlessness. Dyspnea can lead to anxiety, and anxiety can exacerbate dyspnea. Although anxiolytics (e.g., benzodiazepines) are commonly prescribed for anxiety related to dyspnea, the evidence for their effectiveness is not very persuasive (Thomas & von Gunten, 2002). Treatment of anxiety does have a role in a subset of patients for whom it is a significant source of distress, and benzodiazepines can be safely prescribed for those patients at appropriate doses (Thomas & von Gunten, 2002).

NONPHARMACOLOGIC INTERVENTIONS

Smoking Cessation

Patients with COPD and patients who are at risk for COPD should be encouraged to stop smoking. Although the damage may continue to progress, smoking cessation has proved to slow the rate of decline in lung function (Decramer, 2005). As illustrated in Fletcher and Peto (1977), even patients who are in the more severe stages of COPD should be encouraged to stop smoking as they may benefit from decreased symptoms and possible prolongation of life.

Influenza Vaccine

Viral infections are a major cause of COPD exacerbations and are associated with increased mortality. Influenza vaccination has been reported to reduce serious illness and death in COPD patients by 50%. It is imperative for patients with COPD and for patients at risk to receive the influenza vaccine every year, and this is recommended in the GOLD guidelines (GOLD, 2005). Doing so will decrease the frequency of exacerbations and decrease mortality in this already vulnerable population.

Pneumococcal Vaccination

The usefulness of the pneumococcal vaccine has not been clearly shown, although it has been suggested (Rennard, 2004). Because elderly patients are at increased risk of hospitalizations and pneumonia, the pneumococcal vaccine should be also be considered (Rennard, 2004; Sin et al., 2003).

Oxygen

Long-term administration of oxygen (>15 hours per day) has been shown to improve quality of life and increase survival in patients with severe COPD and chronic hypoxemia (Sin et al., 2003). The primary goal is to increase the baseline PaO_2 to at least 8.0 kPa (60 mm Hg) at sea level and rest and/or produce an SaO_2 of at least 90%, which will provide adequate delivery of oxygen to preserve vital organ function (GOLD, 2005).

Other

Pulmonary rehabilitation and exercise are useful interventions to improve dyspnea and physical deconditioning. Other useful interventions can include positioning, relaxation techniques, and patient and family education.

CONCLUSION

The management of pulmonary disease can be complicated. Proper diagnosis is imperative when treating pulmonary disease, as there are many forms of obstructive and restrictive diseases. Although many medications are available, the treatment approach must be personalized since interpatient variability is common. Proper treatment may require the combination of drugs from several classes and the inclusion of nonpharmacologic interventions to treat symptoms, prevent exacerbations, improve quality of life, and reduce mortality.

REFERENCES

American Thoracic Society. (2004). *Standards for the diagnosis and treatment of patients with chronic obstructive pulmonary disease.* Retrieved May 10, 2005, from www.thoracic.org/COPD.
Anderson, R.N. (2002). Deaths: Leading causes for 2000. *National Vital Statistics Report, 50,* 1-85.
Barnes, P. (2000). Chronic obstructive pulmonary disease. *N Engl J Med, 343,* 269-280.
Barnes, P. (2004). Small airways in COPD. *N Engl J Med, 350,* 2635-2637.
Barr, R., Bourbeau, J., Camargo, C., et al. (2005). Inhaled tiotropium for stable chronic pulmonary disease. *Cochrane Database Syst Rev, 2,* CD002876.

Bramen, S. & Peters, S. (2005). COPD: Will early detection and aggressive intervention control disease progression. *CE Today Nurse Prac, 4,* 7-16.

Calverley, P. (2005). The role of corticosteroids in chronic obstructive pulmonary disease. *Semin Resp Crit Care Med, 26,* 235-245.

Centers for Disease Control and Prevention. (2002). Centers for Disease Control and Prevention. *MMWR: Surveill Summ, 51,* SS-6.

Centers for Disease Control and Prevention. (2003). Centers for Disease Control and Prevention: MMWR series on public health and aging. *MMWR: Recomm Rep, 52,* 101-124.

Chan, E. & Welsh, C. (1998). Geriatric respiratory medicine. *Chest, 114,* 1704-1733.

Decramer, M. (2005). Effects of treatments on the progression of COPD: Report of a workshop held in Leuven, 11-12 March 2004. *Thorax, 60,* 343-349.

Doherty, D. (2005). COPD: A contemporary overview. *Clinical Advisor: A Suppl Clin Adv, January,* 2-9.

Dolovich, M., Ahrens, R., Hess, D., et al.; American College of Chest Physicians; American College of Asthma, Allergy, and Immunology. (2005). Device selection and outcomes of aerosol therapy: Evidence-based guidelines. *Chest, 127,* 335-371.

Dransfield, M. & Bailey, W. (2005). Maintenance pharmacotherapy of chronic obstructive pulmonary disease: An evidence-based approach. *Exp Opin Pharmacother, 6,* 13-25.

Fletcher, C. & Peto, R. (1977). The natural history of chronic airflow obstruction. *Br Med J, 1,* 645-648.

Foral, P., Malesker, M., Huerta, G., et al. (2004). Nebulized opioids use in COPD. *Chest, 125,* 691-694.

Global Initiative for Chronic Obstructive Lung Disease (GOLD). (2005). *Global strategy for the diagnosis, management, and prevention of chronic obstructive pulmonary disease.* Bethesda: U.S. Department of Health and Human Services, Public Health Services, National Institutes of Health, National Heart, Lung and Blood Institute.

Hilleman, D., Dewan, N., Malesker, M., et al. (2000). Pharmacoeconomic evaluation of COPD. *Chest, 118,* 1278-1285.

Jennings, A.L., Davies, A.N., Higgins, J.P., et al. (2002). A systematic review of the use of opioids in the management of dyspnea. *Thorax, 57,* 939-944.

Kesten, S. (2001). Chronic obstructive pulmonary disease in a managed-care setting. *Dis Manage Health Outcomes, 9,* 589-599.

Man, S. & Sin, D. (2005). Inhaled corticosteroids in chronic obstructive pulmonary disease: Is there a clinical benefit? *Drugs, 65,* 579-591.

Mannino, D.M., Homa, D.M., Akinbami, L.J., et al. (2002). Chronic obstructive pulmonary disease surveillance—United States, 1971-2000. *MMWR: Surveill Summ, 51,* 1-16.

Minino, A., Arias, E., Kochanek, K., et al. (2002). Deaths: Final data for 2000. *Nat Vital Stat Rep, 50,* 1-119.

National Heart, Lung, and Blood Institute. (2001). *Data fact sheet. Chronic obstructive pulmonary disease (COPD).* Bethesda: U.S. Department of Health and Human Services, Public Health Service, National Institutes of Health.

National Heart, Lung, and Blood Institute. (2002). *2002 Morbidity and mortality: Chartbook on cardiovascular, lung and blood disease.* Bethesda: U.S. Department of Health and Human Services, Public Health Service, National Institutes of Health.

Ram, F. (2005). Efficacy of theophylline in people with stable COPD: A systematic review and meta-analysis. *Respir Med, 99,* 135-144.

Rennard, S. (2004). Treatment of stable chronic obstructive pulmonary disease. *The Lancet, 364,* 794-802.

Sin, D., McAlister, F., Man, S., et al. (2003). Contemporary management of chronic obstructive pulmonary disease: Scientific review. *JAMA, 290,* 2301-2312.

Tashkin, D. (2005). Is a long-acting bronchodilator the first agent to use in stable chronic obstructive pulmonary disease? *Curr Opin in Pulm Med, 11,* 121-128.

Tashkin, D. & Cooper, C. (2004). The role of long-acting bronchodilators in the management of stable COPD. *Chest, 125,* 249-259.

Thomas, J. & von Gunten, C. (2002). Clinical management of dyspnea. *Lancet Oncol, 3,* 223-228.

Tinkelman, D. & Corsello, P. (2003). Chronic obstructive pulmonary disease: The impact occurs earlier than we think. *Am J Managed Care, 9,* 767-771.

Voelkel, N. & Agusti, A. (2004). COPD at the 2004 9th European Pulmonary Summit. *Pulm Pharmacol Ther, 17,* 249-251.

West, J. (2003) *Pulmonary pathophysiology: The essentials* (6th ed.). Philadelphia, Lippincott Williams & Wilkins.

World Health Organization. (2003). *World health report.* Geneva, Author. Retrieved May 10, 2005, fromwww.who.int/mip/2003/other_documents/en/causesofdeath.pdf.

CHAPTER 12

HEPATIC DISEASE

Pamela Sue Spencer

■

This chapter specifically highlights hepatic failure and discusses the crucial role that acetaminophen metabolism plays as a causative agent in toxic liver injury. Distinctively, the liver is a highly vascular and vital organ that has an extensive capacity and operates with complexity within the human body. The liver is involved in numerous biochemical pathways that affect growth, immunological defense, and regulation of homeostasis and is the major site of substance detoxification. As a consequence, it represents the major processing center for medications, environmental toxins, and other substances.

ETIOLOGY AND PATHOPHYSIOLOGY

Cirrhosis of the liver represents the final common pathway of many hepatic disorders characterized by chronic cellular destruction. An intervening stage of increased fibrosis is followed by formation of parenchymal regenerative nodules. It is the nodular distortion of the lobules and vascular network that defines cirrhosis and ultimately plays a critical part in the development of portal hypertension (Fitz, 2003). The cellular and biochemical events leading to this altered growth response and resulting architectural distortion are not well characterized (Yamada, 1998). Cirrhosis accounts for over 40,000 deaths each year in the United States and more than 228,145 years of potential life lost. The average patient with alcoholic liver disease loses 12 years of productive life, a much larger loss than that for heart disease (2 years) and cancer (4 years) (Fitz, 2003).

Causes of Cirrhosis

Common causes are (1) ethanol, (2) chronic hepatitis C virus infection, and (3) chronic hepatitis B virus infection with or without hepatitis D virus infection.

Infrequent causes are (1) primary biliary cirrhosis, (2) primary sclerosing cholangitis, (3) secondary biliary cirrhosis, (4) autoimmune hepatitis, (5) hemochromatosis, and (6) cryptogenic cirrhosis.

Rare causes are (1) Wilson disease, (2) α_1-antitrypsin deficiency, (3) small bowel bypass, (4) methotrexate, (5) amiodarone, (6) methyldopa, (7) cystic fibrosis, (8) sarcoidosis, (9) glycogen storage disease, and (10) hypervitaminosis A.

Malignancy can be a cause of end-stage hepatic disease and is often potentiated by the risk factors associated with hepatitis B, hepatitis C, chronic hepatitis B infection, cirrhosis, hemochromatosis, and ingestion of estrogens and androgens. The progression of disease occurs via direct extension within or from around the liver. Tumors typically alter blood flow within the liver, resulting in the rapid spread of tumor.

In patients with advanced disease, pneumonia, hepatic failure, and hemorrhage are frequently the cause of death. Tamponade can occur within the liver and lead to necrosis and rupture, and ultimately hemorrhage. If left untreated, death can occur in approximately 6 to 8 weeks.

Hepatic failure can also take the form of a rejected liver transplant. Obviously, these patients and families come to palliative care with unique issues. While the end-stage symptoms of cirrhosis and liver failure are the same, the meaning of the illness for the patient and family is important to recognize, explore, and incorporate into the individual plan of care.

Acetaminophen

The majority of medications used in the palliative care setting are metabolized through the liver (Bernard & Bruera, 2000; Kuebler et al., 2003). If used inappropriately, many of these medications can cause liver injury; acetaminophen poisoning is the most common medication cause of liver failure in the United States (Litovitz, Watson, & Klein-Schwartz, 2000). Acetaminophen (N-acetyl-p-aminophenol, paracetamol, or APAP) is the most popular over-the-counter (OTC) analgesic used in the United States and is reported as one of the most common toxic exposures reported to poison control centers nationwide (Hung & Nelson, 2000). Acetaminophen has been available since 1950 and is widely used in its single and compound formulas in both OTC and prescription medications. This drug is used for a variety of pain syndromes in both long-term care and palliative care settings, which can attribute to chronic use.

Acetaminophen use was identified by the American College of Rheumatology (2000) and the American Geriatrics Society (1998) as the analgesic of choice for the treatment and management of osteoarthritis. Numerous studies have identified that the U.S. population is living longer and often experiencing chronic pain syndromes that potentiate an increased vulnerability to drug-induced hepatic injury, while at the same time necessitating medical treatment for pain conditions that warrant aggressive symptom control. Hepatic injury with acetaminophen can occur with chronic use over time at lower doses (<4 g/day), particularly in the presence of other predisposing factors (McClain, Price, Barve et al., 1999). Therefore, the influence of advanced age in conjunction with the management of treating symptoms can pose an increased risk for liver toxicity. Age-related hepatic and renal dysfunction can lead to higher drug concentrations—a result of reduced drug metabolism and excretion capacities (Jakobsson, Klevsgard, & Westergen, 2003).

Causes of Acetaminophen Toxicity

Liver damage from excessive acetaminophen ingestion can occur in four circumstances (Lee, 2003):

- Excessive intake of acetaminophen
- Excessive cytochrome P450 activity due to inductions by chronic alcohol or other drug use
- Decreased capacity for glucuronidation or sulfation
- Depletion of glutathione stores due to malnutrition or chronic alcohol ingestion

A number of other factors can influence the propensity of acetaminophen to cause hepatotoxicity, including comorbid diseases and the patient's age, genetic background, and/or nutritional status. Food and dietary regimens high in protein can enhance the activity of the cytochrome P450 system as it relates to pharmaceutical utilization. Protein can increase the potential for converting a specific drug to its toxic metabolite (Lee, 2003). These metabolites can mediate toxicity close to or within the tissue where they are generated—creating additional tissue injury (Meyer, 2001). Numerous studies have also correlated a strong association between the age of the patient and the number of medications prescribed, all adding to the complexity of pharmaceutical biotransformation (see Chapter 7). It is important for the advanced practice nurse to appreciate that the physiologic changes associated with aging within the liver alter the pharmacokinetics of many drugs, including frequently used analgesics such as acetaminophen (Beckman, 2002). This predisposes the elderly to an increased risk of adverse drug events.

ASSOCIATED SYMPTOMS

Clinical manifestations of end-stage liver disease follow a similar pattern despite the causative etiology. Early indications of disease are often vague and include gastrointestinal symptoms such as anorexia, indigestion, nausea, vomiting, constipation, diarrhea, and complaints of dull, diffuse abdominal pain. The major symptoms that often accompany the early manifestations of this disease occur as a result of hepatic insufficiency and portal hypertension and may lead to the following organ system abnormalities (Isselbacher & Podolsky, 2004):

- **Respiratory** Pleural effusion and limited thoracic expansion due to abdominal ascites interfering with efficient gas exchange and eventual hypoxia
- **Central nervous system** Progressive symptoms of hepatic encephalopathy: lethargy, mental changes, slurred speech, asterixis, peripheral neuritis, paranoia, hallucinations, extreme obtundation, and coma
- **Endocrine** Testicular atrophy, menstrual irregularities, gynecomastia, and loss of chest and axillary hair
- **Skin** Severe pruritus, extreme dryness, poor tissue turgor, abnormal pigmentation, spider angiomas, palm erythema, and possibly jaundice
- **Hepatic** Jaundice, hepatomegaly, ascites, edema of legs, hepatic encephalopathy, and hepatorenal syndrome, comprising the other major effects of full-fledged cirrhosis

Additional symptoms can include a musty (acetone) breath, enlarged superficial abdominal veins, muscle atrophy, pain in right abdominal quadrant that worsens when the patient sits up or leans forward, palpable liver or spleen, and temperature of 101° to 103° F. Bleeding from esophageal varices can occur from an increase in the portal vascularity leading to hypertension and increasing the likelihood of esophageal hemorrhage (Meyer, 2001).

Chronic liver failure caused by acetaminophen toxicity can present with varying complications. Patients may be asymptomatic, with only incidentally detected laboratory test abnormalities, or they may have obvious features of liver involvement. Typically, drug hepatotoxicity begins 1 to 2 months after initiation of a drug, but latency may be longer (Krahenbuhl & Reichen, 2000).

HISTORY AND PHYSICAL EXAMINATION

An extensive patient history is crucial when evaluating for liver pathologies and/or gastrointestinal complaints during any juncture of the disease. Evaluation of suspected liver disease begins with a detailed assessment of risk factors (Kamath, 2001), followed by a clear chronological account of the patient's current situation that includes the onset of the problem, the setting in which it developed, and identification of concomitant manifestations. Identification of factors that alleviate or exacerbate the patient's symptoms is helpful. Additional assessment should query the patient about previous surgeries; abdominal or liver traumas; alcohol ingestion; comorbid pathologies; past or present viral, bacterial, parasitic, or fungal infections; and a family history of illnesses, as this health information is valuable and may influence treatment options. In addition, it is important to include a current list of medications taken, dosages used, allergies, previous drug toxicities, illicit drug use, OTC medications, herbal products, and any drug-drug interactions previously experienced. A study by Bernard and Bruera (2000) identified patients who were admitted to palliative settings and generally prescribed six or seven medications at any given time, contributing to the risk of adverse drug reactions and to drug-to-drug interactions. Many of these patients were prescribed 10 to 20 different medications and had a 20% or greater chance of experiencing a significant adverse drug-to-drug event, which can be fatal.

The patient's general appearance and vital signs may suggest clues to his or her overall condition and stability. Inspection, palpation, and auscultation of the abdomen may disclose signs of abdominal inflammation, scars, abdominal bulges, hernias, or distention; symmetry; and skin color. The liver and spleen are measured, and abdominal percussion identifies the amount of air in the stomach and bowel. Percussion also identifies the presence of abdominal masses and ascites. Many individuals with cirrhosis in the early stage often present with few nonspecific symptoms, making the diagnosis less obvious.

DIAGNOSTICS

Causes of liver injury are diverse, ranging from isolated and clinically silent laboratory abnormalities to dramatic and rapidly progressive liver failure. This spectrum relates in part to the broad range of pathophysiologic processes that can damage the liver and in part to the reserve capacity of the organ, which is large and can mask significant injury. It is estimated that approximately 40% of patients with cirrhosis are asymptomatic. When the diagnosis of end-stage liver disease is confirmed, the diagnosis often is confirmed before the patient seeks palliative care treatment (Fitz, 2003). However, some diagnostics may be appropriate and guide interventions that enhance the patient's diagnosis and comfort. Plasma ammonia levels are often markedly elevated in end-stage liver disease (Kichian & Bain, 2003). The diagnosis of liver injury from acetaminophen toxicity should be confirmed by a serum acetaminophen level, laboratory markers include evaluating the aspartate aminotransferase, alanine aminotransferase, bilirubin, electrolytes, and prothrombin time. The clinician can also order an abdominal ultrasound and computed tomography scan to investigate for suspected biliary obstruction or abdominal masses (Kichian & Bain, 2003).

CONCLUSION

Human illness results from a complex interplay of clinical, biologic, psychologic, and sociologic variables. The clinician's understanding of these diverse yet interacting variables is critical for appropriate treatment of end-stage liver disease (Yamada, 1998). The clinician aids in giving realistic prognostic information and facilitating exchange of information with every patient when discussing appropriate diagnostics in relationship to the goals of care. Skilled, compassionate palliative care clinicians should continue to use their expertise in maintaining safe prescribing practices by reviewing individual patients' medication profiles on a routine basis, which will assist in avoiding adverse drug reactions and toxicities. Some adverse drug events can be minimized by reducing the number of drugs prescribed and by use of a dose interval and route based on known drug pharmacodynamics and pharmacokinetics (Bernard & Bruera, 2000).

REFERENCES

American College of Rheumatology. (2000). Recommendations for the medical management of osteoarthritis of the hip and knee. *Am Rheumatol, 43,* 1905-1915.

American Geriatrics Society. (1998). Clinical practice guidelines and management of chronic pain in older persons. *Geriatrics, 5,* 235-249.

Beckman, M. (2002). The bulk of pain on the shoulders of aging. *Sci Aging Knowl, 16,* 173-186.

Bernard, S.A. & Bruera, E. (2000). Drug interactions in palliative care. *J Clin Oncol, 18,* 1780-1799.

Kichian, K. & Bain, G. (2003). Jaundice, ascites, and hepatic encephalopathy. In D. Doyle, G. Hanks, N. Cherny, & K. Calman (Eds.). *Oxford textbook of palliative medicine* (3rd ed.) pp. 507-519. New York: Oxford University Press.

Fitz, J.G. (2003). Disease of the liver and biliary system. In S.L. Friedman, K.R. McQuaid, & J.H. Grendell (Eds.). *Current diagnosis and treatment in gastroenterology* (pp. 521-535). New York: McGraw-Hill.

Hung, O.L. & Nelson, L.S. (2000). Acetaminophen. In J. Tintinalli, G. Kelen, & S. Stapczynski (Eds.). *Emergency medicine* (pp. 1088-1094). Baltimore: McGraw-Hill.

Isselbacher, K.J. & Podolsky, D.K. (2004). Approach to the patient with gastrointestinal disease. In D.L. Kasper, E. Braunwald, A. Fauci, & S. Hauser (Eds.). *Harrison's principles of internal medicine.* New York: McGraw-Hill.

Jakobsson, U., Klevsgard, R., & Westergen, A. (2003). Old people in pain: A comparative study. *J Pain Symptom Manage, 26,* 625-636.

Kamath, P.S. (2001). A model to predict survival in patients with end stage liver disease. *Hepatology, 33,* 464.

Kichian, S. & Bain, V. (2003). Drug-induced liver disease. *Hepatology, 31,* 201-236.

Krahenbuhl, S. & Reichen, J. (2000). Drug hepatotoxcity. In B.R. Bacon & A.M. Di Bisceglie (Eds.). *Liver disease, diagnosis, and management* (pp. 294-309). New York: Churchill Livingstone.

Kuebler, K. & Varga, J., & Mihelic, R.A. (2003). Why there is no cookbook approach to palliative care: Implications of the P450 enzyme system. *Clin J Oncol Nurs, 7,* 569-572.

Lee, W.M. (2003). Drug-induced hepatotoxicity. *N Engl J Med, 349,* 474.

McClain, C.J., Price, S., Barve, S., et al. (1999). Acetaminophen hepatotoxicity: An update. *Curr Gastroenterol Rep, 1,* 42-49.

Meyer, U.A. (2001). Drugs and toxins—drug handling. In J.L. Boyer, H.E. Blum, K.P. Maier, et al. (Eds.). *Liver cirrhosis and its development* (pp. 236-241). Amsterdam: Kluwer.

Watson, W.A., Litovitz, T.L., Rodgers, G.C., Jr., et al. (2003). 2002 Annual report of the American Association of Poison Control Centers Toxic Exposure Surveillance System. *Am J Emerg Med, 21,* 353-421.

Yamada, T. (1998). *Handbook of gastroenterology.* Philadelphia: Lippincott-Raven.

CHAPTER 13

CHRONIC KIDNEY DISEASE

Michael J. Germain and Debra E. Heidrich

■

DEFINITIONS AND INCIDENCE

Chronic kidney disease (CKD) is defined as kidney damage or impaired renal function that persists for 3 or more months (National Kidney Foundation [NKF], 2002). The severity of the disease is staged based on the level of kidney function as measured by the glomerular filtration rate (GFR) (Table 13-1). In the United States, it is estimated that 80,000 people are diagnosed with CKD annually, 20 million people are living with this disease, and an additional 20 million people are at increased risk (Coresh, Astor, Greene et al., 2003; NKF, 2006; United States Renal Data System [USRDS], 2005). The incidence and prevalence of CKD in the United States have been rising steadily, likely due to the increased prevalence of obesity and type 2 diabetes and an increasingly elderly population.

The most advanced stage of CKD is end-stage renal disease (ESRD). Patients with ESRD require dialysis or transplantation to survive (Zandi-Nejad & Brenner, 2005). In 2003, about 450,000 patients in the United States had ESRD, of whom 325,000 were being treated with dialysis and the remaining 128,000 received a kidney transplant (USRDS, 2005). There were 82,588 deaths attributed to ESRD in 2003, and about 13.5% of these patients were receiving care from a hospice at the time of their deaths (USRDS, 2005).

Risk factors for CKD include diabetes, hypertension, and family history of kidney disease. In addition, African Americans, Hispanics, Pacific Islanders, Native Americans, and people over the age of 65 are at increased risk (NKF, 2006). Cardiac disease is the single greatest cause of mortality in the ESRD population (USRDS, 2005). Older patients with ESRD and CHF have an annual mortality rate of about 60% and an expected survival of less than 6 months. This emphasizes the importance of palliative care and end-of-life planning for this group of patients (Germain & Cohen, 2001).

TABLE 13-1 ■ Stages of Chronic Kidney Disease

Stage	Description	GFR (ml/min/1.73 m^2)
1	Kidney damage with normal or increased GFR	≥90
2	Kidney damage with mild decrease in GFR	60-89
3	Moderate decrease in GFR	30-59
4	Severe decrease in GFR	15-29
5	Kidney failure	<15 or dialysis

Modified from National Kidney Foundation (NKF). (2005). K/DOQI clinical practice guidelines for chronic kidney disease: evaluation, classification, and stratification. *Am J Kidney Dis*, 39(suppl): S1, 2002. Retrieved August 10, 2006 from www.kidney.org/professionals/kdoqi/guidelines_ckd/toc.htm, Table 3.

Patients with chronic renal failure have a high symptom burden. A study by Wiesbord, Fried, Arnold et al. (2005) showed that the median number of symptoms for patients with ESRD receiving chronic hemodialysis was nine, with the severity of each averaging 3 on a scale of 1 to 5. Dry skin, fatigue, itching, and bone and/or joint pain were reported by at least 50% of patients. The overall symptom burden and severity were each correlated directly with impaired quality of life and depression.

Increasing evidence accrued in the past decades indicates that the adverse outcomes of chronic kidney disease, such as kidney failure, cardiovascular disease, and premature death, can be prevented or delayed through early detection and initiation of interventions to slow progression. Methods to slow the progression of CKD include optimal control of hypertension, optimal management of diabetes and hyperlipidemia, avoidance of nephrotoxins, cessation of smoking, and the use of medications that block the production of or effect of angiotensin II (Shaver, 2004).

ETIOLOGY AND PATHOPHYSIOLOGY

The two main causes of chronic kidney disease are diabetes (43%) and hypertension (26%). Other conditions that affect the kidneys are glomerulonephritis, inherited diseases (e.g., polycystic kidney disease), interstitial nephritis and/or pyelonephritis, and secondary glomerulonephritis (e.g., lupus nephritis) (Shaver, 2004). Obstructions due to kidney stones, tumors, or an enlarged prostate gland in men also can lead to kidney damage.

Each human kidney contains about 1 million nephrons, consisting of the renal corpuscle (glomerulus) and renal tubules, that function to maintain homeostatic functions of the body (Kumar, 2004) (Table 13-2). Insult to the kidney causes acute inflammation of glomeruli leading to a cascade of proteinuria, glomerular sclerosis, interstitial fibrosis, and, eventually, permanent nephron damage. In response to a

TABLE 13-2 ■ Renal Homeostatic Functions

Function	Mechanism	Affected Elements
Waste excretion	Glomerular filtration	Urea, creatinine
	Tubular secretion	Urate, lactate, drugs (diuretics)
	Tubular catabolism	
Electrolyte balance	Tubular NaCl absorption	Volume status, osmolar balance
	Tubular K^+ secretion	Potassium concentration
	Tubular H^+ secretion	Acid-base balance
	Tubular water absorption	Osmolar balance
	Tubular calcium, phosphate, magnesium transport	Calcium, phosphate, magnesium homeostasis
Hormonal regulation	Erythropoietin production	Red blood cell mass
	Vitamin D activation	Calcium homeostasis
Blood pressure regulation	Altered sodium excretion	Extracellular volume
	Renin production	Vascular resistance
Glucose homeostasis	Gluconeogenesis	Glucose supply (maintained) in prolonged starvation

From Kumar, J. (2004). Elements of renal structure and function. In T.E. Andreoli, C.C. Carpenter, R.C. Griggs, et al. (Eds.). *Cecil essentials of medicine* (6th ed., p. 235). Philadelphia: Saunders.

reduction in renal function, the remaining nephrons adapt with hyperfiltration. For this reason, patients can lose up to 75% of GFR with no pronounced symptoms (Shaver, 2004). The hyperfiltration causes glomerular capillary hypertension, which leads to glomerular sclerosis and nephron death. The glomerular capillary hypertension is maintained by the renin-angiotensin-aldosterone system (Zandi-Nejad & Brenner, 2005). The kidneys lose their ability to concentrate urine adequately, putting patients at risk for dehydration. As the GFR further declines, the body is unable to rid itself of excess water, salt, and other waste products, and serum urea nitrogen and creatinine levels increase (Molzahn, 2005a). The process of nephron death, hyperfiltration, and additional nephron death means that CKD tends to be progressive. This progression, however, may be slowed with optimal management.

CKD is a common microvascular complication of diabetes. Microangiopathy affecting the afferent and efferent arterioles of the nephron causes glomerulosclerosis. This leads to scarring of the glomerulus, tubules, and interstitium of the kidney and an increase in intraglomerular pressure. Microalbuminuria occurring about 10 to 15 years after the diagnosis of diabetes (preclinical diabetic nephropathy) is an early marker of developing diabetic nephropathy. With progression of the disease, more and more protein is excreted in the urine and renal insufficiency ensues (Barnett & Braunstein, 2004; Molzahn, 2005b).

A sustained systemic high blood pressure leads to nephrosclerosis. There is a direct correlation between the duration and degree of hypertension and the severity of renal damage. Kidney disease can also lead to hypertension. For example, hypertension may result from the kidney's decreasing ability to excrete salt and water when glomeruli are damaged (Molzahn, 2005b). Thus, a vicious cycle occurs as the renal damage causes hypertension and hypertension worsens renal damage.

ASSOCIATED SYMPTOMS

Many people have no symptoms of declining renal function until their kidney disease is advanced, that is, stage 4 or 5. Uremia affects every organ system and is likely due to multiple factors, including retained molecules, deficiencies of important hormones, and metabolic factors (Shaver, 2004). Table 13-3 shows the major manifestations of uremia.

HISTORY AND PHYSICAL EXAMINATION

History includes identification of those patients at high risk for CKD, including patients with any family history of CKD and those with diabetes, hypertension, recurrent urinary tract infections, urinary obstruction, or a systemic illness that affects the kidneys (Snyder & Pendergraph, 2005). The history should also include the onset of any of these high-risk diseases, the treatments used to manage the disease over time, and the effectiveness of these treatments.

Patients with a diagnosis of renal disease may present in various ways. In addition to the signs and symptoms of uremia as presented in Table 13-3, physical findings that might suggest the presence of renal disease include the following:

- Skin: itching from uremia with related excoriations
- Eyes: optic fundi changes or alterations (severe hypertension)
- Ears: hearing loss (associated with hereditary nephritis)

TABLE 13-3 ■ Major Manifestations of the Uremic Syndrome

System	Manifestations
Nervous	**Central** Irritability Insomnia Lethargy Anorexia Seizures Coma **Peripheral** Glove and stocking sensory loss Restless leg Footdrop or wrist drop
Musculoskeletal	Muscle weakness Gout and pseudogout Renal osteodystrophy
Hematologic	Anemia Bleeding disorders Leukocyte dysfunction
Gastrointestinal	Anorexia Nausea Vomiting Disturbance of taste Gastritis Peptic ulcer Gastrointestinal bleeding
Cardiovascular	Cardiomyopathy Arrhythmias Pericarditis Accelerated atherosclerosis
Pulmonary	Noncardiogenic pulmonary edema Pneumonitis Pleuritis
Acid-base/electrolytes	Anion gap acidosis Hyperkalemia Fluid overload Hypocalcemia Hyperphosphatemia Hypermagnesemia
Endocrine/metabolism	Hyperparathyroidism Increased insulin resistance Amenorrhea Impotence Hyperlipidemia
Skin	Pruritus Yellow pigmentation

Data from: Shaver, M.J. (2004). Chronic renal failure. In T.E. Andreoli, C.C. Carpenter, R.C. Griggs, et al. (Eds.). *Cecil essentials of medicine* (6th ed., pp. 301-310). Philadelphia: Saunders.

- Mouth, throat, neck: breath that smells like acetone or ammonia (uremia); distended neck veins (congestive heart failure)
- Chest: pericardial rub (pericarditis); diminished lung sounds (pleural effusion) or rales (congestive heart failure)
- Urinary: enlarged kidneys (polycystic kidney disease); flank pain; enlarged bladder (bladder outlet obstruction)
- Peripheral vascular: peripheral edema; anasarca
- Musculoskeletal: joint pain; arthritis; bone pain; muscle weakness
- Mental status: changes in cognition; asterixis

DIAGNOSTICS

Several diagnostic tests may be required to identify the cause of CKD and to monitor the progression of the disease over time. The following may provide valuable information (Veterans Hospital Administration/Department of Defense [VHA/DoD], 2001):

- Urinalysis
- Quantitative proteinuria
- Complete blood count
- Na^+, K^+, Cl^-, CO_2, blood urea nitrogen, serum creatinine, glucose, Ca^{2+}, PO_4^-, albumin, total protein
- Estimated GFR
- Cholesterol
- Kidney ultrasound
  - To evaluate for urinary tract obstruction
  - To estimate the size of the kidney
  - To evaluate for polycystic kidney disease

The following laboratory data may be helpful to identify complications in stages 3 and 4 CKD (Snyder & Pendergraph, 2005):

- Hemoglobin to identify anemia
- Red blood cell indexes, reticulocyte count, iron studies, and fecal occult blood test to rule out other causes of anemia
- Serum electrolytes to identify hyperkalemia, hyponatremia, and acidosis
- Calcium, phosphorus, and parathyroid hormone levels to identify hypocalcemia, hyperphosphatemia, and secondary hyperparathyroidism
- Serum albumin and total protein levels to identify hypoalbuminemia and decreased levels of immunoglobulins in patients with nephritic levels of proteinuria or signs of malnutrition

INTERVENTIONS

When CKD is diagnosed, it is important for the patient and family to understand the illness and its management, taking into account the nature of the disease in the context of patient and family values and wishes. Aggressive management of CKD involves using interventions to slow or arrest disease progression. As mentioned earlier, these interventions include optimal control of hypertension, optimal management of diabetes and hyperlipidemia, avoidance of nephrotoxins, cessation of smoking, and the use of medications that block the production of or effect of angiotensin II. Angiotensin-converting enzyme inhibitors and angiotensin II receptor blockers lower blood pressure and demonstrate a nephroprotective effect beyond that of their ability to lower blood pressure (Shaver, 2004). Restricting dietary protein may slow CKD progression, but protein malnutrition must be avoided.

Renal impairment affects medication selection and dose. Nephrotoxic drugs should be avoided, and medications eliminated via the urine may require dose reduction. Table 13-4 lists dosage modifications for selected medications when used in patients with renal failure.

Patients with ESRD require kidney replacement therapy to survive, either some form of dialysis (home peritoneal dialysis, home hemodialysis, in-center hemodialysis) or a renal transplantation. Hemodialysis is associated with significant symptom burden, leading some patients, especially the elderly and those with multiple comorbid medical conditions, to decline dialysis. Those who decide to forgo dialysis should be referred to a hospice program and receive maximal palliative care (Moss, 2001).

Offering the patient a trial of dialysis for 3 to 6 months may be an acceptable choice for those with a limited prognosis (Cohen, Germain, & Poppel, 2003).

TABLE 13-4 ■ Drug Dosage in Chronic Renal Failure for Selected Medications

Major Dosage Reduction	Minor or No Dosage Reduction	Avoid Usage
Antibiotics	**Antibiotics**	**Antibiotics**
Aminoglycosides	Erythromycin	Nitrofurantoin
Penicillin	Nafcillin	Nalidixic acid
Cephalosporins	Clindamycin	Tetracycline
Sulfonamides	Chloramphenicol	**Others**
Vancomycin	Isoniazid/rifampin	NSAIDs
Quinolones	Amphotericin B	Aspirin
Fluconazole	Aztreonam/tazobactam	Sulfonylureas
Acyclovir/ganciclovir	Doxycycline	Lithium carbonate
Foscarnet	**Others**	Acetazolamide
Imipenem	Antihypertensives	
Others	Benzodiazepines	
Digoxin	Diphenhydramine	
Procainamide	Haloperidol	
H_2 antagonists	Prochlorperazine	
Metoclopramide	Phenytoin	
Meperidine	Lidocaine	
Codeine	Quinidine	
Propoxyphene	Spironolactone	
	Triamterene	
	Opioids*	

Data from Neely, K.J. & Roxe, D.M. (2000). Palliative care/hospice and the withdrawal of dialysis. *Journal of Palliative Medicine*, 3(1), 57-67; and Shaver, M.J. (2004). Chronic renal failure. In T.E. Andreoli, C.C. Carpenter, R.C. Griggs, et al. (Eds.). *Cecil essentials of medicine* (6th ed., pp. 301-310). Philadelphia: Saunders.
NSAIDs, Nonsteroidal anti-inflammatory drugs.
*Due to the potential for accumulation of active metabolites, dosage reduction or opioid rotation may be required over time.

Box 13-1	Checklist for Dialysis Withdrawal

1. Identify patient who may benefit from withdrawal.
   a. Estimate prognosis; share with patient and family.
   b. Poor quality of life
   c. Pain unresponsive to treatment
   d. Progressive untreatable disease (e.g., cancer, dementia, AIDS, peripheral vascular disease, CHF)
   e. Unable or unwilling to tolerate further dialysis
2. Discuss goals of care with patient and family and review advanced care planning/advanced directives.
3. Ask patient/family if they are satisfied with quality of life on dialysis.
4. Discuss possible treatable symptoms and their palliation.
   a. Rule out depression.
   b. Assess for secondary gain by family.
5. Make explicit that dialysis withdrawal is an option.
6. Reassure that dialysis withdrawal can be a peaceful death.
7. Allow time for discussion.
8. Let the patient and family know the decision is reversible at any time.
9. Once the decision has been made to withdraw from dialysis, outline a plan with the patient and family.
10. Offer options of spiritual/religious support.
11. Discuss location at which patient will be most comfortable in last few days (home, hospice, nursing home, hospital).
12. Stop nonpalliative medications and order palliative medications.
13. Make hospice referral.
14. Reinforce continued availability of clinician.
15. Arrange bereavement services.

Over time, some patients who are on dialysis may elect to stop treatment. Often, this decision is due to (1) failure to thrive despite aggressive intervention, (2) poor quality of life as defined by the patient, or (3) worsening of comorbid complications (amputations, calciphylaxis, stroke, CHF), terminal illness (malignancies, AIDS, etc), or acute catastrophic illness. Death after dialysis withdrawal usually occurs quickly. Studies of patients who withdrew from dialysis showed that the time to death after stopping dialysis was less than 30 days, with a median of 8 to 10 days (Cohen, McCue, Germain et al., 1995; Neely & Roxe, 2000). The presumed immediate cause of death in most of these patients was uremia, which is often described as a painless and peaceful death. However, patients who stop dialysis are at high risk for delirium and accumulation of toxic metabolites of certain medications; these symptoms should be anticipated and appropriately managed. Box 13-1 provides a helpful checklist to use when patients elect to withhold or withdraw from dialysis.

Symptom relief should be a priority for all patients throughout the course of treatment for CKD. Table 13-5 lists medications that may be helpful for common CKD-related symptoms.

CONCLUSION

CKD is an increasingly common disorder in the United States. Although the progression of this disease can be slowed by early intervention, CKD is often diagnosed at a

TABLE 13-5 ■ **Pharmacological Interventions for Common Symptoms of CKD**

Symptom	Treatment	Dosage	Comments
Cramps	Quinine	260-325 mg oral	Limit to three doses daily
	Vitamin E	400 IU oral	
	Carnitine	1000-2000 mg IV during dialysis	Also used for cardiomyopathy and refractory anemia
Restless legs	Clonazepam	0.5-2 mg oral at bedtime as needed	
	Carbidopa-levodopa	25-100 mg oral at bedtime as needed	
	Pergolide	0.05 mg oral daily up to 0.2 mg oral four times daily	
	Bromocriptin	2-20 mg oral at bedtime	
	Gabapentin	100 mg every other day up to 300 mg three times daily	
	Clonidine	0.1-1.0 mg oral at bedtime	
Pruritus	Skin moisturizer		
	Hydrourea cream		
	UVB light		
	H_1 antagonist (any)		
	Activated charcoal	6 g oral four times daily × 8 wk	
	Lidocaine	100 mg IV during dialysis	Potential for seizure
	Ondansetron	4 mg oral twice daily	Expensive
	Plasmapheresis	3-4 exchanges	
Hypotension (intradialytic or persistent)	Alterations to dialysis bath, temperature, sodium, or ultrafiltration		
	Midodrine	2.5-10 mg oral three times daily as needed or predialysis	
	Sertraline	25-50 mg oral predialysis	
	Ketotifen	100 mg IV on dialysis	Mast cell stabilizer, not available in the United States
Fatigue	Methylphenidate	5-10 mg oral AM and noon	

Data from Germain, M.J., & McCarthy, S. (2004). Symptoms of renal disease. In E.J. Chambers, M. Germain, & E. Brown (Eds.). *Supportive care for the renal patient* (pp. 75-95). New York: Oxford University Press.

late stage because signs and symptoms do not become evident until significant kidney damage occurs. Cardiovascular disease is a common complication of CKD and is associated with a high mortality. Patients with ESRD require kidney replacement therapy with either dialysis or a kidney transplant to survive. Patients with CKD experience a high symptom burden throughout the continuum of care and require aggressive palliative symptom management to promote comfort and enhance quality of living.

REFERENCES

Barnett, P.S. & Braunstein, G.D. (2004). Diabetes mellitus. In T.E. Andreoli, C.C. Carpenter, R.C. Griggs, et al. (Eds.). *Cecil essentials of medicine* (6th ed., pp. 621-638). Philadelphia: Saunders.

Cohen, L M., Germain, M.J., & Poppel, D.M. (2003). Practical considerations in dialysis withdrawal: "To have that option is a blessing." *JAMA, 289(16),* 2113-2119.

Cohen, L.M., McCue, J.D., Germain, M., et al. (1995). Dialysis discontinuation: A 'good' death'? *Arch Intern Med, 155(1),* 42-47.

Coresh, J., Astor, B.C., Greene, T., et al. (2003). Prevalence of chronic kidney disease and decreased kidney function in the adult US population: Third National Health and Nutrition Examination Survey. *Am J Kidney Dis, 41(1),* 1-12.

Germain, M.J. & Cohen, L. (2001). Supportive care for patients with renal disease: Time for action. *Am J Kidney Dis, 38(4),* 884-886.

Kumar, J. (2004). Elements of renal structure and function. In T.E. Andreoli, C.C. Carpenter, R.C. Griggs, et al. (Eds.). *Cecil essentials of medicine* (6th ed., p. 229-236). Philadelphia: Saunders.

Molzahn, A.E. (2005a). Management of clients with renal failure. In J.M. Black & J.H. Hawks (Eds.). *Medical-surgical nursing: Clinical management for positive outcomes* (7th ed., pp. 941-972). St. Louis: Elsevier.

Molzahn, A.E. (2005b). Management of clients with renal disorders. In J.M. Black & J.H. Hawks (Eds.). *Medical-surgical nursing: Clinical management for positive outcomes* (7th ed., pp. 913-940). St. Louis: Elsevier.

Moss, A.H. (2001). Shared decision-making in dialysis: The new RPA/ASN guidelines on appropriate initiative and withdrawal of treatment. *Am J Kidney Dis, 37(5),* 1081-1091.

National Kidney Foundation (NKF). (2002). *K/DOQI clinical practice guidelines for chronic kidney disease: evaluation, classification, and stratification.* Retrieved March 26, 2006 from: www.kidney.org/professionals/kdoqi/guidelines_ckd/toc.htm.

National Kidney Foundation (NKF). (2006). *Kidney disease.* Retrieved March 26, 2006 from www.kidney.org/kidneyDisease.

Neely, K.J. & Roxe, D.M. (2000). Palliative care/hospice and the withdrawal of dialysis. *J Palliat Med, 3(1),* 57-67.

Shaver, M.J. (2004). Chronic renal failure. In T.E. Andreoli, C.C. Carpenter, R.C. Griggs, et al. (Eds.). *Cecil essentials of medicine* (6th ed., pp. 301-310). Philadelphia: Saunders.

Snyder, S. & Pendergraph, B. (2005). Detection and evaluation of chronic kidney disease. *Am Fam Physician, 72(9),* 1723-1732.

United States Renal Data System (USDRS). (2005). USRDS 2005 annual data report: Atlas of end-stage renal disease in the United States. National Institutes of Health, National Institute of Diabetes and Digestive and Kidney Diseases, Bethesda, Md. Retrieved March 27, 2006, from: www.usrds.org/atlas.htm.

Veterans Hospital Administration/Department of Defense [VHA/DoD] (2001). *Pre-end-stage renal disease. Clinical practice guidelines.* Retrieved March 28, 2006, from: www.oqp.med.va.gov/cpg/ESRD/ESRD_Base.htm.

Wiesbord, S.D., Fried, L.F., Arnold, R.M., Fine, M.J., Levenson, D.J., Peterson, R.A., & Switzer, G.E. (2005). Prevalence, severity and importance of physical and emotional symptoms in chronic hemodialysis patients. *J Am Soc Nephrol, 16(8),* 2487-2494.

Zandi-Nejad, K. & Brenner, B.M. (2005). Strategies to retard the progression of chronic kidney disease. *Med Clin North Am, 89(3),* 489-509.

CHAPTER 14

NEUROLOGICAL DISEASES
Debra E. Heidrich and Pamela Sue Spencer
■

Several different neurological diseases are seen as primary, and sometime secondary, diagnoses in palliative care settings. This chapter discusses cerebrovascular accidents (CVAs) and five degenerative neurological diseases: Alzheimer's disease (AD), amyotrophic lateral sclerosis (ALS), Huntington's disease (HD), multiple sclerosis (MS), and Parkinson's disease (PD). While each of these diseases is unique, the components of assessment and physical examination are similar. The etiology/pathophysiology, associated symptoms, and treatments of each disease are presented first followed by an overview of assessment and physical examination.

CEREBROVASCULAR ACCIDENTS

Approximately 700,000 people in the United States experience a new or recurrent cerebrovascular accident (CVA) each year, with about 500,000 of these being first attacks. In 2002, about 275,000 people died from stroke, making it the third leading cause of death in the United States (American Heart Association, 2004; Kochanek, Murphy, Anderson et al., 2004). Stroke is also the leading cause of serious, long-term disability in the United States (Centers for Disease Control and Prevention, 2001). Individuals who do not die with the acute event of a CVA tend to stabilize during hospitalization and require intensive rehabilitation therapies. Those who show steady improvement with rehabilitation are likely not terminal but may have some permanent disabilities related to the stroke; those who show continuous decline have a poor prognosis and are candidates for palliative care (National Hospice and Palliative Care Organization [NHPCO], 1996).

Etiology and Pathophysiology of Cerebrovascular Accidents

CVAs may be caused by thrombotic or embolic occlusion of cerebral vessels (ischemic stroke) or a rupture in a blood vessel (hemorrhagic stroke). Approximately 88% are ischemic strokes and most of these are caused by thrombosis (American Heart Association, 2004; Bowman, 2005). Almost all elderly people have some degree of blockage of the arterial supply to the brain, mostly due to arteriosclerotic plaques in one or more feeder arteries. The plaque activates platelets that secrete growth factors, encouraging further proliferation of the plaque. Eventually, these plaques grow large enough to occlude the vessel or may rupture, releasing emboli (Messing, 2003). Hemorrhagic strokes most often result from high blood pressure and cause the most fatalities of all strokes (Bowman, 2005). Risk factors for CVAs include hypertension, cardiovascular disease, atrial fibrillation, diabetes mellitus, cigarette smoking, hyperlipidemia, heavy alcohol use, and obesity (Bowman, 2005).

Regardless of the cause of the stroke, the result is loss of blood supply to the cerebral issues. Within minutes of cerebral ischemia, neurotoxins are released and acidosis develops, causing edema and cell death. With a cerebral hemorrhage, cerebral ischemia is caused by irritation of the cerebral tissues from the surrounding blood.

Symptoms Associated with Cerebrovascular Accidents

The location and extent of the ischemia determine the type and severity of the resulting deficits. These deficits may include the following (Bowman, 2005):

- Motor changes: hemiparesis, hemiplegia, intention tremor, ataxia
- Sensory changes: hemisensory alterations, diffuse sensory loss
- Visual or ocular changes: hemianopia, deviation of eyes, papillary dysfunction, loss of depth perception, cortical blindness, double vision, nystagmus
- Speech changes: dyslexia, dysgraphia, aphasia, dysarthria
- Mental changes: memory deficits, confusion, disorientation, flat affect, shortened attention span, loss of mental acuity
- Miscellaneous changes: nausea and vomiting, apraxia, incontinence, visual hallucinations, tinnitus, hearing loss, vertigo, dysphagia, coma, Horner's syndrome, hiccups, coughing

Depression is common among people living with the consequences of stroke and among their caregivers. In a study of 80 stroke survivors and their spouses, Ostwald (2004) reported that depression and stress in stroke survivors are predicted by functional status and perception of recovery, whereas depression and stress in spousal caregivers are associated with perceived caregiver burden and age.

Treatments for Cerebrovascular Accidents

Rehabilitation after stroke requires an interdisciplinary team, including physicians, nurses, social workers, counselors, physical therapists, occupational therapists, speech therapists, and dieticians. Patients who have had a stroke are at risk of developing another stroke, so it is important to institute measures to prevent a recurrence. Prevention strategies include control of hypertension, control of blood lipids, anticoagulant therapy, and treatment with antiplatelet agents, such as aspirin, clopidogrel, or dipyridamole (Ezekowitz, 2004).

ALZHEIMER'S DISEASE

Alzheimer's disease (AD) is the most common form of dementia. In 2000 there were 4.5 million Americans with AD, and it is estimated that there will be 13.2 million people with AD in 2050 (Hebert, Scherr, Bienias et al., 2003). In 2000, 58,866 people died from AD (Kochanek et al., 2004). It affects about 10% of people over the age of 65, and the incidence increases with aging. It is estimated that about 3% of people 65 to 74 years of age, 20% of those 75 to 84 years old, and 50% of people over the age of 85 have AD (Evans, Funkenstein, Albert et al., 1989). People with AD live an average of 8 years and up to as many as 20 years from the onset of symptoms (U.S. Congress, Office of Technology Assessment, 1987). Factors associated with reduced survival include rapidity of cognitive decline, decreased functional status, history of falls, frontal release signs, and abnormal gait (Hui, Wilson, Bennett et al., 2003; Larson, Shadlen, Wang et al., 2004).

Etiology and Pathophysiology of Alzheimer's Disease

The cause of AD is not known, but it is associated with age and there is some evidence that genetic factors play a role; approximately 10% of cases are familial. Alterations in brain tissue seen in AD include the formation of beta-amyloid neuritic plaques (also called senile plaques) between neurons and neurofibrillary tangles within neurons (Delagarza, 2003; Messing, 2003). Structural changes include a thickening of the leptomeninges, shrunken gyri, widened sulci, enlarged ventricles, hippocampal shrinkage, and generalized atrophy (Black, 2005). Biochemically, there is a 50% to 90% reduction in the activity of choline acetyltransferase, the biosynthetic enzyme of acetylcholine. The severity of the cognitive losses with AD is roughly proportional to the loss of choline acetyltransferase (Mayeux & Chun, 1995). These changes lead to the memory failure, personality changes, and functional disabilities seen in AD, and these structural and chemical changes become more widespread as the disease progresses.

Symptoms Associated with Alzheimer's Disease

Memory disturbances are usually the first sign of AD. Individuals with early AD may become irritable, suspicious, agitated, apathetic, or dysphoric. As the disease progresses, language disturbances and apraxia occur, swallowing may become difficult, and irritability and depression worsen (Black, 2005). These behaviors can place a great deal of both physical and emotional stress on the caregivers and may eventually lead to institutionalization of the patient.

Up to 25% of people with AD become clinically depressed (Mayeux & Chun, 1995). However, depression may be difficult to diagnose due to the cognitive and functional changes associated with the disease.

Malnutrition and weight loss often occur with AD and are associated with mortality risk and cognitive decline (Guerin, Soto, Brocker et al., 2005). Problems contributing to decreased oral intake include anorexia, agnosia, swallowing problems, functional impairment, and social support issues (Feldman & Woodward, 2005). The final stages of AD are characterized by an inability to ambulate independently, inability to dress without assistance, inability to bathe properly, urinary and fecal incontinence, and inability to communicate meaningfully (NHPCO, 1996).

Treatments for Alzheimer's Disease

Medications that inhibit the degradation of acetylcholine are the mainstay of therapy for AD, but they can cause cholinergic side effects, such as nausea, anorexia, vomiting, and diarrhea (Delagarza, 2003). These acetylcholinesterase inhibitors include donepezil (Aricept), galantamine (Reminyl), memantine (Namenda), rivastigmine (Exelon), and tacrine (Cognex) (Delagarza, 2003; Hodgson & Kizior, 2006). Some studies show cognitive improvements with vitamin E and selegine (Eldepryl), but the evidence is not strong (Birks & Flicker, 2003; Tabet, Birks, & Grimley Evans, 2000). These medications should be discontinued when dementia is severe (Delagarza, 2003).

Symptomatic treatments of depression, anxiety, and agitation and of the side effects of medications are important supportive interventions throughout the course of the disease. Nutritional support may be helpful in early and mid-stages of the disease. However, enteral feedings in advanced dementia do not appear to improve outcome and may put the patient at risk for complications (Finucane, Christmas, & Travis, 1999).

AMYOTROPHIC LATERAL SCLEROSIS

Amyotrophic lateral sclerosis (ALS), also known as Lou Gehrig's disease, is a disorder of progressive upper and lower motor neuron degeneration. The incidence of ALS is 0.4 to 1.8 per 100,000, and the prevalence is 4 to 6 per 100,000 people (Black, 2005). The course of ALS is relentless, without remissions, relapses, or even stable plateaus. Death usually occurs within 2 to 5 years of diagnosis, usually due to respiratory complications (Black, 2005; Messing, 2003). Older age at onset and early bulbar symptoms are associated with a shorter life expectancy.

Etiology and Pathophysiology of Amyotrophic Lateral Sclerosis

The cause of ALS is unknown, but about 5% to 10% of cases appear to have a genetic link; others are believed to be sporadic. Many different causes of sporadic ALS have been proposed, including exposure to heavy metals, viral infection, and autoimmune disorders, but there is no strong evidence for any of these theories (Rowland & Shneider, 2001). The pathology of ALS includes the replacement of large motor neuron cell bodies of the anterior horn of the spinal cord by fibrous astrocytes, resulting in gliosis. Abnormal protein aggregation, disorganization of intermediate filaments, and glutamate-mediated excitotoxicity are proposed to be involved in mediating this process (Messing, 2003; Rowland & Shneider, 2001).

Symptoms Associated with Amyotrophic Lateral Sclerosis

Upper motor neuron degeneration causes hyperactive tendon reflexes, Babinski's reflex, and clonus. Lower motor neuron disease leads to weakness, muscle wasting, muscle cramps, and muscle fasciculations (Rowland, 1995). Interestingly, the following functions do not appear to be affected by ALS: cognition, sensation, bladder and bowel control, autonomic function, and extraocular movements. Involvement of the corticobulbar tracts causes dysphagia and dysarthria (Black, 2005; Rowland, 1995).

The functional decline and uncomfortable symptoms of ALS cause distress to both the patient and the family. A study by Adelman and colleagues (2004) showed that caregivers accurately report information about a patient's physical function but that both patients and caregivers overestimated the psychosocial impact of the disease on the other. Caregivers rated patients as having less energy, greater suffering, and greater weariness than the patients indicated for themselves, and patients rated caregivers as more burdened than the caregivers reported for themselves.

Treatment of Amyotrophic Lateral Sclerosis

The only medication approved in the United States for the treatment of ALS is the glutamate antagonist riluzole (Rilutek). In a review of studies on riluzole, Miller and associates (2002) concluded that it probably prolongs survival by about 2 months and may improve bulbar and limb function, but it does not improve muscle strength. A longer survival benefit may be possible if riluzole is started early in the course of the disease (Wicklund, 2005). Many other treatments have undergone trial, including antioxidants, amino acids, neurotrophins, human insulin-like growth factor, creatine, minocycline, selegiline, and amantadine, but either these medications were ineffective or results were inconclusive (Mitchell, Wokke, & Borasio, 2005; Orrell, Lane, & Ross, 2005; Parton, Mitsumoto, & Leigh, 2005; Wicklund, 2005).

Individuals with ALS experience many discomforts that must be addressed to optimize quality of living.

- Muscle cramps can be excruciatingly painful. Use a combination of stretching, massage, and skeletal muscle relaxants to treat this problem (Simmons, 2005). One study showed improvement in spasticity by implementing an exercise program (Drory, Goltzman, Reznik et al., 2001).

- People with bulbar dysfunction are at risk for malnutrition and dehydration as well as aspiration due to dysphagia. Thin liquids are particularly difficult to swallow. Consult with a dietician about use of thickening agents for liquids as well as other food suggestions. Feeding via a gastrostomy tube may improve nutritional status, but the decision to accept artificial feedings is highly individual.

- Excessive drooling due to the inability to swallow secretions is sometimes a problem. Interventions include having suction available or use of an anticholinergic agent (e.g., hyoscyamine, atropine) to dry secretions. If anticholinergics are used, monitor for uncomfortable side effects.

- The dysarthria of bulbar involvement is extremely distressing to individuals. Explore other forms of communication, such as "magic slates," Magna-Doodle slates, or communication boards. Consult with a speech therapist for additional suggestions.

- Dyspnea and respiratory compromise result as the intercostal muscles and diaphragm weaken. Noninvasive positive pressure ventilation (NIPPV) may prolong survival, delay the need for tracheostomy, improve cognitive function, and improve quality of life (Bourke, Bullock, Williams et al., 2003; Simmons, 2005). When NIPPV no longer provides sufficient ventilatory support, some patients may choose tracheostomy and mechanical ventilation. Again, this is a highly individual decision.

HUNTINGTON'S DISEASE

Huntington's disease (HD) is a relentless, noncurable neurological disorder that causes gradual devastating effects to individuals in both mind and body. HD causes profound decline in cognition, behavior, and motor function in an unpredictable manner. The prevalence of HD is estimated at 5 to 8 per 100,000 individuals (SuttonBrown & Suchowersky, 2003), affecting both children and adults of all races and ethnicity around the globe. With no cure available, there is an unwavering need to embrace palliative care as a critical priority for individuals living with HD.

Etiology and Pathology of Huntington's Disease

The main manifestations of HD include choreiform and athetoid movements, accompanied by cognitive and behavioral changes, eventually involving dementia. HD, the most common hereditary cause of chorea, is transmitted in an autosomal dominant pattern, with complete penetrance (Ravina & Hurtig, 2002). Additional features of the inheritance of HD include anticipation, a trend toward earlier onset in successive generations, and paternal descent, which refers to the tendency for anticipation to be most pronounced in individuals who inherit the disease from their father (Yamada, Tsuji, & Takahashi, 2002).

Clinical manifestations usually begin between the ages of 30 to 40 years (Black, 2005). About 6% of the cases start before the age of 21 years (juvenile-onset HD) with an akinetic-rigid syndrome (the Westphal variant). Approximately 28% of cases start after the age of 50 years (late-onset HD). "Senile chorea" is simply chorea in an older person and is considered a diagnosis of exclusion; however, the majority of cases likely have HD (Quinn, 2003).

HD is caused by an anomaly of chromosome 4 and is fully penetrant, so the children of an affected parent have a 50% risk of developing the disease (Harper, 2002). The gene abnormality appears as an excessively long repeat of trinucleotides CAG, the length of which determines not only the presence of the disease but also the age of onset (Adams & Victor, 2001). The pathological process in HD is characterized by severe neuronal loss and gliosis occurring selectively in the caudate nucleus and putamen (basal ganglia), with vulnerability in other regions, such as the deep layers of the cortex (Paulsen, Zhao, Stout et al., 2001). Further studies in HD patients have shown alterations in the metabolic activity in muscle tissue and the basal ganglia. (Gu, Gash, Mann et al., 1996; Lodi, Shapira, Manners et al., 2000). Changes in the concentration of neuropeptides in the basal ganglia have also been found, including decreased substance P, methionine enkephalin, dynorphin, and cholecystokinin and increased somatostatin and neuropeptide Y. Positron emission tomography (PET) has shown reduced glucose utilization in an anatomically normal caudate nucleus (Yamada et al., 2002).

Symptoms Associated with Huntington's Disease

Early signs and symptoms of HD include subtle abnormal eye movements, uncoordinated fine motor movements of the hands and face, clumsiness, impulsiveness, decreased concentration, and increased fluctuations of impulsiveness, anxiety, and restlessness. Poor self-control may also be reflected in outbursts of temper, fits of despondency, alcoholism, or sexual promiscuity. Disturbances in mood, particularly depression, are common (almost half of the patients in some series) and may constitute the most prominent symptoms early in the disease (Adams & Victor, 2001).

As HD progresses, physical, emotional, and cognitive symptoms become more compromised. Speech, walking, swallowing, and motor control also worsen throughout the disease trajectory. In many individuals, the involuntary, forceful, random movements worsen in an unpredictable manner and the patient is seldom still for more than a few seconds (Adams & Victor, 2001). Anxiety, stress, and lack of appropriate amounts of sleep can aggravate chorea involvement, adding to the patient's increased fatigability. Thus, with the progression of HD, signs, symptoms, and functional decline become more debilitating. Surprisingly, during periods of sleep, the chorea movements subside and the individual is able to fully rest. Other clinical features in advanced stages of HD include urinary incontinence, motor instability, and loss of proper swallowing, which causes aspiration and cachexia. The hyperkinetic state combined with abnormalities of muscle and adipose tissue metabolism is the postulated explanation for cachexia (Lodi et al., 2000; Sanberg, Fibiger, & Mark, 1981). Inevitably, complications of functional decline and onset of infections (such as pneumonia and aspiration pneumonia due to impairment of swallowing, choking, and coughing) contribute to the cause of death in these individuals.

Juvenile-onset HD often presents between the ages of 15 to 18 years (Davis, Cheema, Oliver et al., 2005). Early signs and symptoms of juvenile-onset HD include poor school performance, difficulty in comprehending new information, slowness and stiffness, awkwardness in walking, clumsiness and frequent falls, slurred speech, choking and drooling, behavioral changes, personality changes, and slowness in responding. Seizures occur in 25% to 30% of children and usually develop after the first obvious motor abnormalities appear (Huntington Society of Canada, 2000). As the disease progresses, muscles stiffen, causing worsening rigidity. Variable signs and symptoms include weight loss, swallowing difficulties, aggressiveness, mania, hallucinations, and paranoia (Higgins, 2001).

Treatment of Huntington's Disease

There is no cure for HD and currently no treatments that will reverse or halt the progression of this illness. Treatment is aimed at reducing symptoms, preventing complications, and maximizing the individual's ability to function as long as possible throughout the disease trajectory (Davis et al., 2005).

Abnormal movements may be suppressed with medications that block dopamine receptors. Many dopamine antagonists, such as risperidone and olanzapine, have neuroleptic properties, which have the added benefit of controlling psychiatric symptomatology (SuttonBrown & Suchowersky, 2003). Amantadine, tetrabenazine, and other antiparkinsonian medications may also be helpful.

Depression affects 22% of patients the first year after diagnosis and remains high throughout the course of the illness (Harper, 2002; Kirkwood, Su, Conneally et al., 2001). Selective serotonin reuptake inhibitors and tricyclic antidepressants are used for the management of depression and anxiety. Treatment recommendations used specifically for juvenile-onset HD include anticonvulsant medications to help prevent and control seizures (Davis et al., 2005).

MULTIPLE SCLEROSIS

Multiple sclerosis (MS) is an idiopathic inflammatory disease characterized by demyelination of neurons in the central nervous system. MS typically occurs between the ages of 20 to 45 and affects twice as many women as men (Black, 2005; Calabresi, 2004). About 400,000 individuals are living with MS in the United States (National Multiple Sclerosis Society [NMSS], 2005). Although there is no cure for MS, the course tends to include relapses and remissions. MS usually takes one of four clinical courses:

1. *Relapsing-remitting* course (most common form of MS)—characterized by partial or complete recovery after attacks.
2. *Secondary-progressive* course—a relapsing-remitting course that later becomes progressive with only partial recovery after attacks.
3. *Primary-progressive* course—symptoms generally do not remit; even though there are no acute attacks, there is progressive disability.
4. *Progressive-relapsing* course—progressive from the outset, with obvious, acute attacks along with way.

Approximately 95% of people with MS can expect a normal life expectancy. Patients with early symptoms of tremor, difficulty with coordination, difficulty walking, frequent attacks with incomplete recoveries, or more lesions on MRI tend to have a more progressive course (NMSS, 2005).

Etiology and Pathophysiology of Multiple Sclerosis

It is believed that MS involves an autoimmune process. The trigger that initiates this process is not known, but viruses, especially the Epstein-Barr virus and herpes virus, are suspected (NMSS, 2005; Sundstrom, Juton, Wadell et al., 2004; Villoslada et al., 2003). Individuals with a first-degree relative with MS have a much greater risk of developing MS than does the general population, and some common genetic factors have been found in families where more than one person has MS. It may be that genetic susceptibility alters the body's response to a viral infection (Black, 2005; NMSS, 2005).

When this autoimmune process is triggered, plaques form along the myelin sheath of nerves in the central nervous system, leading to demyelination. Inflammation, edema, and death of the myelin-producing cells occur over time. Remissions are probably due to reformation of some myelin when inflammation subsides. Progressive decline occurs due to scarring and destruction of the nerve axons. Although plaques may form anywhere in the white matter of the central nervous system, the optic nerves, cerebrum, and cervical spinal cord are most commonly involved (Black, 2005).

Symptoms Associated with Multiple Sclerosis

Nerve demyelination and axon scarring cause motor changes (e.g., weakness, spasticity, hyperreflexia) and sensory impairment (e.g., impaired vibration and position sense); impaired perception of pain, temperature, or touch; and moderate to severe pain. When nerves of the cerebellum are involved, the patient experiences ataxia, tremors, nystagmus, and dysarthria. Visual disturbances, bulbar signs, and vertigo occur when the cranial nerves or brainstem is affected. Changes in autonomic functioning may cause bowel incontinence, neurogenic bladder, or sexual dysfunction. Patients with MS are also at risk for depression and cognitive abnormalities (Sadiq & Miller, 1995).

Treatments for Multiple Sclerosis

Two biological response modifiers, interferon β-1a and interferon β-1b, and one immunosuppressive agent, glatiramer, are approved for the initial management of MS in the United States. These medications reduce the frequency of relapses. Another medication, mitoxantrone, is an antineoplastic agent and is used in patients with progressive forms of MS. Mitoxantrone can be used for only 2 to 3 years due to the risk of cumulative cardiotoxicity. Also, intravenous IgG, azathioprine, methotrexate, and cyclophosphamide, either alone or in combination with standard therapy, are not Food and Drug Administration approved but have been used to treat MS (Calabresi, 2004).

PARKINSON'S DISEASE

Parkinson's disease (PD) is an idiopathic progressive neurological disorder with six cardinal features: tremor at rest, muscle rigidity, bradykinesia, flexed posture, loss of postural reflexes, and freezing movement (Black, 2005). Approximately 1% of the U.S. population over age 65 is diagnosed with PD (Centers for Disease Control and Prevention, 2005). There is no cure for this very slowly progressive disease. In 2002, 16,959 people died from PD (Kochanek et al., 2004).

Etiology and Pathophysiology of Parkinson's Disease

The etiology of PD is unknown. PD is not thought to be an inherited disease, but the etiology may involve an interaction of environmental and genetic factors (Guttman, Kish, & Furukawa, 2003). In PD, there is selective degeneration of the dopaminergic neurons of the substantia nigra and eosinophilic inclusion bodies (Lewy bodies) in the basal ganglia, brainstem, spinal cord, and sympathetic ganglia (Messing, 2003). Dopamine is the neurotransmitter that enables people to move normally and smoothly; a severe shortage of dopamine in relation to acetylcholine in the basal ganglia leads to the clinical manifestations of PD (Black, 2005).

Symptoms Associated with Parkinson's Disease

As mentioned above, there are six cardinal features of PD. The tremors are most often coarse movements at rest, which disappear with intentional movement. However, some people may have intention tremors as well. The bradykinesia is exhibited in a slow, shuffling gait, a loss of spontaneous facial expression (i.e., a masklike face), drooling from failure to swallow spontaneously, and stooped posture. Muscles become rigid with increased muscle tone. Although PD does not affect intellectual ability, dementia develops in about 15% to 20% of people with PD (Black, 2005).

Treatments for Parkinson's Disease

Classes of medications used for early stage PD include the following (Guttman et al., 2003; Horn & Stern, 2004):

- Monoamine oxidase inhibitors, such as selegiline and rasagiline
- Anticholinergic medications, such as trihexyphenidyl and benztropine
- Antiviral dopaminergic agonist, that is, amantadine
- Dopamine agonists, such as pergolide, ropinirole, and pramipexole
- Levodopa, such as carbidopa/levodopa

There is much debate regarding which drug to choose first in the treatment of PD. Decision-making criteria include the level of disability and age of the patient. Minor symptoms may be treated with amantadine or an anticholinergic drug. These medications should be used with caution in the elderly due to the risk of cognitive and psychiatric side effects. Levodopa is used for symptoms that interfere with daily living or when other medications are no longer working. These medications may be used in combination as the disease progresses. Catechol-O-methyltransferase (COMT) inhibitors are adjunctive medications that enhance the delivery of levodopa. Examples of COMT inhibitors are tolcapone and entacapone. COMT inhibitors are added when breakthrough symptoms occur at the end of the dosing interval.

HISTORY AND PHYSICAL EXAMINATION

History

When obtaining the history, it is important to consider the ability of the patient to provide accurate and complete information. Some neurological diseases impair mentation, resulting in less-than-reliable responses from patients. A family member can assist in providing important details. Be careful to not suggest symptoms. It is important to assess the following:

- History of the neurological disease to date: presenting symptoms, diagnosis, and changes since diagnosis
- Mentation status
  - ▶ Language skills—ability to read, speak, and understand spoken words; for people who have lost the ability to speak, any form of meaningful communication
  - ▶ Memory losses: short-term or long-term
  - ▶ Difficulty concentrating or making decisions
- Functional ability
  - ▶ Weakness, tremors, or abnormal movements
  - ▶ Balance problems
  - ▶ Difficulty chewing or swallowing
  - ▶ Difficulties with self-care activities
- Sensory perception
  - ▶ Changes in ability to see, smell, hear, or taste
  - ▶ Abnormal sensations or pain, such as burning, numbness, tingling, or aching
- Bowel and bladder function
  - ▶ Urinary or bowel incontinence
  - ▶ Urinary retention or hesitancy
  - ▶ Constipation
- Breathing difficulties
- Psychosocial impact of disease
  - ▶ Signs of anxiety, fear, or depression
  - ▶ Patient and family assessment of coping
  - ▶ Strength of social support network

Physical Assessment

The physical assessment identifies the patient's status on the initial visit and is used as a baseline to compare changes over time. In end-of-life care, it is anticipated that the disease will progress, and documentation of these changes is important for monitoring the patient's status. Because documentation of declining patient status is required to maintain hospice support for some patients, even subtle changes are significant. However, not all of the following data are important to monitor in all patients:

- Mental status
  - ▶ Level of consciousness
  - ▶ Orientation
  - ▶ Mood and affect
- Motor function
  - ▶ Muscle strength of major muscle groups. Use a strength scale:
    - ● 5 = Full strength
    - ● 4 = Movement against gravity and some resistance
    - ● 3 = Movement against gravity but not against resistance
    - ● 2 = Movement but not against gravity
    - ● 1 = Trace movement
    - ● 0 = No movement

- ⟩ Muscle groups
  - ● Upper extremity: finger abductors, wrist extensors, wrist flexors, biceps, triceps, and deltoids
  - ● Lower extremity: hip flexors, quadriceps, hamstrings, foot dorsiflexors, and foot plantar flexors
  - ⟩ Muscle tone: any rigidity, spasticity, or flaccidity; any signs of muscle wasting
- ■ Cranial nerve functioning
  - ⟩ Babinski's reflex
  - ⟩ Any akinesia, dystonia, myoclonus, or tremors
- ■ Ability to speak
- ■ Signs of respiratory compromise
- ■ Sensory function
  - ⟩ Ability to sense light touch, pain (pin-prick), and vibration
  - ⟩ Ability to identify numbers traced in the palm of patient's hand (graphesthesia) and ability to identify objects by feel (stereognosis)
  - ⟩ Sensory extinction or inattention
- ■ Deep tendon reflexes

DIAGNOSTICS

Most of the neurological diseases are diagnosed based on symptoms and patient history. Magnetic resonance imaging or computed tomography scanning can confirm a diagnosis of cerebral bleeds (CVA) or show cerebral atrophy in AD or HD. PET studies in people with HD can show changes in metabolism of the caudate that correlate with clinical decline (Feigin, Leenders, & Moeller, 2001; Reynolds, Hellman, Tikofsky et al, 2002). Electromyographic findings assist in the diagnosis of ALS. Genetic testing is an important part of screening and detection of HD.

PSYCHOSOCIAL CONSIDERATONS

These progressive neurological diseases eventually cause individuals to become fully dependent on health care providers and family members for their daily functioning needs. Recommendations include integrating supportive therapy, such as physical therapy, speech therapy, occupational therapy, and nutritional counseling, into the plan of care to optimize the patient's functional capabilities for as long as possible. Additionally, advance directives need to be discussed early in the disease course, as cognitive decline occurs with most of these diseases. Advance directives are a sensitive issue and should be discussed with patients and family members in a supportive environment. A diagnosis of any of these neurological diseases can be overwhelming. It remains central to not only engage in dialogue but to maintain open communication channels. Participating in advance care planning discussions and completing advance directives allow individuals to direct their own plan of care throughout the disease process, including their end-of-life care requests. Although not all future decisions that must be made are predictable, recognizing individuals' concerns, hopes, and goals throughout the illness trajectory will promote a sense of control in decision making. Acknowledging and legitimating patients' concerns communicate respect and lead to a sense of enhanced dignity (Back, Arnold, & Quill, 2003). Finally, emotional and spiritual needs are high priorities with both patients and families experiencing these progressive, incurable illnesses.

REFERENCES

Adams, R. & Victor, M. 2001. Degenerative diseases of the nervous system. In R. Adams & M. Victor (Eds.). *Principles of neurology* (2nd ed., pp. 1122-1125). New York: McGraw-Hill.

Adelman, E.E., Albert, S.M., Rabkin, J.G., et al. (2004). Disparities in perceptions of distress and burden in ALS patients and family caregivers. *Neurology, 62(10),* 1766-1770.

American Heart Association. (2004). *Heart disease and stroke statistics—2005 update.* Dallas, Tex: Author.

Back, A.L., Arnold, R.M., & Quill, T.E. (2003). Hope for the best, and prepare for the worst. *Ann Intern Med, 138(5),* 439-443.

Birks, J. & Flicker, L. (2003). Selegiline for Alzheimer's disease. *Cochrane Database Syst Rev, (1),* CD000442.

Black, J.M. (2005). Management of clients with degenerative neurologic disorders. In J.M. Black & J.H. Hawks (Eds.). *Medical-surgical nursing: Clinical management for positive outcomes* (7th ed., pp. 2161-2187). St. Louis: Elsevier Saunders.

Bourke, S.D., Bullock, R.E., Williams, T.L., et al. (2003). Noninvasive ventilation in ALS: Indications and effect on quality of life. *Neurology, 61(2),* 171-177.

Bowman, L. (2005). Management of clients with stroke. In J.M. Black & J.H. Hawks (Eds.). *Medical-surgical nursing: Clinical management for positive outcomes* (7th ed., pp. 2107-2137). St. Louis: Elsevier Saunders.

Calabresi, P.A. (2004). Diagnosis and management of multiple sclerosis. *Am Fam Physician, 70(10),* 1935-1944.

Centers for Disease Control and Prevention. (2001). Prevalence of disability and associated health conditions among adults—United States, 1999. *MMWR, 50(7),* 120-125.

Centers for Disease Control and Prevention. (2005). *National Center for Health Statistics data on Parkinson's disease.* Retrieved November 5, 2005, from www.cdc.gov/nchs/data/factsheets/Parkinsons.pdf.

Davis, M.P., Cheema, B.I, Oliver, D., et al. (2005). Neurology. In K.K. Kuebler, M.P. Davis, & C.D. Moore (Eds.). *Palliative practices: An interdisciplinary approach* (pp. 269-288). St. Louis: Mosby.

Delagarza, V.W. (2003). Pharmacologic treatment of Alzheimer's disease: An update. *Am Fam Physician, 68(7),* 1365-1372.

Drory, V.E., Goltzman, E., Reznik, J.G., et al. (2001). The value of muscle exercise in patients with amyotrophic lateral sclerosis. *J Neurol Sci, 191(1-2),* 133-137.

Evans, D.A., Funkenstein, H.H., Albert, M.S., et al. (1989). Prevalence of Alzheimer's disease in a community population of older patients: Higher than previously reported. *JAMA, 262(18),* 2551-2556.

Ezekowitz, M. (2004). Medical prevention of secondary stroke: A cardiologist's perspective. *Clin Cardiol, 27(5 Suppl 2),* II36-II42.

Feigin, A., Leenders, K.L., & Moeller, J.R. (2001). Metabolic network abnormalities in early Huntington's disease: A PET study. *J Nuclear Med, 42(11),* 1591-1595.

Feldman, H.H. & Woodward, M. (2005). The staging and assessment of moderate to sever Alzheimer disease. *Neurology, 65(Suppl 3),* S10-S17.

Finucane, T.E., Christmas, C., & Travis, K. (1999). Tube feeding in patients with advanced dementia: A review of the evidence. *JAMA, 282(14),* 1365-1370.

Gu, M., Gash, M.T., Mann, V.M., et al. (1996). Mitochondrial defect in Huntington's disease caudate nucleus. *Ann Neurol, 39(3),* 385-389.

Guerin, O., Soto, M.E., Brocker, P., et al. (2005). Nutritional status assessment during Alzheimer's disease: results after one year (the REAL French Study Group). *J Nutr Health Aging, 9(2),* 81-84.

Guttman, M., Kish, S.J., & Furukawa, Y. (2003). Current concepts in the diagnosis and management of Parkinson's disease. *Can Med Assoc J, 168(3),* 293-301.

Harper, P.S. (2002). Huntington's disease. In P.S. Harper (Ed.). *Major problems in neurology* (3rd ed., pp. 239-242). London: Saunders.

Hebert, L.E., Scherr, P.A., Bienias, J.L., et al. (2003). Alzheimer disease in the U. S. population: Prevalence estimates using the 2000 census. *Arch Neurol, 60(3),* 1119-1122.

Higgins, D.S. (2001). Chorea and its disorders. *Neurol Clin, 19(3),* 707-722.

Hodgson, B.B. & Kizior, R.J. (2006). *Mosby's 2006 drug consult for nurses.* St. Louis: Elsevier Mosby.

Horn, S. & Stern, M.B. (2004). The comparative effects of medical therapies for Parkinson's disease. *Neurology, 63(Suppl 2),* S7-S12.

Hui, J.S., Wilson, R.S., Bennett, M.D., et al. (2003). Rate of cognitive decline and mortality in Alzheimer's disease. *Neurology, 61(10),* 1356-1361.

Huntington Society of Canada. (2000). *A resource for families, health professionals and caregivers.* Ontario, Canada: Author.

Kirkwood, S.C., Su, J.L., Conneally, P.M., et al. (2001). Progression of symptoms in the early and middle stages of Huntington's disease. *Arch Neurol, 58(2),* 273-278.

Kochanek, K.D., Murphy, S.L., Anderson, R.N., et al. (2004). Deaths: Final data for 2002. *Nat Vital Stat Rep, 53(5),* 1-115.

Larson, E.B., Shadlen, M.R., Wang, L., et al. (2004). Survival after initial diagnosis of Alzheimer disease. *Ann Intern Med, 140(7),* 501-509.

Lodi, R., Schapira, A. H., Manners, D., et al. (2000). Abnormal in vivo skeletal muscle energy metabolism in Huntington's disease and dentatorubropallidoluysian atrophy. *Ann Neurol, 48(1),* 72-76.

Mayeux, R. & Chun, M.R. (1995). Dementias. In L.P. Rowland (Ed.). *Merritt's textbook of neurology* (9th ed., pp. 677-685). Baltimore: Williams & Wilkins.

Messing, R.O. (2003). Nervous system disorders. In S.J. McPhee, W.R. Lingappa, & W.F. Ganong (Eds.). *Pathophysiology of disease: An introduction to clinical medicine* (4th ed., pp. 143-188). New York: Lange/McGraw-Hill.

Miller, R.G., Mitchell, J.D., Lyon, M., et al. (2002). Riluzole for amyotrophic lateral sclerosis (ALS)/motor neuron disease (MND). *Cochrane Database Syst Rev, (2),* CD001447.

Mitchell, J.D., Wokke, J.H., & Borasio, G.D. (2005). Recombinant human insulin-like growth factor I (rhIGF-I) for amyotrophic lateral sclerosis/motor neuron disease. *Cochrane Database Syst Rev, (3),* CD002064.

National Hospice and Palliative Care Organization (NHPCO). (1996*). Medical guidelines for determining prognosis in selected noncancer diseases* (2nd ed.). Arlington, Va.: Author.

National Multiple Sclerosis Society (NMSS). (2005). *Multiple sclerosis information sourcebook.* Retrieved November 5, 2005, from www.nationalmssociety.org/sourcebook.asp.

Orrell, R.W., Lane, R.J., & Ross, M. (2005). Antioxidant treatment for amyotrophic lateral sclerosis/motor neuron disease. *Cochrane Database Syst Rev, (1),* CD002829.

Ostwald, S.K. (2004). Stroke is a family affair: The CAReS intervention study [Abstract]. *Geriatr Nurs, 25(1),* 53.

Parton, M., Mitsumoto, H., & Leigh, P.N. (2005). Amino acids for amyotrophic lateral sclerosis/motor neuron disease. *Cochrane Database Syst Rev, (4),* CD003457.

Paulsen, J.S., Zhao, H., Stout, J.C., et al.; Huntington Study Group. (2001). Clinical markers of early disease in persons near onset of Huntington's disease. *Neurology, 57(4),* 658-662.

Quinn, N.P. (2003). Movement disorders. In N.P. Quinn (Ed.). *Clinical neurology* (3rd ed., pp. 225-244). New York: Oxford University Press.

Ravina, B. & Hurtig, H. (2002). Movement disorders in the older adult. In B. Ravina & H. Hurtig (Eds.). *Clinical neurology of the older adult* (pp. 292-303). Philadelphia: Lippincott Williams & Wilkins.

Reynolds, N.C., Hellman, R.S., Tikofsky, R.S., et al. (2002). Single photon emission computerized tomography (SPECT) in detecting neurodegeneration in Huntington's disease. *Nucl Med Comm, 23(1),* 13-18.

Rowland, L.P. (1995). Hereditary and acquired motor neuron diseases. In L.P. Rowland (Ed.). *Merritt's textbook of neurology* (9th ed., pp. 742-749). Baltimore: Williams & Wilkins.

Rowland, L.P. & Shneider, N.A. (2001). Amyotrophic lateral sclerosis. *N Engl J Med, 344,* 1688-1700.

Sadiq, S.A. & Miller, J.R. (1995). Multiple sclerosis. In L.P. Rowland (Ed.), *Merritt's textbook of neurology* (9th ed., pp. 804-825). Baltimore: Williams & Wilkins.

Sanberg, R.R., Fibiger, M.C., & Mark, R.F. (1981). Body weight and dietary factors in Huntington's disease patients compared with matched controls. *Med J Aust, 1(8),* 407-409.

Simmons, Z. (2005). Management strategies for patients with amyotrophic lateral sclerosis from diagnosis through death. *The Neurologist, 11(5),* 257-270.

Sundstrom, P., Juto, P., Wadell, G., et al. (2004). An altered immune response to Epstein-Barr virus in multiple sclerosis: A prospective study. *Neurology, 62(12),* 2277-2282.

SuttonBrown, M. & Suchowersky, O. (2003). Clinical and research advances in Huntington's disease. *Can J Neurol Sci, 30(Suppl 1),* S45-S52.

Tabet, N., Birks, J., & Grimley Evans, J. (2000). Vitamin E for Alzheimer's disease. *Cochrane Database Syst Rev, (4),* CD002854.

U.S. Congress, Office of Technology Assessment. (1987). *Losing a million minds: Confronting the tragedy of Alzheimer's disease and other dementias.* OTA-BA-323. Washington, DC: Government Printing Office.

Villoslada, P., Juste, D., Tintore, M., et al. (2003). The immune response against herpesvirus is more prominent in the early stages of MS. *Neurology, 60(12),* 1944-1948.

Wicklund, M.P. (2005). Amyotrophic lateral sclerosis: Possible role of environmental influences. *Neurol Clin, 23,* 461-484.

Yamada, M., Tsuji, S., & Takahashi, H. (2002). Neuropathology. In D.A. Greenberg, M.J. Aminoff, & R.P. Simon (Eds.). *Clinical neurology* (5th ed., pp. 232-256). New York: McGraw-Hill.

CHAPTER 15

MALIGNANCIES

Debra E. Heidrich and Peg Esper

■

The term *cancer* refers to a group of diseases characterized by uncontrolled growth of abnormal cells, with local tissue invasion and systemic metastasis. It is estimated that 1,399,790 Americans will be diagnosed with cancer in 2006 and 564,830 patients—approximately 1500 a day—are expected to die of malignant disease. Cancer is the second leading cause of death in the United States, accounting for one of every four deaths. The 5-year survival rate for patients diagnosed with cancer between 1995 to 2001 was 65%; this is an increase from 50% between 1974 to 1976. The increased survival is likely due to advances in early detection and treatment (American Cancer Society [ACS], 2006).

According to the National Hospice and Palliative Care Organization (NHPCO, 2006), approximately 46% of the 1,060,000 patients admitted to hospice programs in 2004 had a diagnosis of cancer. While there are potential flaws in using the data on cancer deaths from one report to compare with the number of cancer patients served by hospice programs based on a different report, it is reasonable to conclude that a large majority of patients who die with cancer are admitted to hospice programs. However, the average and median lengths of stay in hospice programs are only 57 days and 22 days, respectively. So, even though many cancer patients are referred to hospice programs, the referrals come late. In order to promote optimal quality of life, patients with advanced cancers require coordinated, individualized interdisciplinary palliative care and appropriate referrals to hospice programs. The question becomes, then, how can the clinician do a better job of identifying those who should be referred for palliative care in a timely manner?

Cancers of the lung, colon and rectum, breast, pancreas, and prostate, as well as non-Hodgkin's lymphoma, have the highest mortality rates, accounting for approximately 60% of all cancer deaths in both males and females (ACS, 2006). These cancers are briefly discussed in this chapter. Among these cancers there is wide variability on survival based on tumor size, histological grade, response to treatment, and number of metastatic sites. In general, larger, poorly differentiated tumors and the presence of distant metastasis are poor prognostic indicators. A referral to a palliative care team is appropriate for all patients with stage IV disease. Also, those patients with other stages of cancer whose diseases progress while on treatment or with short progression-free intervals after completing a course of treatment have a worse prognosis and should be referred for a palliative care team consult.

Figure 15-1 shows the typical dying trajectory for cancer patients. This model is based on a study that monitored the number of independent activities of daily living performed over the last year of the lives of patients with cancer (Lunney, Lynn, Foley et al., 2003). As illustrated in this figure, performance status is a good indicator of length of life for cancer patients—the poorer the performance status, the shorter

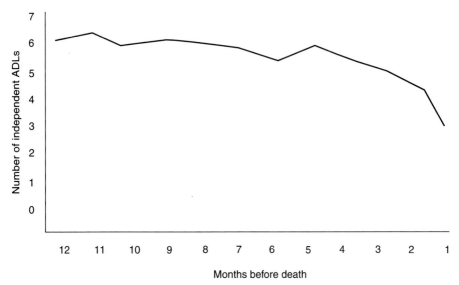

Figure 15-1 Functional decline in patients with advanced cancer at the end of life. (Adapted from Lunney, J.R., Lynn, J., Foley, D.J., et al. [2003]. Patterns of functional decline at the end of life. *JAMA, 289[18], 2387-2392.*)

the survival. Multiple studies of patients enrolled in palliative care programs report that a Karnofsky Performance Status score of 50% suggests a life expectancy of less than 8 weeks (Lamont & Christakis, 2003). Patients with a declining performance status should be referred to a palliative team. Many patients with cancer are likely eligible for hospice care under the admitting criteria of the Hospice Medicare benefit (i.e., a life expectancy of 6 months or less) when their performance status begins to decline.

The symptom profile of the patient also assists in identifying those patients appropriate for palliative care. Dyspnea, dysphagia, xerostomia, anorexia, and cognitive impairment are consistently identified as being associated with decreased length of life (Glare, 2005; Lamont & Christakis, 2003). Interestingly, pain is not predictive of poor survival, although increasing pain is reported to be more common in the last weeks of life (Glare, 2005). Also, increasing pain can be a sign of disease progression and must be evaluated thoroughly and managed optimally.

Predictions of survival by physicians are usually overly optimistic, but there is a correlation between predicted and actual survival up to 6 months. The most precise predictions are for those with less than 4 weeks to live, but predictions beyond 6 months show no relationship to actual survival (Glare, 2005). This helps explain why the median length of stay in hospice programs is only 22 days—physicians are most confident in predicting that a patient is in the last 6 months of life only about 4 weeks before the patient's death.

Patients who should receive palliative care from an interdisciplinary team include those with a cancer diagnosis who have an advanced stage of disease; a tumor that progresses during treatment; a short interval between treatment and tumor progression; a poor functional status; a symptom profile that includes dyspnea, dysphagia, xerostomia, anorexia, and cognitive impairment; or a clinician's prediction of survival of 6 months or less.

ETIOLOGY AND PATHOPHYSIOLOGY

Cancer is now understood to be caused by genetic mutations, including hereditary genetic factors and somatic genetic changes. It likely requires multiple accumulated oncogenic changes for complete transformation to malignancy. These genetic changes may lead to dysregulated growth, silencing of tumor-suppression capabilities, interference with normal cell death (apoptosis), and arresting of cell differentiation (Calvo, Petricoin, & Liotta, 2005). Together, these changes allow cancer cells to become self-renewing, immortal, and undifferentiated, as well as to possess the ability to be invasive. The familial cancers, such as certain retinoblastomas, breast cancers, colon cancers, and Wilms' tumors, involve at least one, if not several, hereditary genetic factors that interact with somatic genetic changes before malignant cells develop. The somatic genetic changes may be caused by viruses, chemical agents (including tobacco), radiation, and ultraviolet light (Yuspa & Shields, 2005).

Cancer is primarily a disease of the older population. One reason for this may be that progression from normal tissue to invasive cancer takes place over 5 to 20 years (Calvo et al., 2005). The fact that many of the cancers of the elderly (e.g., breast, lung, colon, prostate) arise from epithelial tissue is of interest. Because the epithelial tissues tend to be in areas that have undergone continued renewal throughout the life span, it is possible that cancers arise from a cumulative mutational load (Wong & Depinho, 2005).

Metastasis is the process by which malignant cells are released from the primary tumor and travel to regional or distant sites where they adhere and grow. Metastasis is the leading cause of both treatment failure and death for most patients who die of cancer. The process of metastasis formation is called the *metastatic cascade*. A host of factors are involved that allow tumor cells to "detach from the primary tumor, invade the extracellular basement membrane and enter circulation, survive in circulation to arrest in the capillary bed, adhere to a subendothelial basement membrane, gain entrance into the organ parenchyma, respond to paracrine growth factors, proliferate and induce angiogenesis, and evade host defenses" (Stetler-Stevenson, 2005, p. 117).

Common sites of metastasis are the lymph nodes, bone, brain, liver, and lungs. Cancer diagnoses that most often lead to terminal illness are those that metastasize early and therefore are diagnosed at advanced stages. The six leading causes of death due to cancer are discussed below. Table 15-1 outlines the metastatic patterns of these diseases.

Lung Cancer

Accounting for 13% of all new cancers and 29% of all cancer deaths, lung cancer is the predominant cause of cancer deaths across all race, gender, and ethnic groups in the United States. In 2006, an estimated 162,460 Americans will die from lung cancer (ACS, 2006). Squamous cell lung cancers tend to remain more localized than the other cell types and thus have the best chance for surgical cure. The other major cell types—adenocarcinoma and large-cell and small-cell lung cancers—tend to metastasize early and frequently (Murren, Turrisi, & Pass, 2005; Schrump, Altorki, Henschke et al., 2005).

In addition to the common sites of metastasis as outlined in Table 15-1, all cell types of lung cancer are highly likely to metastasize to mediastinal lymph nodes.

TABLE 15-1 ■ **Common Metastatic Sites by Cancer Diagnosis**

Cancer Diagnosis	Lung	Pleura	Brain	Bone	Liver	Adrenal Glands	Lymph Nodes	Skin	Bone Marrow
Lung									
Squamous	—			X	X	X			
Adenocarcinoma	—	XX	XX	XX	XX	XXX	XX		
Large-cell	—	XXX	X	XX	XX	XXX	XX		
Small-cell	—	XXX	X	XX	XXX	XXX	XXX		
Colorectal	XX		X	X	XXX		XXX		
Breast	XXX	XX	XX	XXX	XXX	XX	XXX	X	
Prostate	X			XXX	X		XXX		
Pancreas	XX	XX	X	XX	XXX	XX	XXX		
Non-Hodgkin's lymphoma	XX	X	XX	X	XX	XX	—	X	XX

Data from DeVita, V.T., Hellman, S., & Rosenberg, A. (Eds.). *Cancer: Principles and practice of oncology* (7th ed.). Philadelphia: Lippincott Williams & Wilkins.
XXX, Seen in almost all patients with advanced disease; *XX,* seen in most patients with advanced disease; *X,* seen in many patients with advanced disease.

Other potential sites of metastasis include the pericardium and the pancreas. Lung cancers may also lead to the following paraneoplastic syndromes (Murren et al., 2005; Schrump et al., 2005):

- Hypercalcemia occurs secondary to parathyroid hormone–related protein production and is most common with squamous cell lung cancer.
- The syndrome of inappropriate antidiuretic hormone (SIADH) develops due to ectopic natriuretic factor and is most common with small-cell lung cancer.
- Eaton-Lambert syndrome occurs due to a reduction in acetylcholine released at motor nerve terminals. This syndrome is most common with small-cell lung cancer. Symptoms include proximal muscle weakness, diplopia, bulbar symptoms, dry mouth, impotence, and constipation.
- Ectopic adrenocorticotropic hormone leads to Cushing's syndrome and is seen in small-cell lung cancer. Symptoms include muscle weakness, edema, hypertension, mental changes, glucose intolerance, and weight loss.

The pattern of early and frequent metastasis in lung cancer often translates into patients being diagnosed when the disease has reached an advanced stage. Indeed, 60% of small-cell lung cancers and 40% of non–small-cell lung cancers present in stage IV (Smith & Khuri, 2004). The 5-year survival rate for individuals diagnosed with distant metastasis is only 2.1% (ACS, 2006). Most patients should be referred for palliative care from the time of diagnosis.

Essentially all chemotherapy for advanced lung cancer is palliative in that cure is not the aim. Survival may be prolonged with chemotherapy, but the potential for increased length of life must be balanced against the effect on quality of life, toxicity of the chemotherapy, and costs of treatment. It is important to note that patients who respond best to chemotherapy are those who have not been previously treated with chemotherapy and who have a good performance status. Patients who have disease progression while receiving chemotherapy, relapse soon after completion of chemotherapy, or have a compromised performance status have a much lower potential for favorable outcomes from chemotherapy.

Colorectal Cancer

Colorectal cancer is the third leading cause of cancer deaths for men and for women and is the overall second leading cause of cancer deaths (men and women combined) in the United States. An estimated 55,170 will die of colorectal cancer in 2006, accounting for 10% of all cancer deaths (ACS, 2006). As with all cancers, the stage at diagnosis is the primary determinant of prognosis. The 5-year survival rate for colorectal cancers with distant metastasis is 9.7% (ACS, 2006).

Sites of metastasis include the lymph nodes, liver, lung, brain, bone, and adrenal glands (Libuiti, Saltz, Rustgi et al., 2005). These tumors are also likely to cause obstruction of the bowel, leading to nausea and vomiting and abdominal distention; obstruction of the ureter, causing flank pain, hydronephrosis, and renal failure; and obstruction of the urethra, leading to urinary retention and risk of bladder infection.

Until the past few years, colorectal tumors were considered resistant to most antineoplastic agents. Newer chemotherapy drugs and molecularly targeted therapies are improving survival in colorectal cancer (Wilkes, 2005). There is some controversy regarding the optimal duration of chemotherapy for metastatic disease. It appears that continuation of chemotherapy until clinical deterioration or disease progression has no advantage over a planned discontinuation of therapy after a fixed time (e.g., 3 months or 6 months). Patients with good performance status, good bone marrow reserve, and good organ function appear to benefit more from chemotherapy than do those who do not meet these criteria (Libuiti et al., 2005).

Breast Cancer

In the United States, breast cancer is the most frequent new cancer diagnosis in women and the second leading cause of cancer deaths in women. An estimated 41,430 patients will die from breast cancer in 2006 (ACS, 2006). The mortality rate has declined over the past decade largely due to early detection and the use of aggressive multimodality treatments (Wood, Muss, Solin et al., 2005). The 5-year survival rate for patients with distant metastasis is 26.1% (ACS, 2006). Poor prognostic indicators include stage IV disease, young age, estrogen receptor (ER)–and progesterone receptor (PR)–negative tumors, and tumors with *HER2* overexpression. Stage IV breast cancer is not considered curable. The median survival for patients with metastatic disease is 18 to 24 months. However, many treatments are available to control metastasis and prolong life considerably, and with newer therapies, it is estimated that approximately 10% of patients with metastasis will survive 10 years or longer (Wood et al., 2005).

Women who receive hormonal therapy and chemotherapy following surgery in early-stage disease demonstrate delayed recurrence and improved overall survival compared with those who do not receive chemotherapy (Wood et al., 2005). Women with ER- and PR-positive tumors tend to respond to hormone therapy. Women with ER- and PR-negative tumors and slowly progressive disease with minimal symptoms should be considered for hormone therapy as well. However, women with ER- and PR-negative tumors with rapidly progressive tumors should be considered for chemotherapy (Wood et al., 2005).

Women with ER-positive tumors with metastatic disease should be treated with hormone therapy before chemotherapy is considered (Wilcken, Hornbuckle, & Ghersi, 2003). Tamoxifen is still considered first-line hormonal therapy for premenopausal women with ER-positive metastatic disease. In postmenopausal women with metastasis, the ideal sequencing of hormonal therapy is not clear; tamoxifen, aromatase inhibitors, and fulvestrant are all considered reasonable choices for first-line therapy at this time (Wood et al., 2005). Improvement in bone pain is the best indication of response to hormone therapy in women with metastasis. Hormone therapy is generally continued as long as symptoms are controlled and side effects are tolerated. If hormone therapy is no longer indicated, the dose of the hormone is weaned slowly to prevent a withdrawal response.

When hormone treatment is no longer effective, chemotherapy is usually considered. Improved survival and symptom control may be possible in stage IV disease with combination chemotherapy, even in women who have previously received chemotherapy (Berruti, Sperone, Bottini et al., 2000; Ghersi, Wilcken, & Simes, 2005; Nagourney, Link, Blitzer et al., 2000; Wood et al., 2005). Taxane-containing regimens have fewer side effects than regimens with platinum-containing chemotherapeutic agents (Carrick, Ghersi, Wilcken et al., 2005; Ghersi et al., 2005). Response rates to initial chemotherapy regimens range from 25% to 60%, with a median time to progression of 6 months. Response rates for second- and third-line treatments diminish by half (Wood et al., 2005). The beneficial effect of chemotherapy, when given for symptom control, should be apparent by the second or third treatment. If the symptom being treated is not improving, carefully evaluate the benefits versus the burdens of continuing treatment should be carefully evaluated.

The lymph nodes are the most frequent site of metastasis. Other sites include the bone, lung, liver, pleura, adrenal glands, kidney, brain, skin, and chest wall. Women with ER- and PR-positive tumors are most likely to develop bone metastasis, and those with ER- and PR-negative tumors tend to have liver and other visceral metastasis (Wood et al., 2005). Due to the proximity of tumors to the skin surface, breast tumors may cause skin lesions that can progress to fungating tumor wounds.

Prostate Cancer

Cancer of the prostate is the most frequent cause of cancer in men, with 234,460 new diagnoses expected in 2006. It is the second leading cause of cancer deaths in men. Approximately 27,350 men will die of prostate cancer in 2006. The 5-year survival rate for patients with distant metastasis is 33.5% (ACS, 2006). Again, distant metastasis is not considered curable, but clearly, with a 5-year survival of 33.5%, men are living for years with metastatic prostate cancer.

Prostate cancers are often androgen dependent. Most tumors will respond to hormonal manipulation, providing symptomatic benefits and a moderate survival benefit (Scher, Leibel, Fuks, et al., 2005). However, the side effects of androgen suppression can reduce the quality of life for some patients (Schmitt, Bennett, Seidenfeld et al., 2000). These tumors are also radiosensitive and may be treated with external beam radiotherapy or implanted radioactive seeds. Systemic irradiation (e.g., strontium 89) may be helpful for managing widely metastatic bone pain, but it is more expensive and no more effective than local field radiotherapy for managing bone pain in a localized area (Finlay, Mason, & Shelley, 2005; Oosterhof, Roberts, de Reijke et al., 2003).

Until recently, chemotherapy did not play a role in the management of prostate cancer. Mitoxantrone-based regimens were the first to show palliative benefits in hormone-resistant tumors, but docetaxel-based therapies are also showing promise (Petrylak, Tangen, Hussain et al., 2004; Tannock, de Wit, Berry et al., 2004). Keep in mind that most study subjects showing a good response were less symptomatic and had a good performance status at the initiation of treatment; the benefit and tolerability of chemotherapy regimens in patients with poorer performance status, widely metastatic disease, or some organ system compromise are not known. Clinical trials using vaccines derived from dendritic cells expressing prostatic acid phosphatase are showing promise (Arlen & Gulley, 2005; Vieweg & Dannull, 2005).

Local spread of prostate cancer to the pelvic and abdominal lymph nodes, seminal vesicles, bladder, and peritoneum is common. Frequent sites of metastasis beyond the pelvis are bone (most frequent), lungs, and liver (Scher et al., 2005). Men with prostate cancer are at risk for developing urinary outflow obstruction, leading to urinary frequency, hesitancy, and nocturia; this may progress to urinary retention. They are also at risk for urethral obstruction, causing bladder dilatation, hydronephrosis, and impaired renal function.

Pancreatic Cancer

Although pancreatic cancer ranks eleventh in incidence of new cancers in the United States, it is the fourth leading cause of cancer deaths. In 2006, an estimated 32,300 patients will die from this malignancy. The prognosis for patients with pancreatic cancer is poor. The 5-year survival rate for all stages is just 4.6%, and for those with distant metastasis, the 5-year survival is only 1.8% (ACS, 2006). The disease generally does not display early symptoms. By the time jaundice is present or pain becomes significant enough for an individual to seek medical evaluation, 80% of pancreatic cancers are metastatic (Yeo et al., 2005).

Treatment options are limited. In the rare instance that disease is localized, surgery offers the only potential for cure, but survival after resection is often still limited. Most often, however, surgery is used for palliation of symptoms by relieving or preventing obstructions of the biliary duct and duodenum. The median survival after palliative surgery is about 6 months (Yeo et al., 2005). Chemotherapy does appear to modestly improve survival and to palliate some symptoms (El-Rayes & Philip, 2003; Yeo et al., 2005). Patients in clinical trials with gemcitabine demonstrated less pain, improved functional ability, and weight gain (Burris, Moore, Anderson et al., 1997). Patients showing the best responses to chemotherapy are treated soon after diagnosis, having not previously received chemotherapy, and have a good performance status. Combination chemotherapy with gemcitabine-based protocols is showing promise but needs further evaluation (Reni, Cordio, Milandri et al., 2005). The role of radiation therapy is limited, but some studies show benefit when chemotherapy is combined with radiation, particularly to shrink tumors preoperatively (Yeo et al., 2005). Palliative uses include relief of intestinal obstruction or unresectable biliary obstruction.

Regional metastatic sites include the regional lymph nodes, major vessels, celiac nerve plexus, duodenum, stomach, bile duct, retroperitoneum, spleen, kidney, adrenal glands, and colon. Distant metastasis occurs most often to the liver. Jaundice due to biliary obstruction is common. Additional metastatic sites include lung, bone, and brain

(Yeo et al., 2005). Patients with pancreatic cancer may also develop a sudden onset of diabetes due to destruction of the islet cells.

Non-Hodgkin's Lymphoma

In 2006, approximately 58,870 people will be diagnosed with non-Hodgkin's lymphoma and 18,840 will die of this disease, making it the sixth leading cause of cancer deaths. The 5-year survival rate is 60% (ACS, 2006). Patients over the age of 60 tend to have a poorer prognosis (Fisher, Mauch, Harris et al., 2005).

The major classifications of non-Hodgkin's lymphoma are based on cell-line (B cell or T cell/NK [natural killer] cell) and histological grade (low, medium, and high grade). Each of these types of classification has a significant influence on both treatment options and prognosis. In addition to cell type and histology, the stage of the disease influences the outcome. Although the staging system is different than that for solid tumors, stage IV is, again, the most advanced stage. Patients with diffuse or disseminated involvement of one or more extralymphatic organs, bone marrow involvement, or liver involvement have stage IV disease (Fisher et al., 2005).

Symptoms are related to the organ systems affected by the lymphadenopathy. Abdominal lymphadenopathy causes pain, anorexia, nausea and vomiting, bleeding, diarrhea, and obstruction. Hilar and mediastinal lymphadenopathy lead to cough, dyspnea, chest pain, pleural effusion, and superior vena cava syndrome. Central nervous system lymphoma may cause headache, lethargy, focal neurologic symptoms, seizures, and paralysis. Night sweats, recurrent fevers, and weight loss tend to be poor prognostic indicators (Fisher et al., 2005).

Many patients receive treatment upon diagnosis, because even when cure is not possible, treatment can significantly prolong survival. Patients with low-grade lymphoma who relapse may be retreated with the same or second-line therapy for symptomatic relief. Chemotherapy, radiation therapy, monoclonal antibody therapy, and stem cell transplantation are all potential options depending on the cell type and stage of disease.

COMMON SYMPTOMS OF ADVANCED CANCERS

As noted in Table 15-1, patients with advanced cancers may have multiple sites of metastasis. Keep in mind that almost all cancers can metastasize to almost any site; the sites identified on the chart are the more common metastatic sites. The symptoms commonly experienced by patients when cancer invades these sites are outlined below.

In addition to the following symptoms, all patients with cancer are at risk for pain due to compression of tissues by the tumor itself, leading to local ischemia, nerve compression, and obstruction of organ systems. Tumors may also invade local blood vessels. Oozing from small vessels may cause anemia; invasion of a major vessel may lead to death from exsanguination. Another common symptom of many advanced cancers is cachexia and anorexia (see Chapter 20). In addition to the symptoms caused by the disease itself, the treatments for cancer lead to uncomfortable symptoms, such as nausea and vomiting, diarrhea, anemia, mucositis, fatigue, and chemotherapy-induced peripheral neuropathies.

Lymph Node Metastasis

Lymph node metastasis causes pain from inflammation and swelling. When lymph flow is blocked by a tumor, lymphedema results and the affected area is at risk for infection, massive edema, and pain. Enlarged lymph nodes can also compress organs and surrounding tissues, leading to a risk for superior or inferior vena cava syndrome, spinal cord compression, nerve plexus compression, and obstruction of the bowel, urinary tract, or esophagus.

Bone Metastasis

Bone metastasis causes sharp pain that ranges from moderate to severe in intensity. Bone destruction leads to hypercalcemia and risk for pathological fractures. Patients with extensive bone metastasis are also at great risk for spinal cord compression from vertebral collapse.

Brain Metastasis

Brain metastasis puts the individual at risk for increased intracranial pressure and its accompanying symptoms—headache, vomiting, and change in level of consciousness. Depending on the area of the brain involved, personality changes are possible. Patients with brain metastasis are also at risk for seizure activity.

Liver Metastasis

Liver metastases interfere with the functioning of the liver, leading to impaired drug metabolism, disturbances in hemostasis, malabsorption, pruritus, anorexia, ascites, jaundice, and hepatic encephalopathy. Pain along the right rib margin is caused by the enlarging liver and is often referred around to the back and to the right shoulder.

Lung Tumors and Metastasis

Lung tumors, whether primary or metastatic, put the individual at risk for cough from irritation; dyspnea from effusion, atelectasis, and pneumonia; and wheezing from bronchospasm and obstruction. Hemoptysis results when tumor erodes blood vessels in the lung. Large tumors can compress local organs and tissues: if the esophagus is compressed, the individual experiences dysphagia; neuropathic pain occurs if there is pressure on the brachial plexus.

Adrenal Gland Metastasis

Adrenal gland metastases are often asymptomatic until the tumor size is at least 5 cm. With increasing tumor size, the individual experiences abdominal or back pain, as well as the gradual onset of weakness, lethargy, and anorexia. Hyperpigmentation is observed, especially in buccal mucosa, skin creases, and sites of friction. Nausea, vomiting, and postural hypotension are late signs of adrenal gland metastasis.

Bone Marrow Involvement

Bone marrow involvement by tumor leads to depression in bone marrow function. The result may be infections related to neutropenia, bleeding resulting from thrombocytopenia, and fatigue and dyspnea from anemia.

HISTORY AND PHYSICAL EXAMINATION

A complete history and physical examination of the individual with advanced cancer is essential for disease and symptom treatment planning.

General Assessment

■ Identify and evaluate anorexia/cachexia, weight loss, fatigue level, functional status, pain, temperature, and reports of night sweats.

Cardiac Assessment

■ Evaluate pulse rate and rhythm, heart sounds, and blood pressure.

Respiratory Assessment

■ Assess respiratory rate, effort, and patient reports of dyspnea.
■ Auscultate the lungs to identify any wheezing, rales, crackles, pleural rub, decreased breath sounds, or distant breath sounds.
■ Percuss the chest, noting any dullness over effusions or atelectasis.
■ Observe sputum for hemoptysis and evaluate the color and consistency for signs of infection.
■ Observe the color of nail beds and mucous membranes for signs of cyanosis.

Skin/Mucous Membrane Assessment

■ Identify erythema, skin breakdown, dryness or lesions of mucous membranes, bruising/petechiae, jaundice, hyperpigmentation, and signs of itching.
■ Evaluate any tumor nodules or wounds.

Abdominal Assessment

■ Assess bowel status, bowel patterns, and any problems with nausea or vomiting.
■ Auscultate bowel sounds; percuss abdomen for air, fluid, or consolidation.
■ Palpate lightly to identify presence of lymphadenopathy or enlargement or tenderness of the liver, spleen, or kidneys.
■ Look for signs of bleeding—occult or frank bleeding of upper or lower gastro-intestinal tract, melena, and "coffeeground" emesis.

Genitourinary Tract Assessment

■ Assess urinary output and observe the concentration and color of the urine.
■ Evaluate for hematuria and dysuria.
■ Identify any difficulties with urinary retention.

Musculoskeletal Assessment

■ Evaluate range of motion and muscle strength.
■ Note any lymphedema or sign of infection.
■ Identify the potential for pathological fracture.

Neurologic Assessment

■ Assess motor strength and coordination.
■ Evaluate changes in sensation and mental status.

- Identify signs of increased intracranial pressure—headache, wide pulse pressure, increased blood pressure, and bradycardia.

DIAGNOSTICS

Diagnostic testing should be considered if the identification or confirmation of the underlying cause of uncomfortable symptoms influences the course of action. If, for example, superior vena cava syndrome is suspected but the patient is clearly close to death, interventions to promote comfort (e.g., corticosteroids to reduce inflammation, opioids to treat dyspnea) can be instituted without confirmation of the diagnosis with a radiographic study or computed tomography scan. Likewise, serum aspartate amino-transferase and alanine aminotransferase levels, while supplying chemical evidence of liver dysfunction, are not necessarily helpful in managing symptoms.

- Chest radiographic studies identify bronchial obstruction, atelectasis, pneumonia, pleural effusion, and superior vena cava syndrome.
- Computed tomography scans may show metastasis to brain, liver, lungs, adrenal glands, and abdomen; pleural effusion; superior vena cava syndrome; and spinal cord compression.
- Bone scans show sites of bone metastasis.
- Sputum culture and sensitivity tests assist in selecting the appropriate antiinfective interventions if pulmonary infection recurs or is persistent after empiric antibiotic treatment.
- Blood count and serum chemistries, including complete blood count, calcium, sodium, and glucose, aid in the detection of bone marrow deficiencies and chemical imbalances.

INTERVENTIONS PARTICULAR TO METASTATIC DISEASE

All of the symptoms addressed in Unit IV are potential complications of advanced cancer. Refer to the guidelines provided in Unit IV for management of these symptoms. In addition, the following section presents interventions specifically helpful for symptom management in advanced cancer. These interventions are to be considered in combination with the interventions in Unit IV.

Bone Metastasis

The pain associated with bone metastasis often requires a combination of opioid and nonsteroidal antiinflammatory drugs. More recent data show that bisphosphonates help decrease the risk of skeletal complications and delay their onset in patients with bone metastasis. Zolendronic acid has better efficacy in solid tumors than other bis-phosphonates (Lipton, 2005). Discussion must take place as to whether the benefit warrants the cost associated with these agents and, if initiated, when it is appropriate to discontinue them. Obtaining local control is thought to be paramount to ensuring the patient's quality of life, making surgical intervention to prevent, stabilize, or repair a pathological fracture an alternative that should be considered in some circumstances (Manabe, Kawaguchi, Matsumoto et al., 2005). Radiation therapy is also very helpful for the pain of bone metastasis. It appears that there is no difference in pain relief using high-dose single fractions versus fractionated schedules (Wu et al., 2003). Consider that high-dose single fractions are less disruptive to daily living. Systemic radiopharmaceuticals (e.g., strontium 89) may be considered if the patient has widespread bone metastasis and has a prognosis of at least 3 months. Hormonal manipulation may be helpful for bone pain in patients with breast or prostate cancer.

A less frequently used measure may include embolization of metastatic lesions. This can be done with coils, alcohol, or other agents, resulting in significant pain relief (Kato, Tsuyuki, Kikuchi et al., 2005). Palliation using hyperthermia or cryotherapy continues to be explored (Uchida, Wakabayashi, Okuyama et al., 2004).

Brain Metastasis

Brain metastases are typically treated by one of the following modalities: surgery, whole brain irradiation, stereotactic radiosurgery, chemotherapy, or symptom management. Brain metastasis occurs in approximately 25% of all patients with cancer (Kaal, Niel, & Vecht, 2005). The diagnosis of brain metastasis generally portends an ominous prognosis, with those patients who decline any treatment having an estimated survival of approximately 1 month (Lassman & DeAngelis, 2003). Symptoms associated with brain metastasis are largely dependent on the site of disease within the brain and the degree of associated edema. Headache is noted to be the presenting symptom in approximately half of the patients. Chemotherapeutic strategies to control brain metastasis are very limited because most agents are unable to cross the blood-brain barrier. Progress has been made in glioblastoma and in anecdotal cases of metastatic melanoma to the brain using temozolamide. Whole brain irradiation remains a primary treatment when multiple brain lesions exist. Research continues to identify potential chemotherapeutic agents that may serve as radiation sensitizers in this setting.

Management strategies are best identified with an evaluation of the patient's general clinical status. Aggressive treatment may not be appropriate in patients with declining performance status, multiple brain tumors, significant neurological deficits, and radioresistant histologies such as melanoma, renal cancer, and sarcoma (Pollock, Brown, Foote et al., 2003). Corticosteroids, while having no direct effect on tumors other than lymphomas, are often used for symptom palliation. However, long-term use is not without side effects; these side effects can also prove to diminish the patient's quality of life and include proximal myopathies, bacterial and fungal infections, mood disorders, and blood sugar elevations, to name a few. Dosing may include an initial bolus of dexamethasone 10 mg to 24 mg orally followed by 2 mg to 6 mg orally every 6 hours (Lassman & DeAngelis, 2003).

The prophylactic use of anticonvulsant medications in patients with brain metastasis is no longer thought to be of benefit but is appropriate for patients with a history of seizures. Use of an anticonvulsant agent such as levetiracetan (Keppra) that is not metabolized via the P450 enzyme system is preferred (Barker, 2005).

In the event of a sudden increase in intracranial pressure with risk of herniation— and if reversal of this condition is in the patient's interest—consider admission to an intensive care unit for assisted ventilation, administration of hyperosmolar agents (mannitol), and administration of high-dose intravenous corticosteroids. These intensive measures are rarely appropriate in the palliative care setting because reversal of the disease process is not possible.

Liver Metastasis

The liver is one of the most common sites of metastatic disease (Adam, 2002). A celiac plexus block should be considered for the pain associated with liver metastasis if it persists despite maximal pharmacological management. If the underlying disease process is small-cell lung cancer, chemotherapy may be appropriate after careful evaluation. Before initiating chemotherapy, the individual's previous response to chemotherapy, length of time from last treatment to disease progression, and functional status must be considered.

Corticosteroids are sometimes helpful for anorexia and malaise associated with liver metastasis, and cholestyramine is helpful for pruritus. Short fractionation radiotherapy may provide palliation (10 Gy in two fractions over 2 days) (Bydder, Spry, Christie et al., 2003). A role may exist for the insertion of stents such as self-expanding metallic stents inserted endoscopically in patients with obstructions of the gastrointestinal and biliary tract (Holt, Patel, & Ahmed, 2004). Less data are available regarding the evidence for the use of radiofrequency ablation, cryotherapy, chemoembolization, and octreotide administration, although each may have a role in specific circumstances (Lau, Lo, & Tan, 2003; Parikh, Curley, Fornage et al., 2002; Patel & Jindal, 2001; Sotsky & Ravikumar, 2002; Valiozis, Zekry, Williams et al., 2000). Treat encephalopathy due to liver failure as a terminal event; do not institute unpleasant therapies (e.g., magnesium sulfate enemas and lactulose).

Pleural Effusions

Malignant pleural effusions are common in a number of malignancies and may be seen in any malignancy that involves metastasis to the lungs. Thoracentesis provides relief of the dyspnea and discomfort associated with pleural effusions. However, malignant effusions will almost always recur within a relatively short time frame. Large-bore chest tube placement requires hospitalization and can involve a significant amount of discomfort for patients, making it a less desirable choice in the palliative setting. Sclerotherapy to produce pleurodesis is recommended to decrease the incidence of recurrence. Doxycycline is the agent of choice for this, because it is relatively inexpensive and has reasonably good efficacy (Covey, 2005). More recently, a variety of small-bore tunneled or pigtail catheters have been used as a way to drain pleural fluid and relieve patient symptoms. These tubes are inserted using radiographic guidance in the outpatient setting, and patients can be sent home with the catheter in place. The patient and family are instructed to connect the pleural catheter to a vacuum drainage system at prescribed intervals and as needed. If drainage decreases significantly or stops altogether, the tube may be removed. In many cases, it appears that mechanical pleurodesis occurs (Musani, Haas, Seijo et al., 2004; Putman, Light, Rodriguez et al., 1999; Putman, Walsh, Swisher et al., 2000; Pollak, 2002). A more aggressive procedure involves the use of video-assisted thoracoscopic surgery (VATS). This technique is useful in draining loculated fluid collections but typically involves general anesthesia and a hospital stay of several days (Brega-Massone, Conti, Magnani et al., 2004).

Compression and Obstruction Due to Tumor or Lymphadenopathy

Excessive tumor growth can result in obstruction of airways; obstruction of urinary, gastrointestinal, and biliary passages; as well as compression of lymph and blood vessels. The associated symptoms depend on the site of obstruction.

Obstruction of the urinary system may require the use of stents, urinary catheters, or suprapubic catheters to maintain adequate flow. A surgical procedure to debulk the tumor or bypass the obstruction is an option if the patient is a good surgical candidate. Airway obstruction can be more difficult to manage and is certainly more anxiety producing for patients and families. Endobronchial surgical techniques, radiotherapy, chemotherapy, or embolization procedures should be considered for symptom palliation along with the use of oxygen or humidified air.

Venous compression, as seen in superior vena cava syndrome, may be initially managed with corticosteroids to decrease inflammation and edema. This can be followed by radiation therapy, raising the head of the bed, oxygen therapy, and diuretics (Jacobs, 2003). Measures to control lymphedema will be based on the patient's activity level and prognosis.

CONCLUSION

The care of the patient with advanced cancer and his or her family requires a combination of in-depth knowledge of the underlying disease process and probable symptom progression as well as expertise in symptom management. As with all patients at the end of life, patients with cancer and their families have often experienced years of tiresome and perhaps ineffective treatments, uncomfortable symptoms (many of which are not adequately controlled), and an increasing burden on caregivers. Oftentimes patients and families have lost faith in the health care system. In addition to expertise related to the disease process and progression, the clinician needs to establish and maintain a relationship based on mutual trust and respect.

REFERENCES

Adam, A. (2002). Interventional radiology in the treatment of hepatic metastases. *Cancer Treat Rev, 28(2)*, 93-99.

American Cancer Society (ACS). (2006). *Cancer facts and figures 2006*. Atlanta: Author.

Arlen, P.M. & Gulley, J.L. (2005). Therapeutic vaccines for prostate cancer: A review of clinical data. *Curr Opin Investig Drugs, 6(6)*, 592-596.

Barker, F.G. (2005). Surgical and radiosurgical management of brain metastases. *Surg Clin North Am, 85(2)*, 329-345.

Berruti, A., Sperone, P., Bottini, A., et al. (2000). Phase II study of vinorelbine with protracted fluorouracil infusion as a second- or third-line approach for advanced breast cancer patients previously treated with anthracycline. *J Clin Oncol, 18*, 3370-3377.

Brega-Massone, P.P., Conti, B., Magnani, B., et al. (2004). Minimally invasive thoracic surgery for diagnostic assessment and palliative treatment in recurrent neoplastic pleural effusion. *Thorac Cardiovasc Surg, 52(4)*, 191-195.

Burris, H.A. III, Moore, M.J., Andersen, J., et al. (1997). Improvements in survival and clinical benefits with gemcitabine as first-line therapy for patients with advanced pancreas cancer: A randomized trial. *J Clin Oncol, 15,* 2403-2413.

Bydder, S., Spry, N.A., Christie, D.R., et al. (2003). A prospective trial of short-fractionation radiotherapy for the palliation of liver metastases. *Australas Radiol, 47(3),* 284-288.

Calvo, K.R., Petricoin, E.F., & Liotta, L.A. (2005). Genomics and proteomics. In V.T. DeVita, S. Hellman, & S.A. Rosenberg (Eds.). *Cancer: Principles and practice of oncology* (7th ed., pp. 51-72). Philadelphia: Lippincott Williams & Wilkins.

Carrick, S., Ghersi, D., Wilcken, N., et al. (2005). Platinum containing regimens for metastatic breast cancer. *Cochrane Database Syst Rev, (3),* CD003374.

Covey, A.M. (2005). Management of malignant pleural effusions and ascites. *J Support Oncol, 3(2),* 169-173.

El-Rayes, B.F. & Philip, P.A. (2003). A review of systemic therapy for advanced pancreatic cancer. *Clin Adv Hematol Oncol, 1(7),* 430-434.

Finlay, I.G., Mason, M.D., & Shelley, M. (2005). Radioisotopes for the palliation of metastatic bone pain: A systematic review. *Lancet Oncol, 6(6),* 392-400.

Fisher, R.I, Mauch, P.M., Harris, N.L., et al. (2005). Non-Hodgkin's lymphomas. In V.T. DeVita, S. Hellman, et al. (Eds.). *Cancer: Principles and practice of oncology* (7th ed., pp. 1957-1997). Philadelphia: Lippincott Williams & Wilkins.

Ghersi, D., Wilcken, N., & Simes, J. (2005). Taxane containing regimens for metastatic breast cancer. *Cochrane Database Syst Rev, (2),* CD003366.

Glare, P. (2005). Clinical predictors of survival in advanced cancer. *J Support Oncol, 3(5),* 331-339.

Holt, A.P., Patel, M., & Ahmed, M.M. (2004). Palliation of patients with malignant gastroduodenal obstruction with self-expanding metallic stents: The treatment of choice? *Gastrointest Endosc, 60(6),* 1010-1017.

Jacobs, L.G. (2003). Managing respiratory symptoms at the end of life. *Clin Geriatr Med, 19(1),* 225-239.

Kaal, E.C., Niel, C.G., & Vecht, C.J. (2005). Therapeutic management of brain metastasis. *Lancet Neurol, 4(5),* 289-298.

Kato, Y., Tsuyuki, A., Kikuchi, K., et al. (2005). Dramatic relief of pain by transcatheter arterial embolization for bone metastasis from hepatocellular carcinoma. *J Gastroenterol Hepatol, 20(2),* 326-327.

Lamont, E.B. & Christakis, N.A. (2003). Complexities in prognostication in advanced cancer. *JAMA, 290(1),* 98-104.

Lassman, A.B. & DeAngelis, L.M. (2003). Brain metastases. *Neurol Clin, 21(1),* 1-23.

Lau, T.N., Lo, R.H., & Tan, B.S. (2003). Colorectal hepatic metastases: Role of radiofrequency ablation. *Ann Acad Med, Singapore, 32(2),* 212-218.

Libuiti, S.K., Saltz, L.B., Rustgi, A.K., et al. (2005). Cancer of the colon. In V.T. DeVita, S. Hellman, & S.A. Rosenberg (Eds.). *Cancer: Principles and practice of oncology* (7th ed., pp. 1061-1109). Philadelphia: Lippincott Williams & Wilkins.

Lipton, A. (2005). Management of bone metastases in breast cancer. *Curr Treat Opt Oncol, 6(2),* 161-171.

Lunney, J.R., Lynn, J., Foley, D.J., et al. (2003). Patterns of functional decline at the end of life. *JAMA, 289(18),* 2387-2392.

Manabe, J., Kawaguchi, N., Matsumoto, S., et al. (2005). Surgical treatment of bone metastasis: Indications and outcomes. *Int J Clin Oncol, 10(2),* 103-111.

Murren, J.R., Turrisi, A.T., & Pass, H.I. (2005). Small cell lung cancer. In V.T. DeVita, S. Hellman, & S.A. Rosenberg (Eds.). *Cancer: Principles and practice of oncology* (7th ed., pp. 810-843). Philadelphia: Lippincott Williams & Wilkins.

Musani, A.I., Haas, A.R., Seijo, L., et al. (2004). Outpatient management of malignant pleural effusions with small-bore, tunneled pleural catheters. *Respiration, 71(6),* 559-566.

Nagourney, R.A., Link, J.S., Blitzer, J.B., et al. (2000). Gemcitabine plus cisplatin repeating doublet therapy in previously treated, relapsed breast cancer patients. *J Clin Oncol, 18,* 2245-2249.

National Hospice and Palliative Care Organization (NHPCO). (2006). *Hospice facts and figures.* Retrieved February 20, 2006, from www.nhpco.org/files/public/Facts_Figures_for2004data.pdf.

Oosterhof, G.O., Roberts, J.T., de Reijke, T.M., et al. (2003). Strontium(89) chloride versus palliative local field radiotherapy in patients with hormonal escaped prostate cancer: A phase III study of the European Organisation for Research and Treatment of Cancer, Genitourinary Group. *Eur Urol, 44(5),* 519-526.

Parikh, A.A., Curley, S.A., Fornage, B.D., et al. (2002). Radiofrequency ablation of hepatic metastases. *Semin Oncol, 29(2),* 168-182.

Patel, N.H. & Jindal, R.M. (2001). The role of chemoembolization in the treatment of colorectal hepatic metastases. *Hepatogastroenterology, 48(38),* 448-452.

Petrylak, D.P., Tangen, C.M., Hussain, M.H., et al. (2004). Docetaxel and estramustine compared with mitoxantrone and prednisone for advanced refractory prostate cancer. *N Engl J Med, 351(15),* 1513-1520.

Pollak, J.S. (2002). Malignant pleural effusions: Treatment with tunneled long-term drainage catheters. *Curr Opin Pulm Med, 8(4),* 302-307.

Pollock, B.E., Brown, P.D., Foote, R.L., et al. (2003). Properly selected patients with multiple brain metastases may benefit from aggressive treatment of their intracranial disease. *J Neuro-oncol, 61(1),* 73-80.

Putman, J.B., Light, R.W., Rodriguez, R.M., et al. (1999). A randomized comparison of indwelling pleural catheter and doxycycline pleurodesis in the management of malignant pleural effusions. *Cancer, 86(10),* 1992-1999.

Putman, J.B., Walsh, G.L., Swisher, S.G., et al. (2000). Outpatient management of malignant pleural effusion by a chronic indwelling pleural catheter. *Ann Thorac Surg, 69(2),* 369-375.

Reni, M., Cordio, S., Milandri, C., et al. (2005). Gemcitabine versus cisplatin, epirubicin, fluorouracil, and gemcitabine in advanced pancreatic cancer: A randomized controlled multicentre phase III trial. *Lancet Oncol, 6(6),* 369-76.

Scher, H.I., Leibel, S.A., Fuks, Z., et al. (2005). Cancer of the prostate. In V.T. DeVita, S. Hellman, & S.A. Rosenberg (Eds.). *Cancer: Principles and practice of oncology* (7th ed., pp. 1192-1259). Philadelphia: Lippincott Williams & Wilkins.

Schmitt, B., Bennett, C., Seidenfeld, J., et al. (2000). Maximal androgen blockade for advanced prostate cancer. *Cochrane Database Syst Rev, (2),* CD001526.

Schrump, D.S., Altorki, N.K., Henschke, C.L., et al. (2005). Non-small cell lung cancer. In V.T. DeVita, S. Hellman, & S.A. Rosenberg (Eds.). *Cancer: Principles and practice of oncology* (7th ed., pp. 753-810). Philadelphia: Lippincott Williams & Wilkins.

Smith, W., & Khuri, F.R., (2004). The care of the lung cancer patient in the 21st century: A new age. *Semin Oncol, 31(2 Suppl. 4),* 11-15.

Sotsky, T.K. & Ravikumar, T.S. (2002). Cryotherapy in the treatment of liver metastases from colorectal cancer. *Semin Oncol, 29(2),* 183-191.

Stetler-Stevenson, W.G. (2005). Invasion and metastases. In V.T. DeVita, S. Hellman, & S.A. Rosenberg (Eds.). *Cancer: Principles and practice of oncology* (7th ed., pp. 113-127). Philadelphia: Lippincott Williams & Wilkins.

Tannock, I.F., de Wit, R., Berry, W.R., et al.; TAX 327 Investigators. (2004). Docetaxel plus prednisone or mitoxantrone plus prednisone for advance prostate cancer. *N Engl J Med, 351(15),* 1502-1512.

Uchida, A., Wakabayashi, H., Okuyama, N., et al. (2004). Metastatic bone disease: Pathogenesis and new strategies for treatment. *J Orthop Sci, 9(4),* 415-420.

Valiozis, I., Zekry, A., Williams, S.J., et al. (2000). Palliation of hilar biliary obstruction from colorectal metastases by endoscopic stent insertion. *Gastrointest Endosc, 51(4 Pt 1),* 412-417.

Vieweg, J. & Dannull, J. (2005). Technology insight: vaccine therapy for prostate cancer. *Nature Clin Pract Urol, 2(1),* 44-51.

Wilcken, N., Hornbuckle, J., & Ghersi, D. (2003). Chemotherapy alone versus endocrine therapy alone for metastatic breast cancer. *Cochrane Database Syst Rev, (2),* CD002747.

Wilkes, G.M. (2005). Therapeutic options in the management of colon cancer: 2005 Update. *Clin J Oncol Nurs, 9(1),* 31-43.

Wong, K., & Depinho, R.A. (2005). Telomerase. In V.T. DeVita, S. Hellman, & S.A. Rosenberg (Eds.). *Cancer: Principles and practice of oncology* (7th ed., pp. 105-112). Philadelphia: Lippincott Williams & Wilkins.

Wood, W.C., Muss, H.B., Solin, L.J., et al. (2005). Malignant tumors of the breast. In V.T. De Vita, S. Hellman, & S.A. Rosenberg (Eds.). *Cancer: Principles and practice of oncology* (7th ed., pp. 1415-1477). Philadelphia: Lippincott Williams & Wilkins.

Wu, J.S., Wong, R., Johnston, M., et al.; Cancer Care Ontario Practice Guidelines Initiative Supportive Care Group. (2003). Meta-analysis of dose-fractionation radiotherapy trials for the palliation of painful bone metastases. *Int J Radi Oncol Biol Physics, 55(3),* 594-605.

Yeo, C.J., Yeo, R.P., Hruban, R.H., et al. (2005). Cancer of the pancreas. In V.T. DeVita, S. Hellman, & S.A. Rosenberg (Eds.). *Cancer: Principles and practice of oncology* (7th ed., pp. 945-986). Philadelphia: Lippincott Williams & Wilkins.

Yuspa, S.H. & Shields, P.G. (2005). Etiology of cancer: Chemical factors. In V.T. DeVita, S. Hellman, & S.A. Rosenberg (Eds.). *Cancer: Principles and practice of oncology* (7th ed., pp. 185-191). Philadelphia: Lippincott Williams & Wilkins.

CHAPTER 16

HIV/AIDS

James C. Pace

■

At the end of the year 2003 approximately 790,000 to 1.2 million Americans were living with human immune deficiency virus/acquired immunodeficiency syndrome (HIV/AIDS) and approximately 46 million were living with HIV/AIDS worldwide (World Health Organization, 2003). Prior to the advent of antiretroviral medications (AZT monotherapy first appeared in 1987), HIV/AIDS was viewed as a death sentence—death often occurred less than 1 year after the diagnosis. Once protease inhibitors (PIs) were developed in the mid-1990s, with the concurrent development of highly active antiretroviral therapy (HAART), there were dramatic changes in the trajectory of HIV/AIDS. AIDS-related deaths in the United States declined approximately 70% in the years 1985 through 2001 following the introduction of HAART; death rates from AIDS have only recently begun to show a very slow upward direction due to rapidly developing viral resistance factors (Center for Palliative Care Education, 2003). As a result, post-HAART health care clinicians in HIV/AIDS care have often not been immersed in the historical issues surrounding death and dying as have seasoned clinicians with memories of caring for those with short survival times combined with extremely limited health care options. Since 1997, AIDS has no longer been one of the top 15 causes of death for *all age groups* combined; however, AIDS remains the fifth leading cause of death among all Americans aged 25 to 40, the leading cause of death among African American men in this age group, and the third leading cause of death among African American women in this age group (Center for Palliative Care Education, 2003).

Currently, HIV/AIDS is perceived as a chronic, manageable disease for those who can take HAART. HIV/AIDS continues to have an unpredictable course, however, related to impaired immune competence, side effects of medications, comorbidities, and issues involving the psychosocial and emotional costs of living with HIV/AIDS (Sherman, 2001). As with other chronic disease states, HIV/AIDS constitutes a continuum of health concerns beginning at initial seroconversion and continuing into its terminal stages. Current statistics reveal that in the absence of therapy, this slowly progressive disease has an average course of 10 to 15 years.

AIDS is often a disease of the disenfranchised and marginalized. In 2004, African Americans accounted for 49% of all AIDS cases although they composed only 13% of the population, and 19% of all AIDS cases occurred in Hispanics although they represented only 14% of the U.S. population (Centers for Disease Control and Prevention [CDC], 2004; Ramirez & de la Cruz, 2003). Many of these patient groups lacked access to medical care, mistrusted the health care system, were involved with the health care of family members to the exclusion of personal health status, or were diagnosed with AIDS during hospitalization when HIV infection was far advanced. It is a well-established fact that minority groups are most often diagnosed with HIV/AIDS later in the disease process than are whites and have significantly greater immunosuppression and symptoms (Sackoff & Shin, 2001). If HAART was made available to many in the above-mentioned groups, adherence was often compromised by such issues as poverty, substance abuse, comorbidities, depression, and lack of sustained support systems (Center for Palliative Care Education, 2003; Jordan, Vaughn, & Hood, 2004). It is important to consider the palliative care implications of HIV/AIDS especially in light of the above scenarios and because HAART therapies are losing their antiviral effectiveness for a select few, are refused entirely by some, and are discontinued by many who tire of the associated pill burden of complex HAART therapies and their often unrelenting drug and metabolic side effects.

PATHOPHYSIOLOGY AND NOMENCLATURE

HIV is a retrovirus that has a particular affinity for the body's immune system, particularly infecting macrophages and T-lymphocytes (T cells or CD4 cells). Continual destruction of the body's immune system leaves the body open to more virulent attacks by HIV as well as from opportunistic organisms that would not be able to harm nonimpaired immune systems. Infection with HIV can eventually progress to AIDS. In the term *acquired immunodeficiency syndrome*, "acquired" means that the illness is not usually inherited from a parent, "immunodeficient" describes the condition of altered immune competence, and "syndrome" means that AIDS cannot be defined by a single disease or illness but rather by a collection of possible health insults. HIV and AIDS are not synonymous terms. HIV describes a living virus; AIDS names a syndrome of health care concerns. Being HIV positive refers to the presence of the virus within a person's body irregardless of T-cell count; AIDS describes a profound immunocompromised state where the T-cell count falls below 200 cells (or a percentage of <14%) (see below for details). A person can be HIV positive for decades without showing any symptoms of or being diagnosed with AIDS (Sherman, 2001; Zwolski, 2001). Once infected with HIV by means of exposure to infected blood, semen, or bodily fluids, a person will develop antibodies to HIV that can be detected by a blood test. The development of such antibodies may take anywhere from a few weeks to 6 months after exposure. Once antibodies are detected with an HIV test, the person is then diagnosed as being HIV positive.

In 1993, the CDC developed a revised HIV classification system and an expanded AIDS surveillance definition for adolescents and adults. The CDC system provides a clinically based definition of AIDS that includes categories A, B, and C. These categories are briefly summarized as follows (Zwolski, 2001):

- *Category A* includes patients with acute primary HIV illness (acute retroviral syndrome), asymptomatic HIV infection, or persistent generalized lymphadenopathy.
- *Category B* includes a number of symptomatic conditions that are either directly attributable to HIV infection or have a clinical course or management complicated by the presence of HIV. Examples of these symptomatic conditions include oropharyngeal candidiasis, vulvovaginal candidiasis, constitutional symptoms to include fever and diarrhea, herpes zoster, oral hairy leukoplakia, pelvic inflammatory disease, peripheral neuropathy, and cervical dysplasia.
- *Category C* comprises AIDS indicator conditions, including bronchial, tracheal, pulmonary, or esophageal candidiasis; invasive cervical cancer; cryptococcosis;

cryptosporidiosis; cytomegalovirus disease (CMV, including CMV retinitis); encephalopathy; persistent herpes simplex (HSV); Kaposi's sarcoma; lymphomas (Burkitt's, immunoblastic, primary of brain); *Mycobacterium avium* complex (MAC) and *Mycobacterium tuberculosis; Pneumocystis jiroveci* (formerly *carinii*) pneumonia (PCP); toxoplasmosis of brain; and HIV wasting disease.

TRAJECTORY AND ASSOCIATED CLINICAL SYMPTOMS

Primary HIV infection (acute retroviral syndrome), the period immediately after infection with HIV (2 to 8 weeks), is characterized by high levels of viremia and is accompanied by such symptoms as fever (97%), myalgia or arthralgia (58%), lethargy and malaise (common), lymphadenopathy (70%, particularly in the groin and head and neck), pharyngitis (73%), and an erythematous, nonpruritic, maculopapular rash affecting most often the face or trunk (70%).

Chronic HIV infection is divided into categories based on the CD4 count:

- *Early: CD4 count >500.* Although the virus is actively reproducing at this stage, there is generally a period of clinical latency in terms of visible symptoms. Minor infections may take longer times to heal, depending upon the patient. Patients often report symptoms such as mild diarrhea, cough, fatigue, night sweats, minor skin rashes, weight loss, oral problems, and persistent or recurrent vaginal yeast infections.
- *Middle (intermediate): CD4 count 200 to 500.* Features present in early HIV disease often worsen (e.g., diarrhea, recurrent HSV, oral or vaginal candidiasis). There is an increased incidence of bacterial infections of sinuses, respiratory tract, and skin; there is also an increased disruption of lymphoid tissue.
- *Late (AIDS): CD4 count <200.* Appearance of opportunistic infections—any or a combination of the AIDS indicator conditions as described by CDC (see category C on p. 234). Lymphoid tissue is mostly replaced by fibroid tissue (Sherman, 2001; Zwolski, 2001).

DIAGNOSTICS AND ASSESSMENT

HIV-positive status is tested by means of an ELISA (enzyme-linked immunosorbent assay) (which measures antibody to HIV) and, if reactive, is then confirmed with the Western blot. Once positive status is documented, the clinician looks at various laboratory diagnostic tools for the establishment of a long-term treatment plan that includes medical management combined with nutritional, emotional, and behavioral health supportive care.

- *CD4 cell count or percentage:* A normal CD4 count is 600 to 1200 cells per microliter (or 30% to 60%). AIDS is diagnosed when the CD4 cell count drops below 200 (<14%). At this time, prophylaxis against various opportunistic infections (PCP, cryptococci, MAC) should be initiated (Table 16-1).
- *CD8 count:* These are sometimes called the cytotoxic T cells; the normal count is 420 to 660 cells/mm^3. The CD8 lymphocytes mediate the direct killing of cells infected with HIV. Gradual decline in CD8 cells (as well as CD4 cells) indicates disease progression. In an adult, a count above 400 cells/mm^3 is considered desirable.

TABLE 16-1 ■ **Recommendations for Infection Prophylaxis in HIV/AIDS**

Pathogen	Indication	First Choice
PCP	CD4 <200	TMP-SMX
Toxoplasmosis	CD4 <100	TMP-SMX
MAC	CD4 <50	Azithromycin or clarithromycin
CMV	Secondary prophylaxis	Ganciclovir Valganciclovir Foscarnet Cidofovir
Cryptococcosis	Secondary prophylaxis after history of cryptococcal meningitis	Fluconazole
Tuberculosis	Positive PPD (≥5 mm induration) Recent contact with TB case History of inadequately treated TB	INH
Streptococcus pneumoniae	All patients	Pneumovax
HBV	Antibody HBc negative	HBV vaccine series
Influenza	All patients	Influenza vaccine
HAV	Antibody HAV negative	HAV vaccine series

CMV, Cytomegalovirus; *HAV,* hepatitis A virus; *HBc,* hepatitis B core antibody; *HBV,* hepatitis B virus; *MAC, Mycobacterium avium* complex; *PCP, Pneumocystis jiroveci* (formerly *carinii*) pneumonia; *TB,* tuberculosis; *TMP-SMX,* trimethoprim-sulfamethoxazole.
Adapted from Barlett, J.G. (2005). *A pocket guide to adult HIV/AIDS treatment.* Rockville, Md.: U.S. Department of Health and Human Services Health Resources and Services Administration. Retrieved October 25, 2005, from www.hab.hrsa.gov/tools/HIVpocketguide/index.htm.

■ *Viral load:* Quantitative polymerase chain reaction (PCR) or PCR-DNA (which identifies the amount of HIV RNA or DNA present) provides a measure of viremia. Viral load and CD4 count provide critical markers in the management of HIV disease and in monitoring disease progression. The quantified viral load helps the clinician know when to initiate therapy, evaluate the effectiveness of the antiviral, and change therapy due to viral resistance (failing drug regimen). Viral load measures can vary between undetectable (lower limit of detection is usually between 20 and 400 copies, depending on the laboratory measure chosen) to several million copies. An undetectable viral load does not mean the patient is cured of HIV infection. In addition, there is no direct correlation between CD4 cell count and viral load—a person may have a very low T-cell count and be extremely viremic (that is, having a very high viral load—this being the most fragile and vulnerable of possibilities), have an undetectable viral load and a very high T-cell count (the goal of "curative" therapy), or have any possible combination between these two extremes.

■ *Other laboratory tests* of significance in the treatment plan include routine complete blood cell count to monitor for anemia; renal and liver function tests to monitor the effects of HAART on various organs that metabolize drug;

hepatitis, toxoplamosis, and CMV antibody testing to check for potential disease comorbidities; cholesterol and glucose monitoring to assess metabolic complications of therapy; and annual tuberculosis and VDRL (Venereal Disease Research Laboratory slide) testing as a means of monitoring common infectious diseases (Barlett, 2005).

THERAPEUTIC INTERVENTIONS

Lifestyle Modifications

- *Foods:* A diet tailored to the needs of each client is preferred based on disease progression and calorie and protein needs. Foods are to be fully cooked and properly stored. Patients should avoid raw foods and shellfish due to the presence of bacteria, parasites, and viruses. Bottled water should be used in place of tap water. Kitchen counters must be cleaned before, during, and after food preparation.
- *Personal care:* Patients are urged to not share toothbrushes or razors to minimize the possibility of sharing blood. They should not change pet litter boxes to avoid contact with harmful microorganisms. If caring for pets is necessary, patients should wear gloves when changing cat litter boxes, birdcages, fish tanks, and reptile cages, as well as a mask when cleaning bird cages. Patients are urged to use antibacterial soaps free of fragrances.

Emotional, Spiritual, and Economic Factors

Support systems, including family, friends, faith communities, and support groups as well as individuals' faith and spirituality can be excellent sources of hope, strength, peace, and well-being for clients. Patients' self-concept, body image, current social support, and feelings of isolation should be routinely assessed. Feelings of depression, anxiety, grief, loss, guilt, or hopelessness, as well as drug and alcohol use or dependency, violence in the home, suicidal ideations, and any desire to harm others, should be explored with patients. Economic assessments include the monitoring of food and shelter on an ongoing basis, financial assistance as needed, community resources for medications, and economic entitlements where necessary (Kirton, 2001; Sherman, 2001).

Medications for Routine Use

HAART treatment regimens are complex, usually involving at least three drug combinations to avoid viral resistance patterns. These medications should be prescribed and monitored by experienced health care providers. As of 2005, clinicians have 26 approved antiretroviral drugs from four drug classes from which to construct HAART regimens: nucleoside/nucleotide reverse transcriptase inhibitors (NRTIs or "nukes"), non-nucleoside reverse transcriptase inhibitors (NNRTIs or "non-nukes"), PIs, and the newest product line of fusion/entry inhibitors. The U.S. Department of Health and Human Services (DHHS) has developed guidelines for initiating treatment in therapy-naïve patients that include two NRTIs and either the lopinavir/ritonavir coformulation or efavirenz (DHHS, 2004). (The clinician should visit the DHHS AIDS Information Web site for details on antiretroviral therapies; see the reference list for the Web site address.) Despite drug improvements and advances, the ideal drug combination still does not exist. Currently approved agents continue to exhibit drug-related toxicities, daily pill burden, regimen complexity, suboptimal antiviral activity, and low threshold for the development of drug resistance. In addition, prophylaxis regimens entail daily, two or three times weekly, or weekly dosing of various antibiotics or antifungal agents based on CD4 cell immunocompetence (Kirton, 2001; Murphy, 2003).

PALLIATIVE CARE MANAGEMENT

Treatment goals for people infected with HIV/AIDS include promoting the highest quality of life possible, maximizing functional ability, and alleviating suffering through pain and symptom management throughout the illness trajectory. Palliative care for people with HIV/AIDS begins in the earliest stages of illness and increases in complexity as the disease progresses. Patients with HIV/AIDS may exhibit a multitude of symptoms resulting from a variety of disease processes, side effects of medications, and other therapies. AIDS can be characterized by bouts of severe debilitating illness followed by miraculous-appearing rebounds of apparent health and vitality. Such polarities often make it difficult to describe a traditional model of palliative care for this patient population (Kirton, 2001; Sherman, 2001; Center for Palliative Care Education, 2003).

Palliative care for people who are HIV positive and who are without an AIDS diagnosis includes the "watch and wait" scenario if the T-cell count is robust and the viral load is relatively low (parameters vary according to clinician philosophy and experience). Once the T-cell count drifts below 300 cells (or if the viral load indicates the necessity for antiretroviral drugs even with a higher T-cell count), the patient should receive instructions in current antiretroviral care, complementary and alternative care coordination, and the necessity of adherence to the antiretroviral protocol, as well as the necessity for frequent health care follow-up and continuous exposure to an interdisciplinary care team to coordinate care services as the trajectory evolves.

Palliative care of patients with AIDS includes the notion of seamless care. As patients exhaust options or immunosuppression worsens, clinicians must focus on quality of life issues while managing chronic debilitating conditions, opportunistic infections, and superimposed primary infections. Such issues might entail the need for blood transfusions, ongoing intravenous therapy to prevent complications such as blindness from CMV retinitis, and short-term aggressive curative therapies (often in the acute care setting)—all of which are treated while keeping in mind the overall health care desires of the patient. Hospice referral should be considered when consistent with the patient's goals. The criteria for hospice admission for a patient with HIV/AIDS often include the following guidelines (National Hospice and Palliative Care Organization [NHPCO], 1996): (1) CD4 count <25 cells, (2) persistent viral load >100,000 copies, and (3) presence of at least one of the following: central nervous system lymphoma, progressive multifocal leukoencephalopathy, cryptosporidium infection, wasting (the loss of 33% of lean body mass), MAC bacteremia, visceral Kaposi's sarcoma, renal failure in the absence of dialysis, advanced AIDS dementia complex, or toxoplasmosis. Additionally, the presence of any of the following is further support that a hospice admission is appropriate and should be documented: persistent diarrhea, serum albumin <2.5, concomitant substance abuse, age greater than 50 years, absence of HAART, or congestive heart failure.

In the light of these rather stringent criteria, the primary reason for denial of hospice services entails the patient being on antiretroviral drugs without documented decline in status over time. In some instances, the patient is introduced to HAART as a palliative therapy and actually improves dramatically. In such cases, if the patient warrants further hospice care, a change in the terminal diagnosis from HIV/AIDS to another diagnostic cause, such as wasting or failure to thrive, may be indicated.

SYMPTOM MANAGEMENT AND TREATMENT

In people with HIV/AIDS, there are a number of common symptoms that require palliative interventions to improve quality of life (Center for Palliative Care Education, 2003; Kirton, 2001; Sherman, 2001). Table 16-2 identifies interventions for the most common symptoms seen in patients with HIV/AIDS.

TABLE 16-2 ■ Symptom Management in HIV/AIDS

Fatigue	Treat underlying causes, when possible.
	Obtain a dietary consult.
	Encourage naps, cool room temperatures, warm rather than hot showers and baths, relaxation exercises.
	Consider the use of oral dextroamphetamine.
Anorexia or cachexia	Treat underlying causes, when possible.
	Obtain a dietary consult.
	Make food appealing in appearance.
	Avoid noxious odors.
	Avoid fatty and strong smelling foods.
	Encourage patient to eat whatever food is appealing.
	Provide small, frequent meals with snacks.
	Encourage high protein–high energy liquid supplements.
	Consider appetite stimulants.
Fever	Treat reversible causes, when possible.
	Maintain fluid intake.
	Encourage patient to wear loose clothing and change bed linens frequently if diaphoresis is present.
	Use antipyretics around the clock.
	Consider cool compresses, ice packs, or cooling blankets if these provide comfort and do not lead to chilling.

Data from Center for Palliative Care Education. (2003). *Overview of HIV/AIDS palliative care.* Retrieved October 25, 2005, from www.uwpallcare.org; Department of Health and Human Services (DHHS). (2004). *Panel on clinical practices for treatment of HIV infection. Guidelines for the use of antiretroviral agents in HIV-1 infected adults and adolescents.* Retrieved October 25, 2005, from http://aidsinfo.nih.gov/ContentFiles/AdultandAdolescentGL.pdf; Kirton, C.A. (2001). Guidelines for initiation of antiretroviral therapy. In C.A. Kirton, D. Talotta, & K. Zwolski (Eds.). *Handbook of HIV/AIDS nursing* (pp. 65-82). St. Louis: Mosby; and Sherman, D.W. (2001). Patients with acquired immune deficiency syndrome. In B.R. Ferrell & N. Coyle (Eds.). *Textbook of palliative nursing* (pp. 467-500). New York: Oxford University Press.

Continued

TABLE 16-2 ■ Symptom Management in HIV/AIDS—cont'd

Dyspnea	Treat reversible causes, such as bronchospasm.
	Elevate head of bed.
	Provide humidified oxygen therapy, when appropriate.
	Encourage the use of fans or open windows.
	Remove irritants.
	Teach pursed-lip breathing.
	Encourage frequent mouth care.
	Suppress cough.
	Consider use of nebulized lidocaine for hyperactive gag reflex.
Nausea and vomiting	Treat underlying causes, when possible.
	Use antiemetics.
	If on opioid therapy, consider changing to a different opioid.
Dehydration	Encourage oral fluids, as tolerated.
	Consider intravenous or subcutaneous (hypodermoclysis) fluids.
Constipation	Increase oral fluids, as tolerated.
	Increase dietary fiber, if sufficient oral intake.
	Institute a bowel protocol using stimulant and softening laxatives.
Urinary incontinence	Determine need for intermittent self-catheterization or insertion of indwelling Foley catheter.
	Teach good skin care to prevent skin breakdown.
Cough	Treat underlying causes.
	Use cough suppressants (may include opioids).
Decubitus ulcers	Teach or provide fastidious skin care.
	Consult a wound care specialist, as appropriate.
Delirium, dementia	Assess and treat reversible causes as appropriate (e.g., hydration and electrolyte replacement).
	Evaluate current pharmacotherapeutic agents.
	Institute safety precautions.
	Consider sliding scale haloperidol for delirium; chlorpromazine may be used if haloperidol not effective (newer agents, such as risperidone and olanzapine, have demonstrated effectiveness as well).
Diarrhea	Treat underlying cause, when possible.
	Maintain hydration, replace electrolytes, and increase protein and calorie intake, as tolerated.
	Ensure access to bathroom or commode.
	Maintain good perianal care.
	Administer antidiarrheal medications (see Chapter 26).
Insomnia	Reduce daytime napping.
	Avoid caffeine and alcohol.
	Encourage a warm bath before bed.
	Teach relaxation techniques.
	Promote a dark, quiet environment.
	Consider anxiolytics, antidepressants, or sedatives as appropriate.
Pain or discomfort	Treat pain and other discomforts, recognizing that pain may be multifocal and involve functional as well as psychological morbidities.
	Prevent or treat uncomfortable side effects of opioids or other medications.
Depression, anxiety, fear or spiritual distress	Assess for depression, generalized anxiety disorder, mood disorders, and substance abuse.
	Consider antidepressants.
	Foster support groups, psychological growth, and feelings of self-acceptance and personal worth.
	Assess for fear, loneliness, or spiritual distress.

ADVANCE CARE PLANNING

Advance care planning should be initiated as early in the disease as possible. This process continues throughout the course of the illness because the patient's wishes may change over time. Advanced care planning for the patient with HIV disease should entail a minimum of the following (Sherman, 2001):

1. Foster communication regarding life-preserving measures and wishes.
2. Discuss benefits of social support programs.
3. Have health care power of attorney in place as early as possible.
4. In the event of joint ownership of property, have a will prepared and updated that designates legally binding beneficiaries.
5. Discuss preferences regarding who is to be present at time of death, how the body is to be prepared, and the type of funeral and/or memorial service desired.
6. Discuss where donations should be sent at the time of death, as appropriate.
7. Provide assistance to survivors in terms of bereavement and related support groups.

CONCLUSION

The diagnosis of HIV/AIDS is a physically, emotionally, and spiritually burdensome condition for the patient, the family, and other significant support systems. The use of HAART has greatly increased survival but has introduced drug-related side effects that often compromise quality of life. Overall, those infected with HIV/AIDS are relatively young in age. Palliative care issues include the need for impeccable symptom management, as well as psychosocial and spiritual support to deal with issues related to death, dying, and advance care planning. All of the resources of the interdisciplinary team are vital for maximizing quality of life and palliation of symptoms.

REFERENCES

Barlett, J.G. (2005). *A pocket guide to adult HIV/AIDS treatment.* Rockville, Md.: U.S. Department of Health and Human Services Health Resources and Services Administration. Retrieved October 25, 2005, from www.hab.hrsa.gov/tools/HIVpocketguide/index.htm.

Center for Palliative Care Education. (2003). *Overview of HIV/AIDS palliative care.* Retrieved October 25, 2005, from www.uwpallcare.org.

Centers for Disease Control and Prevention (CDC). (2004). *HIV/AIDS surveillance by race/ethnicity* (through 2004). Retrieved June 30, 2006, from www.cdc.gov/hiv/graphics/minority.htm.

Department of Health and Human Services (DHHS). (2004). Panel on clinical practices for treatment of HIV infection. *Guidelines for the use of antiretroviral agents in HIV-1 infected adults and adolescents.* Retrieved October 25, 2005, from http://aidsinfo.nih.gov/ContentFiles/AdultandAdolescentGL.pdf.

Jordan, W.C., Vaughn, A.C., & Hood, R.G. (2004). African Americans and HIV/AIDS: Cultural concerns. *AIDS Reader, 14(10 Suppl),* S22-S25.

Kirton, C.A. (2001). Guidelines for initiation of antiretroviral therapy. In C.A. Kirton, D. Talotta, & K. Zwolski (Eds.). *Handbook of HIV/AIDS nursing* (pp. 65-82). St. Louis: Mosby.

Murphy, R.L. (2003). Antiretroviral class of 2003: From clinical trials to clinical practice. *AIDS Reader, 13(12 Suppl),* S4.

National Hospice and Palliative Care Organization (NHPCO). (1996). *Medical guidelines for determining prognosis in selected non-cancer diseases* (2nd ed.). Arlington, Va.: Author.

Ramirez, R.R. & de la Cruz, G. (2003). *The Hispanic population in the United States: March 2002.* Washington DC: U.S. Census Bureau, U.S. Dept of Commerce.

Sackoff, J.E. & Shin, S.S. (2001). Trends in immunologic and clinical status of newly diagnosed HIV-positive patients initiating care in the HAART era. *Journal of Acquired Immune Deficiency Syndrome, 28,* 270-272.

Sherman, D.W. (2001). Patients with acquired immune deficiency syndrome. In B.R. Ferrell & N. Coyle (Eds.), *Textbook of palliative nursing* (pp.467-500). New York: Oxford University Press.

World Health Organization. (2003). *Regional HIV/AIDS statistics and features, end of 2003.* Retrieved October 25, 2005 from www.who.int/hiv/pub/epidemiology/imagefile/en/index2.html.

Zwolski, K. (2001). Introduction to HIV: Immunopathogenesis and clinical testing. In C.A. Kirton, D. Talotta, & K. Zwolski (Eds.). *Handbook of HIV/AIDS nursing* (pp. 3-25). St. Louis: Mosby.

UNIT IV

CLINICAL PRACTICE GUIDELINES

CHAPTER 17

ANXIETY

Debra E. Heidrich and Peg Esper

■

DEFINITION AND INCIDENCE

Anxiety is an experience of diffuse apprehension or uneasiness, often accompanied by feelings of uncertainty and helplessness and activation of the autonomic nervous system (Carpenito, 2000). In nursing diagnosis terminology, the source of anxiety is either nonspecific or unknown, contrasting with fear, which occurs when the source of the uneasiness is known (Carpenito, 2000). Since these two nursing diagnoses overlap in terms of defining characteristics and appropriate interventions, the term *anxiety* is used here to describe a symptom associated with apprehension and uneasiness. Everyone feels anxious at times, especially when facing new situations, and particularly when facing a new medical diagnosis of an advanced, progressive disease. Anxiety may be mild, moderate, severe, or extreme. Although mild anxiety can be beneficial, leading people to seek appropriate information and support, increased or sustained anxiety can be detrimental both physiologically and psychologically (Shoemaker, 2005).

Studies of prevalence rates of anxiety are difficult to interpret since the term is neither defined nor measured consistently. Mild to moderate anxiety is common and expected when facing the physical, psychosocial, emotional, and spiritual issues associated with cancer and terminal illnesses (Breitbart, Chochinov, & Passik, 2004; Dinoff & Shuster, 2005; Noyes, Holt, & Massie, 1998; Vachon, 2004). Family caregivers of patients with advanced, progressive illnesses also experience anxiety and at higher levels than the general population (Grov, Dahl, Moum et al., 2005). Most people possess the necessary coping skills to manage lower levels of anxiety. However, in those with borderline coping skills, mild anxiety may progress to severe anxiety. Thus, even mild anxiety, although expected, must be assessed and addressed. Contrary to some beliefs, a high level of anxiety is not inevitable during the terminal phase of illness and should not be expected or tolerated (Breitbart, Chochinov, & Passik, 2004).

Anxiety disorders are syndromes characterized by anxiety that is beyond the norm in intensity, duration, or behavioral manifestations (Noyes, et al., 1998). There are several *DSM-IV* anxiety disorder diagnoses, including acute stress disorder, anxiety disorder due to general medical condition, generalized anxiety disorder, obsessive-compulsive disorder, panic disorder, phobias, and posttraumatic stress disorder (American Psychiatric Association, 1994). Anxiety disorders affect approximately 19 million Americans, or about 6% of the general population (National Institute of Mental Health, 2001). The incidence of anxiety disorders is higher in patients with cancer and those at the end of life than the general population.

Studies examining the prevalence of pathological anxiety in patients with early to advanced stages of various cancer diagnoses show a range from 1% to 44% (Noyes et al., 1998). In addition, Olfson, Shea, Feder et al. (2000) reported that 14.8% of patients seeking primary care in an urban general medicine practice met the criteria for generalized anxiety. So, it appears appropriate to conclude that the prevalence of anxiety is higher in people seeking medical attention than the general, healthy population. Psychiatric disorders, including anxiety, often are unrecognized and untreated in the terminally ill, as a result of several factors (Academy of Psychosomatic Medicine, 1999):

- Difficulty in differentiating symptoms of physical disease from a psychiatric problem
- Belief that many of the symptoms of psychiatric illnesses are normal in the dying process
- Belief that patients at the end of life do not respond to treatment of psychiatric problems
- Barriers associated with accessing trained psychiatrists
- Stigma associated with a psychiatric diagnosis by professionals, family, and patient
- Formal diagnosis of psychiatric complications is not sufficiently emphasized in palliative care

Patients with higher anxiety scores are more likely to request a hastened death and less likely to have a peaceful death (Georges, Onwuteaka-Philipsen, van der Heide et al, 2005; Mystakidou, Rosenfeld, Parpa et al., 2005). This emphasizes the importance of assessing and aggressively managing, Rosenfeld, Parpa anxiety in the palliative care setting.

ETIOLOGY AND PATHOPHYSIOLOGY

Anxiety has many causes—physical, psychosocial, emotional, and spiritual. Anxiety can be a manifestation of a medical problem (e.g., hypoxia) or a symptom of physical discomfort (e.g., dyspnea, pain, nausea). Many practitioners have observed that physical discomfort is often perceived as being worse in the presence of anxiety, creating a snowball effect of a symptom, anxiety, worsening of symptom, and worsening of anxiety.

Anxiety is sometimes a side effect of medications or a symptom of medication or substance withdrawal. Patients with cognitive dysfunction, such as those with Alzheimer's disease or delirium, commonly exhibit anxiety or agitation. Indeed, anxiety can also be an early sign of delirium, so it must be assessed carefully (Caracini, Martini, & Simonetti, 2004).

A host of psychological or emotional concerns may lead to anxiety. Concerns or fears about control of symptoms, addiction to medicines, self-concept and role changes, the dying process, and unresolved family or financial issues are examples of potential issues that may contribute to anxiety in both patients and caregivers. And certainly, anxiety may be a symptom of spiritual distress. Box 17-1 illustrates the wide-ranging causes of anxiety.

Anxiety activates the sympathetic branch of the autonomic nervous system, eliciting the stress or fight-or-flight response. The physiological changes that occur with the stress response are initially adaptive, enhancing the body's ability to perform physically and mentally. However, a sustained stress response can lead to complications due to continued overstimulation of the sympathetic nervous system and physiological exhaustion, including hypertension, palpitations and stress on cardiac functioning, nausea, tissue breakdown, hyperglycemia, impaired psychological functioning,

Box 17-1   The Multiple Causes of Anxiety

ANXIETY AS A SYMPTOM OF A PHYSICAL PROBLEM

- Any unrelieved distressing symptom such as pain or dyspnea
- Underlying somatic process (hypoxia, sepsis)
- Adverse drug reaction such as akathisia (haloperidol), psychosis (corticosteroids), or toxicity (meperidine)
- Medication or substance withdrawal (alcohol, anticonvulsants, benzodiazepines, nicotine, and opioids)
- Actual or impending delirium

MEDICAL PROBLEMS ASSOCIATED WITH ANXIETY SYMPTOMS

- Cardiovascular: angina, arrhythmias, valvular disease, congestive heart failure, myocardial infarction
- Fluid and electrolyte imbalances: dehydration, hyponatremia, hyperkalemia, hypercalcemia, or hypocalcemia
- Endocrine: hyperthyroidism, hypothyroidism, Cushing's syndrome, Addison's disease, hyperparathyroidism, abnormal glucose levels
- Pulmonary: asthma, chronic obstructive pulmonary disease (COPD), dyspnea, hypercapnia, hypoxia, pneumothorax, pulmonary embolism, sleep apnea, pneumonia
- Neurologic: encephalopathy, vertigo, delirium, cerebrovascular accident, multiple sclerosis, transient ischemic attacks, hematoma
- Hematologic/malignancy: any brain metastasis, anemia, pheochromocytoma
- Nutritional: anemia, folate deficiency, vitamin B_{12} deficiency
- Drug or medication side effects: for example, bronchodilators, phenothiazines, corticosteroids, digitalis preparations, anticholinergics, central nervous system stimulants used to counteract the sedative side effects of opioids: caffeine, methylphenidate (Ritalin), amphetamine
- Any infectious process, for example, pneumonia and urinary tract infections

ANXIETY AS A SYMPTOM OF A PSYCHOSOCIAL, EMOTIONAL, OR SPIRITUAL CONCERN

- Normal reaction to a threatening situation
- Indication of an anxiety disorder as defined by *DSM-IV* criteria
- Expression of existential or spiritual suffering

Data from Breitbart, W., Chochinov, M., & Passik, S. (2004). Psychiatric aspects of palliative care. In D. Doyle, G. Hanks, N. Cherny, et al. (Eds.), *Oxford textbook of palliative medicine* (3rd ed., pp. 746-771). New York: Oxford University Press; Hinshaw, D.B., Carnahan, J.M., & Johnson, D.L. (2002). Depression, anxiety, and asthenia in advanced illness. *J Am Coll Surg, 195(2)*, 271-277; Shoemaker, N. (2005). Clients with psychosocial and mental health concerns. In J.M. Black & J.H. Hawks (Eds.), *Medical-surgical nursing: Clinical management for positive outcomes* (7th ed., pp. 523-536). St. Louis: Elsevier Saunders; and Vachon, M.L.S. (2004). The problems of the patient in palliative medicine. In D. Doyle, G. Hanks, N. Cherny, et al. (Eds.), *Oxford textbook of palliative medicine* (3rd ed., pp. 961-985). New York: Oxford University Press.

increased blood coagulation (leading to potential complications like pulmonary emboli), and immunosuppression (Guyton & Hall, 2005).

ASSESSMENT AND MEASUREMENT

Anxiety is manifested in many ways—subjective experiences, observable signs, and physiological changes. These symptoms vary with the intensity of the patient's anxiety (Carpenito, 2000; Dinoff & Shuster, 2005; Shoemaker, 2005). The clinician must use a combination of patient and family interviews, astute observation of anxiety-associated behaviors, anxiety assessment tools, and physical assessment to evaluate the presence and severity of anxiety. It is important to have one-on-one discussions between the clinician and patient and between the clinician and caregiver to elicit subjective experiences associated with anxiety, assess coping styles, and identify changes in behavior that indicate anxiety.

Subjective Experiences Associated with Anxiety

- Apprehension, uneasiness, fear
- Tension or nervousness
- Irritability
- Restlessness
- Loss of control (feelings of helplessness, angry outbursts)
- Increased attention with mild anxiety, difficulty concentrating with increasing anxiety
- Physical discomforts: headaches; pains in neck, back, or chest; nausea; hot or cold flashes

Observable Signs of Anxiety

- Tense posture
- Fidgeting with fingers or clothing
- Frequent sighing
- Dryness and licking of dry lips
- Trembling
- Insomnia
- Changes in communication: quieter or more talkative than usual
- Changes in speech: pitch higher than normal, voice tremors
- Clenched jaw or grinding of teeth

Physiological Signs of Anxiety

- Changes in vital signs: increase in heart rate, respiratory rate, and systolic blood pressure
- Diaphoresis
- Flushing or pallor
- Dry mouth
- Dilated pupils
- Urinary frequency or urgency
- Diarrhea
- Fatigue

TABLE 17-1 ■ Manifestations of Four Levels of Anxiety

Anxiety Level	Physical Manifestations	Emotional Manifestations	Cognitive Manifestations
Mild	Increased pulse and blood pressure	Positive affect	Alert, can solve problem, prepared to learn new information
Moderate	Elevated vital signs, tense muscles, diaphoresis	Tense, fearful	Attention focused on one concern, may be able to concentrate with directions
Severe	Fight-or-flight response, dry mouth, numb extremities	Distressed	Decreased sensory perception, can focus only on details, unable to learn new information
Panic	Continued as in severe level	Totally overwhelmed	Ignores external cues, focused only on internal stimuli, unable to learn

From: Shoemaker, N. (2005). Clients with psychosocial and mental health concerns. In J.M. Black & J.H. Hawks (Eds.). *Medical-surgical nursing: Clinical management for positive outcomes* (7th ed., pp. 523-536). St. Louis: Elsevier Saunders.

The appropriate treatment of anxiety is guided by its severity. The level of anxiety is inferred on the basis of the severity of the patient's subjective feelings, observable signs, and physical symptoms associated with anxiety. As with other subjective symptoms, asking individuals to rate their anxiety on a numeric scale may be helpful. One well-researched tool used in the palliative care setting is the Edmonton Symptom Assessment System (Edmonton Regional Palliative Care Program, 2001). This tool includes a visual analogue scale for rating anxiety from 0 (not anxious) to 10 (worst possible anxiety). Observable signs and physical symptoms of anxiety may also be used to identify the severity of this symptom (Table 17-1).

Individuals with severe or panic levels of anxiety and those with prolonged anxiety require further screening for the presence of clinical anxiety disorders. Consultation with a psychologist or psychiatrist is recommended for patients or caregivers with anxiety disorders.

HISTORY AND PHYSICAL EXAMINATION

Because anxiety is characterized by a variety of subjective feelings, observable behaviors, and physiologic changes and has multiple causes, the history and physical examination must include assessment of physical, psychological, emotional, and spiritual issues.

- General appearance: dress, hygiene, motor activity, facial expression, and speech pattern
- Primary and secondary medical diagnoses, noting those with a potential for complications with anxiety symptoms; for example, bone metastasis and hypercalcemia, lung disease and hypoxia, syndrome of inappropriate antidiuretic hormone (SIADH) and hyponatremia
- Systems review
  - Cardiovascular: tachycardia, increased systolic pressure, angina, facial flushing or pallor, diaphoresis
  - Respiratory: dyspnea, tachypnea, signs of hypoxia

- ▶ Gastrointestinal: nausea, vomiting, diarrhea
- ▶ Musculoskeletal: muscle tension, trembling
- ■ Presence of pain from any source
- ■ Use of any medications associated with anxiety
- ■ Psychoemotional status
  - ▶ Patient and family's understanding of the advanced illness
  - ▶ Present concerns or worries, including those about the illness itself, the symptoms, or the management of symptoms
  - ▶ Stresses affecting the patient or family: any change in health, marital status, family unit, living arrangements, responsibilities, employment, or financial status
  - ▶ Self-appraisal of patient and family adjustment to these changes
- ■ History of substance abuse: alcohol, nicotine, prescription medications, or illicit drugs
- ■ History of an anxiety disorder, depression, or other mental health disorder, including time since diagnosis, treatments, ongoing interventions, and current status
- ■ Presence and severity of anxiety at this time
  - ▶ Feelings of uneasiness, tension, or restlessness
  - ▶ Presence and severity of observable signs or physiologic changes associated with anxiety
- ■ Resources available to manage anxiety: social support, religion, recreational or social activities, support groups, professional assistance
- ■ Spiritual belief system, including spiritual meaning of experiences, beliefs about an afterlife, and existential concerns and questions

DIAGNOSTICS

The appropriate use of diagnostic tests is determined by the suspected underlying cause of the anxiety. If a medical complication is suspected, appropriate diagnostics may include pulse oximetry to assess oxygen saturation; blood chemistries to evaluated abnormalities, such as hyponatremia, hypokalemia, hypercalcemia, or hypocalcemia; chest radiograph to diagnose pneumonia; or urine cultures to verify urinary tract infection. If an anxiety disorder is suspected, the patients may be referred to a psychiatrist for further evaluation and diagnosis.

INTERVENTION AND TREATMENT

Appropriate treatment depends on the underlying cause and level of anxiety. Because anxiety is typically multidimensional, it is helpful to use multiple approaches to manage this symptom.

Treat Physical Causes

- ■ Aggressively treat uncomfortable symptoms, such as pain, dyspnea, and nausea.
- ■ Manage, as feasible and appropriate, medical conditions contributing to anxiety, such as anemia, hypercalcemia, SIADH, and pulmonary compromise.

- Reduce or discontinue medications that may be contributing to anxiety.
- Treat symptoms related to withdrawal.
  - ‣ Medications such as benzodiazepines or opioids must be tapered if no longer necessary for symptom control to prevent withdrawal. Be aware that caregivers sometimes stop giving these medications when the patient is no longer alert.
  - ‣ Consider using a nicotine patch for patients with a history of smoking who stop smoking, whether by choice or due to physical condition.
  - ‣ Consider adding a benzodiazepine to manage the symptoms of alcohol withdrawal for patients with physical dependence on alcohol who are no longer able to swallow. Evaluate the benefits versus potential complications of continuing alcohol via nasogastric or gastrostomy.

Enhance Coping Skills

For mild-to-moderate anxiety
- Listen actively to concerns and fears.
- Encourage to express feelings.
- Convey respect for the individual and acceptance of feelings (e.g., "feelings are neither right nor wrong—they just are").
- Provide information to clarify misconceptions, answer questions, and alleviate concerns. For example, discussing the facts about the extremely low incidence of addiction when opioids are used for pain management may significantly decrease anxiety and pain.
- Clarify information and reinforce teaching frequently.
- Teach relaxation techniques.
- Use complementary therapies, such as music, art, imagery, and massage.
- Assist the individual to identify anxiety-provoking stimuli.
- Assist in developing strategies to prevent or modify an anxiety-provoking situation, if possible.
- Encourage the patient to recognize the onset of anxiety early and intervene before it escalates.
- Refer to counseling services, as appropriate, such as medical social services, pastoral counseling, and financial and estate planning.
- Consider referral to a support group, as appropriate.
- Encourage the patient and caregiver to accept assistance to reduce stress:
  - ‣ Make lists of tasks that can be delegated.
  - ‣ Delegate these tasks to available extended family, worship community, and neighborhood or civic group members.

For severe anxiety
- Provide a safe, calm environment.
  - ‣ Remove as many stressors as possible, including limiting number of people in the room.
  - ‣ Avoid moving the patient from familiar surroundings, if possible.
  - ‣ Encourage the physical presence of a trusted person.
- Communicate in short, simple sentences in a calm tone of voice.
- Do not overload the patient and caregiver with information; the ability to concentrate and learn is impaired.

- Avoid asking the individual to make decisions.
- Allow expression of feelings, without probing or confrontation.
- Consider consultation with a clinical psychiatrist.

Pharmacological Interventions

Although the interventions to enhance coping skills are effective for mild and, to some degree, moderate anxiety, anxiolytic medications are very important in the treatment of prolonged or severe anxiety. If anxiety is interfering with quality of life, a short course of anxiolytic medication may reduce the unpleasant symptoms associated with anxiety and enable the individual to learn new coping skills. Severe anxiety and anxiety disorders often require ongoing pharmacological treatment in addition to psychotherapy. Table 17-2 provides dosage ranges for the medications discussed later.

Benzodiazepines

The benzodiazepines are the most commonly prescribed anxiolytics. These medications work by potentiating gamma-aminobutyric acid, an inhibitory neurotransmitter in the central nervous system (CNS). The result is CNS suppression, especially at the level of the limbic system (Hodgson & Kizior, 2004). The benzodiazepines with a short half-life (e.g., lorazepam) are generally preferred in elderly patients and for short-term management of anxiety. Alprazolam has an intermediate half-life (approximately 14 hours) and is also an effective, widely used anxiolytic. A potential problem with the short-acting benzodiazepines is end-of-dose failure; the medications with a longer half-life, such as clonazepam, may be preferred if breakthrough anxiety is present (Goldberg, 2004). Clonazepam is also a recommended choice in individuals with neurological disorders (Hinshaw, Carnahan, & Johnson, 2002).

Diazepam, clorazepate, flurazepam, and other benzodiazepines with active metabolites should be avoided due to the risk of escalating blood levels, inducing side effects such as slurred speech, somnolence, and confusion. Those individuals exhibiting both anxiety and depression may benefit from the use of an antidepressant. Patients with compromised respiratory function or who are on large doses of opioid analgesics should be evaluated carefully prior to prescribing benzodiazepines secondary to their potential for central respiratory suppression (Hinshaw et al., 2002).

Neuroleptics

The neuroleptic medications are used when the benzodiazepines are not effective or when confusion or hallucinations accompany the anxiety. Be aware that the combination of anxiety with a mental status change is a sign of delirium. Haloperidol is often used to manage severe anxiety on a short-term basis or for treating psychotic episodes. It is not as sedative as agents such as chlorpromazine (Montagnini & Moat, 2004; Paice, 2002). Neuroleptic medications work by suppressing the cerebral cortex, limbic system, and hypothalamus and by blocking CNS dopamine receptors (Hodgson & Kizior, 2004).

Other Anxiolytics

Buspirone is a nonbenzodiazepine anxiolytic. Inhibition of serotonin appears to be the mechanism of action (Thomson Micromedex, 2005). This medication may

TABLE 17-2 ■ Anxiolytics

Drug	Dosage Range (mg/day)	Available Routes*	Half-life (hr)	Comments
Benzodiazepines				
Very short acting				
Midazolam	10-60	IV, subcutaneous	2-7	Used when quick relief is needed
Short acting				
Alprazolam	0.75-4	Oral, SL	9-27	Used in anxiety and panic disorders
Lorazepam	2-4	Oral, SL, IV, IM	10-20	Readily absorbed, moderate price
Intermediate acting				
Chlordiazepoxide	15-100	Oral, IM, IV	24-48	Useful with comorbid seizure disorders
Long acting				
Diazepam	4-40	Oral, IM, IV, PR	24-120	Useful with comorbid seizure disorders
Clonazepam	1.5-20	Oral	30-40	Adjuvant for neuropathic pain
Nonbenzodiazepine				
Buspirone	15-30	Oral	2-11	Will not block withdrawal effects from discontinuation of benzodiazepines
Neuroleptics				
Haloperidol	1-15	Oral, IV, subcutaneous, IM	12-38	Not as sedative as chlorpromazine
Chlorpromazine	50-100	Oral, IM, IV	30	Also useful in hiccups
Olanzapine	5-10	Oral, IM	30-38	Not recommended in Parkinson's disease
Risperidone	1-2	Oral, IM	20	May cause significant hypotension
Antihistamines				
Hydroxyzine	50-100	Oral, IM	3-20	Useful in management of pruritus
Promethazine	12.5-100	Oral, IM, IV, PR	5-14	Also useful to control nausea and vomiting; IV is not the preferred route

Data from Esper, P. & Heidrich, D.E. (2005). Symptom clusters in advanced illness. *Semin Oncol Nurs, 21(1),* 20-28; Goldberg, L. (2004). Psychological issues in palliative care: Depression, anxiety, agitation, and delirium. *Clin Fam Pract, 6(2),* 441-470; Hinshaw, D.B., Carnahan, J.M., & Johnson, D.L. (2002). Depression, anxiety, and asthenia in advanced illness. *J Am Coll Surg, 195(2),* 271-277; Thomson Micromedex. (2005). *Micromedex® healthcare series.* Retrieved September 1, 2005, from http://micromedex.med.umich.edu/mdxcgi/quiklocn.exe?CTL=E:\mdx\mdxcgi\ MEGAT.SYS&SET=1C64C5D24F042200&SYS=19&T=799&D=1&Q=26; and USP DI. (2005). *USP DI® drug information for the health care provider* (25th ed.). Retrieved September 1, 2005, from http://online.statref.com/Document/ Document.aspx?DocId=3449&FxId=6&Scroll=1&Index=0&SessionId=65E26DIZLYGKCYJY.
*Avoid the IM route of administration whenever possible.

take 1 to 2 weeks to reach maximal effectiveness and is generally used for chronic anxiety. The clinician must be cautious when switching to buspirone from a benzodiazepine since buspirone does not block benzodiazepine withdrawal (*USP DI*, 2005).

Antihistamines have also been used for their anxiolytic properties (Goldberg, 2004; Montagnini & Moat, 2004). Hydroxyzine appears to depress the CNS more than diphenhydramine, but both have been used. Some practitioners prefer to use antihistamines if the patient's respiratory status is extremely compromised and there is a concern about respiratory depression from benzodiazepines (Breitbart, Chochinov, & Passik, 2004). However, as the antihistamines tend to have a relatively mild anxiolytic effect, a benzodiazepine or neuroleptic may be required for moderate to severe anxiety even in the presence of a compromised respiratory system (Goldberg, 2004). Antihistamines such as promethazine have been used in patients with chronic obstructive pulmonary disease. Their effect on anxiety is mild and additional agents may be required (Runo & Ely, 2001).

Special Considerations

Patients on longer-term anxiolytics, in particular, benzodiazepines, need to be tapered off of these medications slowly if it appears they are no longer needed. However, many patients require treatment until death to avoid withdrawal symptoms. If stopped abruptly, terminal agitation can occur. This can be treated, if needed, by using rectally administered diazepam, sublingual lorazepam, or subcutaneous midazolam for those patients unable to swallow (Periyakoil, Skultety, & Sheikh, 2005).

Midazolam is an appropriate choice for patients with anxiety and agitation in the final days of life if they are unable to take oral agents or if other agents have not been successful. Initial dosing is generally 0.5 to 1 mg per hour by continuous subcutaneous or intravenous infusion; the dosage may be increased by 25% to 50% hourly as needed to effect comfort (Hanks-Bell, Paice, & Krammer, 2002).

PATIENT AND FAMILY EDUCATION

Providing information is extremely important in the management of anxiety, including explaining aspects of symptom management to alleviate the source of the anxiety, when possible, and discussing the recognition and management of anxiety itself. Both the patient and the family are at risk, because anxiety in one person can exacerbate that in another. Thus, it is important to include both patients and caregivers when providing information.

- Teach accurate symptom assessment and management.
- Correct misconceptions and fears regarding medications (e.g., addiction, respiratory depression, sedation).
- Assist the individual to identify his or her own signs of anxiety.
- Teach relaxation and other stress management techniques.
- Emphasize that anxiety is a symptom that requires treatment (versus a sign of weakness).
- Teach the potential benefit of using many approaches to manage anxiety, including counseling.

- Teach appropriate use of anxiolytic medications and potential side effects.
- Teach patients and caregivers to consult a clinician before stopping any medication.

EVALUATION AND PLAN FOR FOLLOW-UP

Successful intervention for anxiety leads to a resolution or, at least, a decrease in the subjective and objective signs of anxiety. Evaluating the subjective aspects of anxiety includes asking the individual about feelings of uneasiness, apprehension, and helplessness. Use of a numeric scale or anxiety assessment tool as part of initial and ongoing assessments assists in documenting the subjective experience of anxiety and in monitoring for changes over time. Objective signs of anxiety are also monitored to determine the effectiveness of the interventions. In addition to evaluating the effectiveness of medications ordered for anxiety, the patient should be monitored for side effects of these medications.

The potential for anxiety is always present in patients with advanced illness and their caregivers, making ongoing evaluation a necessity. And, since anxiety can change from day to day, the ongoing evaluation process should include not only present anxiety but any anxiety in the past 24 hours or since the last visit or appointment. Be sure to consider that meeting with health care professionals may increase or decrease anxiety, depending on the individual's degree of comfort with his or her clinician. Remember that a high level of anxiety is not inevitable during the terminal phase of illness and should not be expected or tolerated; it must be anticipated, carefully assessed, and appropriately managed.

CASE STUDY   Mr. K. is a 52-year-old man with a new diagnosis of metastatic non–small-cell lung cancer. He lives at home with his wife; his children are married and live out of state. Mr. K. had a history of panic attacks in his late 20s but has not been on any medication for this in over 10 years. His lung cancer was diagnosed after he began coughing up blood. Following two standard and one investigational treatment regimens, he has continued to show progressive disease. He has become weaker and has increasing anorexia. His wife has had to continue her employment in order to maintain their insurance coverage. Mr. K. expressed that he is starting to have difficulty sleeping at night because he "can't stop [his] mind from going in 100 different directions." He is exhausted during the day but states he doesn't like to sleep when his wife is away at work. During his clinic appointment, the clinician has a chance to speak with Mr. K. alone. In reviewing his current problems, it is noted that Mr. K. is quite fidgety and has difficulty maintaining eye contact. As the discussion continues, the clinician explores with Mr. K. the "thoughts" that he has at night that keep him awake. In doing this, the clinician identifies that Mr. K. is afraid of going to sleep and not waking up again. He is also afraid that he'll cough up blood in his sleep and not be able to breathe.

The clinician offers support to Mr. K. and asks if his current symptoms are anything like the previous panic attacks he used to experience. Mr. K. seems almost surprised at the realization that they are, indeed, quite similar. After evaluating the effectiveness of Mr. K.'s previous treatments, the clinician orders oral lorazepam 1 mg twice daily. The clinician also explores additional support systems available to Mr. K. As it turns out, he states that a retired brother-in-law had offered to come over several days a week to keep him company. Mr. K. is encouraged to pursue this and is also offered a social work consult to see if any other arrangements can be made for his wife in regard to her work situation.

Mrs. K. is able to obtain a family medical leave. Mr. K. begins the lorazepam and initially finds that it allows him to sleep better at night, and he even takes an occasional nap during the day. As his disease progresses, however, Mr. K. begins to experience more problems with dyspnea and is coughing up more blood. His anxiety level is not being controlled with lorazepam. Based on his rapidly declining condition, the clinician decides to initiate a subcutaneous infusion of midazolam at 1 mg/hr. Mr. K. is able to obtain good relief of anxiety within 24 hours of initiation of this therapy. As his condition deteriorates he ultimately requires titration up to 4 mg/hr but is without perceptible restlessness or anxiety at the time of his death.

REFERENCES

Academy of Psychosomatic Medicine. (1999). *Psychiatric aspects of excellent end-of-life care* (Position statement). Chicago: Academy of Psychosomatic Medicine. Retrieved November 20, 2005, from www.apm.org/papers/eol-care.shtml.

American Psychiatric Association. (1994). *Diagnostic and statistical manual of mental disorders* (DSM-IV) (4th ed.). Washington, DC: Author.

Breitbart, W., Chochinov, M., & Passik, S. (2004). Psychiatric aspects of palliative care. In D. Doyle, G. Hanks, N. Cherny, et al. (Eds.). *Oxford textbook of palliative medicine* (3rd ed., pp. 746-771). New York: Oxford University Press.

Caracini, A., Martini, C., & Simonetti, F. (2004). Neurological problems in advanced cancer. In D. Doyle, G. Hanks, N. Cherny, et al. (Eds.). *Oxford textbook of palliative medicine* (3rd ed., pp. 702-726). New York: Oxford University Press.

Carpenito, L.J. (2000). *Nursing diagnosis: Application to clinical practice* (8th ed.). Philadelphia: Lippincott.

Dinoff, B.L. & Shuster, J.L. (2005). Psychological issues. In V.T. DeVita, S. Hellman, & S.A. Rosenberg (Eds.). *Cancer: Principles and practice of oncology* (7th ed., pp. 2683-2690). Philadelphia: Lippincott Williams & Wilkins.

Edmonton Regional Palliative Care Program. (2001). *Guidelines for using the Edmonton Symptom Assessment System (ESAS)*. Retrieved on November 20, 2005, from www.palliative.org/PC/ClinicalInfo/AssessmentTools/esas.pdf.

Georges, J.J., Onwuteaka-Philipsen, B.D., van der Heide, A., et al. (2005). Symptoms, treatment and "dying peacefully" in terminally ill cancer patients: A prospective study. *Support Care Cancer, 13(3),* 160-168.

Goldberg, L. (2004). Psychological issues in palliative care: Depression, anxiety, agitation, and delirium. *Clin Fam Pract, 6(2),* 441-470.

Grov, E.K., Dahl, A.A. & Moum, T., et al. (2005). Anxiety, depression, and quality of life in caregivers of patients with cancer in late palliative phase. *Ann Oncol, 16(7),* 1185-1191.

Guyton, A.C. & Hall, J.E. (2005). The autonomic nervous system and the adrenal medulla. In A.C. Guyton & J. E. Hall (Eds.). *Textbook of medical physiology* (11th ed., pp. 697-708). Philadelphia: Saunders.

Hanks-Bell, M., Paice, J., & Krammer, L. (2002). The use of midazolam hydrochloride continuous infusions in palliative care. *Clin J Oncol Nurs, 6(6)*, 367-369.

Hinshaw, D.B., Carnahan, J.M., & Johnson, D.L. (2002). Depression, anxiety, and asthenia in advanced illness. *J Am Coll Surg, 195(2)*, 271-277.

Hodgson, B.B., & Kizior, R.J. (2004). *Saunders nursing drug handbook 2004*. St. Louis: Saunders.

Montagnini, M.L., & Moat, M.E. (2004). Non-pain symptom management in palliative care. *Clin Family Pract, 6(2)*, 395-422.

Mystakidou, K., Rosenfeld, B., Parpa, E., et al. (2005). Desire for death near the end of life: The role of depression, anxiety and pain. *Gen Hospital Psychiatry, 27(4)*, 258-262.

National Institute of Mental Health. (2001). *Facts about anxiety disorder*. Retrieved November 20, 2005, from: www.nimh.nih.gov/publicat/NIMHadfacts.pdf.

Noyes, R., Holt, C.S., & Massie, M.J. (1998). Anxiety disorders. In J.C. Holland (Ed.). *Psycho-oncology* (pp. 548-563), New York: Oxford University Press.

Olfson, M., Shea, S., Feder, A., et al. (2000). Prevalence of anxiety, depression, and substance use disorder in an urban general medicine practice. *Arch Family Med, 9(9)*, 876-883.

Paice, J.A. (2002). Managing psychological conditions in palliative care: Dying need not mean enduring uncontrollable anxiety, depression, or delirium. *Am J Nurs, 102(11)*, 36-43.

Periyakoil, V.S., Skultety, K., & Sheikh, J. (2005). Panic, anxiety, and chronic dyspnea. *J Palliat Med, 8(2)*, 453-459.

Runo, J.R., & Ely, E.W. (2001). Treating dyspnea in a patient with advanced chronic obstructive pulmonary disease. *West J Med, 175(3)*, 197-201.

Shoemaker, N. (2005). Clients with psychosocial and mental health concerns. In J.M. Black & J.H. Hawks (Eds.). *Medical-surgical nursing: Clinical management for positive outcomes* (7th ed., pp. 523-536). St. Louis: Elsevier Saunders.

Thomson Micromedex. (2005). *Micromedex® healthcare series*. Retrieved September 1, 2005 from http://micromedex.med.umich.edu/mdxcgi/quiklocn.exe?CTL=E:\mdx\mdxcgi\MEGAT.SYS&SET=1C6 4C5D24F042200&SYS=19&T=799&D=1&Q=26.

USP DI. (2005). *USP DI® drug information for the health care provider* (25th ed.) Retrieved September 1, 2005, from http://online.statref.com/Document/Document.aspx?DocId=3449&FxId=6&Scroll= 1&Index=0&SessionId=65E26DIZLYGKCYJY.

Vachon, M.L.S. (2004). The problems of the patient in palliative medicine. In D. Doyle, G. Hanks, N. Cherny, et al. (Eds.), *Oxford textbook of palliative medicine* (3rd ed., pp. 961-985). New York: Oxford University Press.

CHAPTER 18

ASCITES

Debra E. Heidrich

■

DEFINITION AND INCIDENCE

Ascites is the abnormal accumulation of fluid in the peritoneal cavity. The majority of patients with ascites have advanced liver disease—usually cirrhosis (Runyon, Montano, Akriviadis et al., 1992). Other nonmalignant diseases associated with ascites include right-sided heart failure, tuberculous peritonitis, nephrotic syndrome, complications of pancreatitis, and chylous ascites from trauma or surgery (Hostetter, Marincola, & Schwartzentruber, 2005; Runyon, 2004). Approximately 10% of patients with ascites have a malignancy as the primary cause (Runyon et al., 1992). Cancer diagnoses most often associated with ascites are ovarian, endometrium, breast, large bowel, stomach, and pancreas (Kichian & Bain, 2004). About 6% of patients entering hospices have ascites (Waller & Caroline, 2000).

Common symptoms associated with ascites include abdominal bloating, abdominal pain, nausea, decreased appetite, and constipation. Large-volume ascites leads to dyspnea and orthopnea. Patients with cirrhosis and ascites have higher variceal pressure than those without ascites and thus are at greater risk for variceal bleeding, which is associated with a high mortality rate (Kravetz, Bildozola, Argonz et al., 2000). The presence of malignancy-associated ascites is a poor prognostic sign, with a 1-year survival rate of 40% (Kichian & Bain, 2004). The median length of survival in a patient with symptomatic malignant ascites is reported to be 1 to 4 months. However, there is some variability in survival based on cancer type; women with breast or ovarian cancer may have a longer survival (Adam & Adam, 2004; Hostetter et al., 2005). Prolongation of survival has been documented in response to aggressive and more-targeted treatment approaches, but few randomized clinical trials exist in these patient populations (Hostetter et al., 2005).

ETIOLOGY AND PATHOPHYSIOLOGY

Ascites with Liver Disease

Common aspects of all postulated mechanisms for the development of ascites in liver disease involve a combination of sodium retention and portal hypertension (Lingappa, 2003). Portal hypertension can arise from hepatic venous outflow blockage caused by nodules and fibrosis in the liver (Wongcharatrawee & Garcia-Tsao, 2001). Three possible effects of portal hypertension are (1) diversion of the vascular volume to the lymphatics, resulting in overloading of the lymphatic drainage and weeping of fluid into the peritoneum; (2) portal-to-systemic shunting causing irritants that are normally cleared by the liver to be released into circulation where they initiate activities that decrease renal perfusion and increase renal tubular sodium resorption; or (3) endothelin-1 secretion, causing renal vasoconstriction, decreased glomerular filtration rate, and sodium retention. Regardless of the causal mechanism involved, depletion of the intravascular volume activates the renin-angiotensin-aldosterone system and vasopressin, causing sodium and water retention, which further contributes to fluid accumulation (Lingappa, 2003).

Ascites with Malignancy

Several mechanisms have been proposed for the development of malignancy-associated ascites. Patients with liver cancer may develop portal hypertension, resulting in ascites formation in much the same way as those with cirrhosis (Kichian & Bain, 2004). In addition, tumors that have seeded the peritoneum may release high levels of vascular endothelial growth factor (VEGF) that increase capillary permeability. Zebrowski, Liu, Ramirez et al. (1999) showed that VEGF protein levels were markedly increased in malignant ascites compared to levels in ascites associated with cirrhosis and that inhibiting VEGF activity decreased endothelial cell permeability in vitro. Further, animal studies show that ascites recurrence can be blocked by inhibiting VEGF expression (Stoelcker, Echtenacher, Weich et al., 2000). When the vascular permeability increases, proteins enter the peritoneal cavity. In mice, proteins in the peritoneal cavity make ascites worse by functionally impairing lymphatic drainage (Nagy, Herzberg, Masse et al., 1989). These proteins also increase the oncotic pressure pulling in more fluids via osmosis. In addition, obstruction or invasion of lymphatic channels by tumors may lead to chylous ascites (Kichian & Bain, 2004).

Effects of Ascites

The accumulation of abnormal amounts of fluid in the peritoneal cavity causes many uncomfortable symptoms. Pain occurs due to stretching or compression of tissues. Also, inflammation from a peritoneal infection may cause severe pain. Increased pressure on the stomach causes early satiety and nausea. Constipation, due to pressure on the bowel, is also a common complication of ascites. Dyspnea may result from pressure on the diaphragm and leakage of ascitic fluid into the pleural space (Kichian & Bain, 2004).

ASSESSMENT AND MEASUREMENT

An observable enlargement of a patient's abdomen is a somewhat late sign of ascites. It has been estimated that 1.5 liters of ascitic fluid must be present before flank dullness is detected and 2 liters must be present before bulging is appreciated on physical examination (Cattau, Benjamin, Knuff et al., 1982; Tabbarah & Casciato, 1990). Patients of short stature may show these physical signs with less fluid accumulation. The earliest signs of ascites are often patient complaints of bloating, abdominal discomfort or pain, and increasing weight or waist size (e.g., clothes do not fit). Patients may also complain of fatigue, inability to sit upright, heartburn, nausea, early satiety, and constipation. As ascites becomes more pronounced, dyspnea and orthopnea may occur. Edema of the legs is also possible with progressive ascites (Kichian & Bain, 2004). Abdominal girth measurement provides a baseline that can be used to monitor worsening ascites, effectiveness of interventions, or recurrence of ascites after treatment.

HISTORY AND PHYSICAL EXAMINATION

Review the Patient's History

Determine the underlying pathophysiology of the ascites (e.g., liver disease, heart disease, renal disease, or cancer).

Assess for Symptoms Associated with Ascites

Ask about onset and severity:
- Weight gain
- Increasing abdominal girth or a change in the way clothes fit
- Indigestion, nausea, and early satiety
- Sensation of fullness or bloating
- Ankle swelling
- Dyspnea
- Constipation
- Urinary frequency

Perform a Physical Examination

- Compare weight to baseline, taking weight loss due to anorexia and cachexia into account.
- Measure abdominal girth.
- Assess abdomen:
  - Note distension with bulging flanks when the patient is supine. This may be difficult to discern if the patient is obese or if less than 2 liters of fluid is present.
  - Percuss abdomen. (Note: percussion may not be sensitive or specific in diagnosing ascites [Cattau et al., 1982].)
    - Note any shifting dullness on percussion with position changes. In the supine patient with ascites, tympany is heard near the umbilicus but dullness is noted when the clinician percusses away from the umbilicus and reaches the level of fluid. When the patient turns to one side, the dullness shifts to the dependent areas.
    - Feel for evidence of a fluid wave (i.e., when flank is tapped on one side, an impulse is felt on the opposite side). Be sure to block transmission of a wave through subcutaneous fat by having an assistant place the medial edges of both hands firmly down the midline of the abdomen.
  - Observe skin across abdomen for signs of tightness or stretch marks.
  - Look for abdominal venous engorgement.
  - Identify changes in umbilicus; may be flattened or everted.
  - Assess for scrotal and/or lower-extremity edema.
  - Assess for associated complications:
    - Note any respiratory changes due to pressure on diaphragm or pleural effusion:
      - Assess rate and depth of respiration.
      - Listen for diminished or absent breath sounds.
    - Assess for dehydration or malnutrition due to nausea and early satiety:
      - Assess hydration of mucous membranes.
      - Assess general nutritional status.

DIAGNOSTICS

Abdominal radiographic studies, ultrasound, and computed tomography scans do verify the presence of free fluid in the abdomen, but these tests are generally not required after a thorough history and physical examination. On radiography, ascites appears with hazy or ground-glass features, distended and separated loops of bowel, and poor definition of abdominal organs (Hostetter et al., 2005; Kichian & Bain, 2004).

Cytology and examination of the protein concentration of the peritoneal fluid are tests that assist in determining the cause of ascites. However, in end-of-life care, the cause is often evident, so a diagnostic paracentesis is rarely required. More commonly, the peritoneal fluid is examined for cell count, Gram stain, and culture to select the appropriate antibiotic intervention when infection is suspected.

INTERVENTION AND TREATMENT

Sodium Restriction and Diuretics

Sodium restriction and diuretics may be effective for ascites caused by increased portal hypertension (e.g., cirrhosis or cancer in the liver) but are rarely effective for other types of malignant ascites (Adam & Adam, 2004). When portal hypertension is contributing to ascites, restrict sodium to 2000 mg/day or less; fluid restriction is not necessary for any cause of ascites unless serum sodium is less than 120 to 125 mmol/L (Runyon, 2004). In end-of-life care, it is important to balance the potential therapeutic effects of sodium and fluid restriction with the quality of living benefits of allowing patients to eat whatever foods taste good to them. As the appetite decreases, the appropriateness of a sodium-restricted diet also decreases.

When diuretic therapy is appropriate, that is, when portal hypertension is contributing to the ascites, spironolactone is more effective than loop diuretics (Kichian & Bain, 2004). However, a combination of spironolactone and loop diuretics (e.g., furosemide) may be even more effective. It may be reasonable to begin with an oral regiment of 100 mg of spironolactone and 40 mg of furosemide. Doses of both diuretics can be increased every 3 to 5 days, maintaining the 100:40 mg ratio, if weight loss and sodium excretion are inadequate (Runyon, 2004). The recommended maximum oral dose of spironolactone is 400 mg/day and of furosemide is 160 mg/day (Sandhu & Sanyal, 2005). Potential complications of diuretics, especially overuse of diuretics, include fluid and electrolyte imbalances, postural hypotension, hepatic encephalopathy, and pre–renal failure (Kichian & Bain, 2004; Sandhu & Sanyal, 2005).

In addition to monitoring for potential complications of diuretic therapy, assess other burdens of these medications. Patients with fatigue and limited mobility may find that diuretic therapy leads to expenditure of energy (e.g., ambulating to the bathroom, getting out of bed to the bedside commode) that might be better used for other activities that contribute to quality of life. Patients experiencing early satiety may find that taking so many medications leaves little room for the intake of more-satisfying food or fluids.

Paracentesis

Paracentesis may be helpful to achieve short-term relief of uncomfortable symptoms, such as abdominal discomfort and dyspnea. Large-volume paracentesis (i.e., up to 5 liters) can be safely performed without replacement of albumin in patients with diuretic-resistant tense ascites (Peltekian, Wong, Lie et al., 1997; Runyon, 2004; Stephenson & Gilbert, 2002). When ascites is related to portal hypertension, this procedure should be followed by diuretic therapy to attempt to prevent reaccumulation. Albumin replacement is recommended if more than 5 liters of ascitic fluid is removed from a patient with ascites caused by portal hypertension to prevent postparacentesis circulatory dysfunction. The dose of albumin is 8 to 10 g/L of fluid removed (Runyon, 2004; Wongcharatrawee & Garcia-Tsao, 2001). The role of albumin replacement after large-volume paracenteses for malignancy-associated ascites is not clear.

Complications of paracentesis include visceral and vascular injury, infection, hypotension, and ascitic fluid leak (Adam & Adam, 2004). Strict sterile technique should be used for the procedure. As with all invasive procedures, paracentesis is contraindicated in patients with low platelet counts.

Ascitic fluid almost always reaccumulates following paracentesis in patients with malignant ascites and in those with diuretic-resistant portal hypertension–related ascites. Repeated removal of fluid can lead to protein deficiencies and electrolyte abnormalities as well as increasing the potential for visceral and vascular injury. To avoid reaccumulation and the need for repeated paracentesis, attempt to control the disease with medications, when appropriate. Consider a long-term drainage device (discussed later) when other measures do not control the ascites.

Medications

In patients with cancer, intracavitary chemotherapy may control ascites and decrease the frequency of paracenteses. However, there are no good prospective studies of this intervention. It appears that this approach is more effective when a tumor has responded to earlier systemic therapy, especially in patients with ascites related to ovarian or breast cancer (Adam & Adam, 2004). A variety of agents have been used in the limited trials that have been done to date, including nitrogen mustard, thiotepa, cisplatin, 5-fluorouracil, doxorubicin, mitomycin C, etoposide, and bleomycin. Although the goal is to decrease the activity of tumor cells, these agents may work by causing sclerosis and adhesions that obliterate the peritoneal cavity, so that there is no space for fluid accumulation (Adam & Adam, 2004). Acute side effects of intracavitary chemotherapy include fever and abdominal tenderness (Waller & Caroline, 2000). In addition, some drug does cross over to systemic circulation, so systemic side effects, such as nausea, vomiting, hair loss, and bone marrow depression, are possible. There is also a high incidence of mechanical bowel obstruction with peritoneal sclerosing associated with intracavitary chemotherapy (Adam & Adam, 2004).

Intraperitoneal triamcinolone hexacetanide, a slowly metabolized corticosteroid, was used in one phase II study of 15 patients with recurrent malignant ascites (Mackey, Wood, Nabholtz et al., 2000). Although 13 of the 15 patients required repeat paracentesis, the interval between paracenteses was extended. Complications included transient abdominal pain, one case of bacterial peritonitis, and a localized herpes zoster infection. Intraperitoneal immunotherapy showed good results in a study of eight patients with malignant ascites due to carcinomatosis (Heiss, Strohlein, Jager et al., 2005). Further investigation is needed to truly evaluate the benefits and burdens of all of these intraperitoneal therapies.

With the new understanding of some of the molecular pathophysiology of ascites, new treatments may be on the horizon. Phase I and II clinical trials of angioinhibitory therapy (anti-VEGF antibodies, anti-VEGF receptor antibodies, tumor necrosis factor, and metalloproteinase inhibitors) and immunomodulators (OK-432, interleukin 2, and beta-interferon) have shown promise (Adam & Adam, 2004).

The administration of octreotide has been cited in case reports to be effective in controlling malignant ascites (Cairns & Malone, 1999; Mincher, Evans, Jenner et al., 2005). A dose of 200 to 400 mcg/day subcutaneously is reported to be effective in some cases of intractable ascites (Waller & Caroline, 2000). There are no studies that compare the benefits and burdens of octreotide versus other therapies, such as implanted peritoneal drainage catheters (discussed below).

Shunts and Drainage Catheters

When repeated paracenteses are required, consider placement of a shunt or a drainage catheter. A transjugular intrahepatic portasystemic stent-shunt (TIPS) allows blood from the portal circulation to flow into the systemic circulation, relieving portal hypertension (Lake, 2000). This intervention may convert a diuretic-resistant ascites into one that is diuretic sensitive (Runyon, 2004). However, the role of TIPS in the treatment of patients with cirrhosis who have ascites is still not clear. It is recommended that it be reserved for patients for whom large-volume paracentesis repeatedly fails and who have relatively good liver function (Sandu & Sanyal, 2005). Peritoneovenous shunts that empty ascitic fluid from the abdomen through a one-way, pressure-sensitive valve to a catheter in the superior vena cava have also been used to relieve ascites. Because of poor long-term patency, excessive complications, and no survival advantage compared to medical therapy in patients with cirrhosis, this intervention is rarely used today (Runyon, 2004).

In the past, peritoneovenous shunts have not been recommended for malignant ascites because of concerns about dumping malignant cells into the circulation and the tendency for the shunts to fail because of occlusion (Hostetter et al., 2005). However, studies support this procedure as being an effective approach to achieve control of ascites and relief of its associated symptoms (Tueche & Pector, 2000; Zanon, Grosso, Apra et al., 2002). Be aware that peritoneovenous shunting has a complication rate of 25% to 40% and the perioperative mortality rate is between 10% and 20% (Adam & Adam, 2004).

Indwelling peritoneal catheters may be used for continuous or intermittent drainage. Tenckhoff and Groshong catheters were the first catheters used for this purpose. This intervention relieves the discomforts of ascites, avoids the complications of repeated paracenteses, and allows the patient or family to drain ascitic fluid at home (Barnett & Rubins, 2002; Lee, Lau, & Yeong, 2000). Over the past few years, small studies and case reports have shown good outcomes using a tunneled, flexible catheter (Pleurx) originally designed for the treatment of recurrent pleural effusions (Iyengar & Herzog, 2002; Richard, Coldwell, Boyd-Kranis et al., 2001; Rosenberg, Courtney, Nemcek et al., 2004).

General Symptom Management

The symptoms associated with ascites, such as abdominal discomfort, anorexia, nausea, constipation, and dyspnea, must be managed while interventions for ascites are implemented. When ascites is controlled, the interventions initiated to manage the associated symptoms may no longer be required and can be discontinued. In the presence of refractory ascites, the clinician must assess for and treat these associated symptoms on an ongoing basis.

PATIENT AND FAMILY EDUCATION

- Teach signs and symptoms to report.
  - Signs of fluid accumulation (e.g., abdominal discomfort or bloating, dyspnea)
  - Signs of infection
- Prepare for paracentesis or indwelling catheter placement, as appropriate.
  - Explain the purpose of the paracentesis.
  - Explain the procedure, potential complications, and follow-up care.
  - Explain that reaccumulation of fluid is likely with paracentesis alone.
- Provide information about diuretic therapy, as appropriate.
- If ascites is caused by liver disease, discuss the "pros and cons" of a low-sodium diet.
- Teach appropriate use of medications and other interventions initiated to treat the symptoms associated with ascites, such as analgesics, antiemetics, and laxatives.

EVALUATION AND PLAN FOR FOLLOW-UP

- Assess abdominal girth after treatment as a measurement of effectiveness.
- Monitor for signs of reaccumulation of fluid.
  - Measure abdominal girth regularly to identify changes.
  - Assess for symptoms associated with fluid accumulation.
  - Monitor weight.
- Following paracentesis or placement of an indwelling catheter
  - Monitor for postural hypotension.
  - Monitor the puncture site for leakage.
  - Monitor vital signs for evidence of infection.
  - Provide site care.

CASE STUDY Mrs. S. is 58 years old and has advanced ovarian cancer. Over the past month, she has noticed an increasing difficulty in fastening the waist closures of pants and skirts. The only pants she can wear now are sweat pants with a drawstring waist. She complains of a poor appetite but has gained about 25 pounds. She states she is always tired and has difficulty lying flat in bed because of shortness of breath, but she is able to sleep if she keeps the head of her bed elevated.

On physical examination, the clinician observes a protruding abdomen when Mrs. S. is standing or sitting and bulging flanks when she is lying. The skin across the abdomen is tight with prominent veins. With percussion, tympany is noted over the umbilicus and dullness is noted at the flanks when Mrs. S. is lying on her back. When the patient lies on her left side, the clinician notes tympany on the right (upper) side and dullness on the left (dependent) side. Her abdominal girth is measured at 144 centimeters.

With the diagnosis of ovarian cancer, the cause of ascites is evident and no diagnostic tests are ordered at this time. Because sodium and fluid restrictions and diuretics are of little value with malignant ascites, paracentesis is performed at the outpatient clinic. About 4 liters of yellow, turbid fluid is removed. Mrs. S. tolerates the procedure well with no signs of postural hypotension. She experiences immediate relief of dyspnea and the generalized abdominal discomfort. Her abdominal girth after the procedure is 105 centimeters. Markings are placed on her abdomen so that her caregiver can monitor the abdominal girth at home. A bowel regimen of two tablets of sennosides 8.6 mg/docusate sodium 50 mg (Peri-Colace/Senokot-S) oral at bedtime is initiated.

Over the next 4 weeks, Mrs. S.'s abdominal girth gradually increases to 124 centimeters and the uncomfortable symptoms return. As repeat paracenteses are anticipated, a Pleurx catheter is placed and 3 liters of yellow, turbid ascitic fluid are removed. The clinician teaches the caregiver how to attach a drainage container to the catheter and to drain up to 2 liters of fluid every 3 days or whenever Mrs. S. reports abdominal fullness. The clinician also explains how to document the amount of drainage on a flow chart and instructs the caregiver to call if there is a change in the color of the drainage; if there is any redness, swelling, or drainage from the catheter insertion site; or if Mrs. S. develops a fever. The caregiver is also shown how to clean the insertion site and change the dressing each time the catheter is connected to drainage.

After 3 weeks of draining 1.5 to 2 liters of ascites fluid every 3 days, the amount of drainage has decreased to an average of 800 ml every 3 days. The clinician instructs the caregiver to try a weekly schedule for draining the catheter unless Mrs. S. reports abdominal fullness. The weekly drainage continues at 1.5 liters. Mrs. S. is eating and drinking very little and is now completely bedbound. Mrs. S. dies at home 2 months after placement of the abdominal drainage catheter with no abdominal distention, no abdominal discomfort, and no dyspnea.

REFERENCES

Adam, R.A. & Adam, Y.G. (2004). Malignant ascites: Past, present, and future. *J Am Coll Surg, 198(6)*, 999-1011.

Barnett, T.D. & Rubins, J. (2002). Placement of a permanent tunneled peritoneal drainage catheter for palliation of malignant ascites: A simplified percutaneous approach. *J Vas Intervention Radiol: JVIR, 13(4)*, 379-383.

Cairns, W. & Malone, R. (1999). Octreotide as an agent for the relief of malignant ascites in palliative care patients. *Palliat Med, 13*, 429.

Cattau, E.L., Benjamin, S.B., Knuff, T.E., et al. (1982). The accuracy of the physical examination in the diagnosis of suspected ascites. *JAMA, 247(8),* 1164-1166.

Heiss, M.M., Strohlein, M.A., Jager, M., et al. (2005). Immunotherapy of malignant ascites with trifunctional antibodies. *Int J Cancer, 117(3),* 435-443.

Hostetter, R.B., Marincola, F.M., & Schwartzentruber, D.J. (2005). Malignant ascites. In V.T. DeVita, S. Hellman, & S.A. Rosenberg (Eds.). *Cancer: Principles and practice of oncology* (7th ed., pp. 2392-2398). Philadelphia: Lippincott, Williams & Wilkins.

Iyengar, T.D. & Herzog, T.J. (2002). Management of symptomatic ascites in recurrent ovarian cancer patients using an intra-abdominal semi-permanent catheter. *Am J Hospice Palliat Care, 19(1),* 35-38.

Kichian, K. & Bain, V.G. (2004). Jaundice, ascites, and hepatic encephalopathy. In D. Doyle, G. Hanks, & N. Cherny, et al. (Eds.). *Oxford textbook of palliative medicine* (3rd ed., pp. 507-520). New York: Oxford University Press.

Kravetz, D., Bildozola, M., Argonz, J., et al. (2000). Patients with ascites have higher variceal pressure and wall tension than patients without ascites. *Am J Gastroenterol, 95,* 1770-1775.

Lake, J.R. (2000). The role of transjugular portosystemic shunting in patients with ascites [letter]. *N Engl J Med, 342(23),* 1745-1747.

Lee, A., Lau, T.A., & Yeong, K.Y. (2000). Indwelling catheters for the management of malignant ascites. *Support Care Cancer, 8,* 493-499.

Lingappa, W.R. (2003). Liver disease. In S.J. McPhee, V.R. Lingappa, & W.F. Ganong (Eds.). *Pathophysiology of disease: An introduction to clinical medicine* (4th ed., pp. 380-419). New York: Lange Medical Books/McGraw-Hill.

Mackey, J.R., Wood, L., Nabholtz, J., et al. (2000). A phase II trial of triamcinolone hexacetanide for symptomatic recurrent malignant ascites. *J Pain Symptom Manage, 19(3),* 193-199.

Mincher, L., Evans, J., Jenner, M.W., et al. (2005). The successful treatment of chylous effusions in malignant disease with octreotide. *Clin Oncol (Royal Coll Radiol), 17(2),* 118-121.

Nagy, J.A., Herzberg, K.T., Masse, E.M., et al. (1989). Exchange of macromolecules between plasma and peritoneal cavity in ascites tumor-bearing, normal, and serotonin-injected mice. *Cancer Res, 49(19),* 5448-5458.

Peltekian, K.M., Wong, F., Lie, P.P., et al. (1997). Cardiovascular, renal, and neurohumoral responses to single large-volume paracentesis in patients with cirrhosis and diuretic-resistant ascites. *Am J Gastroenterol, 92(3),* 394-399.

Richard, H.M., 3rd., Coldwell, D.M., Boyd-Kranis, R.L., et al. (2001). Pleurx tunneled catheter in the management of malignant ascites. *J Vasc Intervention Radiol: JVIR, 12(3),* 373-375.

Rosenberg, S., Courtney, A., Nemcek, A.A., Jr., et al. (2004). Comparison of percutaneous management techniques for recurrent malignant ascites. *J Vasc Intervention Radiol: JVIR, 15(10),* 1129-1131.

Runyon, B.A. (2004). AASLD practice guideline: Management of adult patients with ascites due to cirrhosis. *Hepatology, 39(3),* 841-856.

Runyon, B.A., Montano, A.A., Akriviadis, E.A., et al. (1992). The serum-ascites albumin gradient is superior to the exudates-transudate concept in the differential diagnosis of ascites. *Ann Intern Med, 117(3),* 215-220.

Sandhu, B.S. & Sanyal, A.J. (2005). Management of ascites in cirrhosis. *Clin Liver Dis, 9(4),* 715-732.

Stephenson, J. & Gilbert, J. (2002). The development of clinical guidelines on paracentesis for ascites related to malignancy. *Palliat Med, 16(3),* 213-218.

Stoelcker, B., Echtenacher, B., Weich, H.A., et al. (2000). VEGF/Flk-1 interaction: A requirement for malignant ascites recurrence. *J Interferon Cytokine Res, 20(5),* 511-517.

Tabbarah, H.J. & Casciato, D.A. (1990). Malignant effusions. In C.M. Haskell (Ed.). *Cancer treatment* (pp. 815-825). Philadelphia: Saunders.

Tueche, S.G. & Pector, J.C. (2000). Peritoneovenous shunt in malignant ascites. The Bordet Institute experience from 1975-1998. *Hepato-Gastroenterology, 47,* 1322-1324.

Waller, A. & Caroline, N.L. (2000). *Handbook of palliative care in cancer* (2nd ed.). Boston: Butterworth-Heinemann.

Wongcharatrawee, S. & Garcia-Tsao, G. (2001). Clinical management of ascites and its complications. *Clin Liver Dis, 5(3),* 833-350.

Zanon, C., Grosso, M., Apra, F., et al. (2002). Palliative treatment of malignant refractory ascites by positioning of Denver peritoneovenous shunt. *Tumori, 88(2),* 123-127.

Zebrowski, B.K., Liu, W., Ramirez, K., et al. (1999). Markedly elevated levels of vascular endothelial growth factor in malignant ascites. *Ann Surg Oncol, 6(4),* 373-378.

CHAPTER 19

BOWEL OBSTRUCTION

Debra E. Heidrich and Pamela Sue Spencer

■

DEFINITION AND INCIDENCE

Bowel obstruction is defined as abnormally delayed or blocked transit through the intestinal tract (Ripamonti & Mercadante, 2004; Waller & Caroline, 2000). With obstruction, the motor activities of the small intestine and/or colon, characterized by contractile patterns that serve the requirements of each organ, become impaired (Hasler, 2003). Although not a frequent complication, bowel obstruction occurs more often in the palliative care patient than in patients in other care settings. Malignant bowel obstruction (MBO) occurs in approximately 3% of all patients with cancer, but up to 24% of patients with colon cancer and up to 42% of women with ovarian cancer may develop obstructions (Hirst & Regnard, 2003; Ripamonti & Mercadante, 2004). Less frequently, MBOs are seen with cancers of the pancreas, stomach, endometrium, bladder, and prostate (Waller & Caroline, 2000). One retrospective chart audit showed that 19% of patients with malignant small bowel obstruction also had a large bowel obstruction (Miller, Boman, Shrier et al., 2000). Bowel obstructions are most frequently caused by postoperative adhesions, occurring in about 3.5% of people who have intestinal resection (Dang, Aguilera, Dang et al., 2002; Fazio, Cohen, Fleshman et al., 2006; Ryan, Wattchow, Walker et al., 2004). The incidence of other nonmalignant causes of bowel obstruction is not as well documented. Bowel obstructions may involve the small or large bowel and can be partial or complete. Any site of the gastrointestinal tract may be involved, from the gastroduodenal junction to the rectum and anus (Hirst & Regnard, 2003).

ETIOLOGY AND PATHOPHYSIOLOGY

MBO may be intraluminal due to tumors blocking the bowel, intramural due to tumor infiltration of the intestinal muscles and the accompanying inflammation that occludes bowel, or extramural due to tumors outside the lumen that compress the bowel wall (Davis & Nouneh, 2000; Hirst & Regnard, 2003; Ripamonti & Mercadante, 2004). Adhesions may contribute to malignant obstruction in people who have had previous abdominal surgery (Miller et al., 2000). In addition, patients with cancer may have motility disorders from malignant involvement of intestinal muscle or autonomic nerves. Nonmalignant causes of bowel obstruction include adhesions from previous surgery, incarcerated or strangulated hernias, pseudo-obstruction, and fecal impaction.

Improperly managed constipation may lead to impaction and symptoms of bowel obstruction (Pappagallo, 2001; Ripamonti & Mercadante, 2004). Constipation is a common problem in people with advanced illnesses due to decreased food and fluid intake and decreased mobility. This problem is compounded by the use of medications that contribute to constipation, such as opioids and anticholinergic drugs. An impaction is easily misdiagnosed as clinicians mistake hard abdominal masses of feces for tumors (Hirst & Regnard, 2003).

Pseudo-obstruction presents like a mechanical obstruction but has no anatomic cause (Sutton, Harrell, & Wo, 2006). It is sometimes called adynamic ileus and is defined as a state of inhibited motility in the gastrointestinal tract that may be temporary (reversible) or permanent (Summers, 2003). Although there are many potential causes of pseudoobstruction, the incidence is believed to be rare (Smith, Williams, & Ferris, 2003). In the palliative care setting, the more likely causes of pseudo-obstruction include the following:

- Collagen vascular disease, such as scleroderma
- Primary muscle disease, such as any type of muscular dystrophy
- Endocrine disorders, including diabetes
- Neurological disorders, including Parkinson's disease and paraneoplastic syndromes (e.g., Eaton-Lambert myasthenic syndrome)
- Medications, including opioids, tricyclic antidepressants, phenothiazines, clonidine, antiparkinsonian medications, anticholinergic drugs, and vinca alkaloid chemotherapy agents

When the bowel is obstructed, intestinal contents accumulate proximal to the blockage and the bowel distends. Bowel activity increases in an effort to restore peristalsis, leading to uncoordinated muscle contractions, increased intestinal secretions, and increasing bowel distention. Further, the bacterial flora of the bowel contents increases above normal levels, causing gas production and, again, increasing bowel distention. The increased pressure on the cell walls initiates the inflammatory process, resulting in even more edema and secretions. Hypoxia of the tissues develops as the increased pressure interferes with venous drainage and oxygenation. Death results when third-spacing of fluid causes hypovolemia and renal failure, when the passage of toxins from the intestine into the lymphatics and circulation leads to sepsis, or when these events occur together (Ripamonti & Mercadante, 2004).

Obstructions in the proximal bowel cause vomiting and severe dehydration and electrolyte disturbances but minimal distention. Blockage in the distal bowel causes a large amount of fluid to accumulate in the bowel, third-spacing of fluids and dehydration, abdominal distention, and feculent vomiting (Dang et al., 2002; Hirst & Regnard, 2003). Malignant obstructions may present acutely but are more likely to have a gradual onset over weeks or months (Hirst & Regnard, 2003).

ASSESSMENT AND MEASUREMENT

The assessment of bowel obstruction is based primarily on the presenting symptoms of pain, vomiting, and obstipation (Dang et al., 2002). Abdominal pain is present in about 90% of patients presenting with a bowel obstruction (Hirst & Regnard, 2003). The pain is usually described as colicky, meaning it worsens when the intestines contract in their attempt to restore peristalsis but lessens when the muscles relax. Pain usually presents in the suprapubic region when the obstruction is low in the colon

(Waller & Caroline, 2000). As the distention worsens, so does the pain; it may become constant. Assessment measures include noting the onset, location, and severity of pain, noting whether the pain is intermittent or continuous, and noting any worsening of the pain over time.

Because there is less distention with proximal obstructions (e.g., jejunal or small bowel obstructions), there may be less pain but significantly more vomiting. Vomiting develops later in obstructions of the distal ileum and colon and may be feculent (Dang et al., 2002; Hirst & Regnard, 2003). Assess the amount, color, and odor of emesis. Remember that some patients may have concurrent large and small bowel obstructions.

Dehydration is a concern with high-volume emesis and poor intake, so assessment must include evaluation of hydration status. Assess skin turgor, blood pressure, heart rate, urinary output, and subjective symptoms of dehydration, such as headache and dry mouth.

While patients with complete bowel obstruction are usually obstipated, those with partial or intermittent bowel obstructions may have constipation or diarrhea. Ask about frequency, amount, and consistency of bowel movements. Be aware that what is reported as diarrhea may be overflow of liquefied fecal material (Waller & Caroline, 2000).

Abdominal obstruction can also compromise respiratory function due to pressure on the diaphragm secondary to abdominal distention. Patients with cardiorespiratory problems at baseline are especially vulnerable (Summers, 2003). Assess changes in respiratory rate and effort, as well as any report of dyspnea.

HISTORY AND PHYSICAL EXAMINATION

The diagnosis of bowel obstruction can present challenges for the clinician. Some patients advance from a partial to complete occlusion in an insidious manner, whereas other patients may develop an intermittent obstruction, causing fluctuating symptoms. It is essential that clinicians complete a detailed history, including:

- History of any gastrointestinal disease or surgery (note that this may be unrelated to the terminal illness)
- History of muscular, neurological, endocrine, or collagen disorders that may affect the bowel
- History of receiving a vinca alkaloid chemotherapeutic agent
- Usual bowel patterns and any changes in bowel patterns
- Onset, location, intensity, and duration of pain as well as how the pain has changed over time
- Onset, frequency, and amount of emesis
- Food and fluid intake
- Amount, frequency, and concentration of urine
- Subjective signs of dehydration, especially headache, dizziness, or dry mouth
- Review of all medications, noting those that stimulate the gastrointestinal system, such as laxatives and metoclopramide, as well as those that may decrease peristalsis, like opioids, tricyclic antidepressants, and anticholinergic drugs

A comprehensive physical examination includes assessing the patient's general appearance, signs of hydration, fever, hypotension, and respiratory compromise. Perform a thorough assessment of the abdomen. Note any laparotomy scars or abdominal distention.

Palpate for masses, noting that a fecal impaction can be mistaken for a tumor. Note any tenderness to palpation. Listen to bowel sounds. In early bowel obstruction, bowel sounds may be high pitched and tinkling. Be aware, however, that classic tinkling sounds are actually rare (Twycross & Wilcock, 2001). Bowel sounds may be absent with complete bowel obstruction. Complete a rectal examination to assess rectal tone and the presence of masses, fecal impaction, or liquid stool.

DIAGNOSTICS

When the clinical evaluation suggests obstruction or ileus, radiographic examination is helpful to confirm the diagnosis, differentiate ileus from obstruction, or, at least, contribute to an understanding of the cause (Jenkins, Taylor, & Behrns, 2000). In patients in the end stage of advanced cancer, abdominal films are indicated only when the patient may be a candidate for palliative surgery to relieve the obstruction or to distinguish between mechanical obstruction and severe constipation (Waller & Caroline, 2000). Multislice spiral computed tomography, computed tomography colonography, and magnetic resonance imaging are more accurate than plain radiographs and can determine the extent of intraabdominal cancer, an important factor in determining if a patient is a surgical candidate (Low, Chen, & Barone, 2003; Taourel, Kessler, Lesnick et al., 2003). In addition to radiographic studies, blood chemistries may be obtained to evaluate fluid and electrolyte status.

INTERVENTIONS AND TREATMENT

Treatment decisions should be based on the patient's predicted disease trajectory, current condition, and obstructive involvement. Surgical intervention is the primary approach to the management of bowel obstruction in the general hospital setting. All patients should be evaluated for surgery since those who have surgery are less likely to experience a re-obstruction than are those whose bowel obstructions are managed nonoperatively (Miller et al., 2000). However, many patients with advanced diseases are not good surgical candidates. Also, Miller and colleagues (2000) reported a postoperative morbidity rate of 67% and mortality rate of 13% in patients with MBO. Because of the high morbidity and mortality associated with surgery, it is recommended that a 5-day trial of pharmacological intervention be initiated before considering surgery; if the obstruction does not resolve with pharmacological intervention, then surgery may be an option for the appropriately selected patient (Miller et al., 2000). Factors associated with a poor prognosis with surgery are listed in Box 19-1.

Pharmacological management of bowel obstruction is recommended to control symptoms in patients who are not good surgical candidates and to improve the condition of the bowel in those being prepared for surgery (Mercadante, Ferrera, Villari et al., 2004). One study of 15 patients demonstrated that the combination of metoclopramide 60 mg/day, octreotide 0.3 mg/day, and dexamethasone 12 mg/day, given as a continuous subcutaneous infusion, led to recovery of intestinal transit within 1 to 5 days and resolution of vomiting within 24 hours (Mercadante et al., 2004).

Box 19-1	Indicators of Poor Surgical Outcome in Malignant Bowel Obstruction

ABSOLUTE CONTRAINDICATIONS

Intraperitoneal carcinomatosis with intestinal motility problems
Ascites
Widespread, palpable abdominal masses
Multiple partial bowel obstruction
Previous abdominal surgery that showed diffuse metastatic disease
Involvement of the proximal stomach

RELATIVE CONTRAINDICATIONS

Poor performance status
Patients over 65 years old with cachexia
Previous radiation therapy to the abdomen or pelvis
Low serum albumin
Distant metastasis, pleural effusion, or pulmonary metastasis
Elevated blood urea nitrogen or alkaline phosphatase levels

Adapted from Ripamonti, C. & Mercadante, S. (2004). Pathophysiology and management of malignant bowel obstruction. In D. Doyle, G. Hanks, N. Cherny, & K. Calman (Eds.). *Oxford textbook of palliative medicine* (3rd ed., pp. 496-506). New York: Oxford University Press.

It is proposed that these medications are an effective combination because of the antiemetic and prokinetic effects of metoclopramide, the antisecretory effect of octreotide (decreases intestinal secretions contributing to bowel distention), and the antiinflammatory effect of dexamethasone (decreases intestinal wall edema).

Opioids may be given to treat the abdominal pain. In addition, anticholinergic medications, such as glycopyrrolate or hyoscine butylbromide, may be helpful for colicky pain due to their ability to relax smooth muscle (Davis & Nouneh, 2000; Hirst & Regnard, 2003; von Gunten & Muir, 2002). In the presence of complete obstruction, stimulant laxatives may exacerbate pain and should be discontinued.

Metoclopramide, as mentioned, is a good antiemetic and increases gastrointestinal motility. Increased gastrointestinal motility may be especially helpful if the patient has a partial obstruction or if a motility disorder caused or contributed to the obstruction. As with stimulant laxatives, in complete obstruction, this stimulation may worsen colicky pain and metoclopramide should be discontinued (Hirst & Regnard, 2003; von Gunten & Muir, 2002). Haloperidol is another good medication for nausea and vomiting (Davis & Nouneh, 2000; Hirst & Regnard, 2003; von Gunten & Muir, 2002). Dexamethasone may be included in the plan of care for its antiemetic and antiinflammatory properties.

As discussed, octreotide decreases the amount of gastrointestinal secretions. It may be used alone or in combination with anticholinergic agents such as scopolamine to decrease distention, pain, cramping, nausea, and vomiting (Cowan & Palmer, 2002; Mercandante, Ripamonti, Casucci et al., 2000; Mystakidou, Tsilika, Kalaidopoulou et al., 2002).

Long-acting octreotide, given as a monthly intramuscular injection, may be an option for patients requiring long-term administration (Matulonis, Seiden, Roche et al., 2005). Octreotide is an expensive medication. More research is needed to determine if the costs of this medication make it appropriate for first-line therapy or if other, less-expensive medications to control the symptoms of obstruction should undergo a trial first.

There are times, however, when pharmacological measures fail, leading to intractable vomiting. When this occurs, nasogastric decompression and parenteral hydration are preferable to the suffering produced by unremitting emesis (Waller & Caroline, 2000).

Enteral stents may be used as a less-invasive alternative to surgery for the palliation of unresectable bowel obstructions or to manage symptoms until surgery is scheduled (Baron, Rey, & Spinelli, 2002; Del Piano, Ballare, Montino et al., 2005; Vazquez-Iglesias, Gonzalez-Conde, Vasques-Millan et al., 2005).

Nausea and vomiting interfere with the oral administration of medications to treat the symptoms of obstruction as well as all other medications. Review all medications, discontinue medications that are no longer needed at this time, and select an appropriate alternative route of administration for those medications that are needed for symptom control. Alternative routes may include the sublingual, rectal, transdermal, subcutaneous, or intravenous routes.

PATIENT AND FAMILY EDUCATION

The symptoms of bowel obstruction are extremely uncomfortable and frightening and negatively impact quality of living. Patients and family members need to be kept informed about the potential cause of the symptoms, the interventions that will be used to control symptoms until a definitive diagnosis is made, and the treatment options (including benefits and burdens of each). Instruct the patient and family on the dose and administration of all new medications as well as changes in routes of administration of routine medications required because of nausea and vomiting. Prepare patients and family members for any surgical interventions or invasive procedures. Instruct the patient and family regarding signs and symptoms of recurring or worsening obstruction and encourage them to report these symptoms immediately. The fear of a recurring obstruction may increase anxiety in both the patient and family. Provide emotional support and make referrals to other members of the interdisciplinary team, including the social worker, chaplain, or counselor.

EVALUATION AND PLAN FOR FOLLOW-UP

"The goal of medical management is to decrease pain, nausea, and secretions into the bowel so to eliminate the need for a nasogastric (NG) tube and IV hydration" (von Gunten & Muir, 2002, p. 740). If the pharmacological management of the obstruction is effective, some patients may tolerate being tapered from the analgesics, antiemetics, antisecretory medications, and corticosteroids; other patients will need to be maintained on these medications for the remainder of their lives.

Recurrence of bowel obstruction and multiple bowel obstructions are possible in patients with advanced cancer who have had a previous obstruction. Monitor for any new onset of symptoms and institute symptomatic therapies immediately.

CASE STUDY   Mr. J. is 72 years old and has metastatic colon cancer. He had a colectomy with anastomosis 3 years ago followed by chemotherapy. Liver metastasis was diagnosed 6 months ago. He is at home with an interdisciplinary hospice team providing care to him and his wife. His current medications include controlled-release oxycodone 20 mg by mouth every 12 hours for abdominal pain related to his enlarged liver, 5 mg of immediate-release oxycodone by mouth as needed for breakthrough pain, and a combination stimulant/softener laxative.

Mr. J. reports that he is having intermittent sharp pains in his abdomen. Two days ago he had a very small bowel movement of soft stool. He has not vomited but says he feels nauseated and has no appetite. He has had only sips of fluids in the past 24 hours. Upon physical examination, the clinician notes slight abdominal distention, high-pitched bowel sounds, no palpable abdominal masses, and a small amount of soft stool in the rectum. A partial bowel obstruction is suspected. Mr. J. states that he does not want to go back to the hospital unless it is absolutely necessary.

After consultation with the patient, family, and surgeon, a decision is made to treat the potential obstruction pharmacologically at home and to evaluate the effectiveness. Because Mr. J. is still able to swallow and has not had any vomiting, he is started on a regimen of oral metoclopramide 10 mg every 8 hours to treat nausea and increase bowel motility, dexamethasone 8 mg every 8 hours to decrease inflammation in the bowel, and hyoscyamine 0.25 mg every 4 hours for 24 hours and then every 4 hours as needed to treat the colicky pain. His oxycodone regimen is continued and an additional stool softener is added to his bowel protocol.

After 24 hours on the new regimen, Mr. J. reports a decrease in the sharp abdominal pains, although he feels "twinges" on occasion, and no nausea. After 72 hours, he is eating small amounts of soft foods and is able to take in fluids throughout the day. He reports a moderate-size soft bowel movement. The dexamethasone is tapered to 4 mg every 8 hours and he does not require any hyoscyamine after 7 days.

Mr. J. eventually becomes unable to swallow medications, although he is still able to sip some fluids. Although weak, he does not appear to be imminently dying and there is concern about recurrent bowel obstruction and management of his pain. Rectal administration versus subcutaneous infusion of an opioid, metoclopramide, and dexamethasone is discussed as options with Mr. and Mrs. J. Mr. J. does not want his wife to have to give him suppositories around the clock. Hypodermoclysis at a rate of 100 ml/hr of {2/3} normal saline is initiated to maintain hydration and a subcutaneous infusion of metoclopramide 1.5 mg/hr, dexamethasone 0.5 mg/hr, and hydromorphone 0.1 mg/hr (approximately 75% of the equianalgesic dose of oxycodone) is started. Nursing visits are scheduled daily for the first 3 days of therapy to ensure that Mr. J. is tolerating the infusion and that Mrs. J. is comfortable with instructions regarding both the hypodermoclysis and the ambulatory infusion pump with the medications. When Mr. J. becomes too weak to use a urinal, a urinary catheter is placed to ensure continuous drainage. Over the next 3 weeks, the hydromorphone dosage is titrated up to 1 mg/hr due to reports of pain. He remains lethargic but able to communicate until 24 hours before he dies peacefully at home.

REFERENCES

Baron, T.H., Rey, J., & Spinelli, P. (2002). Expandable metal stent placement for malignant colorectal obstruction. *Endoscopy, 34(10)*, 823-830.

Cowan, J.D. & Palmer, T.W. (2002). Practical guide to palliative sedation. *Curr Oncol Reports, 4(3)*, 242-249.

Dang, C., Aguilera, P., Dang, A., et al. (2002). Acute abdominal pain: Four classifications can guide assessment and management. *Geriatrics, 57(3)*, 30-42.

Davis, M.P. & Nouneh, C. (2000). Modern management of cancer-related intestinal obstruction. *Curr Oncol Reports, 2(4)*, 343-350.

Del Piano, M., Ballare, M., Montino, F., et al. (2005). Endoscopy or surgery for malignant GI outlet obstruction? *Gastrointestin Endosc, 61(3)*, 421-426.

Fazio, V.W., Cohen, Z., Fleshman, J.W., et al. (2006). Reduction in adhesive small-bowel obstruction by Seprafilm adhesion barrier after intestinal resection. *Diseases of the Colon and Rectum, 49(1)*, 1-11.

Hasler, W. (2003). Motility of the small intestine and colon. In T. Yamada & D.H. Alpers (Eds.). *The textbook of gastroenterology* (4th ed., pp. 220-239). Philadelphia: Lippincott, William, & Wilkins.

Hirst, B. & Regnard, C. (2003). Management of intestinal obstruction in malignant disease. *Clinical Med, 3(4)*, 311-314.

Jenkins, J.T., Taylor, A.J., & Behrns, K.E. (2000). Secondary causes of intestinal obstruction; rigorous preoperative evaluation is required. *Am Surgeon, 66(7)*, 662-666.

Low, R.N., Chen, S.C., & Barone, R. (2003). Distinguishing benign from malignant bowel obstruction in patients with malignancy: Findings at MR imaging. *Radiology, 228(1)*, 157-165.

Matulonis, U.A., Seiden, M.V., Roche, M., et al. (2005). Long-acting octreotide for the treatment and symptomatic relief of bowel obstruction in advanced ovarian cancer. *J Pain Symptom Manage, 30(6)*, 563-569.

Mercadante, S., Ferrera, P., Villari, P., et al. (2004). Aggressive pharmacological treatment for reversing malignant bowel obstruction. *J Pain Symptom Manage, 28(4)*, 412-416.

Mercadante, S., Ripamonti, C., Casucci, A., et al. (2000). Comparison of octreotide and hyoscine butylbromide in controlling gastrointestinal symptoms due to malignant inoperable bowel obstruction. *Support Care Cancer, 8(3)*, 188-191.

Miller, G., Boman, J., Shrier, I., et al. (2000). Small-bowel obstruction secondary to malignant disease: An 11-year audit. *Can J Surg, 43(5)*, 353-358.

Mystakidou, K., Tsilika, E., Kalaidopoulou, O., et al. (2002). Comparison of octreotide administration vs conservative treatment in the management of inoperable bowel obstruction in patients with far advanced cancer: A randomized, double-blind, controlled clinical trial. *Anticancer Res, 22(2B)*, 1187-1192.

Pappagallo, M. (2001). Incidence, prevalence, and management of opioid bowel dysfunction. *Am J Surg, 182(5A Suppl)*, 11S-18S.

Ripamonti, C. & Mercadante, S. (2004). Pathophysiology and management of malignant bowel obstruction. In D. Doyle, G. Hanks, N. Cherny, et al. (Eds.). *Oxford textbook of palliative medicine* (3rd ed., pp. 496-506). New York: Oxford University Press.

Ryan, M. D., Wattchow, D., Walker, M., et al. (2004). Adhesional small bowel obstruction after colorectal surgery. *Aus N Z J Surg, 74(1)*, 1010-1012.

Smith, D.S., Williams, C.S., & Ferris, C.D. (2003). Diagnosis and treatment of chronic gastroparesis and chronic intestinal pseudo-obstruction. *Gastroenterol Clin North Am, 32(2),* 619-658.

Summers, R.W. (2003). Approach to the patient with ileus and obstruction. In T. Yamada, D.H. Alpers, L. Laine, et al. (Eds.). *The textbook of gastroenterology* (4th ed., pp. 829-843). Philadelphia: Lippincott Williams, & Wilkins.

Sutton, D.H., Harrell, S.P., & Wo, J.M. (2006). Diagnosis and management of adult patients with chronic intestinal pseudoobstruction. *Nutr Clin Pract, 21(1),* 16-22.

Taourel, P., Kessler, N., Lesnik, A., et al. (2003). Helical CT of large bowel obstruction. *Abdom Imag, 28(2),* 267-275.

Twycross, R.G. & Wilcock, A. (2001). Alimentary symptoms: Obstruction. In R. Twycross & A. Wilcock (Eds.). *Symptom management in advanced cancer* (3rd ed., pp. 111-115). Oxford: Radcliffe Medical Press.

Vazquez-Iglesias, J.L., Gonzalez-Conde, B., Vazquez-Millan, M.A., et al. (2005). Self-expandable stents in malignant colonic obstruction: Insertion assisted with a sphincterotome in technically difficult cases. *Gastrointestin Endosc, 62(3),* 436-437.

von Gunten, C. & Muir, J.C. (2002). Fast facts and concepts #45: Medical management of bowel obstruction. *J Palliat Med, 5(5),* 739-740.

Waller, A. & Caroline, N.L. (2000). *Handbook of palliative care in cancer* (2nd ed.). Boston: Butterworth-Heinemann.

CHAPTER 20

CACHEXIA AND ANOREXIA

Peg Esper

■

DEFINITION AND INCIDENCE

Cachexia, a complex syndrome associated with metabolic changes, fat and muscle wasting, loss of appetite, and involuntary weight loss, is common with many progressive diseases. The true incidence of cachexia is difficult to determine because studies use inconsistent criteria for defining cachexia and because some studies report the incidence based on all patients with a particular disease while others include only patients with an advanced stage of the disease. It is estimated that cachexia occurs in about 80% of patients with advanced cancer, 33% of patients with acquired immunodeficiency syndrome, 20% of those with congestive heart failure, and up to 50% of patients with chronic hypoxemia associated with chronic lung disease (Anker, Ponikowski, Varney et al., 1997; Castillo-Martinez, Orea-Tejeda, Rosales et al., 2005; Davis & Dickerson, 2000; Schols, Soeters, Dingemans et al., 1993; Wanke, 2000). The complex metabolic changes associated with cachexia are characterized by increased energy expenditures that are unaffected by caloric intake. In comparison, starvation leads to energy conservation and is reversed by caloric intake. Thus, cachexia is not synonymous with starvation. Cachexia is correlated with decreased quality of life and decreased survival in all disease populations. An estimated 30% of oncology patients die due to the effects of cachexia (Illman, Corringham, Robinson et al., 2005; Strasser & Bruera, 2002).

ETIOLOGY AND PATHOPHYSIOLOGY

Although the syndrome of weight loss, loss of appetite, and profound weakness has long been recognized in patients with advanced diseases, there is not yet a complete understanding of or agreement on the factors that contribute to its cause. Cancer cachexia was previously thought to be the result of excessive use of nutrients by tumors and decreased energy intake on the part of the individual. Research involving a number of wasting syndromes has now identified several overlapping mechanisms that mediate cachexia, including metabolic alterations, neurohormonal alterations, and changes in anabolic processes (Andreas, 2005; Anker, Steinborn, & Strassberg, 2004; Esper & Harb, 2005; Strasser, 2003; Wouters, Creutzbergt, & Schols, 2002).

Proinflammatory cytokines such as interleukin 1, interleukin 6, interferon γ, and tumor necrosis factor α are likely involved in mediating the cachexia syndrome. These substances may (1) interfere with appetite signals in the hypothalamus, causing anorexia; (2) increase the metabolic rate by inducing thermogenesis and muscle wasting; (3) interfere with lipid storage; and (4) contribute to muscle protein loss and increased energy expenditure (Davis, 2002; Illman et al., 2005; Inui, 2002, McCarthy, 2003;

Strasser, 2003; Winter, 2002). Dietary supplementation does not reverse this process. Thus, the cachexia syndrome may be viewed as a chronic inflammatory condition rather than a nutritional aberration (McCarthy, 2003).

In addition to the metabolic syndrome of cachexia, there are other problems that may contribute to a decreased appetite and weight loss (Strasser, 2003; Strasser & Bruera, 2002):

- Alterations in oral intake (stomatitis, early satiety, nausea and vomiting, bowel obstruction, pain, etc.)
- Alterations in gastrointestinal absorption (autoimmune syndromes, severe diarrhea)
- Protein loss (ongoing drainage of pleural effusions or ascitic fluid, renal failure)
- Catabolic states (infections, renal failure, hyperthyroidism, congestive heart failure)
- Functional loss of muscle mass (prolonged bed rest, hormonal insufficiencies, aging)

ASSESSMENT AND MEASUREMENT

Patients must be assessed for potentially reversible causes of weight loss or lack of appetite before the diagnosis of cachexia-anorexia syndrome can be made. Consider the following factors (Ross & Alexander, 2001):

- Radiation or chemotherapy treatments
- Severe, untreated pain
- Constipation
- Adjustment disorder, depression, or cognitive failure
- Mechanical obstruction of alimentary canal by tumor
- Oral disorders such as *Candida* infection or poorly fitting dentures
- Appetite-reducing medications

Weight may be monitored using scales, although the rapidly falling numbers may be a source of distress to some patients. Appetite is a subjective experience that may be measured by using a visual analog or numerical scale. By asking a patient to indicate a number between 0 and 10, where 10 represents an excellent appetite and 0 means no appetite at all, it is possible to monitor the patient's status and the results of interventions.

HISTORY AND PHYSICAL EXAMINATION

A thorough history includes the following information (Montagnini & Moat, 2004):

- Review of current illness including treatments
- Review of past or concurrent illnesses such as diabetes mellitus
- History of weight loss
- Exploration of dietary and fluid intake, taste changes, food aversions and preferences
- Exploration of current symptom profile, including pain, nausea, dysphagia, bowel habits, fatigue
- Review of functional status
- Review of medications
- Psychological distress, body image

A thorough physical examination includes the following:
- Oral cavity: fungal, bacteria, or viral infection; stomatitis; mucositis; xerostomia; or direct tumor involvement
- Abdomen: masses, bowel sounds
- Skin: dehydration, areas of redness or breakdown

DIAGNOSTICS

Cachectic patients will probably show evidence of a low serum albumin level, decreased total protein levels, anemia, and increased serum triglyceride level, glucose levels, and lactic acidosis. However, these laboratory investigations are generally considered to be nonspecific, too variable, and not helpful in diagnosing or monitoring anorexia and cachexia in people with a terminal illness (Nelson & Walsh, 2002).

Depending on the stage of illness and treatment goals, it may be appropriate to monitor easily reversible problems such as electrolyte and metabolic imbalances (sodium, potassium, magnesium, and calcium levels). More elaborate evaluations such as the use of extensive dietary intake monitoring and skinfold thickness measurements should be reserved for clinical trials. Radiologic investigations may be helpful to rule out treatable problems such as bowel obstruction and constipation.

INTERVENTION AND TREATMENT

With the palliative care goal of improving quality of life, treatment must be aimed at treating any reversible conditions, minimizing symptoms that affect appetite, implementing measures to improve appetite, and educating patients and families about the potential benefits and limits of treatment interventions (Waller & Caroline, 2000). When patients lose weight and family members are distressed about the failing appetites of their loved ones, clinicians must understand that their responses cannot be simply to find ways to introduce more nutrients into patients. This approach has not been successful and may actually create harm (Strasser, 2003).

Preventative Measures

Preventative interventions for the metabolic syndrome of cachexia remain elusive and will ultimately hinge on a better understanding of its pathophysiological processes. Medications that interfere with the inflammatory processes induced by cytokines may hold some promise but are currently investigational. Because cachexia has been shown to have a significant effect on psychological and physiological well-being as well as survival, further research is critical.

Supportive Measures

- Ensure good mouth care.
- Maintain pleasant surroundings with small meals of favorite foods.
- Refer to a nutritionist, if available.
- Choose oral support rather than parenteral intervention.
- Encourage patients and families to think of food as a comfort measure. Advise offering favorite foods without worrying about nutritional value.

Enteral and Parenteral Supplemental Feeding

Enteral feeding may be considered for some patients who have an appetite but are unable to eat as a result of obstruction (e.g., patients with head and neck or esophageal cancer). Side effects of this method may include aspiration pneumonia and diarrhea.

If the underlying problems in cachexia were simply disorders in the patient's ability to eat enough or absorb what was eaten, then total parenteral nutrition would be the answer. However, research has shown that total parenteral nutrition does not improve overall condition or function. Parenteral feeding is not typically recommended in the palliative care setting and is associated with a number of comorbidities, including infection and hepatic and renal problems (Dixon & Esper, 2002).

Pharmacological Intervention

Research into drug therapy continues, but results have been somewhat disappointing and the medications can be expensive. The following may be considered for patients who wish this intervention (Dixon & Esper, 2002; Montagnini & Moat, 2004; Strasser & Bruera, 2002):

- *Progestational agents:* megestrol acetate, 160 to 800 mg/day orally. Although there is no clear evidence that this drug improves quality of life, research has shown that it can definitely improve appetite and can increase nonfluid weight in some patients. It is generally well tolerated but may increase the risk of thromboembolic complications, mild edema, vaginal spotting in women, and impotence in men. Progestational agents can be very expensive.
- *Corticosteroids:* dexamethasone, starting at 4 to 8 mg/day orally. This drug has been less effective than megestrol acetate in improving appetite, and benefits may be short lasting. Side effects may include immunosuppression, weakness, and osteoporosis. However, corticosteroids are less expensive than progestational agents.
- *Prokinetic agents* such as metoclopramide, 10 mg orally before meals, may improve gastric emptying and decrease nausea.
- *Cannabinoids,* specifically delta-9-tetrahydrocannabinol (dronabinol), an active compound of marijuana, have been formulated into oral medications. The drug is marketed as Marinol in the United States and Nabilone in Canada. Cannabinoids may be better tolerated in younger patients. Altered mentation is a potential side effect. Dosages are generally 5 to 15 mg/day when taken orally. Sedation, a common side effect, can be avoided by taking the medication at night.

Future Therapy

Research into the specific causes of cachexia in chronic and end-stage diseases attempts to identify those targets that contribute to the loss of lean muscle mass. One pathway under review is the ubiquitin-proteasome pathway. This pathway has been linked with the muscle wasting seen in cachexia. Targets that inhibit nuclear factor-κB, such as thalidomide, resveratrol, and eicosapentaenoic acid, may prove useful (Davis, 2002; Illman et al., 2005; Tisdale, 2005). Additional studies are evaluating the use of anticytokine-targeted biologics including those that block tumor necrosis factor alpha (TNF-α) and interleukin-6 (Illman et al., 2005). These studies are ongoing and further research is required.

PATIENT AND FAMILY EDUCATION

The symptoms of anorexia and cachexia can be devastating for patients and families, representing a visible sign of illness. The ability to eat is so closely associated with health and well-being that many people have great difficulty accepting that adequate nutrition is no longer possible. It is essential to explain to patients and families that most people with advanced diseases lose weight because of complex metabolic problems that cannot be changed, not because they are not eating (Waller & Caroline, 2000). Eating more or using enteral or parenteral supplements will not make a difference and may lead to more distress.

EVALUATION AND PLAN FOR FOLLOW-UP

Regular assessment and coaching of patients and families are essential to support their ability to cope. Keep both the patient and family informed to enable them to make informed decisions about trying various interventions.

CASE STUDY

Mr. B. is a 68-year-old man with metastatic hormone-refractory prostate cancer. He has not been seen for 8 weeks, as he was receiving radiation therapy for a metastatic lesion at T8 that was impinging on the spinal cord. He has undergone 4 weeks of treatment, which was completed 10 days ago.

Upon entering the examination room, the clinician notes that Mr. B. looks quite gaunt and much frailer than when last seen in clinic. His weight has decreased 30 pounds, from 196 to 166 pounds, since his last clinic visit. As part of the review of systems, Mr. B. identifies the following symptoms:
- Food "doesn't taste right"
- Mild dysphagia and epigastric discomfort
- Low-level nausea present most of the time
- Back pain with a pain score of 4 of 10
- Difficult bowel movements [small quantities of hard stool]
- Complaint of generalized weakness and fatigue

Physical examination includes the following significant findings:
- Skin dry with poor skin turgor, erythema over the mid-back
- White patches covering the buccal mucosa
- Tenderness to palpation over the epigastric region
- Hypoactive bowel sounds
- Trace edema of the lower extremities
- No focal neurological findings

Current medications include

- Dexamethasone taper (currently at 0.75 mg orally twice daily)
- Oxycontin 20 mg orally every 12 hours
- Oxycodone 5 to 10 mg orally every 4 hours as needed (using approximately twice daily)
- Senokot one tablet daily orally
- Atenolol 50 mg/day orally

Mr. B. and his wife are very concerned that he has lost this much weight and they are looking for guidance. Mr. B. expresses that he is not interested in undergoing any additional treatment for his prostate cancer as he feels the radiation "took too much out of me."

Based on a comprehensive evaluation, the clinician concludes that Mr. B.'s issues with anorexia and cachexia are multifactorial in etiology. Oral thrush is common for patients on long-term corticosteroids. It is likely that he has some lack of appetite specifically related to this condition. He may also have some mild esophagitis related to both the candidiasis and the radiation therapy he just completed. His weight loss could cause his dentures to be ill fitted (if he is using dentures). He may have some gastrointestinal irritation from the corticosteroid that causes his mild nausea. It also appears that his fluid status is suboptimal, along with his bowel management.

The clinician discusses the findings with the patient and his wife. They are encouraged to begin the following recommendations with the goal of improving Mr. B.'s physical comfort and sense of well-being:

- Nystatin suspension 5 ml (swish and swallow) three times daily for 10 days
- Omeprazole 20 mg/day orally
- Megestrol acetate (800 mg/20 ml) 20 ml/day orally
- Increase Senokot to two tablets twice daily orally
- Increase fluid intake as tolerated
- Begin small frequent feedings with a nutritional shake twice daily
- Return for a clinic appointment in 2 weeks

When Mr. B. is seen 2 weeks later, he indicates that he is feeling much better. He notes that his taste began to improve almost immediately when the nystatin was initiated. He also notes that 2 to 3 days after starting the megestrol, he found that he was actually feeling hungry again. He has gained 10 pounds since last seen in clinic and has no increased edema. He notes that the discomfort in the epigastric area has also disappeared. His bowel movements have been softer and occurring on a daily basis. He indicates that he stopped the nutritional shakes since he is eating better. His last dose of dexamethasone was 1 week ago.

On examination, his oral thrush has resolved, bowel sounds are normoactive, and skin turgor has improved. Overall, Mr. B. is more animated and appears stronger. The clinician recommends that Mr. B. discontinue the omeprazole since he is no longer taking the dexamethasone. Mr. is also told that he may stop the megestrol at this time.

Over the next 6 months, Mr. B.'s condition slowly deteriorates. He reports no appetite, weight loss, and generalized weakness. There are no clinical signs of gastrointestinal distress or constipation. The clinician concludes that the weight loss and anorexia are part of the cachexia syndrome associated with the advancing disease process. The clinician gently informs the patient and his wife that medications like megestrol and dietary supplementation will not reverse this process and reinforces that comfort is the primary goal at this time. The discussion also includes the fact that this process is not "starvation" and that often trying to eat more makes the patient more uncomfortable. The clinician encourages Mr. B. to eat those foods that taste good to him; the clinician also provides support for Mrs. B. as she allows him to eat small amounts of food and watches her husband continue to lose weight.

REFERENCES

Andreas, S. (2005). Neurohormonal activation as a link to systemic manifestations of chronic lung disease. *Chest, 128(5)*, 3618-3624.

Anker, S.D., Ponikowski, P., Varney, S., et al. (1997). Wasting as independent risk factor for mortality in chronic heart failure. *Lancet, 349(9058)*, 1050-1053.

Anker, S.D., Steinborn, W., & Strassberg, S. (2004). Cardiac cachexia. *Ann Med, 36(7)*, 518-529.

Castillo-Martinez, L., Orea-Tejeda, A., Rosales, M.T., et al. (2005). Anthropometric variables and physical activity as predictors of cardiac cachexia. *Int J Cardiol, 99(2)*, 239-245.

Davis, M.P. (2002). New drugs for the anorexia-cachexia syndrome. *Curr Oncol Report, 4(3)*, 264-274.

Davis, M.P. & Dickerson, D. (2000). Cachexia and anorexia: Cancer's covert killer. *Support Care Cancer, 8(3)*, 180-187.

Dixon, S.W. & Esper, P. (2002). Anorexia, cachexia, and nutritional support. In K.K. Kuebler, & P. Esper (Eds.). *Palliative practices from A to Z for the bedside clinician* (pp. 13-22). Pittsburgh: ONS Press.

Esper, D.H. & Harb, W.A. (2005). The cancer cachexia syndrome: A review of metabolic and clinical manifestations. *Nutr Clin Pract, 20(4)*, 369-376.

Illman, J., Corringham, R., Robinson, D., Jr., et al. (2005). Are inflammatory cytokines the common link between cancer-associated cachexia and depression? *J Support Oncol, 3(1)*, 37-50.

Inui, A. (2002). Cancer anorexia-cachexia syndrome: Current issues in research and management. *CA: Cancer J Clin, 52(2)*, 72-91.

McCarthy, D.O. (2003). Rethinking nutritional support for persons with cancer cachexia. *Biol Res Nurs, 5(1)*, 3-17.

Montagnini, M.L. & Moat, M.E. (2004). Non-pain symptom management in palliative care. *Clin Fam Pract, 6(2)*, 395-396-422.

Nelson, K.A. & Walsh, D. (2002). The cancer anorexia-cachexia syndrome: A survey of the Prognostic Inflammatory and Nutritional Index (PINI) in advanced disease. *J Pain Symptom Manage, 24(4)*, 424-428.

Ross, D.D. & Alexander, C.S. (2001). Terminally ill patients: Part I—Fatigue, anorexia, cachexia, nausea and vomiting. *Am Family Physician, 64(5)*, 807-814.

Schols, A.M., Soeters, P.B., Dingemans, A.M., et al. (1993). Prevalence and characteristics of nutritional depletion in patients with stable COPD eligible for pulmonary rehabilitation. *Am Rev Respir Dis, 147(5)*, 1151-1156.

Strasser, F. (2003). Eating-related disorders in patients with advanced cancer. *Support Care Cancer, 11(1)*, 11-20.

Strasser, F. & Bruera, E.D. (2002). Update on anorexia and cachexia. *Hematol Oncol Clin N Am, 16(3)*, 589-617.

Tisdale, M.J. (2005). The ubiquitin-proteasome pathway as a therapeutic target for muscle wasting. *J Support Oncol, 3(3),* 209-217.

Waller, A. & Caroline, N. (2000). *Handbook of palliative care in cancer* (2nd ed.). Boston: Butterworth-Heinemann.

Wanke, C.A. (2000). Weight loss and wasting remain common complications in individuals infected with human immunodeficiency virus in the era of highly active antiretroviral therapy. *Clin Infect Dis, 31(3),* 803-805.

Winter, S.M. (2002). Terminal nutrition: Framing the debate for withdrawal of nutritional support in terminally ill patients. *Am J Med, 109(9),* 723-726.

Wouters, E.F., Creutzberg, E.C., & Schols, A.M. (2002). Systemic effects of COPD. *Chest, 121(Suppl 5),* 127S-130S.

CHAPTER 21

CONSTIPATION

Debra E. Heidrich

■

DEFINITION AND INCIDENCE

Constipation is an extremely common problem among palliative care patients. Patients with constipation often experience abdominal discomfort, cramping, and distention as well as nausea. Unresolved constipation leads to fecal impaction—a large amount of hard, dry feces that accumulates in the rectum and sigmoid colon and cannot be evacuated—and, potentially, obstipation, a functional bowel obstruction from constipation or impaction. Patients who associate constipation with the use of opioids or other medications may discontinue or decrease these medications, leading to uncontrolled symptoms and additional discomfort. As such, proper and timely management is crucial.

In the general population, the incidence of constipation may range from 5% to 20%. Studies of patients with advanced cancer and other terminal illness indicate the incidence of constipation ranges from 32% to 87% (Potter, Hami, Bryan et al., 2003; Sykes, 1998, 2004; Wirz & Klaschik, 2005). Some of this variation is likely due to the proportion of the study population using opioids. However, Sykes (1998) reported that 64% of hospice patients who were not receiving opioid analgesia had constipation. Other factors contributing to the range in the reported incidence of constipation include variations in the primary diagnoses, ages, and settings of the study participants. In addition, constipation is likely underdiagnosed (Sykes, 2004).

A general definition of constipation is the passage of small amounts of hard, dry stool less often than three times a week (Folden, Backer, Maynard et al., 2002). However, constipation has different meanings to different people (Mercadante, 2002; Sykes, 2004). Patients may report constipation if feces are hard and dry; if there is straining, difficulty, or discomfort in expelling stool; or if stools are less frequent than normal for them.

ETIOLOGY AND PATHOPHYSIOLOGY

Normal bowel function requires the interaction of many body systems to break down food, allow proper absorption and transport of fluids and nutritional elements, and move the remaining food residue through the gastrointestinal (GI) tract to form feces for excretion. These processes are mediated by an interaction of the sympathetic and parasympathetic nervous systems affecting motor, secretory, and endocrine activities (Carroll, 2005). The urge to defecate occurs when the rectum fills with stool. The voluntary relaxation of the external sphincter allows for defecation (Carroll, 2005). Alterations in any of these body systems or physiological processes negatively affect bowel functioning.

Many factors contribute to constipation in patients with advanced progressive illnesses, including the following.

Immobility

Patients with little to no activity cannot maintain normal bowel motility. Defecation requires upright posture and strong abdominal, diaphragmatic, and anal muscles (Folden et al., 2002). Individuals with generalized fatigue and weakness and those who cannot sit on a toilet or bedside commode are at great risk for constipation.

Diet and Hydration

Patients with terminal illnesses often find it difficult to eat and drink adequate amounts of food and fluid for a variety of reasons (see Chapter 20, Cachexia and Anorexia). Low-residue diets may lack the necessary bulk to propel the feces through the bowel. The resulting constipation worsens when there is inadequate fluid intake; as a result, more water is reabsorbed from the colon and hard, dry stool is produced.

Medications

- *Opioids* bind with opioid receptors in the GI tract, leading to (1) a decrease in intestinal, gastric, biliary, and pancreatic secretions, (2) a decrease in propulsive movements due to inhibition of acetylcholine release that relaxes the intestinal musculature, and (3) an increase in internal anal sphincter tone. The net effects of stimulation of the GI opioid receptors are a decrease in stool hydration and an increase in transit time in the colon, leading to constipation (Klaschik, Nauck, & Ostgathe, 2003; Sykes, 2004). Some opioids cause more constipation than others and some individuals seem to be more sensitive to the constipating effects of opioids than others. In a study of laxative use in 49 subjects on opioids, Mancini, Hanson, Neumann et al. (2000) noted that patients on morphine required more laxative than did those on methadone. Another study of 1836 patients receiving long-acting opioid therapy found that those using transdermal fentanyl had less constipation than those using controlled-release oxycodone or controlled-release morphine (Staats, Markowitz, & Schein, 2004).
- *Anticholinergic drugs* and other medications with anticholinergic effects (e.g., tricyclic antidepressants, phenothiazines, some antipsychotics, antiparkinsonian agents) slow peristalsis, increasing the risk of constipation.
- *Other medications* contributing to constipation include antacids containing calcium or aluminum, iron supplements, diuretics, antihypertensives, calcium channel blockers, and antidiarrheal medications (Hodgson & Kizior, 2004; Sykes, 2004). In addition, overuse of laxatives can lead to a weakening of the defecation reflexes, inhibiting natural bowel functioning.

Chemical Imbalances

- *Hypercalcemia.* A high serum calcium level likely depresses the contractility of the muscle walls of the GI tract. In addition, polyuria with hypercalcemia may lead to dehydration, further contributing to constipation (Bower & Cox, 2004; White, 2005).
- *Hypokalemia* can also lead to constipation or, in some situations, paralytic ileus, which probably results from the unresponsiveness of hyperpolarized GI smooth

muscle (White, 2005). A common cause of hypokalemia is administration of thiazide diuretics without potassium replacement.

Pressure and Compression of Intestines

Cancer patients with tumor in the abdomen require more laxatives than do other patients on opioid therapy (Mancini et al., 2000). Patients with ascites, abdominal or pelvic tumors, or enlarged lymph nodes are at risk for abnormalities in digestion and elimination. A partial bowel obstruction from tumor growth either inside the intestinal lumen or due to compression from outside the lumen slows motility, contributing to constipation and potentially leading to a complete obstruction (Sykes, 2004). Patients with a history of abdominal surgery are also at risk for the development of adhesions. These adhesions can decrease intestinal lumen size, interfering with transit time in the bowel; partial and complete bowel obstructions are possible.

Changes in the Innervation of the Gastrointestinal Tract

Constipation has been noted in many patients with motor disorders, such as spinal cord lesions and neurological diseases. This constipation is likely the result of visceral neuropathy and a disturbance in the nerve supply of the colon that slows the colonic transit time. In addition, patients who have neurological diseases may experience failure of the puborectalis and anal sphincter muscles to relax, causing intractable constipation (Mercadante, 2002). The innervation of the intestinal tract can also be interrupted by surgery. A history of abdominal surgery provides helpful information for assessing constipation. Neuropathy is a complication of some cancer chemotherapy agents, in particular, the vinca alkaloids. Although constipation is a well-documented side effect of these medications in patients undergoing active treatment, the long-term effects are not clear. Patients who received high cumulative doses of the vinca alkaloids may be at risk for persistent constipation (Mercadante, 2002).

The elderly may experience sensory changes affecting bowel functioning. In particular, rectal insensitivity may lead to a decrease in the urge to defecate (Sykes, 2004). When the urge to defecate is ignored, the anal muscles become weakened, resulting in a risk for constipation and impaction.

Psychosocial Concerns

Under conditions of fear, anxiety, stress, and depression, epinephrine is released as a sympathetic stress response. Epinephrine decreases peristalsis, leading to a risk for constipation. However, the stress response can also increase intestinal mucus formation and cause pain and cramping. Thus, some patients, when stressed, have alternating bouts of diarrhea and constipation. Patients who are embarrassed about using bedpans or bedside commodes may ignore the need to defecate to preserve their privacy. In addition, those who are confused, lethargic, weak, or in pain may not respond to the defecation reflex. As noted, this inattention to the urge to defecate can result in weakened anal muscles.

ASSESSMENT AND MEASUREMENT

Constipation is identified via patient report of infrequent or absent bowel movements, difficulty or pain in defecating, incomplete defecation, or hard, dry stool. Although patients may associate symptoms such as abdominal pain, bloating, flatulence, nausea, malaise, and headache with constipation, these symptoms are not specific to constipation (Sykes, 2004). Stool amount, consistency, and frequency and the length of time since the last bowel movement are important assessment data.

It is important to identify the patient's definition of constipation. Some may report constipation if a day passes without a bowel movement despite the lack of other symptoms. This may or may not indicate actual constipation. "Normal" bowel habits can range from a bowel movement one to three times a week to daily or several daily bowel movements.

HISTORY AND PHYSICAL EXAMINATION

When performing the history and physical examination, be sensitive to the fact that many people are at least uncomfortable, if not extremely embarrassed, by questioning about bowels and bowel functioning. Maintain an environment as conducive to patient privacy as possible during history taking and examination.

General Assessment

- Patient's medical history and presence of any disease affecting bowel function
- Fluid and food intake, including amounts and types of fluids and food
- Hydration status: skin turgor, condition of mucous membranes, urinary output, orthostatic blood pressure measurements
- Current medications, especially any opioids, tricyclic antidepressants, anticholinergics, sedatives, antiemetics, antipsychotics, antihypertensives, antacids, and diuretics
- Activity level and ability to use a toilet or bedside commode

History Related to Complaint of Constipation

- Normal bowel patterns and history of any constipation problems
- Patient's definition or description of "constipation"
- Date of the last bowel movement as well as the amount, color, and consistency of stool
- Any discomfort or bleeding with bowel movements
- Interventions the individual uses or has used to prevent or relieve constipation, including medications, enemas, or any special teas, juices, or foods
- Patient's evaluation of the effectiveness or side effects of these interventions
- Any use of manual manipulation, such as the application of anal pressure or digital removal of stool

Gastrointestinal Assessment

- Reports of abdominal pain or cramping
  - ▶ Note: The pain of constipation may be mistaken for pain related to the disease and "treated" with additional opioids instead of treating the problem of constipation

(Sykes, 2004). Do not withhold opioids from patients with pain and constipation; perform a thorough assessment to determine the potential cause of pain and treat it appropriately.

- Reports of nausea or vomiting
- Abdominal assessment
  - Distention
  - Bowel sounds
    - Increased activity occurs in early intestinal obstruction
    - Decreased or absent bowel sounds, which may indicate ileus or peritonitis
    - High-pitched tinkling sounds, indicating fluid and air under tension in a dilated bowel
    - Rushes of high-pitched sounds with abdominal cramping, which indicate intestinal obstruction (Bickley & Szilagyi, 2003)
  - Masses and areas of tenderness on palpation
  - Ascites or trapped air that may be noted with percussion

Rectal Examination

- Inspect the rectum for fissures, tears, hemorrhoids, fistulas, or tumors.
- Perform a digital examination to identify stool or tumors in the rectum.
- Avoid digital examination if the patient is neutropenic or thrombocytopenic or has known tumors.

Psychoemotional Assessment

- Assess the patient's ability to maintain privacy for toileting.
- Evaluate the patient's stress and anxiety level.
- Assess for confusion or dementia.

DIAGNOSTICS

As with all symptom evaluation in palliative care, radiographic and laboratory procedures should be performed only when confirmation of the underlying problem will change the course of treatment. If the cause of constipation can be identified on the basis of the medical diagnosis, treatments, or other presenting symptoms, confirmation by radiography or blood work may not be necessary to determine an appropriate course of treatment.

- An abdominal film may differentiate between constipation and obstruction (Mercadante, 2002). It is performed only if there is persistent doubt and is rarely necessary (Sykes, 2004). (See Chapter 19, Bowel Obstruction.)
- Barium studies may be useful in distinguishing between a paralytic ileus and mechanical obstruction (Mercadante, 2002).
- Radiographic studies of colonic transit time, although useful in some settings to determine which areas of the bowel are not functioning, are rarely well tolerated by patients with advanced illness (Mercadante, 2002; Sykes, 2004).
- Serum electrolyte levels will identify hypercalcemia or hypokalemia.

INTERVENTION AND TREATMENT

Prophylactic Interventions

The goal of care is to prevent constipation rather than to wait for it to develop. The appropriateness of the following interventions to prevent constipation is determined by the individual's performance status, mental status, and ability to eat and drink.

- Encourage activity to stimulate natural bowel functioning when pain and fatigue do not interfere. Encourage range of motion and isometric exercises to maintain some muscle strength for patients who are unable to get out of bed (Folden et al., 2002).
- Encourage adequate oral fluid intake. The 1.5 to 2 liters per day required to maintain good hydration is often not tolerated by patients with advanced illnesses.
- Encourage patients to drink warm fluids (e.g., coffee, teas, juices) with or after meals because they stimulate the bowel. Be aware that caffeine may have a mild diuretic effect.
- Encourage foods high in bulk and fiber for patients with normal appetites (Folden et al., 2002).
  - ‣ The amount of fiber required to treat constipation is often not tolerated by patients with advanced illness, and dietary changes alone are generally not sufficient. The dietary emphasis for the terminally ill should be on identifying patient likes and desires versus providing fiber and bulk (Sykes, 2004).
- Maintain a consistent time for defecation, usually after a meal (Folden et al., 2002).
- Instruct caregivers to respond quickly to patient requests to defecate.
- Encourage the use of a toilet or bedside commode so the patient can maintain an upright position. If the patient is unable to sit when defecating, a left-side-lying position is recommended (Folden et al., 2002).
- Allow the patient privacy during toileting. Use of a raised toilet seat and bathroom handrails increases the individual's independence and promotes safety and privacy (Folden et al., 2002).
- Make appropriate changes in medications that are contributing to constipation.
  - ‣ Discontinue nonessential medications.
  - ‣ When the offending medication is required for symptom control, consider a change to a medication with the potential for fewer side effects. For example, as noted earlier, methadone or fentanyl *may* be less constipating for some, but not necessarily all, individuals, and the secondary amine tricyclic antidepressants (e.g., desipramine and nortriptyline) may be less constipating than the tertiary amine tricyclic antidepressants (e.g., amitriptyline) (Lussier & Portenoy, 2004).

Laxatives

Despite the maximal use of prophylactic interventions, many patients with terminal illness require laxatives to treat and prevent constipation (Sykes, 2004). There is little research to guide the appropriate choice of laxatives or combinations of laxatives.

Consider the characteristics of the patient's constipation when selecting a laxative: hard stool requires a softener; soft, difficult-to-pass stool requires a stimulant (Klaschik et al., 2003). Likewise, the patient's response to the laxative regimen will guide titration or changes in the doses and types of laxatives used: too much softening leads to fecal leakage and incontinence; too much stimulant causes abdominal cramping (Sykes, 2004).

Patients for whom the cause of constipation cannot be eliminated will require routine use of laxatives. Low doses of laxatives are best given at night; higher doses may need to be divided, usually into morning and evening doses. Patients receiving opioid therapy almost always require the routine use of a combination of stimulant and softening laxatives.

Laxative agents differ according to active ingredients and mechanism of action. The following discussion outlines the mechanisms of action for the various types of laxatives, examples of each type, and starting doses.

Lubricant Laxatives

Lubricant laxatives penetrate the stool to soften it and to lubricate the surface of the stool. In addition, they prevent some absorption of water from the intestinal tract, which also helps to keep the stool soft (Klaschik et al., 2003; Sykes, 2004). Lubricant laxatives are less palatable than are many other types of laxatives. Also, because of the risk for aspiration pneumonia, oral liquids are avoided in pediatrics and in patients with dysphagia. The onset of action is approximately 6 to 8 hours after oral administration. Mineral oil (e.g., Fleet Mineral Oil Enema, Liqui-Doss, Milkinol) is the most frequently used lubricant laxative. The oral dose is 15 to 30 ml per day. Mineral oil enemas are generally 4 ounces. There are many home remedies that use a lubricating substance, such as petroleum jelly. For example, some hospice programs recommend two frozen 1/2-teaspoon-size balls of petroleum jelly (rolled in sugar to make them more palatable) for constipation. This intervention is usually reserved for patients who do not get a good response from other laxatives and enemas. Note that there is no research on this intervention.

Bulk-Forming Laxatives

Bulk-forming laxatives provide material that resists bacterial breakdown (nondigestible methylcellulose, psyllium, or polycarbophil), which enhances stool bulk. This increases the volume of the stool, dilating the intestinal wall, and stimulates bowel motility. These laxatives also provide substrates for bacterial growth, promoting increased transit time via fermentation (Klaschik et al., 2003; Sykes, 2004). Because of the water-binding capacity of these products, patients must take them orally with 6 to 8 ounces of water or juice and maintain adequate overall fluid intake—at least 1.5 to 2 liters per day. *Bulk-forming laxatives should be avoided if fluid intake is not adequate* or if there is a suspicion of intestinal stricture or bowel obstruction (Waller & Caroline, 2000). Most bulk-forming laxatives take 12 to 72 hours to produce results. Examples include the following:

- Methylcellulose powder (e.g., Citrucel), 3 to 4 g/day orally
- Psyllium (e.g., Natural Fiberall, Metamucil), 3 to 4 g/day orally
- Polycarbophil (e.g., Fiberall, FiberCon), 3 to 4 g/day orally

Emollients and Surfactants

The detergent action of emollient laxatives increases water penetration into fecal matter (Sykes, 2004). They produce softer, moister fecal material. These laxatives are rarely sufficient alone for opioid-induced constipation since the longer transit time caused by the opioids counteracts the benefits of the softeners. Time to action is 12 to 72 hours after administration. Docusate sodium (Colace) 100 to 300 mg/day orally is the most commonly used emollient laxative.

Saccharine Laxatives

The saccharine laxatives create an osmotic gradient in the lumen and prevent water absorption from the small intestine. The oral doses required for opioid-induced constipation often lead to bloating, cramping, and diarrhea (Klaschik et al., 2003; Sykes, 2004). These laxatives pull water from the body and can lead to dehydration. However, glycerin suppositories act in the distal colon and have minimal side effects. Oral agents take 12 to 72 hours to work; suppositories stimulate bowel movements in 15 to 30 minutes. Examples include the following:
- Lactulose (e.g., Cephulac, Duphalac), 15 ml twice daily orally
- Sorbitol, 30 ml/day orally
- Glycerin, one suppository, per rectum

Saline Osmotic Laxatives

The poorly absorbed salts of saline laxatives produce an immediate osmotic gradient. In addition to the influx of fluids secondary to osmosis, the magnesium salts may stimulate the secretion of cholecystokinin, which stimulates motility (Sykes, 2004). Again, these medications pull in body fluids, leading to the potential for dehydration (Klaschik et al., 2003). Oral preparations take 30 minutes to 3 hours to work. Saline enemas are generally effective within 15 minutes. Examples include the following:
- Magnesium citrate, 120 to 240 ml/day orally
- Magnesium hydroxide (e.g., Milk of Magnesia), 2 to 4 g/day orally
- Sodium biphosphate–sodium phosphate (e.g., Fleet Enema, one daily per rectum; Fleet Phospho-Buffered Saline Soda, 20 to 30 ml/day orally)

Macrogol Osmotic Laxatives

The macrogol laxatives bind with the oral fluids with which they are administered and hydrate harden stool, leading to an increase in stool volume and dilation of the bowel wall, which triggers the defecation reflex (Klaschik et al., 2003). These medications were originally marketed for use in high doses as bowel-cleansing agents before GI procedures; in smaller doses, they are used to treat constipation. Because microgols bind only with the orally administered fluids, water is not drawn from the body. Therefore, these medications have a lesser potential for causing dehydration than the other osmotic agents. Also, because these substances do not undergo fermentation in the GI tract like saccharine does, there is no gas production and its associated discomforts. When used to treat constipation, it may take 2 to 3 days for the initial effect, but with regular use, the frequency of bowel movements is usually once per day (Klaschik et al., 2003). Studies show polyethylene glycol is effective for constipation in the palliative care setting (Wirz & Klaschik, 2005). Some programs use these agents as the drug of choice for treating opioid-induced constipation (Klaschik et al., 2003). However, more research is needed to determine if they are truly a better than combinations of standard stimulants plus laxatives. An example of a macrogol is polyethylene glycol (e.g., MiraLax), 17 g (approximately 1 heaping tablespoon) in at least 125 ml of water.

Stimulant Laxatives

Stimulant laxatives increase GI motility by stimulating the myenteric plexus of the intestinal smooth muscle (Sykes, 2004). The absorption of water and electrolytes in the colon is reduced with the use of stimulant laxatives. Stimulants may cause cramping, electrolyte disturbances, and dehydration. Castor oil is a very potent stimulant and is rarely used because of the negative side effects. Aloe extracts and cascara sagrada are not recognized as safe and effective laxatives by the Food and Drug Administration (Department of Health and Human Services, 2002).

Depending on availability, stimulant laxatives may be given by mouth as pills or liquids or by rectum as suppositories or enemas. In addition to the effect of the medication being given, the use of the rectal route may initiate defecation by stimulation of the anocolonic reflex (Sykes, 2004).

The rectal route is considered second-line therapy for use when the oral route is insufficient. This route of administration is not pleasant for the patient or the caregivers giving the medication. All effort should be made to maintain routine bowel movements with oral medication. Examples of stimulant laxatives, with starting doses, include the following:

- Senna (Senokot, Senolax), 15 mg/day orally (Senna teas are also available at some health food stores)
- Bisacodyl (oral: Correctol, Dulcolax, Feen-A-Mint, 10 mg/day orally; suppository: Bisco-Lax, Fleet Laxative)

Combination Laxatives

Combining two or more types of laxatives with different mechanisms of action may produce synergistic effects. A combination of a stimulant and a softener is recommended for patients receiving opioid therapy; others may benefit from this combination as well. There are several combination laxatives available on the market, although the same effect can be obtained by taking the two medications separately. Examples of combination laxatives include the following:

- Bisacodyl–docusate sodium (Modane Plus)
- Senna–docusate sodium (Senokot-S; Peri-Colace)

Other Medications with Laxative Effects

Prokinetic agents have been investigated for the treatment of constipation. The subcutaneous infusion of metoclopramide is noted to be effective in the treatment of narcotic bowel syndrome (Bruera, Brenneis, Michaud et al., 1987). Further investigations comparing metoclopramide with standard laxative therapies are needed to determine its role as an oral laxative (Sykes, 2004).

Opioid-induced constipation has also been treated with opioid antagonists. The goal is to antagonize peripheral opioid receptors in the GI tract without antagonizing the central opioid receptors—that is, reversal of constipation without reversal of analgesia.

Naloxone given orally was the first opioid antagonist investigated for this use. It was believed that the first-pass hepatic metabolism of naloxone would leave very little available to antagonize central opioid receptors (Sykes, 2004). However, in the few limited studies, a high proportion of subjects either experienced withdrawal or required increased opioid doses to control pain (Liu & Wittbrodt, 2002). Currently, methylnaltrexone, a derivative of the opioid antagonist naltrexone, is being investigated for use in treating opioid-induced constipation. Methylnaltrexone does not cross the blood-brain barrier, so it should not induce a withdrawal response. Initial studies are promising (Yuan, Foss, O'Connor et al., 2000; Yuan, 2004). However, more research is needed to evaluate effectiveness and to compare it with other treatments for constipation.

Guidelines for Using Laxatives

Unfortunately, there is no "gold standard" for the management of constipation. Each patient's situation is different in terms of the factors contributing to constipation, and these contributing factors may change over time in the same patient. The most common error in the management of constipation is the failure to titrate laxatives to an effective dose (Ogle & Hopper, 2005).

Before initiating laxative therapy, rule out bowel obstruction and then disimpact the bowel, if necessary. Begin laxative therapy as outlined in Figure 21-1. The initial selection of the laxative regimen is based on the patient's medical history, current medications, and physical examination. If there is soft stool in the rectum that is difficult to eliminate, begin with a stimulant laxative; if there is a small amount of hard, dry stool in the rectum, initiate therapy with an emollient laxative; if there is little to no stool in the rectum, the patient may require a combination of a softener and a laxative. Patients receiving opioids require a combination of a stimulant laxative and an emollient softener.

The goal is for the patient to have a regular, comfortable bowel movement. Assess the usual frequency of bowel movements to determine what is normal for an individual; often this will be daily, but for some patients "normal" may be up to 2 to 3 days between bowel movements. Note that if an additional intervention is required to produce a bowel movement, the routine doses of softener and stimulant laxatives must be adjusted. If an "extra" intervention is required every 2 days, the regimen should be changed. Additional adjustments in laxatives will be required as the disease progresses, due to changes in food and fluid intake, use of medications that affect the bowel, changes in activity level, and decline in muscle strength.

PATIENT AND FAMILY EDUCATION

Patients and families require information on the importance of reporting constipation, the appropriate use of the prophylactic interventions, and the appropriate use of laxatives.

- Discuss the importance of reporting bowel functioning, including frequency, amount, and consistency of stools and any discomfort associated with defecation, to the health care team.
- Teach patients who are able to do so to participate in exercise activities or isometric abdominal and pelvic exercises.

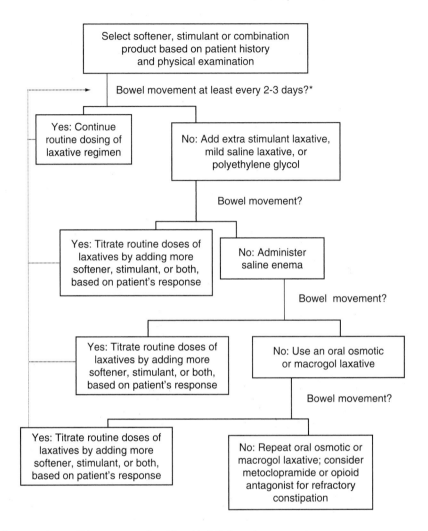

Figure 21-1 Laxative therapy protocol.

*Some patients will be most comfortable with daily bowel movements.

- Instruct the patient to take in at least eight glasses of fluid each day and to increase the bulk in the diet, both as tolerated by the patient.
- Encourage the use of warm liquids with meals to stimulate bowel functioning.
- Discuss the importance of responding immediately to the urge to defecate with both the patient and the caregivers.
- Discuss the benefit of maintaining an upright position for defecation; encourage the use of a toilet or bedside commode.
- Caregivers may require instruction on proper transfer techniques for assisting the patient out of a bed or chair to a bedside commode.
- Teach the appropriate dosing and schedule of laxative medications. Those that require 6 hours or longer to work are best dosed at night.

- Encourage the patient and family to report any cramping, bloating, stool leakage, or diarrhea associated with taking the prescribed laxatives.
- Discuss the importance of avoiding the bulk-forming laxatives for patients taking opioids and for those whose fluid intake is limited.

EVALUATION AND PLAN FOR FOLLOW-UP

The effectiveness of the interventions to manage constipation is determined by reassessing the patient's bowel status. Ask about the frequency, amount, and consistency of stools and about any discomfort or difficulty passing stool. It is also important to ask about the effectiveness of laxatives to determine appropriate changes in the plan of care.

Assessment of bowel status must be a part of the ongoing, routine evaluation of the patient to determine if the prescribed regimen continues to be effective over the course of the patient's care. Patients with advanced illnesses will experience changes in the disease process, fluid intake, activity level, and prescribed medications that will affect the bowels and necessitate modifications in the care plan.

CASE STUDY

Mr. R. has metastatic lung cancer and a history of congestive heart failure. He received treatment with combination chemotherapy 6 months ago, and he tolerated it well. However, the cancer progressed and he was referred for home hospice care. Mr. R. has a poor appetite and states that he feels nauseated if he eats more than a few bites of food. He keeps a 1-quart pitcher of water at his bedside and reports drinking the entire quart over the course of a day. He also drinks a small glass of orange juice with breakfast. He is able to walk to the bathroom with the assistance of his wife. Mr. R. reports that he has not had a bowel movement in 3 days despite taking Metamucil every day. He is complaining of abdominal bloating and cramping.

Mr. R.'s medications include the following: sustained-release oxycodone 40 mg twice daily, immediate-release oxycodone 10 mg every 1 to 2 hours for breakthrough pain or dyspnea, ibuprofen 400 mg four times daily, furosemide 40 mg/day, and digoxin 0.125 mg/day.

On physical examination, the clinician notes that there is no stool in the rectum and that bowel sounds are hyperactive. The constipating effects of the opioids and the need to use both a stimulant and a softener laxative are discussed with the patient. The clinician also explains that the bulk-forming laxatives are not a good choice at this time because these medications may actually cause constipation if fluid intake is less than 8 cups each day. The patient is instructed to take magnesium citrate, 120 to 240 ml over ice, as tolerated. Two hours later, Mr. R. reports that he has passed a small amount of hard feces and feels there is more stool in the rectum. A bisacodyl (Dulcolax) suppository is administered to empty the rectum of stool. The patient is then started on a regimen of sennosides: 8.6 mg and docusate sodium 50 mg

(Peri-Colace, Senokot-S), two tablets at bedtime. He also is instructed to take magnesium hydroxide (Milk of Magnesia), 30 ml at bedtime, if more than 2 days pass without a bowel movement and to inform the clinician if he needs to use the Milk of Magnesia more than once a week.

This regimen works well for Mr. R. for about a month. Then he reports needing to take the Milk of Magnesia every 2 days. Mrs. R. also states that the patient gets short of breath walking to the bathroom and, in general, his activity level has decreased. The clinician instructs the patient to increase the Peri-Colace to three tablets at bedtime. On physical assessment, the clinician notes that the patient is slightly dehydrated with no peripheral edema and the clinician instructs Mr. R. to discontinue the furosemide. The clinician also discusses the energy-saving benefits of a bedside commode and, with the patient's and wife's permission, orders one for the patient.

Mr. R. continued to have bowel movements of soft, formed stool every 1 to 2 days up until 3 days ago. He is now bed-bound, taking in only sips of fluids, and having some difficulty swallowing pills. The Peri-Colace is discontinued. The clinician monitors for bowel sounds, abdominal distention, and the presence of stool in the rectum. The following day, some stool is noted in the rectum, and the clinician administers a Dulcolax suppository with good results. Mr. R. dies peacefully 2 days later, with no sign of abdominal distention or discomfort.

REFERENCES

Bickley, L.S. & Szilagyi, P.G. (2003). The abdomen. In L.S. Bickley & P.G. Szilagyi (Eds.). *Bates' guide to physical examination and history taking* (8th ed., pp. 317-366). Philadelphia: Lippincott, Williams & Wilkins.

Bower, M. & Cox, S. (2004). Endocrine and metabolic complications of advanced cancer. In D. Doyle, G. Hanks, N.I. Cherny, et al. (Eds.). *Oxford textbook of palliative medicine* (3rd ed., pp. 687-702). New York: Oxford University Press.

Bruera, E., Brenneis, C., Michaud, M., et al. (1987). Continuous subcutaneous infusion of metoclopramide for treatment of narcotic bowel syndrome. *Cancer Treat Rep, 71(11),* 1121-1122.

Carroll, R.G. (2005). Anatomy and physiology review: The elimination system. In J.M. Black & J.H. Hawks (Eds.). *Medical-surgical nursing: clinical management for positive outcomes* (7th ed., pp. 766-774). St. Louis: Elsevier Saunders.

Department of Health and Human Services. (2002). Status of certain additional over-the-counter drug category II and III active ingredients. *Federal Register, 67(90),* 31125-31127.

Folden, S.L., Backer, J.H., Maynard, F., et al. (2002). *Practice guidelines for the management of constipation in adults.* Glenview, Ill.: Association of Rehabilitation Nurses.

Hodgson, B.B. & Kizior, R.J. (2004). *Nursing drug handbook 2004.* St. Louis: Saunders.

Klaschik, E., Nauck, F., & Ostgathe, C. (2003). Constipation—Modern laxative therapy. *Support Care Cancer, 11(11),* 679-685.

Liu, M. & Wittbrodt, E. (2002). Low-dose oral naloxone reverses opioid-induced constipation and analgesia. *J Pain Symptom Manage, 23(1),* 48-53.

Lussier, D. & Portenoy, R.K. (2004). Adjuvant analgesics in pain management. In D. Doyle, G. Hanks, N.I. Cherny, et al. (Eds.). *Oxford textbook of palliative medicine* (3rd ed., pp. 349-378). New York: Oxford University Press.

Mancini, I.L., Hanson, J., Neumann, C.M., et al. (2000). Opioid type and other clinical predictors of laxative dose in advanced cancer patients: A retrospective study. *J Palliat Med, 3(1),* 49-56.

Mercadante, W. (2002). Diarrhea, malabsorption, and constipation. In A. Berger, R. Portenoy, & D. Weissman (Eds.). *Principles and practice of palliative and supportive oncology* (2nd ed., pp. 233-249). Philadelphia: Lippincott, Williams & Wilkins.

Ogle, K.S. & Hopper, K. (2005). End-of-life care for older adults. *Primary Care: Clin Office Pract, 32(3),* 811-828.

Potter, J., Hami, F., Bryan, T., et al. (2003). Symptoms in 400 patients referred to palliative care services: Prevalence and patterns. *Palliat Med, 17(4),* 310-314.

Staats, P.S., Markowitz, J., & Schein, J. (2004). Incidence of constipation associated with long-acting opioid therapy: A comparative study. *South Med J, 97(2),* 129-134.

Sykes, N. (2004). Constipation and diarrhoea. In D. Doyle, G. Hanks, N.I. Cherny, & K. Calman (Eds.). *Oxford textbook of palliative medicine* (3rd ed., pp. 483-496). New York: Oxford University Press.

Sykes, N.P. (1998). The relationship between opioid use and laxative use in terminally ill cancer patients. *Palliat Med, 12(5),* 375-382.

Waller, A. & Caroline, N.L. (2000). *Handbook of palliative care in cancer* (2nd ed.). Boston: Butterworth-Heinemann.

White, B. (2005). Clients with electrolyte imbalances. In J.M. Black & J.H. Hawks (Eds.). *Medical-surgical nursing: Clinical management for positive outcomes* (7th ed., pp. 223-245). St. Louis: Elsevier Saunders.

Wirz, S. & Klaschik, E. (2005). Management of constipation in palliative care patients undergoing opioid therapy: Is polyethylene glycol an option? *Am J Hospice Palliat Care, 22(5),* 375-381.

Yuan, C. (2004). Clinical status of methylnaltrexone, a new agent to prevent and manage opioid-induced side effects. *J Support Oncol, 2(2),* 111-117.

Yuan, C., Foss, J.F., O'Connor, M., et al. (2000). Methylnaltrexone for reversal of constipation due to chronic methadone use: A randomized controlled trial. *JAMA, 283(3),* 367-372.

CHAPTER 22

COUGH

Jennifer Fournier

■

DEFINITION AND INCIDENCE

Cough is defined as an explosive expiratory maneuver that, under normal conditions, serves to protect the airways and lungs by clearing inhaled material, excessive mucus, and abnormal substances (Berkow & Fletcher, 1992; Canning, 2006; McCool, 2006). In certain disease states, cough can become excessive, nonproductive, distressing, and potentially harmful to the airway mucosa, and it can be a factor in the spread of infection (Irwin, Boulet, Cloutier et al., 1998; Leach, 2004). Cough is one of the most common symptoms for which the general population seeks medical attention (Beckles, Spiro, Colice et al., 2003; Estfan & LeGrand, 2004; Irwin et al., 1998; Irwin & Madison, 2001; Morice, Kastelik, & Thompson, 2001).

Advanced, progressive diseases that are frequently associated with cough include chronic pulmonary disease, lung cancer, congestive heart failure, and acquired immune deficiency syndrome. In addition, 3% to 35% of people taking angiotensin-converting enzyme (ACE) inhibitors are reported to have cough (Dicpinigaitis, 2006). Cough is also a symptom of other conditions for which patients with advanced illnesses are susceptible, such as the common cold and pneumonia. Few data are available regarding the frequency and severity of cough in the palliative care setting. One study of patients with chronic lung disease and lung cancer in the last year of life showed that 59% of these patients report cough and 46% state that the cough is very distressing (Edmonds, Karlsen, Kahn et al., 2001).

Because cough serves a protective function, an ineffective cough puts patients at risk for complications such as pneumonia and atelectasis (Leach, 2004). Patients with advanced diseases may have difficulty coughing productively due to cachexia and frailty (Estfan & LeGrand, 2004). Also, patients with weakened muscles due to neurological diseases such as cerebrovasular accident, amyotrophic lateral sclerosis, and multiple sclerosis are often not able to cough effectively.

ETIOLOGY AND PATHOPHYSIOLOGY

Pathophysiology

Involuntary cough is a complex process, and it involves the activation and interaction of several subtypes of vagal afferent nerves, including rapidly adapting receptors, mechanoreceptors, C-fibers, and the brainstem. The rapidly adapting receptors are most prevalent in the larynx, main carina, and branching points in the tracheobronchial tree and are activated by chemical (e.g., smoke), inflammatory (e.g., histamine), and mechanical (e.g., foreign body) stimuli, causing bronchospasm and mucus secretion.

Bronchospasm and mucus secretion, in turn, stimulate the mechanoreceptors and C-fibers. The cough reflex is integrated in the brainstem where motor output to the larynx, bronchial tree, and respiratory muscles initiates the cough reflex (Canning, 2006; Dicpinigaitis, 2003; Dicpinigaitis & Gayle, 2003; Leach, 2004). An esophageal-tracheobronchial reflex (also mediated by vagal innervation) is thought to cause cough associated with gastroesophageal reflux disease (GERD) from acid reflux that triggers receptors in the lower esophagus (Irwin & Madison, 2001; Poe & Kallay, 2003).

Voluntary cough is mediated via the cortex. Patients can consciously induce cough to clear the airways (Leach, 2004). The ability to initiate cough is especially helpful for patients whose disease process impairs the spontaneous cough reflex.

The cough reflex initiates a deep inspiration (inspiration phase), followed by closure of the glottis and build-up of intrathoracic pressure (compressive phase). Then, the respiratory muscles contract against the closed glottis resulting in forceful expulsion of air and other material as the glottis opens (expiratory phase) (Estfan & LeGrand, 2004; McCool, 2006; Waller & Caroline, 2000).

Etiologies and Complications of Cough

There are multiple causes of cough (Table 22-1). Patients with a chronic cough and a normal chest radiograph, who do not smoke, and who are not receiving treatment with ACE inhibitors should be evaluated for upper airway cough syndrome (formerly called postnasal drip syndrome), asthma, nonasthmatic eosinophilic bronchitis, and/or GERD (Irwin, Baumann, Bolser et al., 2006). Aspiration caused by pharyngeal dysfunction is another potential cause of cough.

TABLE 22-1 ■ Causes of Cough

Acute (< 3 wk)	Subacute (3 to 8 wk)	Chronic (> 8 wk)
Upper respiratory tract infection (e.g., common cold, bacterial sinusitis)	Postinfectious: Pneumonia Pertussis Bronchitis	UACS Asthma Nonasthmatic eosinophilic bronchitis
Lower respiratory tract infection (e.g., bronchitis)	New onset or exacerbation of UACS, asthma, GERD, chronic bronchitis	GERD Chronic bronchitis Bronchiectasis
Pneumonia		Nonbronchiectatic suppurative airway disease (bronchiolitis)
Exacerbation of asthma, COPD, heart failure		Lung tumors
Pulmonary emboli		ACE inhibitors
Environmental irritant		Smoking
		Chronic interstitial lung disease
		Aspiration

Data from Estfan, B., & LeGrand, S. (2004). Management of cough in advanced cancer. *Journal of Supportive Oncology, 2(6)*, 523-527; and Irwin, R.S., Baumann, M.H., Boulet, L.P., et al. (2006). Diagnosis and management of cough executive summary. ACCP evidence-based clinical practice guidelines. *Chest, 129(Suppl 1)*, 1S-23S.

ACE, Angiotensin-converting enzyme; *COPD*, chronic obstructive pulmonary disease; *GERD*, gastroesophageal reflux disease; *UACS*, upper airway cough syndrome (formerly postnasal drip syndrome).

Box 22-1	Complications of Cough*

- Cardiovascular: hypotension, arrhythmias
- Constitutional: sweating, anorexia, fatigue
- Gastrointestinal: gastroesophageal reflux, herniations
- Genitourinary: urinary incontinence
- Musculoskeletal: strain to rupture of rectus abdominus muscles, diaphragmatic rupture, rib fracture
- Neurological: cough syncope, dizziness, headache, stroke
- Ophthalmologic: rupture of subconjunctival veins
- Psychosocial: self-consciousness
- Respiratory: dyspnea, exacerbation of asthma, laryngeal or tracheobrachial trauma
- Skin: petechiae and purpura, disruption of surgical wounds

Data from Irwin, R.S. (2006). Complications of cough: ACCP evidence-based clinical practice guidelines. *Chest, 129(Suppl 1),* 54S-58S.
*Selected complications. For a more comprehensive listing, see the reference.

The pressures, velocities, and energy required to clear the airways put patients at risk for multiple complications (Box 22-1). Clinicians must be aware of the profound impact cough can have on quality of life and aggressively work to eliminate, or at least minimize, cough.

Emergent Conditions Associated with Cough

Superior vena cava (SVC) syndrome is an emergent condition that may present with cough along with dyspnea, hoarseness, dizziness, lethargy, blurred vision, dysphagia, and/or headache. Patients with lung cancer (especially small cell), lung metastasis, and lymphomas are at risk for this syndrome (Beckles et al., 2003). Physical examination may reveal facial and upper extremity edema, arm vein distention, and dilated collateral veins over chest wall, shoulders, and arms (Beckles et al., 2003; Storey & Knight, 2003). Cough can also be a symptom of cardiac tamponade. With this syndrome, cough is accompanied by chest pain, dyspnea, dizziness, orthopnea, and weakness. Patients with lung cancer, breast cancer, leukemia, and lymphoma are at highest risk for cardiac tamponade (Storey & Knight, 2003).

ASSESSMENT AND MEASUREMENT

Both subjective and objective measures should be used to evaluate cough. Subjective measures include patient diaries, visual analog scales, symptom distress scales (these usually measure multiple symptoms and may be disease specific), and general or cough-specific quality of life instruments (Irwin, 2006). Diaries require a motivated patient to maintain for any length of time. Visual analog scales are frequently used and, although they have not been psychometrically tested, they are recommended because they are commonly used and valid and they are likely to yield results that are different from but complementary to results of subjective instruments (Irwin, 2006).

There are three subjective instruments that have undergone extensive psychometric testing: breathlessness, cough, and sputum scale (BCSS), cough quality-of-life questionnaire (Dyspepsia Quality-of-Life Questionnaire [DQLQ]), and the Leicester

Cough Questionnaire (LCQ). All three of these instruments use Likert-type scales for patient evaluation; the BCSS has 3 items, the DQLQ has 28 items, and the LCQ has 19 items (French, Irwin, Fletcher et al., 2002; Irwin, 2006). There are several disease-specific scales that include measurement of cough. Most of these have not been as extensively studied but have shown good reliability and validity in small studies. For example, the Lung Cancer Cough Questionnaire (LCCQ) and the Lung Cancer Wheezing Questionnaire (LCWQ) were used in a pilot study to measure these symptoms in patients with lung cancer (Chernecky, Sarna, & Waller, 2004). Use of one of these rating scales may assist clinicians with monitoring cough over time and with evaluating treatment.

Objective measures of cough used in palliative care settings most often involve clinician evaluation of frequency, character, and sputum production. More precise measures that may be used by a consulting pulmonologist for difficult-to-control cough include 24-hour counts of coughing either with an observer (labor intensive) or a monitoring device, use of pharmacological tussigenic challenges to assess the effect of therapy on cough, comparison of airway inflammation indexes in induced sputum samples, and comparison of exhaled nitric oxide levels (Irwin, 2006).

HISTORY AND PHYSICAL EXAMINATION

The etiology of a cough can be determined in 80% of patients with advanced progressive illnesses by a thorough history and physical examination (Waller & Caroline, 2000).

General History

- Primary disease and any association between this disease and cough, such as chronic pulmonary obstructive disease (COPD) or lung cancer
- Comorbidities, such as GERD, cerebrovasular accident, pulmonary conditions, cardiac conditions, or asthma
- Allergies, such as to medications, foods, pets, dust, pollen, or mold
- Smoking history, measured in years multiplied by packs per day
- Exposures to substances or infections that may affect the respiratory system, such as asbestos, chemical exposure at work, second-hand smoke, or people with respiratory infections
- Past surgeries, such as thoracic, thyroid, or esophageal operations
- Chemotherapy exposure, including class of drug, dose, and length of treatment
- Radiation therapy, including site, length of treatment, and time since treatment
- Current medications, noting any recent changes in medications or use of ACE inhibitors
- Recent changes in weight, appetite, sleep, voice, activity tolerance, or energy level

Cough Evaluation

- Character of cough, such as barking, hacking, brassy, honking, dry, wet, paroxysmal, frequency, intensity
- Sputum production, including onset, color, volume, tenacity, and any changes over time
- Pain related to cough, including location, severity, and management

- Aggravating factors, such as inspiration, activity level, and eating
- Alleviating factors, including rest, positioning, and medications
- Influence of positioning (lying, upright) on cough
- Temporal patterns, such as constant, nocturnal, only during day, or variable
- Effect of cough on quality of life

Physical Examination

- Overall appearance
- Level of anxiety
- Vital signs, especially respiratory rate and depth, and the presence of fever
- Skin color (ashen, flushed, pink, cyanotic) and character (cool, hot, diaphoretic, presence of edema or finger clubbing)
- Breath sounds: wheezing, rales, rhonchi, crackles, pleural friction rubs, diminished, or absent. Begin and end auscultation at the lung bases to detect atelectasis that may clear with full inspiration (Berry, 2002).
- Upper airways: nasal drainage, throat irritation, or sinus congestion
- Neck: vein distention, deviated trachea, edema, masses, or enlarged lymph nodes
- Chest: shape, vein distention, accessory muscles, retractions, or abnormal percussion sounds
- Abdomen: distention, masses, enlarged organs, tenderness, or abnormal sounds

DIAGNOSTICS

Diagnostic studies are used when the etiology is not evident based on the history and physical examination, when empiric interventions for the presumed etiology fail, or when a precise diagnosis will change the planned course of treatment. The clinician must always evaluate the potential benefits and burdens of diagnostic tests.

Chest radiograph is the primary diagnostic tool when the history and physical examination do not clearly define the reason for cough. A chest radiograph is helpful to identify cough-associated problems such as pulmonary malignancy, pneumonia, pulmonary effusion, SVC syndrome, cardiomegaly or congestive heart failure, and cardiac tamponade. Other potential diagnostic procedures to evaluate cough include the following (Estfan & LeGrand, 2004; Irwin et al., 2006; Irwin & Madison, 2001; Martinez-Garcia, Perpina-Tordera, Roman-Sanchez et al., 2005; Olson, 2001; Poe & Kallay, 2003; Saad, Marrouche, Saad et al., 2003; Storey & Knight, 2003; Waller & Caroline, 2000):

- Echocardiogram to assist in diagnosing cardiac tamponade and left heart failure
- Computed tomography scanning to detect bronchiectasis, tumors, or pulmonary vein stenosis
- Barium swallow to observe for fistulas, aspiration, or reflux; bedside swallow to detect dysphagia; and spirometry to detect asthma
- Methacholine challenge test for bronchial hyperreactivity to diagnose asthma
- Empiric treatment with a proton-pump inhibitor to "diagnose" GERD. (This is more cost-effective, easily tolerated, and readily available than a 24-hour ambulatory esophageal pH monitoring test [Poe & Kallay, 2003].)

The Joint Commission on Accreditation of Healthcare Organizations (JCAHO) Hospital Core Measures for community-acquired pneumonia requires that blood cultures be drawn before initiating antibiotics for patients hospitalized for pneumonia (JCAHO, 2002). This requirement remains somewhat controversial because, although there is evidence to suggest that those who have blood cultures drawn before antibiotics have a lower mortality, there is no good evidence that it is the act of drawing a blood sample that improves outcomes (Barlow, Lamping, Davey et al., 2003). For patients in palliative care settings, the benefits of blood cultures in determining a course of treatment must be balanced with the burdens of the discomfort and costs associated with blood cultures.

The presence or absence of sputum, characteristics of the sputum, and symptoms associated with the cough may assist in determining its cause (Table 22-2). Bronchitis, pneumonia, and heart failure tend to lead to a productive cough. Coughs due to bronchospasm, pleural effusion, or ACE inhibitors are usually nonproductive. Although the color of the sputum may provide a hint as to cause of the cough, sputum color is due to the concentration of cellular debris, predominantly white cells, present in any inflammatory condition, and is not necessarily indicative of bacterial infection (Slovis & Brigham, 2004). The role of sputum culture and sensitivity in the evaluation of pneumonia is controversial. Some guidelines suggest extensive etiologic testing in all patients, and others recommend sputum studies only if a drug-resistant pathogen is suspected (Pimentel & Mcpherson, 2003). Sputum cultures are recommended for diagnosis and monitoring of tuberculosis (Irwin et al., 2006).

INTERVENTION AND TREATMENT

Treating the Cause

The underlying cause of cough should be treated when possible and when the treatment of the underlying cause will improve quality of living. For example, antibiotics for pneumonia are important to treat the discomforts of cough, dyspnea, and fever as well as to preserve life. In situations when treating pneumonia will not improve quality of living, a decision (in consultation with the patient, family, and interdisciplinary team) may be made to provide aggressive symptom management but not antibiotics.

Pharmacological Treatment

Cough serves a protective mechanism and should not be suppressed unless it is excessive, interferes with sleep and rest, causes discomfort, or otherwise interferes with quality of living. Cough can be triggered by more than one cause and therefore may require more than one treatment at a time (Estfan & LeGrand, 2004; Hanak, Hartman, & Ryu, 2005; Irwin & Madison, 2001). Consider maximal pharmacological treatment to bring the quickest and most complete response (Irwin & Madison, 2000).

Table 22-3 identifies the initial pharmacological treatments for cough due to several different causes based on evidence-based clinical practice guidelines from the American College of Chest Physicians. These should be used as the first-line therapies for these conditions.

Additional medications that may be used to suppress cough include the following:

- Guaifenesin, 200 to 400 mg every 4 hours, not to exceed 2400 mg/day, inhibits cough reflex sensitivity in patients with temporary hypersensitive cough receptors by increasing sputum production and decreasing viscosity. It should not be

Cause	Character of Cough	Sputum	Associated Symptoms
ACE inhibitor-induced	Dry, hacking		Tickling or scratchy sensation in throat
Asthma	Dry, hacking; made worse by cold air, exercise, laughing, allergy exposure; cough may be worse at night	May have thick mucoid sputum, especially at end of an attack; brown plugs may indicate aspergillosis	Episodic wheezing and dyspnea
Bronchitis	Productive cough	Mucopurulent; may develop hemoptysis	
Bronchiectasis	May initially be dry, but eventually productive of large amounts of sputum	Mucopurulent; may be blood streaked	Breath may have a fetid odor
Cancer	Dry to productive	Hemoptysis is common (frank blood or streaked)	
CHF	Often dry, may be worse at night	May progress to frothy pink sputum if pulmonary edema	Dyspnea on exertion or orthopnea
GERD	Cough worse at night or early in the morning		Substernal burning, indigestion, regurgitation, early morning hoarseness, choking bitter taste in mouth
Laryngitis	Dry, hacking		Hoarseness
Postinfection	Dry		Cough lasting 3-8 wk after an acute respiratory infection
Postnasal drip	Productive	Mucoid or mucopurulent	Tickle in throat, frequent clearing of throat
Pneumonia, viral	Dry, hacking		High fever, chills, malaise, headache, dyspnea; develops 1-2 days after flu-like symptoms At risk for superimposed bacterial pneumonia
Pneumonia, bacterial	Productive	Mucoid or purulent: *Streptococcus pneumoniae*—rusty or yellow; may be blood streaked *Klebsiella*—sticky, red, and gelatinous (common in chronic alcoholism)	High fever, chills, dyspnea, pleuritic chest pain; often preceded by upper respiratory tract illness
Tuberculosis	Productive	May develop hemoptysis	Weight loss

Data from Bickley, L.S. & Hoekelman, R.A. (1999). An approach to symptoms. In *Bates' guide to physical examination and history taking* (7th ed., pp. 43-103). Philadelphia: Lippincott, Williams & Wilkins; Lederman, M.M. (2004). Infections of the lower respiratory tract. In T.E. Andreoli, C.C. Carpenter, R.C. Griggs, et al. (Eds.). *Cecil essentials of medicine* (6th ed., pp. 861-870). Philadelphia: Saunders; Robinson, D. (2003). Cough. In P.S. Kidd, D.L. Robinson, & C.P. Kish (Eds.). *Family nurse practitioner certification review* (2nd ed., pp. 158-160). St. Louis: Mosby; Slovis, B.S., & Brigham, K.L. (2004). Approach to the patient with respiratory disease. In T.E. Andreoli, C.C. Carpenter, R.C. Griggs, et al. (Eds.). *Cecil essentials of medicine* (6th ed., pp. 177-180). Philadelphia: Saunders; and Slovis, B.S., & Brigham, K.L. (2004). Obstructive lung disease. In T.E. Andreoli, C.C. Carpenter, R.C. Griggs, et al. (Eds.). *Cecil essentials of medicine* (6th ed., pp. 193-200). Philadelphia: Saunders.

TABLE 22-3 ■ Initial Pharmacological Treatments for Selected Causes of Cough

Cause of Cough	Initial Pharmacological Treatments	Examples
ACE inhibitor–induced cough	Discontinue ACE inhibitor, if possible; may repeat trial at a later date	Theophylline* Sulindac Indomethacin
	Agents of various mechanism to suppress cough if cessation of ACE inhibitor not an option	Amlodipine Nifedipine Ferrous sulfate
Asthma	Inhaled bronchodilator + inhaled corticosteroid	Albuterol Beclomethazone dipropionate
Bronchiectasis	Bronchodilator	Albuterol or ipratropium bromide
Bronchitis, acute†	Antitussive medication β$_2$-Agonist bronchodilator (if wheezing)	Dextromethorphan Albuterol
Bronchitis, chronic	Antibiotics only in presence of an acute exacerbation‡ β$_2$-Agonist bronchodilator and/or anticholinergic bronchodilator	Albuterol Ipratropium bromide
Bronchitis, nonasthmatic eosinophilic	Inhaled corticosteroid Bronchodilator	Beclomethazone dipropionate Albuterol or ipratopium bromide
Chronic upper airway congestion syndrome§	Antihistamine + decongestant	Brompheniramine Pseudoephedrine
Common cold	Antihistamine + decongestant ± antiinflammatory	Brompheniramine Pseudoephedrine Naproxen
GERD	Proton pump inhibitor and/or H$_2$ antihistamine ± prokinetic	Omeprazole Famotidine Metoclopramide
Lung tumors	Centrally acting cough suppressant	Dihydrocodeine or hydrocodone
Postinfectious cough	Bronchodilator	Ipratopium

Data from Irwin, R.S., Baumann, M.H., Boulet, LP., et al. (2006). Diagnosis and management of cough executive summary. ACCP evidence-based clinical practice guidelines. *Chest, 129(Suppl 1)*, 1S-23S.
ACE, Angiotensin-converting enzyme; *GERD*, gastroesophageal reflux disease.
*All example medications show efficacy versus placebo for ACE inhibitor–induced cough.
†Routine antibiotics are not recommended for acute bronchitis.
‡Prophylactic antibiotics are not recommended for chronic bronchitis.
§Formerly called postnasal drip syndrome.

used in patients already suffering from increased secretions or ACE inhibitor cough (Dicpinigaitis & Gayle, 2003; Wynne, et al. 2002).

- Hydrocodone (5 to 10 mg orally every 4 to 6 hours), codeine (10 to 20 mg orally every 4 to 6 hours), and dextromethorphan (10 to 30 mg orally every 4 hours, maximum 120 mg/day) are centrally acting antitussives (Estfan & LeGrand, 2004; Waller & Caroline, 2000; Wynne et al., 2002). Antitussives should not be used for chronic coughs related to asthma or emphysema because they will raise airway resistance (Dicpinigaitis & Gayle, 2003).
- Benzonatate, 100 mg orally every 8 hours (may increase to every 4 hours, maximum dose 600 mg/day), deadens the afferent stretch receptor sites in the airways. Side effects may include gastrointestinal upset, sleepiness, pruritus, dizziness, rash, headache, and constipation (Estfan & LeGrand, 2004; Wynne et al., 2002).
- Lidocaine, 1 to 2 ml of 1% to 2% solution via a nebulizer up to four times a day, is reported to be effective when other measures fail, but there are no controlled clinical trials to support the use of this intervention. Patients must not take anything by mouth for 1 hour post–nebulized lidocaine, to prevent aspiration.
- Prednisone, 40 to 60 mg/day orally, 10 to 14 days and then slowly tapered to the lowest dose or dexamethasone 4 mg/day orally may decrease inflammation, reduce bronchospasm, or reduce edema (Storey & Knight, 2003; Waller & Caroline, 2000; Wynne et al., 2002).

For thick secretions that are difficult to expectorate, albuterol 0.5 ml in 2.5 ml of saline via nebulizer helps to loosen secretions (Waller & Caroline, 2000). Adequate fluid intake also helps to lessen the viscosity of secretions.

An anticholinergic, such as hyoscyamine, 0.125 to 0.25 mg sublingually every 4 to 6 hours as needed, or glycopyrrolate, 1 to 2 mg orally two or three times daily or 0.1 to 0.2 mg intravenously every 4 to 6 hours as needed, may decrease cough and secretions due to aspiration and at end-of-life (Estfan & LeGrand, 2004; Kee & Hayes, 2003; Waller & Caroline, 2000). Symptoms of cardiac tamponade can be managed with analgesics, anxiolytics, and oxygen when patients are nearing the end of life. Steroids may be helpful in reducing the edema of SVC syndrome (Storey & Knight, 2003).

Nonpharmacological Treatment
Physiotherapy and Breathing Techniques

- Encourage an effective cough in patients who have difficulty raising secretions. Have the patient sit upright, take a deep breath and hold it for 2 to 3 seconds, and then cough.
- Manually or mechanically assisted cough may reduce respiratory complications in patients with neuromuscular diseases and expiratory muscle weakness (McCool & Rosen, 2006). Consult a respiratory or physical therapist. Avoid using this technique in patients with airflow obstruction, such as those with COPD.
- Expiratory muscle training may be helpful to people with neuromuscular weakness (McCool & Rosen, 2006).
- Huffing may assist patients with COPD and cystic fibrosis to clear sputum (McCool & Rosen, 2006).

- Patients with cystic fibrosis may benefit from chest physiotherapy and drainage, or alternatively, using a device designed to oscillate gas in the airway (McCool & Rosen, 2006).

Interventional Therapies

- Radiation therapy can be effective in relieving tumor-induced cough in patients who have an expected prognosis that is sufficiently long (Storey & Knight, 2003). Short-course radiotherapy (one or two fractions) has been shown to be effective in decreasing symptoms in non–small-cell lung cancer patients. Longer courses should be reserved for patients with good performance status and longer life expectancy (Macbeth, Toy, Coles et al., 2001).
- Thoracentesis followed by pleurodesis or use of an indwelling pleural drainage catheter (e.g., Pleurx) relieves cough and dyspnea associated with malignant pleural effusions. Talc, bleomycin, and doxycycline are the most commonly used chemical sclerosing agents (Covey, 2005).
- Pericardiocentesis can provide quick relief of symptoms of cardiac tamponade, when appropriate, based on expected prognosis. Pericardial window with drainage and sclerosis can prevent recurrence in the patient who is a good surgical candidate (Storey & Knight, 2003).

Lifestyle Changes

- Smoking cessation, even after lung cancer diagnosis, decreases cough over time. Be aware that cough may temporarily increase after quitting due to the return of cilial action and the ability to expectorate toxins from the lungs (Brunton, Carmichael, Colgan et al., 2004; Dweik, 2002; Garces, Yang, Parkinson et al., 2004; Wynne et al., 2002). Clinicians should provide smoking cessation support and guidance and discuss the use of medications to lessen the effects of nicotine withdrawal.
- Patients with GERD should follow an antireflux diet that includes no more than 45 grams of fat per day and no coffee, tea, soda, chocolate, mints, citrus products, or alcohol. They should also stop smoking and limit vigorous exercise that increases intraabdominal pressure (McCool & Rosen, 2006).
- Care should be taken with feeding the patient with dysphagia. The patient should be well rested before meals. Place the patient in a high-Fowler's position while eating and maintain a semi-Fowler's position for 30 minutes after meals. Keep suction equipment within reach and be prepared to perform a Heimlich maneuver. A dietary consult may be helpful to provide instruction on foods and liquids that are less likely to be aspirated by patients with dysphagia, such as thickened beverages.

PATIENT AND FAMILY EDUCATION

Patients need to be reminded that cough is a protective mechanism and should not be suppressed without careful consideration and that self-treatment for cough should not exceed 1 week without seeking professional advice. Encourage patients and caregivers to discuss alternative or home remedies for cough with the clinician before starting these therapies so that they can be evaluated for any potentially harmful consequences or side effects. Instruct patients and caregivers on the proper use of medications and other interventions.

When appropriate, teach patients to keep a cough diary or to use a visual analog scale to rate the severity and frequency of cough as a means to monitor the effectiveness of interventions. Encourage the patient to notify the clinician if the interventions are not effective, if the patient is experiencing any untoward effects, or if the patient develops a fever or worsening of cough.

Teach patients and caregivers to wash hands frequently, to avoid people with infectious respiratory symptoms, and to get an annual influenza vaccine. Remind patients to cover their mouth and nose when coughing and to promptly wash hands afterward.

Encourage patients to take in adequate fluids to keep secretions loose. If the patient has a chronic cough related to GERD, provide verbal and written instructions about appropriate dietary recommendations.

Instruct patients and caregivers on the benefits of smoking cessation and the appropriate use of medications to prevent nicotine withdrawal.

EVALUATION AND PLAN FOR FOLLOW-UP

The most important measure of the success of treatment for cough is the patient's subjective evaluation. The use of visual analog scales to rate severity and frequency of cough assists in evaluating the effectiveness of interventions over time. The goal is to maximize patient comfort while promoting optimal respiratory functioning.

CASE STUDY Mr. T., a 72-year-old man with stage IV lung cancer, was admitted to hospice home care when his oncologist sadly informed him that the chemotherapy was doing more harm than good and that there was no more curative treatment available. One week later, he arrived at the hospice inpatient unit alert and experiencing cough, dyspnea on exertion, and heightened anxiety. He is accompanied by Mrs. T. and their three grown children.

The interdisciplinary team works with Mr. T. to manage his anxiety and dyspnea with lorazepam and his cough with hydrocodone syrup. Two days after admission, the nursing assistant reports to the advanced practice nurse that Mr. T.'s voice sounded hoarse after his morning bath and that he was coughing more and his face looks a little swollen. Further examination shows distended neck veins, facial and bilateral upper extremity edema, and a worsening cough. A clinical diagnosis of superior vena cava syndrome is made based on these symptoms. After consultation with Mr. T. and his family, a radiation therapy consult is obtained and two radiation treatments are ordered to begin immediately. The clinician also orders dexamethasone 4 mg orally every day. Two days after radiation therapy, Mr. T.'s symptoms of superior vena cava syndrome are subsiding and he reports less cough, dyspnea, and anxiety. Mr. T. is discharged back home, where the home care staff would assume the care of Mr. T. and his family.

REFERENCES

Barlow, G.D., Lamping, D.L., Davey, P.G., et al. (2003). Evaluation of outcomes in community-acquired pneumonia: A guide for patients, physicians, and policy-makers. *Lancet Infect Dis, 3(8),* 476-488.

Beckles, M.A., Spiro, S.G., Colice, G.L., et al. (2003). Initial evaluation of the patient with lung cancer: Symptoms, signs, laboratory tests, and paraneoplastic syndromes. *Chest, 123(1),* 97S-104S.

Berkow, R. & Fletcher, A.J. (Eds.). (1992). *The Merck manual of diagnosis and therapy* (16th ed.). Rathway, N.J.: Merck Research Laboratories.

Berry, P.H. (2002). Cough. In K.K. Kuebler, P.H. Berry, & D.E. Heidrich (Eds.), *End-of-life care: Clinical practice guidelines* (pp. 235-241). Philadelphia: Saunders.

Brunton, S., Carmichael, B.P., Colgan, R., et al. (2004). Acute exacerbation of chronic bronchitis: A primary care consensus guideline. *Am J Managed Care, 10,* 689-696.

Canning, B.J. (2006). Anatomy and neurophysiology of the cough reflex. ACCP evidence-based clinical practice guidelines. *Chest, 129(Suppl 1),* 33S-47S.

Chernecky, C., Sarna, L., & Waller, J.L. (2004). Assessing coughing and wheezing in lung cancer: A pilot study. *Oncol Nurs Forum, 31(6),* 1095-1101.

Covey, A.M. (2005). Management of malignant pleural effusions and ascites. *J Support Oncol, 3(2),* 169-173, 176.

Dicpinigaitis, P.V. (2003). Cough reflex sensitivity in cigarette smokers. *Chest, 123,* 685-688.

Dicpinigaitis, P.V. (2006). Angiotensin-converting enzyme inhibitor-induced cough. ACCP evidence-based clinical practice guidelines. *Chest, 129(Suppl 1),* 169S-173S.

Dicpinigaitis, P.V. & Gayle, Y.E. (2003). Effect of guaifenesin on cough reflex sensitivity. *Chest, 124,* 2178-2181.

Dweik, R.A. (2002). Recurrent episodes of purulent phlegm. In J.K. Stoller, E.D. Bakow, & D.L. Longworth (Eds.). *Critical diagnostic thinking in respiratory care: Case-based approach* (pp. 49-55). Philadelphia: Saunders.

Edmonds, P., Karlsen, S., Kahn, S., et al. (2001). A comparison of the palliative care needs of patients dying from chronic respiratory diseases and lung cancer. *Palliat Med, 15(4),* 287-295.

Estfan, B. & LeGrand, S. (2004). Management of cough in advanced cancer. *J Support Oncol, 2(6),* 523-527.

French, C.T., Irwin, R.S., Fletcher, K.E., et al. (2002). Evaluation of a cough-specific quality-of-life questionnaire. *Chest, 121(4),* 1123-1131.

Garces, Y.I., Yang, P., Parkinson, J., et al. (2004). The relationship between cigarette smoking and quality of life after diagnosis. *Chest, 126(6),* 1733-1741.

Hanak, V., Hartman, T.E., & Ryu, J. H. (2005). Cough-induced rib fracture. *Mayo Clin Proc, 80(7),* 879-882.

Irwin, R.S. (2006). Assessing cough severity and efficacy of therapy in clinical research. ACCP evidence-based clinical practice guidelines. *Chest, 129(Suppl 1),* 232S-237S.

Irwin, R.S., Baumann, M.H., Bolser, D.C., et al. American College of Chest Physicians (ACCP). (2006). Diagnosis and management of cough executive summary. ACCP evidence-based clinical practice guidelines. *Chest, 129(Suppl 1),* 1S-23S.

Irwin, R.S., Boulet, L-P., Cloutier, M.M., et al. (1998). Managing cough as a defense mechanism and as a symptom: A consensus panel report of the American College of Chest Physicians. *Chest, 114(Suppl 1),* 133S-181S.

Irwin, R.S. & Madison, M.J. (2000). Anatomical diagnostic protocol in evaluating chronic cough with specific reference to gastroesophageal reflux disease. *Am J Med, 108(4A),* 126S-130S.

Irwin, R.S. & Madison, M.J. (2001). Symptom research on chronic cough: A historical perspective. *Ann Intern Med, 134(9),* 809-814.

Joint Commission on Accreditation of Healthcare Organizations (JCAHO). (2002). *A comprehensive review of development and testing for national implementation of hospital core measures.* Retrieved March 22, 2006, from www.jointcommission.org/NR/rdonlyres/48DFC95A-9C05-4A44-AB05-1769D5253014/0/AComprehensiveReviewofDevelopmentforCoreMeasures.pdf.

Kee, J.L. & Hayes, E.R. (2003). *Pharmacology: A nursing process approach* (4th ed.). Philadelphia: Saunders.

Leach, R.M. (2004). Palliative medicine and non-malignant, end-stage respiratory disease. In D. Doyle, G. Hanks, N. Cherny, et al. (Eds.). *Oxford textbook of palliative medicine* (3rd ed., pp. 895-916). New York: Oxford University Press.

Macbeth, F., Toy, E., Coles, B., Melville, A., et al. (2001). Palliative radiotherapy regimens for non-small cell lung cancer. *Cochrane Database System Rev,* CD002143.

Martinez-Garcia, M.A., Perpina-Tordera, M., Roman-Sanchez, P., et al. (2005). Quality of life in patients with clinically stable bronchiectasis. *Chest, 128,* 739-745.

McCool, F.D. (2006). Global physiology and pathophysiology of cough. ACCP evidence-based clinical practice guidelines. *Chest, 129(Suppl 1),* 48S-53S.

McCool, F.D. & Rosen, M.J. (2006). Nonpharmacological airway clearance therapies. ACCP evidence-based clinical practice guidelines. *Chest, 129(Suppl 1),* 250S-259S.

Morice, A.H., Kastelik, J.A., & Thompson, R. (2001). Cough challenge in the assessment of cough reflex. *J Clin Pharmacol, 52,* 365-375.

Olson, J. (2001). *Clinical pharmacology made ridiculously simple.* Miami: MedMaster.

Pimentel, L. & McPherson, S.J. (2003). Community-acquired pneumonia in the emergency department. A practical approach to diagnosis and management. *Emerg Med Clin North Am, 21(2),* 395-420.

Poe, R.H. & Kallay, M.C. (2003). Chronic cough and gastroesophageal reflux disease: Experience with specific therapy for diagnosis and treatment. *Chest, 123(3),* 679-684.

Saad, E.B., Marrouche, M.D., Saad, C.P., et al. (2003). Pulmonary vein stenosis after catheter ablation of atrial fibrillation: Emergence of a new clinical syndrome. *Ann Inter Med, 138(8),* 634-639.

Slovis, B.S. & Brigham, K.L. (2004). Approach to the patient with respiratory disease. In T.E. Andreoli, C.C. Carpenter, R.C. Griggs, et al. (Eds.). *Cecil essentials of medicine* (6th ed., pp. 177-180). Philadelphia: Saunders.

Storey, P. & Knight, C.F. (2003). *UNIPAC four: Management of selected non-pain symptoms in the terminally ill* (2nd ed.). New Rochelle, N.Y: Mary Ann Liebert.

Waller, A. & Caroline, N.L. (2000). *Handbook of palliative care* (2nd ed., pp. 245-251). Boston: Butterworth Heinemann.

Wynne, A.L., Woo, T.M., & Millard, M. (2002). *Pharmacotherapeutics for nurse practitioner prescribers.* Philadelphia: F.A. Davis.

CHAPTER 23

DEHYDRATION

Kim K. Kuebler and Valarie A. Pompey

■

The issues surrounding dehydration and the implementation of hydration in the palliative and end-of-life care setting to date have been somewhat controversial. The traditional standard of medical care has been to provide routine hydration, whereas the traditional hospice model has promoted the concept of not administering parenteral fluid during the dying or terminal phase of incurable illness, based on the experience that artificial hydration causes potentially uncomfortable symptoms in the dying patient (Walker, 2002). Evidence can be found to support both approaches of care. It is important, however, for the clinician to consider dehydration as a contributing factor in the exacerbation of patient symptoms (Walker, 2002). The use of hydration can be a simple and powerful intervention when combating various symptoms arising from the concomitant manifestations that result from dehydration. Symptoms such as delirium, agitation, somnolence, and dizziness can be resolved with simple, cost-effective hydration. At end-of-life, the benefits of artificial hydration must be balanced by the potential burdens of providing fluids, such as increased secretions, the discomfort of needle sticks, and the physical barrier between patient and family caused by adding tubes. The decision to provide or withhold artificial hydration is based on careful evaluation of the patient's condition and goals. Artificial hydration should not be routinely administered or routinely denied.

DEFINITION AND INCIDENCE

A discussion of the definition and incidence of dehydration must include the symptoms that frequently accompany and are influenced by dehydration. Dehydration may cause a cluster of many symptoms, such as delirium, xerostomia, agitation, myoclonus, somnolence, dizziness, constipation, and fatigue (Huang & Ahronheim, 2002; Waller & Caroline, 2000). Many of these symptoms are discussed elsewhere in this text; the focus of this practice protocol is on briefly describing the role of dehydration in associated symptoms that ultimately influence patient-related quality of life.

Dehydration should be considered under the broader rubric of fluid deficit and defined as the overall reduction of water content within the human body, but particularly from within the intracellular space (Sarhill, Walsh, Nelson et al., 2001). Dehydration is always hypernatremic, while fluid depletion, which is loss of intravascular water and sodium deficit, may be isotonic, hypertonic/hypernatremic, or hypotonic/hyponatremic (Sarhill et al., 2001; Sarhill, Mahoud, Christie et al., 2003). Dehydration is a common condition that occurs in the dying and terminally ill patient as a result of diminished fluid intake, nausea/vomiting, cachexia, anorexia, and diaphoresis (Huang & Ahronheim, 2002). Dehydration may also be the result of drying medications such as opioids, anticholinergics, and diuretics. If not resolved, it can increase the incidence of pressure ulcers, confusion, and renal failure, resulting in an accumulation of active drug metabolites. Accumulation of drug metabolites can further prompt multiple symptoms, such as restlessness, myoclonus, seizures, and hyperalgesia (Walker, 2002).

When describing dehydration, the clinician should also consider the terms *fluid deficit, hypovolemia,* and *volume depletion. Dehydration* does not adequately describe, for example, *fluid deficit,* which is defined as the loss of water with or without accompanying electrolytes, particularly sodium (Beers & Berkow, 2000; Sarhill et al., 2001; Sarhill, 2003). Volume depletion occurs from loss of extracellular fluid (especially intravascular) and is accompanied by a normal, decreased, or increased plasma serum level (Beers & Berkow, 2000; Leaf, 1984; Sarhill et al., 2001). Dehydration occurs when intracellular water is lost. This leads to transmembrane water migration from the intravascular compartment under osmotic pressure and increased plasma sodium concentration (Sarhill et al., 2001; Sarhill et al., 2003).

ETIOLOGY AND PATHOPHYSIOLOGY

To dehydrate is to lose predominantly intracellular water (Feig & McCurdy, 1977; Sarhill et al., 2001). Total body water averages 60% of body weight in young adult males and 50% in young adult females (Sarhill et al., 2001). The total body water decreases with age and accounts for 50% in elder men and 45% in elder women (Sarhill et al., 2001). Because serum sodium and its associated anions account for more than 90% of the solute in extracellular fluid, the plasma sodium concentration is a good indicator of plasma osmolarity (Guyton & Hall, 2001).

In isotonic fluid deficit, there is a depletion of both sodium and water. The serum sodium level is within normal limits (135 to 148 mEq/L) despite a fluid volume deficit. Examples of this deficit can be seen in blood loss and loss of gastrointestinal fluids such as diarrhea, vomiting, or nasogastric suctioning (Sarhill et al., 2001). In hypernatremic dehydration, there is a water loss alone, and in fluid volume deficit, there is water loss in excess of serum sodium. Therefore, serum sodium is concentrated ($\geq$145 mEq/L) as a result of lower fluid volume. Hyponatremic fluid deficit occurs with excessive loss of sodium along with some fluid volume loss, leading to a serum sodium level of less than 130 mEq/L (Guyton & Hall, 2001).

As disease becomes debilitating and the dying process approaches, patients lose their ability or desire to drink fluids. The lack of fluid intake may lead to an isotonic depletion of water and sodium or, possibly, a tendency toward hypernatremic dehydration. In studies of persons experiencing dehydration at end-of-life, more than half had normal or near-normal serum sodium concentrations (Burge, 1993; Ellershaw, Sutcliffe, & Saunders, 1995; Waller, Hershkowitz, & Adunsky, 1994). It must be noted, however, that the results of these studies cannot be generalized because of small sample sizes, potentially biased selection criteria, and missing data (Viola, Wells, & Peterson, 1997).

Patients with dehydration may demonstrate low blood pressure with dizziness and syncope, decreased skin turgor, dry mucous membranes, low-grade fever, decreased urine output, and weight loss. A complaint of thirst is common although not universal. Because the serum is more concentrated, laboratory data may show elevated hemoglobin, hematocrit, and blood urea nitrogen levels (Guyton & Hall, 2001).

Many of the patients in the studies noted did not have isotonic volume depletion but appeared to have a hypertonic/hypernatremic dehydration. Hypernatremia is possible with a prolonged decrease in fluid intake, as may be seen in the terminally ill; it also occurs in the presence of excessive diaphoresis and with diabetes insipidus. The signs and symptoms are the same as those of isotonic dehydration, except that thirst is almost universal, because even slight increases in sodium concentration (as little as 2 mEq/L above normal) activate the thirst mechanism (Guyton & Hall, 2001; Sarhill et al., 2001; Sarhill et al., 2003). As the sodium level increases, anxiety and restlessness may also be present.

The sensation of thirst is important to fluid balance. The presence of thirst or dry mouth has been reported in 25% to 64% of cancer patients initiated to a palliative care service (Morita, Tsunoda, Inoue et al., 1999; Ventafridda, DeConne, Ripamonti et al., 1990). The incidence of thirst is increased to 61% to 87% in the final week of life (Conill et al., 1997; Ellershaw et al., 1995). In dehydration, patients experience thirst due to either dry mucous membranes or increased serum sodium levels and are stimulated to drink to replace the fluid loss. It is important to note, however, that the presence of thirst does not necessarily indicate dehydration. Many medications, such as opioids, phenothiazines, antihistamines, antidepressants, and anticholinergics, can cause the sensation of thirst despite adequate hydration. Thus, thirst alone is not a good indicator of a patient's hydration status.

The elderly are at an increased risk for dehydration, in part because of a decrease in the sense of thirst that accompanies the normal aging process. A lack of thirst may also be the result of a coexistent inability to respond physiologically to thirst from disease or disability (Morita, Tei, Tsunoda et al., 2001; West, 1993). In addition, the elderly are susceptible to the development of dehydration or hypovolemia as a result of chronic use of medications such as diuretic therapy, which can be responsible for significant water and vital electrolyte depletion (Sarhill et al., 2001).

Confusion, agitation, and restlessness are often associated with dehydration and may result from one of several of the following mechanisms. Dehydration directly affects the body's blood volume and circulatory reserve and can cause confusion and restlessness in non–terminally ill patients as well as those with an advanced illness (Fainsinger, Mac Cachern, Miller et al., 1994; Fainsinger & Bruera, 1994; Pereira & Bruera, 1997; Sarhill et al., 2001). In addition, the decreased circulatory volume may lead to decreased renal perfusion and eventual renal failure. In persons receiving opioids, poor renal perfusion may cause accumulation of opioid metabolites, leading to confusion, myoclonus, and nausea (Bruera, Franco, Maltoni et al., 1995; Caraceni & Grassi, 2003). Constipation, pyrexia, and electrolyte imbalance result from dehydration and can further contribute to disorientation, agitation, and neuromuscular irritability (Fainsinger & Bruera, 1994; Steiner & Bruera, 1998).

Providing fluids to persons who are dehydrated may alleviate many of the symptoms of dehydration and assist in flushing waste products and medication metabolites from the circulation. Providing fluids to persons whose kidneys cannot eliminate the additional fluid may lead to discomfort from fluid overload, with symptoms of edema, ascites, pulmonary congestion, and nausea and vomiting.

ASSESSMENT AND MEASUREMENT

The determination of a patient's hydration status is difficult in patients who have multiple problems associated with advanced diseases. Consideration of the following factors, as well as the signs and symptoms of dehydration identified in Box 23-1, may assist the clinician to discern an appropriate diagnosis for dehydration:

- Severely restricted oral intake
- Decreased urine output in patients who do not have preexisting renal failure
- Poor skin turgor, dry mouth, and postural hypotension, noting that dehydration is not the only cause of these symptoms
- Changes in laboratory findings such as elevated urea, creatinine, hematocrit, sodium, and plasma protein levels

It is important to note that the presence of edema is not a good indicator of the patient's hydration status. Edema in the advanced cancer population is often the result of low serum albumin level or tumor blockage of the venous or lymphatic systems. Patients taking corticosteroids may also experience edema. Despite excessive fluid in the interstitial spaces, there may be inadequate intravascular fluid.

HISTORY AND PHYSICAL EXAMINATION

History

- Review history of the terminal illness and any coexisting medical conditions that may affect urinary elimination or the ability to ingest fluids.
- Review intake and output. An estimate from the patient or caregiver may provide sufficient information, or the clinician may instruct the patient and family caregivers to record intake and output.

Box 23-1	Signs and Symptoms of Dehydration

- Confusion
- Restlessness
- Delirium
- Myoclonus
- Seizures
- Constipation
- Nausea and vomiting
- Decreased glomerular filtration rate (may also be the result of renal failure)
- Presence of decubitus ulcers
- Higher-than-normal systolic blood pressure
- Tachycardia at rest
- Thready pulse
- Dry mouth, multiple tongue furrows
- Delayed capillary refill
- Orthostatic blood pressure changes
- Increased body temperature
- Weight loss
- Hypoactive deep tendon reflexes
- Flattened neck veins

- Assess for a change in weight.
- Review history of any recent infection causing fever.
- Review history of any condition causing fluid loss, such as nausea or vomiting, diarrhea, or fistulas or/draining wounds.
- Review patient reports of headache, fatigue, muscle weakness, or anorexia, noting onset and any correlation with decreased fluid intake.
- Assess for the onset and severity of any mental status changes, such as restlessness, confusion, or delirium.
- Assess the use of diuretics, including frequency of administration, last dose, and urine output after last dose.

Physical Examination

- Skin and mucous membranes
  ‣ Body temperature
  ‣ Skin condition, noting skin turgor and any dryness or pruritus
  ‣ Alterations in skin integrity, such as decubitus ulcers, draining wounds, or fistulas
  ‣ Oral mucosa, noting dryness and presence of furrows or fissures
- Cardiovascular system
  ‣ Heart rate, noting strength and any tachycardia
  ‣ Blood pressure, including measurement of orthostatic changes
  ‣ Capillary refill
  ‣ Neck veins, noting any flattening
- Genitourinary system
  ‣ Urinary output and urinary retention
  ‣ Pain or discomfort on urination
- Gastrointestinal system
  ‣ Nausea or vomiting
  ‣ Diarrhea or constipation
- Neurological system
  ‣ Deep tendon reflexes
  ‣ Presence of myoclonus and/or seizures
  ‣ Mental status changes
- Musculoskeletal system
  ‣ Fatigue
  ‣ Muscle weakness

DIAGNOSTICS

Diagnostic procedures provide data that assist in the evaluation and monitoring of hydration and renal status. The following diagnostic procedures should be performed when the data from them influence the course of treatment (Sarhill et al., 2001).

- Blood pressure
- Hematocrit and plasma albumin
- Plasma sodium
- Plasma pH

- Urine sodium
- Urine osmolarity
- Blood urea nitrogen–to–plasma creatinine ratio
- Urinary output (normal is 1 ml/kg of body weight per hour, or approximately 1500 ml/day)

INTERVENTION AND TREATMENT

Once the evaluation is complete and the determination is made that dehydration exists, the decision should be made whether to provide hydration. As mentioned previously, decisions about providing hydration at end-of-life remain controversial. However, the clinician should consider the patient's overall medical condition and goals as well as the perspectives of family members when choosing specific interventions. Providing fluids may be directed by the patient's and family's cultural, religious, or moral convictions (Kedziera, 2001).

Many concerns remain regarding the benefits and risks of providing hydration at end-of-life. There is little research involving dying patients to support either position. Traditionally, hospice providers have argued against hydration in the terminally ill because it interferes with the natural dying process and may cause discomfort or complications, including the following (Dalal & Bruera, 2004; Vena, Kuebler, & Schrader, 2005):

- Cardiopulmonary overload leading to increased secretions, edema, cough, and/or choking
- Increased risk of aspiration
- Increased need for suctioning
- Incontinence
- Discomfort associated with repeated needle sticks
- Increased risk for infection related to intravenous lines and central venous catheter devices
- Increased risk for thrombosis related to central venous catheter lines

However, questions remain. Does providing hydration impede the dying process? Should providing fluids to the dying be considered a basic comfort measure that ensures a dignified end by reducing concomitant symptoms? Data do not support that the provision of hydration prolongs the dying process to a meaningful degree (Vena et al., 2005). Some potential advantages of hydration include the following:

- Prevention or alleviation of neurotoxicity from medications commonly used at end-of-life
- Alleviation of uncomfortable symptoms such as constipation, nausea and vomiting, thirst, and dry mouth (xerostomia)
- Prevention or alleviation of uncomfortable symptoms of confusion, agitation, and neuromuscular irritability (Dalal & Bruera, 2004; Vena et al., 2005).

Methods for the replacement of fluids, when the oral route is no longer feasible, include enteral via feeding tubes, rectal via proctoclysis, and parenteral via intravenous or subcutaneous (hypodermoclysis [HDC]) infusions (Kedziera, 2001).

Enteral Hydration

Enteral hydration is the preferred route for nutrition and hydration because it is safer, simpler, and less costly than parenteral routes, and it provides a normalized physiological response to food and fluid (Dalal & Bruera, 2004). One major disadvantage with enteral hydration is that as the patient become weaker, there is a risk of aspiration. Common types of enteral "lines" include nasogastric, gastrostomy, and jejunostomy. Some disadvantages that may occur as death approaches include the following:

- Discomfort
- Potential for a brief hospitalization for line placement
- Agitation in an already confused patient
- Complications associated with insertion
- Infection
- Aspiration
- Potential for the need to restrain patients to prevent them from pulling on tubes

Proctoclysis

Proctoclysis is the administration of fluids via the rectal route and may be a viable alternative in the home care setting when life expectancy is limited to days. Fluid replacement by proctoclysis is relatively risk free, inexpensive, and easy to administer. When choosing this route, thought should be given to whether family members are willing to assume the physical care associated with this approach (Kedziera, 2001). Disadvantages with protoclysis include the following:

- Abdominal cramping and discomfort
- Rectal leakage
- Reluctance of family members to administer fluids
- Immobility due to length of time needed to administer fluids (typically 6 to 8 hours).

Intravenous Hydration

In the acute care setting, hydration is considered routine and involves the utilization of the intravenous route (Lawlor, 2002). Disadvantages to use of this route may include the following (Kuebler & McKinnon, 2002; Lawlor, 2002):

- Difficulty finding venous access
- Invasive and uncomfortable
- Phlebitis
- Need for frequent site change
- Infection and thrombosis in central lines
- Decreased mobility
- Cost
- Complexity for use in the home setting

Hypodermoclysis

HDC is the administration of fluids via a subcutaneous infusion. This intervention is performed through the use of a butterfly needle (typically a 25-gauge needle) to infuse isotonic fluids into the subcutaneous tissue (Frisoli, de Paula, Feldman et al., 2000; Lawlor, 2002). HDC was widely used in the 1940s and 1950s and slowly fell out of favor with the introduction of hypertonic and electrolyte-free solutions. These fluids resulted in severe adverse reactions, so this intervention was abandoned for many years (Frisoli et al., 2000; Lawlor, 2002).

In the palliative care setting, HDC offers many advantages to patients who might otherwise have difficulty reversing dehydration by oral replacement. It is believed that HDC offers far more benefits of fluid replacement than the traditional intravenous route due to the following factors (Kuebler & McKinnon, 2002; Lawlor, 2002; Moriarty & Hudson, 2001):

- No need for venous access
- Easy for family members to administer using a subcutaneous injection (butterfly needle)
- May be stopped and started without a concern of thrombus development
- No need for hospitalization
- Subcutaneous sites last for several days
- Simple and easy to maintain
- Greater patient mobility and comfort
- Inexpensive
- Less likely to cause edema or fluid overload

In the absence of large volume losses, 1 liter of fluid per 24 hours is usually sufficient to maintain renal function in the patient population with advanced cancer and to prevent potential problems related to overhydration (Kuebler & McKinnon, 2002; Lawlor, 2002). The process of initiating HDC is outlined in Box 23-2.

As death approaches, the clinician should evaluate the benefit versus burden of providing hydration. Less noninvasive choices may be ideal and allow family members to continue to participate in care giving until the end. Simple and effective techniques that are often forgotten include the use of the following (Kedziera, 2001):

- Water or emollients to moisten lips
- Small, frequent sips of fluid (including sports replacement drinks) or ice chips
- Fine mist spray to moisten mouth
- Fans or air conditioners in hot humid weather to decrease amount of insatiable loss

Because of the lack of conclusive and comprehensive scientific data, considerations on whether to start or stop hydration should include the patient's right to autonomy. Ethical and moral precepts of "due no harm," the "doctrine of double effect," and the maintenance of comfort and dignity when death is imminent should help guide clinicians in assisting patients and families to make choices that ultimately result in a "good death."

Box 23-2	**Initiating Hypodermoclysis**

Select an insertion site. Preferred sites include the upper chest (avoid breast tissue), upper back, abdomen, back of upper arms, and upper thighs. Seek fatty areas.

Cleanse the skin over the selected site with alcohol or chlorhexidine.

Gently pinch a well-defined amount of tissue and insert a small needle (25- or 23-gauge butterfly) at a 45-degree angle into the subcutaneous space.

Dress the site with a transparent dressing.

Select a hypotonic or isotonic solution such as $2/3$, $1/3$, or plain normal saline solution, with or without hyaluronidase.

Begin infusions slowly (50 to 75 ml/hr) to determine tolerance. Most patients tolerate 50 to 100 ml/hr

PATIENT AND FAMILY EDUCATION

The prevention and management of dehydration are important in the palliative setting because they can help reduce untoward symptoms. Establishing a patient-specific plan of care is an important opportunity to learn what the patient's and family's expectations are as they relate to providing hydration in the dying process. These conversations provide the clinician with important information on how to plan the patient's care as well as to determine if there is a need for additional disciplines to support the patient and family during the terminal phase. Hydration is often an important issue for family members, who need education and support to understand the benefits and burdens of this intervention.

Patients who experience acute dehydration as a result of vomiting, diarrhea, or polyuria often experience distressing thirst and would benefit from rehydration. However, patients and families who prefer to avoid exogenous hydration for whatever reason should be respected for their informed decisions. The aim of hydration in the palliative care setting is comfort, not the return to a normal fluid and electrolyte balance (Twycross, 1997). Patients and their families should be helped to understand that hydration is a temporary intervention to help relieve distressing symptoms that interfere with the quality of life.

EVALUATION AND PLAN FOR FOLLOW-UP

Ongoing assessment is essential for patients receiving hydration in order to discern their level of comfort. If symptoms improve with hydration and the patient's quality of living is improved, the intervention is maintained. If symptoms do not improve or the patient shows signs and symptoms of fluid overload, hydration is either lessened or discontinued. Clinicians should keep an open mind about the utilization of hydration and recognize the options for fluid replacement (e.g., intravenous, HDC). Respecting the patient's and family's wishes on providing hydration may be the most important intervention offered during the terminal phase. Comfort is the goal in palliative care, and hydration is an easy intervention to address the multiple issues that are associated with dehydration.

CASE STUDY

Mr. B., a 75-year-old man, presents to the clinic for his follow-up evaluation after completing his radiation therapy for metastatic prostate cancer to bone. He complains of fatigue, weakness, dyspnea, and a poor appetite. The clinician performs a physical examination and finds that Mr. B. is febrile with an oral temperature of 101.5 °F; an increased heart rate of 122; slow, shallow breaths with a respiratory rate of 14; and his blood pressure is 188/94 mm Hg. Further evaluation reveals poor skin turgor, pale mucous membranes, delayed capillary refill, and diminished pedal pulses. The clinician orders a complete blood cell count and a comprehensive metabolic profile that includes measuring serum calcium. Mr. B. provided the clinician with a history of his intake of food and fluid over the past 48 hours, which included several cups of black coffee, cola, and soups. The clinician prescribes a nutritional consultation for Mr. B. and sends him to the infusion suite for a liter of normal saline while she waits for his laboratory results. She further investigates Mr. B.'s home situation and learns that he had been taking care of his wife, who recently underwent exploratory surgery. The clinician contacts the local home care agency to follow-up with Mr. B. at home to evaluate his physical status and to provide an infusion of another liter of normal saline the following day.

REFERENCES

Beers, M. & Berkow, R. (Eds.). (2000). *The Merck manual of geriatrics* (pp. 561-568). Rahway, N.J.: Merck Research Laboratories.

Bruera, E., Franco, J., Maltoni, M., et al. (1995). Changing pattern of agitated impaired mental status in patients with advanced cancer: Association with cognitive monitoring, hydration and opioid rotation. *J Pain Symptom Manage, 10(4)*, 287-291.

Burge, F. (1993). Dehydration symptoms of palliative care cancer patients. *J Pain Symptom Manage, 8(7)*, 454-464.

Caraceni, A. & Grassi, L. (Eds.). (2003). *Delirium: Acute confusional states in palliative medicine* (pp. 132-133). New York: Oxford University Press.

Conill, C., Verger, E., Henriquez, I., et al. (1997). Symptom prevalence in the last week of life. *J Pain Symptom Manage, 14(6)*, 328-331.

Dalal, S. & Bruera, E. (2004). Dehydration in cancer patients: To treat or not to treat. *J Support Oncol, 2(6)*, 467-487.

Ellershaw, J., Sutcliffe, J., & Saunders, C. (1995). Dehydration and the dying patient. *J Pain Symptom Manage, 10(3)*, 192-197.

Fainsinger, R. & Bruera, E. (1994). The management of dehydration in terminally ill patients. *J Pain Symptom Manage, 10(3)*, 55-59.

Fainsinger, R. MacCachern, T., Miller, M., et al. (1994). The use of hypodermoclysis for rehydration in terminally ill cancer patients. *J Pain Symptom Manage, 9(5)*, 298-302.

Feig, P. & McCurdy, D. (1977). The hypertonic state. *N Engl J Med, 297(26)*, 1444-1454.

Frisoli Jr, A., de Paula, A.P., Feldman, D., et al. (2000). Subcutaneous hydration by hypodermoclysis: A practical and low cost treatment for elderly patients. *Drugs Aging, 16(4)*, 313-319.

Guyton, A. & Hall, J. (Eds.). (2001). *Pocket companion to the textbook of medical physiology* (10th ed). Philadelphia: Saunders.

Huang, A. & Ahronheim, J. (2002). Issues in nutrition and hydration. In A. Berger, R. Portenoy, & D. Weissman (Eds.), *Principles and practice of palliative care and supportive oncology* (2nd ed., pp. 956-967). Philadelphia: Lippincott Williams & Wilkins.

Kedziera, P. (2001). Hydration, thirst and nutrition. In B.R. Ferrell & N. Coyle (Eds.). *Textbook of palliative nursing* (pp 156-163). New York: Oxford University Press.

Kuebler, K. & McKinnon, S. (2002). Dehydration. In K. Kuebler, P. Berry, & D. Heidrich (Eds.). *End-of-life care: Clinical practical guidelines* (pp. 243-251). Philadelphia: Saunders.

Lawlor, P.G. (2002). Delirium and dehydration: Some fluid for thought? *Support Care Cancer, 10(6)*, 445-540.

Leaf, A. (1984). Dehydration in elderly (editorial). *N Engl J Med 311(12)*, 791-792.

Moriarty, D. & Hudson, E. (2001). Hypodermoclysis for rehydration in the community. *Br J Commun Nurs 6(9)*, 437-443.

Morita, T., Tei, Y., Tsunoda, J., et al. (2001). Determinants of the sensation of thirst in terminally ill cancer patients. *Support Care Cancer, 9(3)*, 177-186.

Morita, T., Tsunoda, J., Inoue, S., et al. (1999). Contributing factors to physical symptoms in terminally-ill cancer patients. *J Pain Symptom Manage, 18*, 338-346.

Pereira, J. & Bruera, E. (1997). *The Edmonton aid to palliative care* (pp. 58-60). Edmonton, Canada: Division of Palliative Care, University of Alberta, Edmonton.

Sarhill, N., Mahoud, F.A., Christie, R., et al. (2003). Assessment of nutritional status and fluid deficits in advanced cancer. *Am J Hospice Palliat Care 20(6)*, 465-473.

Sarhill, N., Walsh, D., Nelson, K., et al. (2001). Evaluation and treatment of cancer-related fluid deficits: Volume depletion and dehydration. *Support Care Cancer, 9(6)*, 408-419.

Steiner, N. & Bruera, E. (1998). Methods of hydration in palliative care patients. *J Palliat Care, 14(2)*, 6-13.

Twycross, R. (1997). Dehydration. In *Symptom management in advanced cancer* (pp. 170-172). Oxon, UK: Radcliffe Medical Press.

Vena, C., Kuebler, K., & Schrader, S. (2005). The dying process. In K. Kuebler, M. Davis, & C. Moore (Eds.). *Palliative care practices: An interdisciplinary approach* (pp. 340-341). St. Louis: Elsevier Mosby.

Ventafridda, V., DeConne, F., Ripamonti, C., et al. (1990). Quality of life during a palliative care programme. *Ann Oncol 1(6)*, 415-420.

Viola, R., Wells, G., & Peterson, J. (1997). The effects of fluid status and fluid therapy on the dying: A systematic review. *J Palliat Care, 13(4)*, 41-52.

Walker, P. (2002). Hydration. In A. Elsayem, L. Driver, & E. Bruera (Eds.). *The M.D. Anderson symptom control and palliative care handbook* (2nd ed., pp. 77-81). Houston: The University of Texas Health Science Center at Houston.

Waller, A. & Caroline, N. (2000). *Handbook of palliative care in cancer.* Boston: Butterworth Heinemann.

Waller, A., Hershkowitz, M., & Adunsky, A. (1994). The effect of intravenous fluid infusion on blood and urine parameters of hydration and on state of consciousness in terminal cancer patients. *Am J Hospice Palliat Care, 11(6)*, 22-27.

West, C. (1993). Ischemia. In V. Carrieri-Kohlman, A. Lindsey, & C. West (Eds.). *Pathophysiological phenomena in nursing* (pp. 1-45). Philadelphia: Saunders.

CHAPTER 24

DELIRIUM AND ACUTE CONFUSION
Catherine Vena

■

DEFINITION AND INCIDENCE

Patients in palliative care likely are of an advanced age, experience severe exacerbations of chronic illnesses, and use multiple medications—all of which put them at risk for changes in mental and cognitive function. Frequently, the new onset of behavior labeled as "confusion" is indicative of the acute syndrome of delirium. Delirium is a serious neuropsychiatric complication that, unlike dementia, is potentially reversible. It must be properly diagnosed and promptly treated in the palliative care setting (Friedlander, Brayman, & Breitbart, 2004). The presence of delirium is associated with increased mortality and morbidity including prolonged hospital stays, functional decline, long-term care placement, and, in the case of the imminently dying, a distressing and uncomfortable death (Breitbart & Strout, 2000; Ely, Margolin, Francis et al., 2001c; Inouye, Rushing, Foreman et al., 1998; Marcantonio, Simon, Bergmann et al., 2003; McCusker, Cole, Abrahamowicz et al., 2002; Pitkala, Laurila, Strandberg et al., 2005).

Descriptions of behaviors commonly noted in delirious patients can be found in medical writings from the time of Hippocrates to the present (Clary & Krishnan, 2001). Despite this history, terminology has been inconsistent, overlapping, poorly defined, and often adapted to the discipline or specialty observing the condition. Historically, terms such as *organic brain syndrome, acute secondary psychosis, exogenous psychosis,* and *sundown syndrome* have been used synonymously with *delirium* (Lipowski, 1990). A review of the recent literature reveals a continuing use of a variety of terms to characterize delirium, including *acute brain failure, acute confusional state, terminal restlessness or agitation,* and *ICU psychosis* (Barber, 2003; Cacchione, Culp, Laing et al., 2003; Maluso-Bolton, 2000; McGuire, Basten, Ryan et al., 2000; Travis, Conway, Daly et al., 2001). The American Psychiatric Association (APA) first established the term "delirium" and defined diagnostic criteria in 1980 (APA, 1980). Increasingly, practitioners from various disciplines have adopted the term. To prevent miscommunication among health care professions, the clinician must always carefully characterize the mental and cognitive status of patients and use the term "delirium" when appropriate.

The most recent diagnostic criteria for delirium from the *Diagnostic and Statistical Manual of Mental Disorders (DSM-IV-TR)* are listed in Box 24-1. Based on these criteria, delirium may be defined as an acute and fluctuating organic brain syndrome characterized by global cerebral dysfunction that includes disturbances in attention, level of consciousness, and basic cognitive functions (thinking, perception, and memory)

The author would like to acknowledge Kim K. Kuebler and Debra E. Heidrich for their contributions that remain unchanged from the first edition of this textbook.

Box 24-1	*DSM-IV-TR* Diagnostic Criteria for the Diagnosis of Delirium

Disturbance of consciousness with reduced ability to focus, sustain, or shift attention

Change in cognition or the development of a perceptual disturbance that is not better accounted for by a preexisting, established, or evolving dementia

Disturbance develops in a short period of time and fluctuates over the course of the day

Evidence from history, physical examination, or laboratory findings that the disturbance

Is the physiological consequence of a general medical condition

Developed during substance intoxication or medication use

Developed during or shortly after a withdrawal syndrome

Has more than one etiology (e.g., more than one medical condition or a general medical condition plus substance intoxication or medication side effect)

Data from American Psychiatric Association (2000). *Diagnostic and statistical manual of mental disorders* (4th ed., text revision). Washington, DC: Author.

(APA, 2000). Other features commonly associated with delirium include increased or decreased psychomotor activity, disturbances in the sleep-wake cycle, and emotional lability (Burns, Gallagley, & Byrne, 2005). Delirium is frequently unrecognized by clinicians or misdiagnosed (Laurila, Pitkala, Strandberg et al., 2004). The fact that demented, depressed, and anxious patients may develop delirium makes the diagnosis additionally difficult (Insel & Badger, 2002). The diagnosis of delirium is primarily clinical and requires careful observation and a thorough history. Because the signs and symptoms of delirium are nonspecific, the clinician must look for a constellation of findings, identify the rapidity of onset, and assess for associated medical and environmental risks to determine an appropriate diagnosis.

Key Features of Delirium

Disturbance of Consciousness

Disturbance of consciousness refers to impairments in attention and the ability to be aware of and sustain attention to the environment (APA, 1999b). Attention is typically fluctuating and may present as a change in the level of consciousness that does not reach the level of stupor or coma. Patients may demonstrate slowed or inadequate reactions to stimuli or manifest distractibility. Individuals may be unable to follow conversations or complete simple tasks, may have slow response time, may be unable to maintain eye contact, or may fall asleep between stimuli. Increasing stimuli (touch, sound) may be needed to elicit a response. Conversely, patients may be hyperalert and overattentive to cues or objects in the environment. The ability to focus can be assessed by the patient's ability to complete a particular task such as spelling the word "world" backward, subtracting serial 7s, or listing the days of the week in reverse order (Tune, 2000).

Change in Cognition

Many aspects of cognitive function are impaired in delirium, including orientation, memory, language, thinking, and perception (APA, 1999b; Tune, 2000). Disorientation usually manifests relevant to time or place, with time disorientation being the first to be affected. Disorientation to other persons occurs commonly, but disorientation to self is very rare. Short-term memory deficits are the most evident memory impairments. Immediate memory (over a period of seconds) is demonstrated by the digit span (a healthy older adult should be able to repeat at least five) while anterograde memory (over a period of minutes) is demonstrated by the ability to remember three objects after 5 to 10 minutes (Burns et al., 2005; Goy & Ganzini, 2003). However, because these tests also reflect attention, severe deficits in this area will affect results. Language disturbances include a lack of fluency and spontaneity (long pauses and use of repetitious phrases), a tendency to ramble and switch from topic to topic, and difficulty finding the correct word to use in conversation or naming objects (anomia). Thinking is usually disorganized as evidenced by incoherent speech, deficits in logic, and responses that are irrelevant to questions asked. Perceptual disturbances may include misinterpretations, illusions, or hallucinations. Visual misperceptions and hallucinations are most common, but auditory, tactile, gustatory, and olfactory misperceptions or hallucinations can also occur. The individual with delirium may have the delusional conviction that the hallucination is real and exhibit emotional and behavioral responses consistent with the hallucination's content.

Acute Onset and Fluctuating Course

The features of confusion that develops over a short period and fluctuates over the course of the day are important defining criteria for delirium. Symptoms develop over hours or days but are likely to be intermittent in presentation and severity. A typical presentation is worsening of symptoms at night with lucid periods during the day where the patient may function normally (Cole, 2004). Noting the onset of the disturbances in consciousness or cognition assists in differentiating delirium from other syndromes that cause mental status changes, such as dementia.

Etiological Evidence

An important criterion for the diagnosis of delirium is evidence that the changes are a physiological consequence of an underlying medical condition, substance or medication intoxication or withdrawal, or combination of these factors. In palliative and end-of-life care, it may be difficult to identify the exact cause of delirium. An individual may have several potential causes at any one time (see "Etiology and Pathophysiology"). The challenge for the clinician is to identify which of the potential causes is the most likely and then determine the appropriate approach to this problem.

Additional Features of Delirium

Although not required for the diagnosis of delirium, a variety of other features often accompany delirium; these include sleep-wake disturbances, psychomotor activity changes, and emotional lability. The clinician should assess for these symptoms and monitor patients for any changes over time to prevent or at least minimize distress for both patients and their caregivers (Breitbart, Gibson, & Tremblay, 2002).

Sleep-Wake Disturbances

Disturbances in sleep patterns include daytime sleepiness, nocturnal insomnia, disturbed sleep continuity, and excessive dreaming. Some patients may experience a complete reversal of the sleep-wake cycle characterized by diurnal sleep periods and nighttime agitation and insomnia, whereas others may have fragmentation of the circadian sleep-wake cycle characterized by short periods of sleep and waking across the 24-hour day (Burns et al., 2005; Trzepacz, Mittal, Torres et al., 2001).

Psychomotor Activity

Patients with delirium may also exhibit disturbed psychomotor activity. Continuing research has indicated that there are several subtypes of delirium based on motor activity. These include a hyperactive-hyperalert subtype, a hypoactive-hypoalert subtype, and a mixed subtype that features components of the other two (Camus, Burtin, Simeone et al., 2000; Meagher & Trzepacz, 2000; Ross, Peyser, Shapiro et al., 1991). Patients with hyperactive-hyperalert delirium show evidence of sympathetic nervous system overactivity manifested in restlessness or agitation. This subtype is the most commonly recognized probably due to the expected presentation of agitation and/or inappropriate behavior (Inouye, Foreman, Mion et al., 2001). Characteristics of hyperactive-hyperalert delirium include plucking at bedclothes, wandering, verbal or physical aggression, increased alertness to stimuli, psychosis, and mood lability. Hypoactive-hypoalert patients appear lethargic and drowsy, respond slowly to questions, and do not initiate movement. This type of delirium is characterized by withdrawal from people and usual activities and decreased responsiveness to stimuli. Because they are quiet and withdrawn, the delirium in these patients is often overlooked or attributed to dementia, depression, or senescence (Casarett, Inouye, & American College of Physicians, 2001; Inouye et al., 2001). Differentiating delirium from normal aging processes, dementia, or depression requires careful and repeated assessment. A patient with a mixed subtype shows alternating periods of both types of behavior. Periods of lethargy may be seen as clinical improvements, when in fact the delirium may be continuing and increasing in severity (Clary & Krishnan, 2001; Milisen, Foreman, Godderis et al., 1998). A complete assessment of all symptoms of delirium is required before a change in behavior can be labeled as an improvement.

Emotional Disturbance

Patients with delirium may exhibit emotional disturbances. Anxiety, fear, depression, irritability, anger, euphoria, and apathy are common, with anxiety being the prevailing emotion. The delirious patient may be emotionally labile, rapidly and unpredictably shifting from one emotional state to another (APA, 1999b).

Prodromal and Subsyndromal Signs of Delirium

Some patients have prodromal symptoms such as restlessness, anxiety, irritability, distractibility, or sleep disturbance that progress to overt delirium over 1 to 3 days (APA, 1999b). Recently, Cole and colleagues described a condition known as subsyndromal delirium (SSD) (Cole, McCusker, Dendukuri et al., 2003). The symptoms of SSD are similar to prodromal symptoms, but the patient never progresses to overt delirium. Patients with SSD have the same risk factors and similar outcomes as those with delirium. These findings suggest that delirium is a spectrum disorder in which increasing numbers of symptoms are associated with increasingly adverse consequences. Patients noted to be exhibiting one or more prodromal symptoms or who report feeling "mixed up," having difficulty judging the passing of time, and having difficulty thinking or concentrating should be assessed for potentially reversible causes of delirium, and appropriate interventions should be initiated.

Prevalence and Outcomes

Researchers have found that the prevalence of delirium ranges from 10% to 80% depending on the population and setting. The palliative care clinician is likely to encounter patients with delirium in a variety of practice settings. In the acute care environment, delirium has been noted in 10% to 30% of general medical and postsurgical patients (Samuels & Neugroschl, 2005; Wise, Hilty, Cerda et al., 2002; Goy & Ganzini, 2003), 40% to 80% of critical care patients (Ely, Inouye, Bernard et al., 2001b; Ely et al., 2001c), and 25% to 50% of cancer inpatients (Fann & Sullivan, 2003). Delirium has also been described in 20% to 45% of patients newly admitted to rehabilitation or skilled nursing facilities (Marcantonio et al., 2003; Pitkala et al., 2005; Samuels & Neugroschl, 2005). From 80% to 90% of terminally ill patients will develop delirium as death approaches (Gagnon, Charbonneau, Allard et al., 2002; Lawlor et al., 2000; Massie, Holland, & Glass, 1983).

The consequences of delirium, including medical and psychosocial morbidity, can be severe for both patients and caregivers. A significant number of patients who recover from delirium remember the episode and report distress from the experience, including anxiety, helplessness, and fear (Breitbart et al., 2002; Laitinen, 1996; Schofield, 1997). Caring for patients with hyperactive delirium has obvious stresses for both families and nurses; however, hypoactive delirium is also stressful, especially for families who regret premature separation from a patient who can no longer communicate (Casarett et al., 2001). Delirium robs patients and families of valuable time. Therefore, because delirium episodes are potentially reversible even in advanced stages of disease, prompt diagnosis and treatment are essential for improving outcomes and quality of life in patients with chronic and advanced illnesses (Lawlor, Fainsinger, & Bruera, 2000).

ETIOLOGY AND PATHOPHYSIOLOGY

Multiple causes have been identified in the development of delirium. Although delirium can occur in a previously healthy person, it is by far more common in people with premorbid conditions. Furthermore, the etiology of delirium is most likely multifactorial. Inouye's Multifactorial Model for Delirium, consisting of predisposing factors (vulnerability) and precipitating factors (insults), provides a useful framework for predicting individual susceptibility for the development of delirium as well as for identifying potential factors that may have precipitated delirium (Inouye, 1998). Many potential predisposing and precipitating factors associated with delirium are listed in Box 24-2.

Very little is known about the underlying pathophysiological mechanisms of delirium, but analysis of symptomatology and known precipitating factors has lead to at least two explanatory models (Breitbart & Cohen, 2000). In the first model, delirium is seen as a global and nonspecific disorder of the brain characterized by generalized dysfunction in cerebral metabolism. The second model proposes that derangements in specific neurotransmitter systems precipitate brain pathology. There is evidence to support both models. Delirium probably represents a variety of disorders in which either specific or multiple interacting neurotransmitter systems (Table 24-1) are impaired as a result of aberrant metabolic activity, hypoxia, or exogenous agents (Samuels & Neugroschl, 2005).

Box 24-2	Common Risk Factors for Development of Delirium in Palliative and End-of-Life Care

PREDISPOSING FACTORS

Demographic
Older age
Male gender

Lifestyle
Drug or alcohol dependence

General Health
Frailty
Impairments in perception (vision, hearing)
Poor nutritional status
Insufficient sleep
Depression

Chronic Illness
Neurological disorder (e.g., dementia, Parkinson's disease, multiple sclerosis, stroke)
AIDS
Cancer
Endocrine disorder (hypothyroidism or hyperthyroidism, Cushing's disease)
Organ system failure (renal, hepatic)

PRECIPITATING FACTORS

Environment
Physical restraint or immobility
Unfamiliar surroundings
Sensory overload or deprivation
Admission to intensive care unit

Disease Related
Metabolic abnormalities (hypercalcemia, hyponatremia, uremia)
Anemia
Hypoxemia
Infection or sepsis
Liver failure
Acute neurological disorder (hemorrhage, infection, metastasis, edema)

Physical Discomfort
Constipation
Urinary retention
Dyspnea
Pain
Sleep disturbance

Data from Burns, A., Gallagley, A., & Byrne, J. (2005). Delirium. *J Neurol Neurosurg Psychiatry, 75,* 362-367; Clary, G.L. & Krishnan, K.R. (2001). Delirium: Diagnosis, neuropathogenesis, and treatment. *J Psychiatric Pract, 7(5),* 310-323; Friedlander, M.M., Brayman, Y., & Breitbart, W.S. (2004). Delirium in palliative care. *Oncology (Huntington), 18(12),* 1541-1550; discussion 1551-1543; Inouye, S.K. (1998). Delirium in hospitalized older patients: Recognition and risk factors. *J Geriatr Psychiatry Neurol, 11,* 118-125; Johnson, M.H. (2001). Assessing confused patients. *J Neurol Neurosurg Psychiatry, 71(Suppl 1),* i7-i12; Samuels, S.C. & Neugroschl, J.A. (2005). Delirium. In B.J. Sadock & V.A. Sadock (Eds.). *Kaplan & Sadock's comprehensive textbook of psychiatry* (8th ed., pp. 1054-1067). Philadelphia: Lippincott Williams & Wilkins; and Tune, L.E. (2000). Delirium. In C.E. Coffey & J.L. Cummings (Eds.). *Textbook of geriatric neuropsychiatry* (2nd ed., pp. 441-452). Washington, DC: American Psychiatric Press, Inc.

Box 24-2	**Common Risk Factors for Development of Delirium in Palliative and End-of-Life Care—cont'd**

PRECIPITATING FACTORS—cont'd

Emotional or Spiritual
Anxiety
Guilt
Spiritual distress or unfinished business

Medications
Polypharmacy
Anticholinergics
Opioids (especially meperidine)
Steroids
Chemotherapeutic and immunotherapeutic agents
Sedatives-hypnotics (benzodiazepines, barbiturates)
H_2 blockers
Phenothiazines

Medication Withdrawal
Alcohol
Benzodiazepines
Nicotine
Opioids
Steroids

ASSESSMENT AND MEASUREMENT

Because of differences in presentation and fluctuation of symptoms, delirium is difficult to detect. In fact, research has shown that clinicians caring for patients do not recognize delirium in a majority of cases (Inouye et al., 2001; Laurila et al., 2004). Because diagnosis depends on recognition of a constellation of symptoms in a temporal context, systematic evaluation of vulnerable patients is warranted. Many delirium assessment scales have been developed, some intended for clinical practice and others for research (APA, 1999b). Several review articles are available to provide an overview of the variety of instruments available for detecting, diagnosing, and rating delirium (Hjermstad, Loge, & Kaasa, 2004; Schuurmans, Deschamps, Markham et al., 2003a; Smith, Breitbart, & Platt, 1995). In general, the steps to a comprehensive plan for early detection and monitoring of delirium include regular screening for the presence of cognitive dysfunction, confirmation of diagnosis, and evaluation of severity over time (Cook, 2004, Hjermstad et al., 2004, Milisen, Steeman, & Foreman, 2004; Schuurmans et al., 2003a). The following section discusses those tools most often used in clinical practice.

Screening Instruments

Screening instruments identify the presence of cognitive impairment but are not diagnostic of delirium. They are very helpful for identifying those patients who require additional evaluation. These scales may also be useful for monitoring improvement or deterioration in cognitive status in patients with delirium.

TABLE 24-1 ■ Possible Neurochemical Changes in Delirium

System and Function	Alteration	Precipitating Factors	Sequelae
Cholinergic System Attention, arousal, memory, rapid eye movement sleep	↓ Acetylcholine (ACh)	Hypoxia, hypoglycemia, thiamine deficiency, anticholinergic medication, increased cytokines	Decreased ability to focus, maintain, or shift attention Impaired cognition
Dopamine System Movement, memory, motivation, emotional response, perception Dopamine has a reverse-parallel relationship with cholinergic system (decreases in ACh are associated with increases in dopamine)	↑ Dopamine	Opioids, hypoxia, hypoglycemia	Increased motor activity, perceptual impairments, stereotypical behaviors, mood alteration
γ-Aminobutyric Acid (GABA) System Major inhibitory neurotransmitter	↑ GABA activity	Hepatic failure, elevated serum ammonia levels, benzodiazepine intoxication	Hypoactive-hypoalert features
	↓ GABA activity	Benzodiazepine, alcohol withdrawal	Hyperactive-hyperalert features
Serotonin System Modulation of pain, mood, sleep, emotion, cognition, memory, and attention; precursor of melatonin	↓ Serotonin (5-hydroxytryptamine [5-HT])	Reduced tryptophan (5-HT precursor) availability secondary to illness or surgery (catabolic states, stress)	Impaired memory, somnolence, hypoactive-hypoalert features
	↑ Serotonin	Liver failure, multiple serotonin agonist use	Cognitive dysfunction, tremor, restlessness, sleep disturbance hyperactive-hyperalert features

Data from Balan, S., Leibovitz, A., Zila, S.O., et al. (2003). The relation between the clinical subtypes of delirium and the urinary level of 6-SMT. *J Neuropsychiatry Clin Neurosci, 15(3),* 363-366; Clary, G.L. & Krishnan, K.R. (2001). Delirium: Diagnosis, neuropathogenesis, and treatment. *J Psychiatric Pract, 7(5),* 310-323; Flacker, J.M. & Lipsitz, L.A. (1999). Neural mechanisms of delirium: Current hypotheses and evolving concepts. *J Gerontol. Series A, Biological Sciences and Medical Sciences, 54A(6),* B239-B246; Lewis, M.C. & Barnett, S.R. (2004). Postoperative delirium: The tryptophan dysregulation model. *Medical Hypotheses, 63(3),* 402-406; Michaud, L., Burnand, B., & Stiefel, F. (2004). Taking care of the terminally ill cancer patient: Delirium as a symptom of terminal disease. *Ann Oncol, 15(Suppl 4),* iv199-iv203; Samuels, S.C. & Neugroschl, J.A. (2005). Delirium. In B.J. Sadock & V.A. Sadock (Eds.). *Kaplan & Sadock's comprehensive textbook of psychiatry* (8th ed., pp. 1054-1067). Philadelphia: Lippincott Williams & Wilkins; Trzepacz, P.T. (2000). Is there a final common neural pathway in delirium? Focus on acetylcholine and dopamine. *Semin Clin Neuropsychiatry, 5(2),* 132-148; and van der Mast, R.C., & Fekkes, D. (2000). Serotonin and amino acids: Partners in delirium pathophysiology? *Semin Clin Neuropsychiatry, 5(2),* 125-131.

Mini-Mental State Examination

This is one of the most frequently used tools for the clinical evaluation of cognitive changes. It assesses orientation, instantaneous recall, short-term memory, attention, constructional capacities, and use of language (oral and written). A score of less than 24 of a possible 30 indicates cognitive impairment. Because the Mini-Mental State Examination is widely used in practice and research, data are available to support use of scores to rate the severity of impairment as follows: 24 to 30, no impairment; 18 to 23, mild impairment; and 0 to 17, severe impairment (Tombaugh & McIntyre, 1992).

NEECHAM Confusion Scale

This scale was designed for rapid and unobtrusive assessment and monitoring of acute confusion by the bedside nurse (Neelon, Champagne, Carlson et al., 1996). It can detect changes in mental status as well as physiological and behavioral manifestations of delirium, including those indicative of hypoactive-hypoalert delirium. A score of less than 25 of a possible 30 indicates the presence of cognitive impairment. Repeated measures can be used to monitor changes in mental status (Csokasy, 1999; Milisen et al., 1998; Rapp, 2001).

Delirium Observation Screening Scale

Like the NEECHAM, the Delirium Observation Screening Scale (DOS) was developed to assist nurses in early recognition of delirium based on observations during regular care (Schuurmans, Shortridge-Baggett, & Duursma, 2003b). The 25-item scale, based on *DSM-IV* criteria for delirium, assesses disturbances in consciousness; attention and concentration; thinking, memory, and orientation; psychomotor activity, sleep-wake pattern; mood; and perception. A reduced, 13-item version of the DOS shows promising results (Schuurmans, Donders, Shortridge-Baggett et al., 2002). The DOS is most applicable to inpatient versus outpatient settings since the scale needs to be administered over three consecutive shifts.

Nursing Delirium Screening Scale

The Nursing Delirium Screening Scale was developed for clinical use as a continuous delirium assessment instrument in busy inpatient units (Gaudreau, Gagnon, Harel et al., 2005). The scale contains five items (disorientation, inappropriate behavior, inappropriate communication, illusions or hallucinations, and psychomotor retardation). Each item is rated on a 0-to-2 scale on each of three shifts. Scores above 2 on any shift indicate the possibility of delirium.

Diagnostic Instruments

Diagnostic instruments are used along with the clinical and cognitive evaluation to make a formal diagnosis of delirium. The following are two examples of diagnostic tools.

Confusion Assessment Method

This valid and reliable tool was designed for efficient and effective detection of delirium (Inouye, van Dyck, Alessi et al., 1990). The four core *DSM-IV* criteria for delirium can be assessed by nonpsychiatric clinicians in less than 5 minutes. A version of the Confusion Assessment Method (CAM) for critical care patients (CAM-ICU) is also available (Ely et al., 2001b, 2001c). The CAM is useful to confirm delirium in patients who score less than 25 on the NEECHAM Confusion Scale or less than 24 on the Mini-Mental State Examination (Rapp, 2001).

Delirium Rating Scale–Revised-98

This scale, a delirium-specific tool, is a revision of the Delirium Rating Scale (DRS) (Trzepacz, 1999; Trzepacz et al., 2001). The DRS-R-98 contains 16 items: 3 are diagnostic in accordance with DSM-IV criteria, and 13 are severity-based on common symptoms found in delirious patients. The scale yields a total score (maximum of 46) that is diagnostic of delirium and a severity score (maximum of 39) that can be used to rate severity of symptoms over time. Higher severity scores indicate increased delirium.

Delirium Symptom Severity Rating Scales

Delirium symptom severity rating scales are designed to rate the severity of this syndrome. After delirium is diagnosed, these tools are useful for monitoring the effectiveness of interventions.

Memorial Delirium Assessment Scale

This scale was designed to quantify the severity of delirium symptoms for use in clinical intervention studies (Breitbart, Rosenfeid, Roth et al., 1997); it is also useful when assessing delirium in clinical populations (Lawlor et al., 2000). The Memorial Delirium Assessment Scale assesses arousal and level of consciousness, cognitive functioning (memory, attention, orientation, disturbances in thinking), and psychomotor activity. Completion requires about 10 minutes. Scores range from 0 to 30, with higher scores indicating more severe delirium.

Delirium Rating Scale–Revised-98

See earlier description.

Delirium Index

The Delirium Index was developed to specifically measure changes in the severity of symptoms in patients already diagnosed with delirium (McCusker, Cole, Bellavance et al., 1998; McCusker, Cole, Dendukuri et al., 2004). The measure is based on direct observation of the patient and does not rely on information from family members, other care providers, or documentation in the medical record. The Delirium Index contains seven items (each scored between 0 and 3) that yield scores between 0 and 21. Symptom domains include attention, thought, consciousness, orientation, memory, perception, and psychomotor activity. Higher scores indicate increased severity.

Objective Evaluation

Few objective measures are available to detect delirium. Of these, the electroencephalogram (EEG) is the most promising (Katz, Mossey, Sussman et al., 1991; Smith et al., 1995). EEG characteristics of delirium include a slowed rhythm, generalized theta or delta slow-wave activity, and loss of reactivity of the EEG to eye opening and closing. These are paralleled by quantitative EEG findings of increased absolute and relative slow-wave (theta and delta) power, reduced ratio of fast-to-slow band power, reduced mean frequency, and reduced occipital peak frequency. In alcohol and sedative withdrawal, EEG findings may include attenuation of voltage and prominence of beta activity (Katz, Curyto, TenHave et al., 2001). Although these EEG changes are important diagnostic signs of delirium, the absence of abnormalities does not necessarily rule out delirium (Smith et al., 1995). Given that EEG administration requires specialized expertise in obtaining and interpreting data, this evaluation may not be readily available to patients in many settings. Especially in end-of-life care, there is a limited role for the use of an EEG.

HISTORY AND PHYSICAL EXAMINATION

A thorough history and physical examination assist the clinician to identify the presence of delirium, determine potential causes of the delirium, and monitor the severity of this syndrome.

History

Review the recent history of the patient's mental status changes, including both patient and caregiver observations:

- Note reported changes in arousal, level of consciousness, orientation, and cognition.
- Note onset of changes and any fluctuation over the course of a day, asking specifically about changes at night.

Review the medical history:

- Note the primary palliative or terminal diagnosis as well as coexisting medical conditions.
- Note diseases that directly affect the central nervous system and those associated with organ system failure.

Review medications (Boxes 24-2 and 24-3):

- Note medications directly associated with delirium.
- Note medications with a potential for toxicity if given in high doses or in the presence of renal or hepatic dysfunction.
- Note any recently discontinued or refused medications with a potential for a withdrawal response.

Assess for a history of substance abuse.
Assess for a history of psychiatric disorders, including depression.
Assess sleeping patterns and signs of sleep deprivation.

Box 24-3	Drugs with High Anticholinergic Activity

Cimetidine
Prednisolone
Theophylline
Tricyclic antidepressants
Digoxin or lanoxin
Nifedipine
Chlorpromazine
Furosemide
Ranitidine
Isosorbide dinitrate
Warfarin
Dipyridamole
Codeine
Captopril

Data from Burns, A., Gallagley, A., & Byrne, J. (2005). Delirium. *J Neurol Neurosurg Psychiatry, 75,* 362-367; and Tune, L. E. (2001). Anticholinergic effects of medication in elderly patients. *J Clin Psychiatry, 62(Suppl 21),* 11-14.

Physical Examination

The clinician should use one of the screening tools discussed to identify patients with mental status or cognitive changes and a diagnostic tool to confirm the diagnosis of delirium. In addition, a targeted physical examination is essential for identifying the potential cause(s) of the delirium.

- Mental status (Box 24-4)
  - Consciousness
  - Cognition
- General survey
  - Vital signs, especially fever and hyperpnea
  - Skin color, especially pallor, cyanosis, jaundice
  - Skin turgor
  - Pruritus
- Respiratory system
  - Dyspnea or hypoxia
  - Cough or congestion
- Gastrointestinal system
  - Pain or discomfort
  - Bowel patterns, including signs of constipation or obstruction
  - Nausea and vomiting

Box 24-4	Tests for Cognitive Function

1. Attention
Subtraction of 7s or 3s from 100
Counting from 20 backward
Reciting months of year backward
2. Orientation
Date, day of the week, time of day
Name and location of place
Identification of familiar persons
3. Memory
Ability to recall three words and three objects after 5 minutes
Digit span
Description of recent events
4. Abstract thinking
Definitions of common words
Interpretation of a simple proverb
Similarities and differences
5. Speed and dynamics of thought
Word fluency
Ask the patient to say as many single words that begin with "F" as possible within 1 minute
6. Perception
Description of the surroundings
Interpretation of photographs or pictures

Modified from Johnson, M.H. (2001). Assessing confused patients. *J Neurol Neurosurg Psychiatry, 71(Suppl 1)*, i7-i12.

- Genitourinary system
  - ‣ Pain or discomfort
  - ‣ Urinary output
  - ‣ Signs of retention or obstruction
- Musculoskeletal system
  - ‣ Pain or discomfort
  - ‣ Weakness or agitation

Environmental and Psychoemotional Assessment

The following assessment variables are best evaluated by an interdisciplinary team approach involving the advanced practice nurse (APN), social worker, and spiritual counselor. The family's observations are very important when assessing the cause of delirium and should be included in a complete assessment of the following variables:

- Signs of anxiety, fear, or guilt
- Potential of "unfinished business"—interpersonal, financial, or spiritual
- Depression (see Chapter 25)
- Signs of spiritual distress
- Potential for sensory overload or sensory deprivation

DIAGNOSTICS

The following diagnostic tests assist in identifying an underlying medical cause of delirium. The extent to which any diagnostic work-up is conducted is dependent on the treatment goals and wishes of the patient and family and as well as the status of the patient's disease trajectory. As patients approach end-of-life, tests are appropriate only when they directly influence the treatment plan. For example, laboratory work to confirm hypercalcemia is necessary only if the patient's quality of living will be enhanced by treating the hypercalcemia and if the diagnosis cannot be made on the basis of the underlying medical diagnosis and associated symptoms. Tests include the following:

Basic

- Complete blood count
- Blood chemistry (electrolytes, glucose, calcium, blood urea nitrogen, creatinine, aspartate aminotransferase, alanine aminotransferase, lactate dehydrogenase)
- Blood gases or oxygen saturation
- Blood, urine, or other cultures
- Serum drug levels (digoxin, theophylline, cyclosporine)
- Urine drug screen

Additional tests—as indicated by patient prognosis and clinical condition

- EEG
- Brain imaging to assess for acute or subacute structural pathology

INTERVENTION AND TREATMENT

It may be possible to reverse delirium even in advanced illness, with the exception of possibly the last 24 to 48 hours of life (Breitbart & Cohen, 2000; Casarett et al., 2001).

When the potential cause of delirium is identified and it is consistent with patient and family treatment goals, the focus of intervention is on reversal of the delirium. When the cause of delirium cannot be identified or cannot be reversed, the focus of care is on comfort. Given the distressing nature of symptoms for both the patient and family, adequate management of symptoms in either case is paramount.

Manage the Underlying Causes of Delirium

- Treat increased intracranial pressure—dexamethasone, 16 to 40 mg/day orally, in the morning (Maity, Pruitt, Judy et al., 2004).
- Treat hypoxia: oxygen therapy.
- Treat infection: appropriate antiinfective agents.
- Correct metabolic abnormalities, as appropriate.
  - Hypercalcemia
    Mild: hydrate by using oral, parenteral, or subcutaneous fluids (hypodermoclysis). *Moderate or severe:* consider administering a bisphosphonate (e.g., pamidronate disodium) if it will improve the quality of living.
  - Hyponatremia due to syndrome of inappropriate antidiuretic hormone
    Mild: encourage moderate alcohol intake (e.g., glass of sherry before meals) and dietary sodium intake (Waller & Caroline, 2000).
    Moderate: demeclocycline, 300 mg orally twice daily (Waller & Caroline, 2000); fluid restriction is often not an issue in palliative care, but consider restricting to 1 L/day.
    Severe: unless chronic hyponatremia is symptomatic, infusion of hypertonic saline is not warranted. The patient with acute, symptomatic hyponatremia is at risk for the development of cerebral edema, cerebral herniation, and death. Depending on the patient's disease trajectory and patient and family goals for care, admission to an acute care facility for infusion therapy and monitoring may be appropriate (Smith, McKenna, & Thompson, 2000).
- Treat physical discomforts (e.g., constipation, dyspnea, pain, and pruritus).
- Address psychoemotional discomforts (e.g., anxiety, depression, and spiritual distress).
  - Be aware that patients with major depression are at greater risk of suicide when experiencing delirium (Waller & Caroline, 2000).
- Treat dehydration, as appropriate (see Chapter 23).
- Modify medication regimen.
  - Limit the use of anticholinergic drugs or decrease the number of drugs with anticholinergic properties (Box 24-2).
  - If accumulation of opioid metabolites is suspected, consider opioid rotation and hydration.
  - Be careful not to stop benzodiazepines abruptly.
  - Taper corticosteroids to lowest effective dose (do not discontinue abruptly).
- Treat withdrawal syndrome: resume the responsible drug and then taper slowly.

Nonpharmacological Treatment

Nonpharmacological strategies that may be instituted by the clinician are based on known risk factors for delirium (Inouye, Bogardus, Charpentier et al., 1999; Inouye, Bogardus, Williams et al., 2003; Lundstrom, Edlund, Karlsson et al., 2005; Weber, Coverdale, & Kunik, 2004). These interventions can be initiated in any setting and are

particularly valuable in allowing families to take an active role in maintaining patient comfort (Casarett et al., 2001).
- Provide orientation clues.
  ‣ Orient frequently to time and place.
  ‣ Encourage familiar persons to be present and keep familiar objects close by.
  ‣ Keep a calendar and clock visible; open shades during the day and darken the room at night but use a night-light.
  ‣ Provide cognitively stimulating activity several times a day (discuss current events, structured reminiscence).
  ‣ If the patient is experiencing illusions or hallucinations, gently correct misconceptions while reassuring the patient that he or she is safe.
- Use strategies to promote sleep and rest (see Chapter 8).
- Avoid too little or too much environmental stimulation.
  ‣ Encourage use of patient's visual and hearing aids.
  ‣ Keep a calm environment (noise reduction).
  ‣ Provide adequate lighting during the day and only minimal lighting at night.
- Reduce immobility.
  ‣ Avoid use of restraints. Keep the patient safe through supervision.
  ‣ Provide for mobility during the day (ambulation, time out of bed, or, for critically ill patients—range of motion).

Pharmacological Management
Antipsychotic Agents
- First line (except in cases of alcohol or benzodiazepine withdrawal)—haloperidol as follows (Cook, 2004; Kuebler, Varga, & Davis, 2005; Michaud, Burnand, & Stiefel, 2004):
  ‣ *Mild symptoms:* 0.5 to 5 mg orally twice or three times daily.
  ‣ *Moderate to severe symptoms* (especially severe agitation): 0.5 to 5 mg intravenously or subcutaneously; repeat every 1 to 4 hours until symptoms are controlled, using the more frequent interval for most severe agitation. When calmed, the patient can be maintained with oral or subcutaneous doses. Doses generally do not exceed 20 mg per 24 hours.
- Second line: atypical agents as follows (Schwartz & Masand, 2002):
  ‣ Olanzapine 2.5 to 5 mg orally at bedtime. May be increased to 20 mg/day if symptoms persist.
  ‣ Rispiradone 0.25 to 0.5 mg orally twice daily. May be increased to 4 mg/day if symptoms persist (0.25 to 0.5 mg orally every 4 hours).
  ‣ Quetiapine 25 to 50 mg orally twice daily. May be titrated up every 1 to 2 days to 100 mg orally twice daily. For agitation or refractory symptoms, 25 to 50 mg orally every 4 hours may be given.
  ‣ These agents (especially quetiapine) should be considered first line in delirious patients with dopamine deficiency: Lewy body dementia, Parkinson's disease, and other movement disorders (Samuels & Neugroschl, 2005).

Benzodiazepines
- Benzodiazepines used as an adjunct to antipsychotics:
  ‣ The use of benzodiazepines for treatment of delirium is controversial. The general consensus is that they should be avoided with the exception of delirium due to

alcohol or sedative withdrawal or in presence of seizures (Cook, 2004; Meagher, 2001). However, in cases where symptoms, particularly agitation, are refractive to neuroleptic therapy, judicious addition of a short-acting benzodiazepine to therapy is warranted.

- ‣ Lorazepam (1 to 2 mg intravenously or subcutaneously every 1 to 4 hours) is the drug of choice due to its short half-life and lack of active metabolites (APA, 1999b).
- ■ Benzodiazepines used for delirium associated with withdrawal:
  - ‣ In palliative care populations, short-acting agents are preferred (Mayo-Smith, Beecher, Fischer et al., 2004).
  - ‣ Lorazepam, 1 to 4 mg intravenously every 5 to 15 minutes, or lorazepam, 1 to 4 mg intramuscularly every 30 to 60 minutes, until calm, and then every hour can be used as needed to control agitation.
  - ‣ Once symptoms are controlled, maintain lorazepam at 1 to 2 mg orally twice to four times daily until delirium clears. Be aware that symptoms may persist for 6 to 12 months after the withdrawal of alcohol (Mayo-Smith et al., 2004).

Terminal Sedation

Sedation may be required for agitation unresponsive to the preceding interventions (Vena, Kuebler, & Schrader, 2005). Depending on the severity and response of the patient to treatment, therapy may be intermittent or continuous.

- ■ *Intermittent:* chlorpromazine suppository, 12.5 to 50 mg orally, per rectum, intramuscularly, or intravenously, every 4 to 12 hours. Titrate to 600 mg/day as necessary. This phenothiazine neuroleptic may assist in clearing the sensorium and is very sedating. One advantage of chlorpromazine is its ease of administration in the home care environment.
- ■ *Continuous*
  - ‣ Midazolam intravenously or subcutaneously, initial bolus of 0.5 to 2 mg, followed by 0.5 to 6 mg/hr. Titrate to 15 to 20 mg/hr.
  - ‣ Phenobarbital intravenously or subcutaneously, initial bolus of 100 to 200 mg, followed by 600 to 1200 mg/day with a maximum dosage of 2500 mg/day. Consider the drug's long half-life, interindividual variability in pharmacokinetics, and high potential for drug interaction when prescribing and titrating (Cheng, Roemer-Becuwe, & Pereira, 2002; Stirling, Kurowska, & Tookman, 1999). Monitor carefully for respiratory depression.
  - ‣ Propofol intravenously, 2.5 to 5 mcg/kg/min (approximately 10 mg/hr). Titrate to effect by increments of 10 mg every 10 to 20 minutes. Maximum dosage is 200 mg/hr. Propofol should not be infused for longer than 5 days without providing a drug holiday to safely replace estimated or measured urine zinc loss.

PATIENT AND FAMILY EDUCATION

The experience of delirium is frightening to both the patient and the family. Both need reassurance that the delirium may be reversible and that the symptoms can be managed. Because caregiving itself is stressful, information may need to be given in small doses and at repeated intervals.

- Teach family caregivers about the condition.
    - ▶ Several examples of educational handouts are readily available for those caregivers who might benefit from written information (APA, 1999a; Gagnon et al., 2002; Torpy, Lynm, & Glass, 2004).
    - ▶ Explain the causes of delirium and the interventions being initiated to reverse it.
- Teach the family the following interventions.
    - ▶ Report changes in the patient's mental status or complaints of feeling confused or unable to concentrate.
    - ▶ Gently correct patient illusions or hallucinations and reassure that the environment is safe (e.g., there are no spiders on the walls).
    - ▶ Provide orientation clues.
    - ▶ Refer to the time of day often (e.g., "It looks like we're going to have a lovely fall day").
    - ▶ Keep the environment familiar. If the patient is unable to be at home, take familiar objects to the inpatient facility.
    - ▶ Have familiar persons at the bedside.
    - ▶ Have a visible clock and calendar and mark off days on the calendar.
- Keep a calm, yet pleasantly stimulating environment:
    - ▶ Provide calm music that is pleasing to the patient.
    - ▶ Use soft lighting. Provide daily sunlight exposure when possible.
    - ▶ Minimize disturbances.
    - ▶ Encourage people to talk with the patient.
- Teach appropriate administration of all medications (e.g., neuroleptics, benzodiazepines, or barbiturates for delirium symptoms).
- Teach the importance of maintaining the pain regimen even if the patient is not able to ask for medications or to communicate pain.

If sedation is required to manage the patient's agitation, discuss the pros and cons of this intervention with the family. In the presence of terminal agitation, the time before sedation may be the last time the family sees the patient awake. Encourage the family to say their good-byes and to address unfinished business while the patient can potentially respond. Reinforce with the family that the patient can likely hear even when sedated and that it is important to continue to share supportive thoughts and feelings and to share good-byes even when the patient cannot respond.

EVALUATION AND PLAN FOR FOLLOW-UP

Patient status is monitored for improvement or decline in the symptoms of delirium. One of the delirium severity rating scales will be helpful for assessing and documenting these changes. When delirium cannot be reversed, the goal is comfort. The patient is monitored to ensure that distressing symptoms, such as illusions, hallucinations, restlessness, and agitation, are optimally managed.

After the treatment of delirium related to medication side effects, the clinician needs to use caution in the selection of medications for control of other symptoms that may emerge over time. The offending class of medication should not be used in the future, if possible. If that class of medication is required for comfort, the medication should be started at a low dose and the patient monitored frequently for early signs of delirium.

CASE STUDY

Mr. J. is a 69-year-old man with renal cell cancer status post right nephrectomy and radiotherapy. Two years after initial treatment, metastatic lesions were found in his right lung, right pelvis, and femur. He completed radiotherapy for the bone metastases but was not considered a candidate for biologic therapy. He has elected palliative care at home under the direction of a home care hospice team. He is cared for at home by his daughter. Mr. J.'s main problems include pain and occasional anxiety. His current medications include sustained-release morphine 60 mg twice daily with immediate-release morphine 15 mg orally for breakthrough pain; ibuprofen 400 mg orally four times daily, Senokot-S 2 tablets twice daily, and lorazepam 0.5 mg orally as needed.

During the regular interdisciplinary team conference, Mr. J.'s nurse reports that he has become increasingly withdrawn over the past 3 days and is sleeping most of the time. Mr. J. was responsive to verbal stimuli, able to take fluids and oral medications, and did not appear to be in discomfort. However, the presence of noisy, rattling respirations was distressing to his daughter. Because the nurse considered the patient to be near death, hyoscyamine (Levsin) 0.125 mg was ordered sublingually every 4 hours to control excessive secretions. The following morning, Mr. J.'s daughter calls the hospice distraught over her father's poor night. She reports that he has been constantly trying to get out of the bed, talking incoherently and, contrary to his usual demeanor, is aggressive and belligerent. She reports administering lorazepam three times during the night without any calming effect.

The team's clinician makes a visit to assess the situation. Upon arrival at the home, Mr. J. is resting quietly in the bed. His daughter is fatigued and frustrated. "I can't believe he is so quiet now. Last night was a nightmare." Upon assessment, the clinician finds that Mr. J. is lethargic but responds to verbal stimuli. He tends to "fall asleep" during her questions. His Mini-Mental State Examination score is 10/30. His skin is hot and dry, with poor skin turgor. His oral mucosa is dry and crusted with purulent sputum. His daughter reports that he "caught a cold" a few days ago, apparently from his grandson, who visited last week. His symptoms included a sore throat, nasal congestion, productive cough (yellow-green sputum), upper chest discomfort, general malaise, and mild shortness of breath. Mr. J.'s oral temperature is 101.4° F, blood pressure 130/84 mm Hg, pulse 104, and respirations 24. His pulse oximetry reading is 91%. Auscultation of the lungs reveals upper airway congestion, but bases are clear. His abdomen is soft, and bowel sounds are hypoactive. The daughter reports that he had a bowel movement yesterday. He is voiding without difficulty, but fluid intake has been low in the last 2 days, and his urine is dark amber.

The clinician concludes that Mr. J.'s clinical picture and symptom presentation indicate delirium. Mr. J.'s underlying vulnerability for development of delirium include his age and advanced metastatic disease. In this case, the clinician believes that the acute onset of bronchitis, dehydration, and the addition of an anticholinergic medication were precipitating factors. The clinician discusses treatment options with the daughter, including the possibility that this episode of delirium could possibly be reversed with treatment of the bronchitis, hydration, and change in medications. In the event that the decision is made not to treat the bronchitis or the treatment is not effective, measures are available to control the agitation. Mr. J.'s daughter elects a treatment plan that will seek to correct the underlying causes. The plan includes the following:

Bronchitis: azithromycin 500 mg orally ASAP followed by 250 mg orally for 4 days; acetaminophen 650 mg orally every 4 hours as needed for fever; guiafenesin 200 mg orally every 4 hours while awake, once able to take oral fluids.

Dehydration: 1000 ml of 5% dextrose in normal saline subcutaneously over next 24 hours as tolerated. Increase oral hydration to at least 1.5 liters per day as sensorium improves.

Delirium: Discontinue hyoscyamine and lorazepam. Begin haloperidol 0.5 mg orally three times daily. Call if patient exhibits agitation or restlessness.

The following afternoon, the clinician returns to reassess Mr. J. His daughter reports that he slept peacefully during the night. Mr. J. is lethargic but less somnolent; his Mini-Mental State Examination score is 23/30. He is afebrile and skin turgor has improved. He has a congested cough but is able to clear his airway. Sputum remains purulent. He is taking fluids well by mouth, and his urine is clear yellow. He denies having pain.

REFERENCES

American Psychiatric Association (1980). *Diagnostic and statistical manual of mental disorders* (3rd ed.). Washington, DC: Author.

American Psychiatric Association (1999a). *Delirium: Patient and family guide.* Retrieved September 10, 2005, from www.psych.org/psych_pract/treatg/patientfam_guide/Delirium.pdf.

American Psychiatric Association (1999b). Practice guideline for the treatment of patients with delirium. *Am J Psychiatry, 156(5 Suppl),* 1-20.

American Psychiatric Association (2000). *Diagnostic and statistical manual of mental disorders* (4th ed., text revision). Washington, DC: Author.

Barber, J.M. (2003). Pharmacologic management of integrative brain failure. *Crit Care Nurs Q, 26(3),* 192-207.

Breitbart, W. & Cohen, K. (2000). Delirium in the terminally ill. In H.M. Chochinov & W. Breitbart (Eds.), *Handbook of psychiatry in palliative medicine* (pp. 75-90). New York: Oxford University Press.

Breitbart, W., Gibson, C., & Tremblay, A. (2002). The delirium experience: Delirium recall and delirium-related distress in hospitalized patients with cancer, their spouses/caregivers, and their nurses. *Psychosomatics, 43(3),* 183-194.

Breitbart, W., Rosenfeld, B., Roth, A., et al. (1997). The Memorial Delirium Assessment Scale. *J Pain Symptom Manage, 13(3),* 128-137.

Breitbart, W. & Strout, D. (2000). Delirium in the terminally ill. *Clin Geriatr Med, 16(2),* 357-372.

Burns, A., Gallagley, A., & Byrne, J. (2005). Delirium. *J Neurol Neurosurg Psychiatry, 75,* 362-367.

Cacchione, P.Z., Culp, K., Laing, J., et al. (2003). Clinical profile of acute confusion in the long-term care setting. *Clin Nurs Res, 12(2),* 145-158.

Camus, V., Burtin, B., Simeone, I., et al. (2000). Factor analysis supports the evidence of existing hyperactive and hypoactive subtypes of delirium. *Int J Geriatr Psychiatry, 15(4),* 313-316.

Casarett, D.J., Inouye, S.K., & American College of Physicians-American Society of Internal Medicine End-of-Life Care Consensus Panel. (2001). Diagnosis and management of delirium near the end of life. *Ann Intern Med, 135(1)*, 32-40.

Cheng, C., Roemer-Becuwe, C., & Pereira, J.L. (2002). When midazolam fails. *J Pain Symptom Manage 23(2)*, 256-265.

Clary, G.L. & Krishnan, K.R. (2001). Delirium: Diagnosis, neuropathogenesis, and treatment. *J Psychiatric Pract, 7(5)*, 310-323.

Cole, M., McCusker, J., Dendukuri, N., et al. (2003). The prognostic significance of subsyndromal delirium in elderly medical inpatients. *J Am Geriatr Soc, 51(6)*, 754-760.

Cole, M.G. (2004). Delirium in elderly patients. *Am J Geriatr Psychiatry, 12(1)*, 7-21.

Cook, I.A. (2004). *Guideline watch: Practice guideline for the treatment of patients with delirium.* Arlington, Va.: American Psychiatric Association.

Csokasy, J. (1999). Assessment of acute confusion: Use of the Neecham Confusion Scale. *Appl Nurs Res, 12*, 51-55.

Ely, E.W., Gautam, S., Margolin, R., et al. (2001a). The impact of delirium in the intensive care unit on hospital length of stay. *Intensive Care Med, 27(12)*, 1892-1900.

Ely, E.W., Inouye, S.K., Bernard, G.R., et al. (2001b). Delirium in mechanically ventilated patients: Validity and reliability of the confusion assessment method for the intensive care unit (CAM-ICU). *JAMA, 286(21)*, 2703-2710.

Ely, E.W., Margolin, R., Francis, J., et al. (2001c). Evaluation of delirium in critically ill patients: Validation of the confusion assessment method for the intensive care unit (CAM-ICU). *Crit Care Med, 29(7)*, 1370-1379.

Fann, J.R. & Sullivan, A.K. (2003). Delirium in the course of cancer treatment. *Semin Clin Neuropsychiatry, 8(4)*, 217-228.

Friedlander, M.M., Brayman, Y., & Breitbart, W.S. (2004). Delirium in palliative care. *Oncology (Huntington), 18(12)*, 1541-1550; discussion 1551-1543.

Gagnon, P., Charbonneau, C., Allard, P., et al. (2002). Delirium in advanced cancer: A psychoeducational intervention for family caregivers. *J Palliat Care, 18(4)*, 253-261.

Gaudreau, J.-D., Gagnon, P., Harel, F., et al. (2005). Fast, systematic, and continuous delirium assessment in hospitalized patients: The nursing delirium screening scale. *J Pain Symptom Manage, 29(4)*, 368-375.

Goy, E. & Ganzini, L. (2003). Delirium, anxiety, and depression. In R.S. Morrison & D. Meier (Eds.), *Geriatric palliative care* (pp. 286-303). New York: Oxford University Press.

Hjermstad, M., Loge, J.H., & Kaasa, S. (2004). Methods for assessment of cognitive failure and delirium in palliative care patients: Implications for practice and research. *Palliat Med, 18(6)*, 494-506.

Inouye, S.K. (1998). Delirium in hospitalized older patients: Recognition and risk factors. *J Geriatr Psychiatry Neurobiol, 11*, 118-125.

Inouye, S.K., Bogardus, S.T., Jr., Charpentier, P.A., et al. (1999). A multicomponent intervention to prevent delirium in hospitalized older patients. *N Engl J Med, 340(9)*, 669-676.

Inouye, S.K., Bogardus, S.T., Jr., Williams, C.S., et al. (2003). The role of adherence on the effectiveness of nonpharmacologic interventions: Evidence from the delirium prevention trial. *Arch Intern Med, 163(8)*, 958-964.

Inouye, S.K., Foreman, M.D., Mion, L.C., et al. (2001). Nurses' recognition of delirium and its symptoms: Comparison of nurse and researcher ratings. *Arch Intern Med, 161(20)*, 2467-2473.

Inouye, S.K., Rushing, J.T., Foreman, M.D., et al. (1998). Does delirium contribute to poor hospital outcomes? A three-site epidemiologic study. *J Gen Intern Med, 13(4)*, 234-242.

Inouye, S.K., van Dyck, C.H., Alessi, C., et al. (1990). Clarifying confusion: The confusion assessment method. *Ann Intern Med, 113*, 941-948.

Insel, K.C. & Badger, T.A. (2002). Deciphering the 4 d's: Cognitive decline, delirium, depression and dementia—A review. *J Adv Nurs, 38(4)*, 360-368.

Katz, I.R., Curyto, K.J., TenHave, T., et al. (2001). Validating the diagnosis of delirium and evaluating its association with deterioration over a one-year period. *Am J Geriatr Psychiatry, 9(2)*, 148-159.

Katz, I.R., Mossey, J., Sussman, N., et al. (1991). Bedside clinical and electrophysiological assessment: Assessment of change in vulnerable patients. *Int Psychogeriatr, 3(2)*, 289-300.

Kuebler, K., Varga, J., & Davis, M. (2005). Medications by disorder. In K. Kuebler, M. Davis, & C.D. Moore (Eds.). *Palliative practices: An interdisciplinary approach* (pp. 418-441). St. Louis: Elsevier Mosby.

Laitinen, H. (1996). Patients' experience of confusion in the intensive care unit following cardiac surgery. *Intensive Crit Care Nurs, 12(2)*, 79-83.

Laurila, J.V., Pitkala, K.H., Strandberg, T.E., et al. (2004). Detection and documentation of dementia and delirium in acute geriatric wards. *Gen Hosp Psychiatry, 26(1)*, 31-35.

Lawlor, P.G., Fainsinger, R.L., & Bruera, E.D. (2000). Delirium at the end of life: Critical issues in clinical practice and research. *JAMA, 284(19)*, 2427-2429.

Lawlor, P.G., Gagnon, B., Mancini, I.L., et al. (2000). Occurrence, causes, and outcome of delirium in patients with advanced cancer: A prospective study. *Arch Intern Med, 160(6)*, 786-794.

Lawlor, P.G., Nekolaichuk, C., Gagnon, B., et al. (2000). Clinical utility, factor analysis, and further validation of the memorial delirium assessment scale in patients with advanced cancer: Assessing delirium in advanced cancer. *Cancer, 88(12)*, 2859-2867.

Lipowski, A.J. (1990). *Delirium: Acute confusional states.* New York: Oxford University Press.

Lundstrom, M., Edlund, A., Karlsson, S., et al. (2005). A multifactorial intervention program reduces the duration of delirium, length of hospitalization, and mortality in delirious patients. *J Am Geriatr Soc, 53(4)*, 622-628.

Maity, A., Pruitt, A.A., Judy, K.D., et al. (2004). Cancer of the central nervous system. In M.D. Abeloff, J.O. Armitage, J.E. Niederhuber, et al. (Eds.). *Clinical oncology* (3rd ed., pp. 1347-1431). Philadelphia: Elsevier/Churchill Livingstone.

Maluso-Bolton, T. (2000). Terminal agitation. *J Hospice Palliat Nurs, 2(1)*, 9-20.

Marcantonio, E.R., Simon, S.E., Bergmann, M.A., et al. (2003). Delirium symptoms in post-acute care: Prevalent, persistent, and associated with poor functional recovery. *J Am Geriatr Soc, 51(1)*, 4-9.

Massie, M.J., Holland, J., & Glass, E. (1983). Delirium in terminally ill cancer patients. *Am J Psychiatry, 140(8)*, 1048-1050.

Mayo-Smith, M.F., Beecher, L.H., Fischer, T.L., et al.; Working Group on the Management of Alcohol Withdrawal Delirium, Practice Guidelines Committee, American Society of Addiction Medicine. (2004). Management of alcohol withdrawal delirium. An evidence-based practice guideline. *Arch Intern Med, 164(13)*, 1405-1412.

McCusker, J., Cole, M., Abrahamowicz, M., et al. (2002). Delirium predicts 12-month mortality. *Arch Intern Med, 162(4)*, 457-463.

McCusker, J., Cole, M., Bellavance, F., et al. (1998). Reliability and validity of a new measure of severity of delirium. *Int Psychogeriatr, 10(4)*, 421-433.

McCusker, J., Cole, M.G., Dendukuri, N., et al. (2004). The delirium index, a measure of the severity of delirium: New findings on reliability, validity, and responsiveness. *J Am Geriatr Soc, 52(10)*, 1744-1749.

McGuire, B.E., Basten, C.J., Ryan, C.J., et al. (2000). Intensive care unit syndrome: A dangerous misnomer. *Arch Intern Med, 160(7)*, 906-909.

Meagher, D.J. (2001). Delirium: Optimising management. *BMJ, 322*, 144-149.

Meagher, D.J. & Trzepacz, P.T. (2000). Motoric subtypes of delirium. *Semin Clin Neuropsychiatry, 5(2)*, 75-85.

Michaud, L., Burnand, B., & Stiefel, F. (2004). Taking care of the terminally ill cancer patient: Delirium as a symptom of terminal disease. *Ann Oncol, 15(Suppl 4)*, iv199-iv203.

Milisen, K., Foreman, M.D., Godderis, J., et al. (1998). Delirium in the hospitalized elderly: Nursing assessment and management. *Nurs Clin North Am, 33(3)*, 417-439.

Milisen, K., Steeman, E., & Foreman, M.D. (2004). Early detection and prevention of delirium in older patients with cancer. *Eur J Cancer Care, 13(5)*, 494-500.

Neelon, V.J., Champagne, M.T., Carlson, J.R., et al. (1996). The Neecham Confusion Scale: Construction, validation, and clinical testing. *Nurs Res, 45(6)*, 324-330.

Pitkala, K.H., Laurila, J.V., Strandberg, T.E., et al. (2005). Prognostic significance of delirium in frail older people. *Dement Geriatr Cogn Disord, 19(2-3)*, 158-163.

Rapp, C.G. (2001). Acute confusion/delirium protocol. *J Gerontol Nurs, 27(4)*, 21-33.

Ross, C.A., Peyser, C.E., Shapiro, I., et al. (1991). Delirium: Phenomenologic and etiologic subtypes. *Int Psychogeriatr, 3(2)*, 135-147.

Samuels, S.C. & Neugroschl, J.A. (2005). Delirium. In B.J. Sadock & V.A. Sadock (Eds.). *Kaplan & Sadock's comprehensive textbook of psychiatry* (8th ed., pp. 1054-1067). Philadelphia: Lippincott Williams & Wilkins.

Schofield, I. (1997). A small exploratory study of the reaction of older people to an episode of delirium. *J Adv Nurs, 25(5)*, 942-952.

Schuurmans, M.J., Deschamps, P.I., Markham, S.W., et al. (2003a). The measurement of delirium: Review of scales. *Res Theory Nurs Pract, 17(3)*, 207-224.

Schuurmans, M.J., Donders, A.R., Shortridge-Baggett, L.M., et al. (2002). Delirium case finding: Pilot testing of a new screening scale for nurses. *J Am Geriatr Soc, 50*, S3.

Schuurmans, M., Shortridge-Baggett, L., & Duursma, S. (2003b). The delirium observation screening scale: A screening instrument for delirium. *Res Theory Nurs Pract, 17(1)*, 31-50.

Schwartz, T. & Masand, P. (2002). The role of atypical antipsychotics in the treatment of delirium. *Psychosomatics, 43(3)*, 171-174.

Smith, D.M., McKenna, K., & Thompson, C. (2000). Hyponatraemia. *Clin Endocrinol, 52(6)*, 667-678.

Smith, M.J., Breitbart, W.S., & Platt, M.M. (1995). A critique of instruments and methods to detect, diagnose, and rate delirium. *J Pain Symptom Manage, 10(1)*, 35-77.

Stirling, L.C., Kurowska, A., & Tookman, A. (1999). The use of phenobarbitone in the management of agitation and seizures at the end of life. *J Pain Symptom Manage, 17(5)*, 363-368.

Tombaugh, T.N. & McIntyre, N.J. (1992). The Mini-Mental State Examination: A comprehensive review. *J Am Geriatr Soc, 40*, 922-935.

Torpy, J.M., Lynm, C., & Glass, R.M. (2004). JAMA patient page. Delirium. *JAMA, 291(14)*, 1794.

Travis, S.S., Conway, J., Daly, M., et al. (2001). Terminal restlessness in the nursing facility: Assessment, palliation, and symptom management. *Geriatr Nurs, 22(6)*, 308-312.

Trzepacz, P.T. (1999). The Delirium Rating Scale: Its use in consultation-liaison research. *Psychosomatics, 40(3)*, 193-204.

Trzepacz, P.T., Mittal, D., Torres, R., et al. (2001). Validation of the Delirium Rating Scale-Revised-98: Comparison with the delirium rating scale and the cognitive test for delirium. *J Neuropsychiatry Clin Neurosci, 13(2)*, 229-242.

Tune, L.E. (2000). Delirium. In C.E. Coffey & J.L. Cummings (Eds.). *Textbook of geriatric neuropsychiatry* (2nd ed., pp. 441-452). Washington, DC: American Psychiatric Press, Inc.

Vena, C., Kuebler, K., & Schrader, S.E. (2005). The dying process. In K. Kuebler, M. Davis, & C.D. Moore (Eds.). *Palliative practices: An interdisciplinary approach* (pp. 335-377). St. Louis: Elsevier Mosby.

Waller, A. & Caroline, N.L. (2000). *Handbook of palliative care in cancer* (2nd ed.). Boston: Butterworth-Heinemann.

Weber, J.B., Coverdale, J.H., & Kunik, M.E. (2004). Delirium: Current trends in prevention and treatment. *Intern Med J, 34(3)*, 115-121.

Wise, M.G., Hilty, D.M., Cerda, G.M., et al. (2002). Delirium (confusional states). In M.G. Wise & J.R. Rundell (Eds.). *The American Psychiatric Publishing textbook of consultation-liaison psychiatry* (2nd ed., pp. 257-272). Washington, DC: American Psychiatric Publishing, Inc.

CHAPTER 25

DEPRESSION

Peg Esper

■

DEFINITION AND INCIDENCE

The term "depression" can be used to describe an emotional state that may be as simple as minor mood alterations or as major as a pathological inability to function or cope with life (Breitbart, Dickerson, Shuster et al., 2002). Reactive, or situational, depression is a common and expected response to a life-threatening disease. Reactive depression is generally self-limiting and resolves as the individual uses education, support, and other coping resources to face the threat against well-being.

A depressed mood becomes a problem for patients when it is prolonged or severe and interferes with daily functioning. Depressed mood related to an identifiable psychosocial stressor that exceeds what would be normally expected or that impairs social or occupational functioning may fit the *Diagnostic and Statistical Manual of Mental Disorders, Fourth Edition (DSM-IV)* criteria for an Adjustment Disorder with Depressed Mood (Strain, 1998). Although less specific than the criteria for Major Depressive Disorder, this diagnosis does allow for identification of early or temporary depressed states and can assist in obtaining appropriate treatment.

Major Depressive Disorder is a serious medical condition that disrupts an individual's mood, behavior, thought processes, and physical health (American Psychiatric Association, 2000a). The *DSM-IV* criteria for this diagnosis are listed in Box 25-1.

Many studies document the prevalence of depression in various populations. However, these studies are somewhat difficult to compare since the researchers do not always differentiate among reactive depression, adjustment disorders, and major depressive disorders. The incidence of depressive symptoms in cancer patients varies among studies, but it is thought to be as high as 25% for significant mood disturbance (Goy & Ganzini, 2003). Depression is seen in equal proportions in patients without cancer who have terminal diagnoses (Waller & Caroline, 2000).

The data on incidence of major depressive episodes in persons with advanced cancer show less variability than do the preceding studies, probably because the criteria for major depression are well defined. Approximately 5% to 15% of patients with advanced cancer have a major depressive disorder (Hinshaw, Carnahan, & Johnson, 2002).

The author would like to acknowledge Kim K. Kuebler for her contributions that remain unchanged from the first edition of this textbook.

Box 25-1	Criteria for Major Depressive Episode

At least five of the following symptoms have been present most of the day, or almost every day, for at least 2 weeks. At least one of the symptoms must be item 1 or 2.
1. Depressed mood (feeling sad or empty; appears tearful)
2. Markedly decreased interest or pleasure in all, or almost all, activities
3. Significant weight loss
4. Insomnia or hypersomnia
5. Psychomotor agitation or retardation
6. Fatigue or loss of energy
7. Feelings of worthlessness, or excessive or inappropriate guilt
8. Diminished ability to think or concentrate, or indecisiveness
9. Recurrent thoughts of death (not just fear of dying), recurrent suicidal ideation, or suicide attempt

From American Psychiatric Association (2000a). Major depressive disorder: A patient and family guide. Washington, DC; Author: American Psychiatric Association (2000b). Practice guidelines for the treatment of patients with major depression (2nd ed.). Washington, DC: Author.

ETIOLOGY AND PATHOPHYSIOLOGY

Recent research into the etiology of depression has found what appears to be complex bidirectional relationships among neural, endocrine, and immune systems (Illman, Corringham, Robinson et al., 2005). These data lend support for a theory of cytokine-mediated depression. Interleukin-6 has been specifically identified as higher in individuals with acute depressive conditions (Illman et al., 2005). Overactivity of the hypothalamic-pituitary-adrenal axis has also been implicated in the development of depression. This combination is believed to have an overall immunosuppressive effect on the patient (Hinshaw et al., 2002).

There are a number of risk factors associated with a diagnosis of depression (Goldberg, 2004; Hinshaw et al., 2002; Paice, 2002):
- Older age
- Diagnosis with a chronic or life-threatening illness
- Unmanaged symptoms, especially pain
- Lack of social support
- Self-concept disturbance, due to changes in body image or ability to carry out roles
- History of substance use
- Personal or family history of depression
- Difficulty in expressing emotions
- Spiritual or existential distress
- Use of medications with depressive side effects, including antihypertensives, benzodiazepines, corticosteroids, neuroleptics, amphotericin B, and certain chemotherapy agents
- Disease-related metabolic changes, nutritional deficiencies, systemic infections, hypercalcemia, the syndrome of inappropriate antidiuretic hormone, hypothyroidism or hyperthyroidism, and adrenal insufficiency

ASSESSMENT AND MEASUREMENT

As individuals face end-of-life, the emotions that accompany the dying process can be overwhelming. The terminally ill experience multiple losses and naturally grieve these losses. Although reactive depression is normal, it is nonetheless distressing and should not be ignored. It is extremely important that the clinician assess for signs of a depressed mood and determine the severity of the patient's depression—from mood change to adjustment disorder to major depression—and provide for the appropriate management for all levels of depression.

Assessment of Depression

The problem often cited when assessing major depression in persons with advanced diseases is that many of the somatic symptoms of depression (e.g., weight loss, fatigue, sleeping alterations) overlap with the symptoms of the disease process itself. Thus, the clinician must focus on the psychological symptoms of depressed mood, decreased interest in activities, inability to concentrate, feelings of worthlessness or excessive guilt, and recurrent death wishes as potential signs of depression (Goldberg, 2004; Nelson, 2002). In a major depression, these symptoms are present every day or almost every day for at least 2 weeks.

Major depression may be classified as mild, moderate, or severe on the basis of the severity of the symptoms. Mild depressive episodes have minimal symptoms and minor functional impairment. Moderate depression is characterized by symptoms that exceed the minimum and a greater degree of functional impairment. Severe episodes of depression involve the presence of several symptoms in excess of the minimum, and these symptoms markedly interfere with social or occupational functioning (American Psychiatric Association, 2000b).

It is often helpful to use a screening tool to assist in identifying the presence and, to some degree, the severity of depressed mood states. Information from one of the following assessment tools assists the clinician in identifying those persons who require a more detailed evaluation of their depressed mood and incorporating an instrument that best fits the practice setting.

- Beck Depression Inventory: The patient is asked a series of 21 questions that are scored to determine depression (Beck & Steer, 1987). This tool is based on the *DSM* criteria for depression.
- Hospital Anxiety and Depression (HAD) scale: This 14-item self-report tool excludes most of the somatic symptoms of depression that are often symptoms of advanced disease and takes about 5 to 7 minutes to complete (Zabora, 1998). This tool cannot distinguish between depression and sadness (Carroll, Callies, & Noyes, 1993).
- Geriatric Depression Scale: This tool is designed specifically for assessing depression in the elderly. It is a 30-item subjective questionnaire that excludes somatic complaints, focusing on the psychosocial symptoms of depression (Koenig, Meador, & Cohen, 1988).
- In evaluating effectiveness of measurement tools to screen for and evaluate ongoing depression, the measure with the best sensitivity, specificity, and positive predictive value in a study conducted by Lloyd-Williams, Spiller, and Ward (2003) was identified to be the act of asking the patient, "Are you depressed?" (Nelson, 2002).

■ Distress Thermometer: The National Comprehensive Cancer Network (NCCN) recommends use of a symptom distress thermometer that includes a 0-to-10 rating scale for any kind of distress that the individual is feeling. The patient places a mark on the thermometer in response to the question, "How distressed have you been in the past week?" A mark of 5 or higher should be further evaluated by the clinician (NCCN, 2005).

Assessment of Suicide Risk

Although suicide is relatively uncommon among cancer patients, this population has a risk of committing suicide twice that of the general population (Hinshaw et al., 2002). Essentially all persons in palliative care programs have one of the risk factors for suicide: advanced disease and poor prognosis; a suicide assessment is essential for all persons with depressed mood states.

The clinician must assess for additional factors associated with a higher risk for suicide (Goldberg, 2004; Waller & Caroline, 2000):

■ Uncontrolled symptoms, including pain, fatigue, and emotional suffering
■ Feelings of hopelessness and despair
■ Men are at greater risk than women
■ Higher incidence in oral, pharyngeal, or lung cancer or AIDS
■ Delirium
■ History of substance abuse, psychiatric disorder, or suicide attempt
■ Familial history of suicide
■ Social isolation
■ Recent death of a loved one

It is essential that the clinician assess the seriousness of suicidal intent by asking patients whether they have ever considered taking their own lives. Further questioning is then necessary to determine whether the individual has a plan for self-harm, to establish the specificity of the plan, and to determine whether the patient has the means to carry it out. Mental health experts emphasize that any patient who has devised a plan and a means to commit suicide should be immediately referred for a thorough psychiatric evaluation. The assessment for suicide risk is ongoing. It is especially important to reevaluate the severely depressed patient who is frequently undergoing treatment for depression. A patient without the energy to follow through on a suicidal act while severely depressed may indeed have the energy as the depression lessens.

HISTORY AND PHYSICAL EXAMINATION

The patient's feelings of hopelessness, worthlessness, or suicidal ideation must be fully explored along with a thorough physical assessment of the somatic responses to depression (Breitbart et al., 2002; Goldberg, 2004; Hinshaw et al., 2002; Mystakidou, Rosenfeld, Parpa et al., 2005). Changes in heart rate and respiratory rate may indicate anxiety, which often accompanies depression.

The clinician must identify other potential causes for the patient's somatic complaints, as well as disease-, symptom-, or medication-related causes of the depressive symptoms. A thorough assessment includes identification of uncontrolled symptoms, metabolic abnormalities, endocrine abnormalities, and medications associated with depressive symptoms.

INTERVENTION AND TREATMENT

The clinician must utilize the entire team when caring for persons with depressive symptoms. The supportive care of the nurse, social worker, spiritual counselor, and primary care physician may be sufficient to address the distress associated with a depressed mood. However, a clinical psychiatrist should be consulted when caring for the individual with major depression (American Psychiatric Association, 2000b).

Optimal therapy for major depression is often a combination of supportive psychotherapy, cognitive-behavioral techniques, and pharmaceutical management. For mild major depression, psychotherapy alone, antidepressant medication alone, or a combination of the two may be used. Moderate and severe major depressions often require the combination of psychotherapy and antidepressant medications. Short-term interventions for mild depression include active listening, offering verbal support, providing information to assist the individual in coping with the situation, identifying past strengths, and supporting previously successful ways of coping. The importance of incorporating spiritual support when appropriate should not be under-rated. For the individual at risk for suicide, it is essential to consult a skilled psychiatrist, maintain a supportive relationship, and focus on improved quality of living (Goldberg, 2004; Goy & Ganzini, 2003; Hinshaw et al., 2002; Nelson, 2002; American Psychiatric Association, 2000b).

For individuals with a high risk of suicide, the clinician must take steps to ensure safety. Supervision, either in the patient's residence or in a facility, may be required 24 hours a day. Objects or medications that may be used for self-harm must also be removed from the environment.

Antidepressant medications are effective in the treatment of depression. There are several different classes of antidepressant medications, whose effectiveness is comparable among and within classes. Medication selection is based on anticipated side effects, patient preference, quantity and quality of clinical trial data, and medication costs. Based on these considerations, the following medications can be considered: selective serotonin reuptake inhibitors (SSRIs), desipramine, nortriptyline, bupropion, and venlafaxine (American Psychiatric Association, 2000b). The elderly are particularly prone to the orthostatic hypotensive and anticholinergic side effects of tricyclic antidepressants and tend to have fewer side effects if one of the antidepressants listed is used (Goldberg, 2004). The axiom "start low and go slow" is certainly appropriate when titrating antidepressants in the elderly. Table 25-1 lists some of the more frequently used antidepressants by class and indicates the prevalence of various side effects. In June 2005, the Food and Drug Administration (FDA) issued a Public Health Advisory regarding the potential suicidality in adults taking antidepressant medications. It is clear that clinicians must use sound clinical judgment in placing individuals on any medication and that in situations such as this, where an increased risk of suicide may exist, patients must be followed carefully for clinical changes suggestive of worsening symptoms. This includes closer monitoring when doses are increased or agents changed as well as when first initiated (FDA, 2005).

TABLE 25-1 ■ Antidepressants

Drug	Dosage (mg/day)	Effect*						Comments
		Anticholinergic Effects	Sedation	Orthostatic Effects	Sexual Effects	GI Upset	Agitation/ Insomnia	
Tricyclics‡								
Amitriptyline (Elavil)	100-300	++++	++++	++++	+++	+	None	Used for neuropathic pain/hypnotic
Desipramine (Norpramin)	100-300	++	++	++	+++	+	+	
Doxepin (Sinequan)	100-300	++++	++++	++++	+++	+	None	
Imipramine (Tofranil)	100-300	++++	+++	++++	+++	+	None	
Nortriptyline (Pamelor)	50-200	++	++	++	+++	+	None	"Therapeutic window" plasma level; must be within 50-150 ng/ml efficacy
Selective Serotonin Reuptake Inhibitors‡								
Citalopram HBr (Celexa)	20-60	None	+	None	++++	+++	+	
Fluoxetine (Prozac)	10-80	None	None	None	+++	+++	+++	Used for neuropathic pain/hypnotic
Paroxetine (Paxil)	20-60	+	+	None	+++	+++	+	
Sertraline HCl	50-200	None	+	None	+++	++++	++	

Serotonin/Norepinephrine Reuptake Inhibitors§

Drug	Dosage (mg/day)						Comments
Venlafaxine HCl (Effexor)	37-375	None	+	+	+++	++	"Therapeutic window" plasma level; must be within 50-150 ng/ml for efficacy

Norepinephrine/Dopamine Reuptake Inhibitors||

Drug	Dosage (mg/day)						Comments
Bupropion HCl (Wellbutrin)	150-450	None	None	None	+++	++++	

Other Antidepressants¶

Drug	Dosage (mg/day)						Comments
Maprotiline HCl (Ludiomil)	150-225	++	++	++	+	None	
Mirtazapine (Remeron)	15-45	None	None	None	+	None	
Nefazodone HCl (Serzone)	300-600	None	+	None	++	+	
Trazodone HCl (Desyrel)	200-600	+	++++	+++	++	None	

*Prevalence: ++++, very high; +++, high; ++, moderate; +, low.

†All tricyclics cause slowed cardiac conduction; have the propensity to lower seizure threshold; 2000 mg can be a fatal overdose in adults; some tricyclics have established therapeutic plasma levels; moderately priced.

‡The lower dosages are most appropriate for depressed symptoms; no need to titrate as the tricyclics; caution warranted when coprescribed with other medications that undergo extensive hepatic metabolism, especially in the elderly; costly.

§Side effects similar to those of the SSRIs; daily dosing for extended-release capsules, twice-daily and thrice-daily dosing for tablets; should be considered when a trial of SSRIs has been ineffective; costly.

||Sustained-release form given twice daily; tablets thrice daily; avoid use in patients with a history of seizure disorders; most activating antidepressant available; costly.

¶Moderate to costly medications; often good for depression mixed with insomnia.

Psychostimulants are another class of medications used for the treatment of depression in the terminally ill. These medications enhance mood, decrease fatigue, and stimulate appetite, leading to an overall improved sense of well-being. Unlike the antidepressants, which tend to require several days to weeks to achieve therapeutic effect, the psychostimulants generally have a more immediate onset of action. Potential adverse side effects include tremor, tachycardia, insomnia, nightmares, and psychosis (Breitbart et al., 2002; Hinshaw et al., 2002; Rozans, Dreisbach, Lertora et al, 2002; Waller & Caroline, 2000). These medications are generally started at low doses and titrated upward for desired effect or until untoward side effects occur. Dextroamphetamine is usually started at 2.5 to 5 mg orally daily. The starting dose for methylphenidate is 5 mg orally in the morning and 2.5 mg orally at noon.

Anxiety often accompanies depression. Cognitive-behavioral interventions, active listening, and psychosocial support, alone or in combination with administration of benzodiazepines, are helpful in managing this symptom. See Chapter 17 for a more detailed discussion.

Complementary interventions also play a role in the treatment of depression. These interventions can improve mood and outlook, decrease feelings of hopelessness and helplessness, and decrease anxiety (Goldberg, 2004; Hinshaw et al., 2002). Chapter 32 addresses the use and benefits of complementary therapies in end-of-life care. The clinician should consider the following for patients who have depressed mood states:

- Pet therapy
- Art therapy
- Color therapy
- Music therapy
- Guided imagery
- Aromatherapy

PATIENT AND FAMILY EDUCATION

Depression, like many psychiatric illnesses, is often perceived as an embarrassment or a disgrace. Patients and families need support and education about the diagnosis of depression, with emphasis that it is not a sign of weakness or a character flaw. Some persons find written information helpful, such as the *Major Depressive Disorder: A Patient and Family Guide* (American Psychiatric Association, 2000a).

The following information must be included in the teaching plan for the patient and family:

- Take medications as prescribed, noting that antidepressants may not produce the full therapeutic benefit for a few weeks.
- Report any untoward side effects of the medications so that they can be addressed.
- Report any worsening of symptoms.
- Keep a record of the depressive symptoms to assist in evaluating the effectiveness of interventions.
- Use the interdisciplinary team for support and information.

EVALUATION AND PLAN FOR FOLLOW-UP

Early detection and ongoing assessment of depression are important considerations for the clinician caring for patients at end-of-life. Timely interventions are not always possible, and thoughtful consideration should be given to the appropriate medications that can be used to improve patient outcomes.

CASE STUDY Mr. G. is a 42-year-old man with metastatic melanoma. He has completed three cycles of treatment with a combination therapy that he has tolerated quite well. His major complaints had been fatigue and mild anorexia. Before starting a fourth cycle of treatment, he experienced some visual disturbances, so an MRI of the brain was performed. MRI showed that he had developed two new metastatic sites of disease in the brain. One lesion was identified as being very close to his optic nerve, and the other was located more centrally in the brain. The tumor near the optic nerve was surgically resected, leaving Mr. G. with minimal visual sequelae, but the other lesion was deemed inoperable and treated with stereotactic radiosurgery.

The clinician saw Mr. G. in the clinic after he completed the stereotactic radiosurgery. He was on a steroid taper to be completed later in the week. Mr. G. is a little quiet during the visit and, when asked about this, he states he feels he is just tired from his stay in the hospital. On the review of systems, his only complaints are some mild fatigue and anorexia. The physical examination today does not reveal any significant findings, and his laboratory studies show only a slight anemia of 12.2 mg/dl. His weight is down 10 pounds from his visit 4 weeks earlier. Residual fatigue is often seen following radiation therapy, and suggestions to help with the patient's weight loss are discussed. The clinician notices that the patient's wife appears frustrated and questions whether there is something else that needs to be addressed. The wife indicates that her husband has become very distant and short-tempered with everyone at home. She also states that he is not going to bed until very late at night and then wants to sleep off and on all day. She is tearful and says that she feels like he is pushing everyone away from him right now.

Mr. G. has central nervous system involvement by disease, but it was already determined during the examination that he has no specific neurological symptoms that day. However, the clinician realizes that Mr. G. was not quite "himself" during the visit. The patient and his wife have had a very supportive relationship during previous clinic appointments. When Mr. G. is asked to comment on his wife's concerns, he is unable to make eye contact and states that he is just concerned about recovery from his treatment. Following a review of what can be expected, this does not appear to be the whole story. The clinician asks Mr. G., "Are you depressed?" Mr. G. then broke out in sobs and admitted that he is just tired of everything. He does not want to think about the cancer and the fact that it will likely end his life sooner rather than later. He gets angry with himself for being short with his family and says that he feels all alone. Mr. G. acknowledges that he probably is depressed.

Patients taking corticosteroids may have mood swings and can be psychologically labile. To determine how much of Mr. G.'s symptoms might be related solely to the use of corticosteroids, it is noted as part of this assessment that his symptoms have been worsening despite having been on regularly decreasing doses of steroid medication. Although there may be an association with his current emotional state and steroid use, there still appears to be an underlying issue with depression.

Support is offered to Mr. and Mrs. G. and they are assured that this is not an abnormal response to everything Mr. G. is dealing with right now. He is referred for some counseling and the entire family is encouraged to speak with someone outside of the situation. Mr. G. agrees to counseling and to a trial of an antidepressant medication. Mr. G begins with bupropion hydrochloride 100 mg twice daily for 3 days; the dosage is then increased to 100 mg three times daily because Mr. G. has also expressed frustration in the past with his difficulties in trying to stop smoking. A follow-up is scheduled in 2 weeks.

After 1 week, Mr. G. calls and indicates that his mood seems to be improved and that he and his family are scheduled to have their first counseling session in a couple of days. He notes that he really has not wanted a cigarette since his neurosurgical procedure and does not know if that really has anything to do with the antidepressant medication. He is quite concerned, however, that over the last 48 hours he has had a significant problem with insomnia and feels very agitated in the evening. The decision is made to change Mr. G.'s antidepressant to citalopram hydrobromide (Celexa) 20 mg/day orally. The following week when he comes to the clinic, both he and his wife indicate that things are much improved. Mr. G. notes that the insomnia is no longer present and that he feels he is coping a little better. The patient was able to be maintained at the 20 mg/day dosage with adequate control of his depression and minimal side effects.

REFERENCES

American Psychiatric Association (2000a). *Major depressive disorder: A patient and family guide.* Washington, DC: Author.

American Psychiatric Association (2000b). *Practice guidelines for the treatment of patients with major depression* (2nd ed.). Washington, DC: Author.

Beck, A. & Steer, R. (1987). *Beck Depression Inventory (BDI) manual.* San Antonio, Tex.: The Psychological Corporation, Harcourt Brace Jovanovich.

Breitbart, W., Dickerson, E.D., Shuster, J.L., et al. (2002). Depression. In K.K. Kuebler & P. Esper (Eds.). *Palliative care practices from A to Z for the bedside clinician* (pp. 85-88). Pittsburgh: Oncology Nursing Society Press.

Carroll, B., Callies, A., & Noyes, R. (1993). Screening for depression and anxiety in cancer patients using the hospital anxiety and depression scale. *Gen Hosp Psych,* 15, 69-74.

Food and Drug Administration. (2005). *FDA reviews data for antidepressant use in adults.* Retrieved August 8, 2005, from www.fda.gov/bbs/topics/ANSWERS/2005/ANS01362.html.

Goldberg, L. (2004). Psychological issues in palliative care: Depression, anxiety, agitation, and delirium. *Clin Fam Prac, 6(2),* 441-470.

Goy, E. & Ganzini, L. (2003). End-of-life care in geriatric psychiatry. *Clin Geriatr Med, 19(4),* 841-56, vii-viii.

Hinshaw, D.B., Carnahan, J.M., & Johnson, D.L. (2002). Depression, anxiety, and asthenia in advanced illness. *J Am Coll Surg, 195(2),* 271-277.

Illman, J., Corringham, R., Robinson, D., Jr., et al. (2005). Are inflammatory cytokines the common link between cancer-associated cachexia and depression? *J Suppl Oncol, 3(1),* 37-50.

Koenig, H., Meador, K., & Cohen, H. (1988). Self-rated depression scales and screening for major depression in the older hospitalized patient with medical illness. *J Am Geriatc Soc, 36,* 699-706.

Lloyd-Williams, M., Spiller, J., & Ward, J. (2003). Which depression screening tools should be used in palliative care? *Pall Med, 17(1),* 40-43.

Mystakidou, K., Rosenfeld, B., Parpa, E., et al. (2005). Desire for death near the end of life: The role of depression, anxiety and pain. *Gen Hosp Psych, 27(4),* 258-262.

National Comprehensive Cancer Network (2005). *NCCN Clinical Practice Guidelines in Oncology.* Retrieved August 31, 2005, from www.nccn.com/professionals/physician_gls/PDF/distress.pdf

Nelson, J.E. (2002). Palliative care of the chronically critically ill patient. *Crit Care Clin, 18(3),* 659-681.

Paice, J.A. (2002). Managing psychological conditions in palliative care: Dying need not mean enduring uncontrollable anxiety, depression, or delirium. *Am J Nurs, 102(11),* 36-43.

Rozans, M., Dreisbach, A., Lertora, J.L., et al. (2002). Palliative uses of methylphenidate in patients with cancer: A review. *J Clin Oncol, 20(1),* 335-339.

Strain, J.J. (1998). Adjustment disorders. In J.C. Holland (Ed.). *Psycho-oncology* (pp. 509-517). New York: Oxford University Press.

Waller, A. & Caroline, N. (2000). *Handbook of palliative care in cancer* (2nd ed.). Boston: Butterworth-Heinemann.

Zabora, J.R. (1998). Screening procedures for psychosocial distress. In J.C. Holland (Ed.). *Psycho-oncology* (pp. 653-661). New York: Oxford University Press.

CHAPTER 26

DIARRHEA

Debra E. Heidrich

■

DEFINITION AND INCIDENCE

Diarrhea is defined as an increase in stool volume and liquidity, resulting in the passage of three or more loose or unformed stools per day (Carpenito, 2000; Rogers, 2005; Sykes, 2003). This symptom, however, is somewhat subjective: some may report three soft stools in a day as diarrhea, but others may report only stools that are liquid and occur in large volume. Diarrhea is often associated with abdominal cramping and rectal urgency (Carpenito, 2000; Levy, 1991). Uncontrolled diarrhea can lead to fluid and electrolyte imbalances, resulting in lethargy, weakness, and orthostatic hypotension. In addition, persistent diarrhea may lead to malnutrition, impaired skin integrity, altered sleeping patterns, social isolation, anxiety, and self-concept disturbances.

Approximately 7% to 10% of persons with advanced cancer report diarrhea (Sykes, 2003; Waller & Caroline, 2000), and 50% or more of those with human immunodeficiency virus (HIV) disease may experience this symptom (Cohen, West, & Bini, 2001; Sykes, 2003). The number of acquired immunodeficiency virus (AIDS) patients admitted to the hospital for uncontrolled diarrhea has decreased with the use of highly active antiretroviral therapy. A review of data from the state of New York in 1998 revealed that of the 15,000 persons with AIDS admitted to hospitals, 2.8% had a diarrheal diagnosis (Anastasi & Capili, 2000). This study did not indicate the number of persons with AIDS who experience diarrhea that is not severe enough to warrant hospitalization. Even mild to moderate diarrhea can have debilitating effects. Sanchez, Brooks, Sullivan et al. (2005) reported that although the incidence of bacterial diarrhea in patients with HIV disease decreased over the decade of 1992 to 2002, there is still an increased incidence over the general population and the risk of diarrhea increases with increased severity of HIV disease.

Most diarrhea is acute, lasting only a few days, and is generally due to infection or overuse of laxatives. Diarrhea that lasts longer than 3 weeks is considered chronic and is usually due to organic disease (Sykes, 2003).

ETIOLOGY AND PATHOPHYSIOLOGY

The three most common causes of diarrhea in persons with advanced cancer are laxative overdose, fecal impaction with overflow diarrhea, and partial bowel obstruction (Sykes, 2003; Mercadante, 2002). Other common causes are radiation enteritis, medications, and steatorrhea. In persons with AIDS, infection is often the cause, although the pathogen is not always identifiable.

Any condition that increases secretion within the gastrointestinal (GI) tract, interferes with reabsorption from the GI tract, increases the motility of the GI tract, or causes excretion of mucus, fluids, or blood can cause diarrhea. These correspond with the general mechanisms of diarrhea: secretory, osmotic, hypermotile, and exudative (Lingappa, 2003). Diarrhea in the terminally ill often involves more than one mechanism. The pathophysiological characteristics of these mechanisms are discussed later. Table 26-1 includes many of the conditions that lead to diarrhea in the palliative care setting, the pathophysiological mechanism(s), descriptors that may be helpful in determining the type and cause of this symptom, and suggested interventions.

TABLE 26-1 ■ Causes, Character, and Treatment of Diarrhea

Cause	Mechanism(s)	Descriptors	Treatment
Cancer-Related Diarrhea			
Endocrine-producing tumor	Secretory via production or stimulation of secretagogues	High volume, watery Associated with abdominal cramping	Encourage or replace fluids, as needed Control diarrhea: antidiarrheals Inhibit intestinal secretion (if severe): octreotide, clonidine Treat pain: anticholinergics
Obstruction	Exudative and hypermotility	Alternating constipation and diarrhea, often with mucus and blood; colicky pain	Reduce inflammation: steroids Treat pain: anticholinergics Control diarrhea: cautious use of antidiarrheals
Biliary or pancreatic obstruction	Osmotic due to fat malabsorption	Steatorrhea: large volume, pale, foul odor; feces floats in toilet	Decrease dietary fat Treat fat malabsorption: pancreatic enzymes, famotidine
Cancer Treatment–Related Diarrhea			
Chemotherapy	Secretory due to damage to villi, inhibiting absorption; hypermotility due to irritation	High volume, watery; may be explosive Associated with colicky pain	Encourage or replace fluids, as needed Slow motility: antidiarrheals Inhibit intestinal secretion (if severe): octreotide, clonidine Treat pain: anticholinergics

Data from Benson, C.A., Kaplan, J.E., Masur, H., et al. (2004). *Treating opportunistic infections among HIV-infected adults and adolescents: Recommendations from CDC, the National Institutes of Health, and the HIV Medicine Association/Infectious Diseases of Society of America.* Retrieved November 15, 2005, from www.cdc.gov/mmwr/preview/mmwrhtml/rr5315a1.htm; Bickley, L.S. (2004). The abdomen. In L.S. Bickley, *Bates' guide to physical examination and history taking* (8th ed., pp. 355-386). Philadelphia: Lippincott; Mercadante, W. (2002). Diarrhea, malabsorption, and constipation. In A. Berger, R. Portenoy, & D. Weissman (Eds.). *Principles and practice of palliative and supportive oncology* (2nd ed., pp. 233-249). Philadelphia: Lippincott Williams & Wilkins; Levy, M.H. (1991). Constipation and diarrhea in cancer patients. *Cancer Bull, 43*, 412-422; Rogers, H.M. (2005). Management of clients with intestinal disorders. In J.M. Black & J.H. Hawks (Eds.). *Medical-surgical nursing: Clinical management for positive outcomes* (7th ed., pp. 807-855). St. Louis: Elsevier Saunders; Sykes, N. (2003). Constipation and diarrhoea. In D. Doyle, G. Hanks, N.I. Cherny, et al. (Eds.). *Oxford textbook of palliative medicine* (3rd ed., pp. 483-496). New York: Oxford University Press; and Woodruff, R. & Glare, P. (2003). AIDS in adults. In D. Doyle, G. Hanks, N.I. Cherny, et al. (Eds.). *Oxford textbook of palliative medicine* (3rd ed., pp. 847-880). New York: Oxford University Press.

TABLE 26-1 ■ Causes, Character, and Treatment of Diarrhea—cont'd

Cause	Mechanism(s)	Descriptors	Treatment
Cancer Treatment–Related Diarrhea—cont'd			
Radiation therapy ■ Acute	Secretory (due to inflammation and bile salt malabsorption), osmotic, and hypermotility due to effects of bile salts	High volume, watery, explosive; Associated with abdominal cramping; Usually self-limiting	Encourage or replace fluids, as needed; Treat inflammation: nonsteroidal anti-inflammatory drugs; Absorb bile salts: cholestyramine; Slow motility: antidiarrheals
Radiation therapy ■ Chronic (may occur 5 to 15 years after treatment)	Ischemic enteritis, ulcerations, or impaired cellular functioning; may be secretory and/or osmotic	Depends on mechanism; generally high volume and watery	Encourage or replace fluids, as needed; Control diarrhea: antidiarrheals; Absorb bile salts: cholestyramine
Surgery ■ Gastrectomy	Secretory, osmotic, and hypermotility due to "dumping syndrome" and potential for bile salt malabsorption	High volume with undigested food; Associated with nausea, vomiting, flatulence, and colicky pain	Frequent, small meals; Control diarrhea: antidiarrheals; Bile salt malabsorption: cholestyramine; Treat pain: simethicone for gas pain; anticholinergics for colicky pain
Surgery ■ Ileal resection	Secretory, osmotic, and hypermotility due to poor reabsorption of bile salts	High volume with undigested food	Frequent, small meals; Control diarrhea: antidiarrheals; Bile salt malabsorption: Cholestyramine; Treat pain: simethicone for gas pain; anticholinergics for colicky pain
Surgery ■ Short bowel syndrome	Osmotic due to decreased fluid absorption	Depends on length of bowel resected: loose to watery	Increase bulk of stool: bulk-forming laxatives; Slow motility: antidiarrheals
Infection-Related Diarrhea			
Noninflammatory infections (e.g., viruses, *Escherichia coli*, *Staphylococcus aureus*)	Secretory due to stimulation of secretagogues via endotoxins	Often self-limiting; Watery, without pus or mucus; Associated with periumbilical cramping, nausea, and vomiting; Temperature normal or slightly elevated	If prolonged: Treat infection, when possible; Encourage or replace fluids, as necessary; Control diarrhea: antidiarrheals, using bismuth subsalicylate (Pepto-Bismol) as first choice, if required; Treat pain: anticholinergics
Inflammatory infections (e.g., *Shigella, Salmonella, Campylobacter* spp., invasive *E. coli*)	Secretory	Loose to watery, often with blood, pus, or mucus; Associated with lower abdominal cramping, rectal urgency, and fever	Treat infection, when possible; Encourage or replace fluids, as necessary; Control diarrhea: antidiarrheals; Treat pain: anticholinergics

Continued

TABLE 26-1 ■ Causes, Character, and Treatment of Diarrhea—cont'd

Cause	Mechanism(s)	Descriptors	Treatment
Infection-Related Diarrhea—cont'd			
Cryptosporidiosis	Secretory	High volume, watery, explosive; associated with abdominal cramping, fever, and vomiting	Treat immunosuppression: antiretroviral therapy Treat infection: nitazoxamide or paramomycin Encourage or replace fluids, as necessary Control diarrhea: antidiarrheals Treat pain: anticholinergics
Other Treatment-Related Diarrhea			
Overuse of laxatives	Depends on type(s) of laxative; usually osmotic or hypermotility	Frequent, loose stools	Discontinue or decrease dose of laxatives
Impaction	Exudative	Rectal leakage with too much softener; cramping with too much stimulant Small amounts of dark, mucuslike liquid; rectal pressure	Perform disimpaction Begin or adjust laxative protocol
Enteral supplements or feedings	Osmotic due to hyperosmolality of supplement or due to lactose intolerance	Large volume and watery Associated with abdominal cramping, distension, and flatulence Low stool pH	Dilute supplement with water and gradually increase strength Consider using bulk-forming agents Evaluate need for lactose-free supplement
Celiac plexus block	Hypermotility due to suppression of sympathetic nervous system	Moderate to large volume, loose stool May be self-limiting	Slow motility: antidiarrheals; anticholinergics
Anxiety	Hypermotility and secretory of lower gastrointestinal tract via parasympathetic stimulation	Generally moderate to large volume; loose stool Stool may contain mucus	Treat anxiety: address psychosocial concerns; Teach relaxation techniques; Evaluate need for anxiolytic
Medication	Often secretory	Secretory is generally large volume; but diarrhea character may vary with offending medication	Stop offending medication, when possible

Pathophysiological Characteristics of Secretory Diarrhea

The lining of the walls of the small intestine includes small pits, called the *crypts of Lieberkühn*, that lie between the intestinal villi. The crypts produce the four cell types of villi: enterocytes, goblet cells, enteroendocrine cells, and Paneth cells. The mucus of the goblet cells lubricates and protects the surfaces of the bowel lumen. The enterocytes of the crypts secrete large quantities of water and electrolytes, and those of the villi reabsorb water and electrolytes along with the products of metabolism. The enteroendocrine cells secrete hormones into the bloodstream, and the Paneth cells produce antimicrobial peptides and growth factors (Lingappa, 2003). Active secretion that overwhelms the absorptive processes of the GI tract leads to diarrhea that generally persists with fasting (Mercadante, 2002). Substances that increase bowel secretions (secretagogues) include vasoactive intestinal polypeptide, calcitonin, serotonin, bradykinin, substance P, prostaglandins, and gastrin (Levy, 1991; Lingappa, 2003; Mercadante, 2002). Conditions that lead to the production of one or more of these secretagogues include the following:

- Inflammation in the bowel wall causes the release through the cyclooxygenase pathway of prostaglandins, which stimulate bowel secretions. In addition, the inflammation interferes with the absorption process, further contributing to diarrhea (Mercadante, 2002). This is the likely mechanism for the diarrhea associated with acute radiation enteritis, chemotherapy, and infection.
- Two infections that lead to significant fluid and electrolyte losses from secretory diarrhea are cryptosporidiosis and pseudomembranous colitis. *Cryptosporidium* sp., a common cause of diarrhea in the AIDS population, attaches to the intestinal epithelium. It damages the enterocytes, leading to impaired absorption and enhanced secretion within the intestinal tract (Rogers, 2005). The diarrhea of cryptosporidiosis is profuse and watery and is associated with abdominal cramping, fever, and vomiting (Woodruff & Glare, 2003). Pseudomembranous colitis is caused by colonization with *Clostridium difficile* after antibiotic therapy. *C. difficile* produces toxins that damage the mucosa, leading to a secretory diarrhea (Rogers, 2005). Symptoms begin within 1 week to 1 month of starting antibiotic therapy.
- Certain tumors, including small-cell lung cancer, ganglioneuroma, pheochromocytoma, carcinoma of thyroid, malignant carcinoids, and gastrinomas, produce one or more of these secretagogue substances (Mercadante, 2002).
- The inability to reabsorb bile acids from the small intestine leads to diarrhea via the secretory effect of these substances on the mucosa of the colon and their osmotic effect in the colon. The result is diarrhea that is watery and explosive (Mercadante, 2002; Sykes, 2003). Ileal resection, gastrectomy with vagotomy, and postirradiation enteritis may interfere with bile acid reabsorption.
- Some medications, such as caffeine, theophylline, antacids, some antibiotics, and poorly absorbable osmotic laxatives, also cause secretory diarrheas via direct simulation of secretions or secondary to irritation of the epithelial cells (Mercadante, 2002).

Pathophysiological Characteristics of Osmotic Diarrhea

The small bowel is highly permeable to sodium and water transport but not to solute. When large amounts of nonabsorbable sugar (e.g., lactulose and sorbitol) are ingested, the ability of the GI tract to compensate may be overwhelmed, resulting in diarrhea from the osmosis of fluid into the lumen. The diarrhea due to carbohydrate malabsorption is characterized by a low pH, high content of carbohydrates, high stool osmolality, and flatulence. Other substances that cause osmotic diarrhea are magnesium, sulfate, and poorly absorbed salts, including bile salts. The pH of diarrhea caused by one of these latter substances is usually normal (Mercadante, 2002).

Persons with lactose intolerance and those receiving high-carbohydrate supplements or enteral feedings are at risk for osmotic diarrhea. The sorbitol in sugar-free elixirs and enteral feedings is often overlooked as a cause of this symptom (Sykes, 2003). The overuse of osmotic laxatives is also a cause of diarrhea for some persons with advanced disease.

Malabsorption of fat is another cause of osmotic diarrhea. Most dietary intake of fat is absorbed in the small intestines and only small amounts of lipids enter the colon. The absorption of fat from the small intestines is dependent on pancreatic enzymes to break down the fats and bile salts to make the fat particles soluble. Pancreatic cancer or resection of the pancreas may cause a deficiency of pancreatic enzymes, leading to malabsorption of fat and steatorrhea. Biliary tract obstruction, terminal ileal resection, and cholestatic liver disease cause a decrease in bile salt formation, again contributing to malabsorption of fat and steatorrhea (Mercadante, 2002). Steatorrhea is characterized by loose, pale, foul-smelling feces. The feces may be greasy in appearance and tend to float in the toilet, making them difficult to flush.

Pathophysiological Characteristics of Diarrhea Due to Hypermotility

When GI tract motility is abnormally stimulated, bowel contents are moved through the intestines too quickly to prevent adequate absorption, leading to diarrhea. Several factors may contribute to GI hypermotility.

Parasympathetic stimulation enhances GI motility and leads to diarrhea. Both the small and the large intestines receive parasympathetic stimulation from the vagus and the hypogastric plexus. Stimulation of the sympathetic nervous system inhibits activity of the GI tract and generally acts to balance parasympathetic activity. Sympathetic innervation originates in the celiac, superior mesenteric, inferior mesenteric, and hypogastric ganglia (Rogers, 2005). If sympathetic activity is blocked, leaving the parasympathetic activity unopposed, hypermotility and diarrhea may result. This is the likely mechanism for the diarrhea associated with celiac plexus block (Mercadante, 2002).

- Irritation of the small or large bowel may stimulate an increase in peristaltic activity. In addition to causing increasing secretions in the GI tract, food poisoning and infections may directly irritate the small bowel and increase motility. This is generally considered a protective mechanism to rid the body of the irritative substance. Ulcerative colitis and tumors of the large bowel may similarly increase the motility of the large bowel due to direct irritation.
- Medications that increase bowel motility, including stimulant laxatives and cholinergics (e.g., metoclopramide), may also lead to diarrhea.

Pathophysiological Characteristics of Exudative Diarrhea

The presence of serum proteins, blood, or excessive amounts of mucus in the bowel contributes to diarrhea.

- Excessive proteins may be seen with bowel obstruction. The obstruction increases intestinal capillary pressure and causes serum proteins to leak into the intestinal lumen. This has an osmotic effect and pulls in more fluids, leading to diarrhea.
- Tumors of the bowel or any GI ulceration may cause bleeding into an intestinal lumen. Blood, like serum proteins, has an osmotic effect.
- The large intestine has many crypts of Lieberkühn lined with epithelial cells. The primary purpose of these epithelial cells is to secrete mucus. Normally, this mucus serves to lubricate the bowel lumen and soften the stool. In the presence of abnormal stimulation, as may occur with tumors, partial or complete bowel obstruction, or impactions, excessive amounts of mucus may be secreted.

Diarrhea in AIDS Patients

Most diarrheas in AIDS patients are due to infection. Although some pathogens are those that also infect immunocompetent patients, most are opportunistic infections. Cytomegalovirus and cryptosporidiosis are the most common forms of diarrhea in HIV-infected patients, but other protozoan, viral, fungal, and bacterial infections are also seen in this population (Cohen et al., 2001).

ASSESSMENT AND MEASUREMENT

A thorough assessment and physical examination of the patient are required to identify the causes of diarrhea and guide appropriate intervention. Measurement of the severity of diarrhea is based on the number and quantity of loose stools per day and any associated symptoms. The National Cancer Institute developed a grading tool for diarrhea severity related to cancer treatment on a 0-to-4 scale (Table 26-2).

TABLE 26-2 ■ Common Toxicity Criteria for Diarrhea

	GRADE				
	0	1	2	3	4
Symptoms	None	Increase of <4 stools per day over baseline; mild increase in ostomy output compared to baseline	Increase of 4 to 6 stools per day over baseline; IV fluids indicated for less than 24 hr; moderate increase in ostomy output compared to baseline; not interfering with activities of daily living	Increase to 7 or more stools per day over baseline; incontinence; IV fluids for 24 hr or longer; hospitalization; severe increase in ostomy output compared to baseline; interfering with activities of daily living	Life-threatening consequences (e.g., hemodynamic collapse)

Modified from National Cancer Institute. (2003). *Common terminology criteria for adverse events version 3.0.* Bethesda, Md.: Author. Retrieved November 14, 2005, from http://ctep.cancer.gov/forms/CTCAEv3.pdf.

This scale is useful in categorizing responses to treatment for research purposes and could be used in the clinical setting. However, many patients and health care practitioners use the number of diarrhea stools per day as a "rating scale." The rating scale used must be clear to all persons since a 4 on the NCI scale is very different from having four diarrhea stools in 1 day.

The character and amount of diarrhea provide clues regarding the underlying cause.

- Disorders of the small intestine or proximal colon tend to cause large amounts of diarrhea that is light in color and watery or greasy. Undigested food may be present, but blood usually is not.
- Disorders of the left side of the colon or rectum tend to cause small amounts of diarrhea that is dark in color and contains mucus or blood. This diarrhea may also be accompanied by a sense of rectal urgency (Mercadante, 2002).
- Stools that are pale and fatty and have an offensive odor indicate steatorrhea and fat malabsorption.
- Diarrhea that follows several days of constipation suggests fecal impaction or partial obstruction (Mercadante, 2002; Sykes, 2003).
- Osmotic diarrheas tend to stop with fasting, whereas diarrhea that persists after a 2- or 3-day fast suggests a secretory process. Hypermotility disorders are suspected when osmotic and secretory diarrhea is ruled out (Levy, 1991).
- General history
  - ▶ Terminal diagnosis and its potential effect on bowel functioning or risk of infection

    Bowel tumors

    Immunosuppression
  - ▶ History of chronic bowel diseases (e.g., ulcerative colitis)
  - ▶ History of food intolerances or allergies, especially intolerance of milk or milk products due to lactase deficiency
  - ▶ Recent history of chemotherapy
  - ▶ Recent or past history of radiation therapy
  - ▶ Recent food and fluid intake, including alcohol consumption
  - ▶ Current medications:

    Laxatives (excessive stimulative laxatives cause colic and urgency; excessive softening leads to fecal leakage) (Sykes, 2003)

    Antibiotics

    Any new medication
- Diarrhea history
  - ▶ Duration (how long diarrhea has been present)
  - ▶ Whether diarrhea was preceded by constipation
  - ▶ Frequency (number of diarrhea stools in 24 hours)
  - ▶ Timing (times of day when diarrhea is worse or absent):

    Association with intake of food or fluids

    Wakening of the patient from sleep
  - ▶ Quantity (size of diarrhea stools):

    Consistency (e.g., semiformed, unformed, liquid)

    Color (light or dark)

    Other characteristics (e.g., foul odor, tendency to float in toilet)

Discomfort (e.g., location of associated pain—periumbilical colicky pain often indicates small intestinal origin, whereas left-sided lower abdominal pain may indicate lower colon or rectal origin)
■ Physical examination
▸ Auscultate bowel sounds:
Hyperactivity with most diarrheas
Intestinal obstruction indicated by high-pitched sounds accompanied by abdominal cramping (Bickley, 2004)
▸ Palpate abdomen for fecal or tumor mass
▸ Note any ascites or abdominal distension
▸ Examine the rectum for tone, presence of feces in ampulla, or signs of rectal discharge
▸ Assess the presence of fever, indicative of an infectious process
▸ Note any signs of dehydration:
Postural hypotension
Poor skin turgor
Decreased urine output
▸ Assess nutritional status (in advanced diseases, it may be difficult to determine whether the cause of poor nutritional status is related more to terminal illness or to malabsorption of nutrients)

DIAGNOSTICS

Often, a careful history and clinical examination identify the cause of diarrhea and further diagnostic evaluation is not necessary. If information is not sufficient, examination of the stool for pus, blood, fat, and ova and parasites, as well as stool culture, may be appropriate (Mercadante, 2002; Sykes, 2003). Guaiac-positive diarrhea indicates an exudative mechanism, such as chronic radiation colitis, cancerous tumor, or infectious diarrhea.

Bowel obstructions are often diagnosed on the basis of findings from the patient's history and physical examination. Abdominal radiography to confirm a bowel obstruction is generally not necessary in palliative care settings. If a surgical intervention for the bowel obstruction is a consideration, radiography is appropriate.

Calculating the stool osmolality anion gap (stool osmolality anion gap = stool osmolality − 2 [stool sodium + stool potassium]) can assist in determining whether the diarrhea is osmotic or secretory:

■ If the stool osmolality anion gap is more than 50 mmol/L, the diarrhea is osmotic.
■ If the stool osmolality anion gap is less than 50 mmol/L, the diarrhea is secretory.

In addition to calculation of the anion gap, the presence of secretory agents in the serum, such as vasoactive protein, gastrin, and calcitonin, may indicate a secretory diarrhea (Levy, 1991).

Endoscopy, biopsy, or barium radiography may be necessary to determine the cause of inflammatory processes (Levy, 1991). The patient's physical status and ability to tolerate the procedure, as well as the likelihood of identifying a treatable cause of the diarrhea, are important considerations when determining the appropriateness of these invasive, uncomfortable procedures.

INTERVENTION AND TREATMENT

Appropriate interventions are aimed at treating reversible causes of diarrhea, preventing complications, promoting comfort, and improving quality of living.

General Measures

Discontinue any laxatives and begin a clear liquid diet to promote bowel rest. It is helpful to avoid very hot and very cold foods, as well as any milk products. Gradually, add semisolids such as bananas, rice, applesauce, and crackers or plain toast. The diet can be advanced as tolerated. Encourage a gluten-free diet to reduce abdominal cramping, and avoid fatty foods, whole grain products, and fresh fruits and vegetables.

Monitor hydration status by tracking intake and output. Most diarrhea in palliative care other than HIV-associated diarrhea is rarely of sufficient amount or duration to require rehydration (Sykes, 2003). When rehydration is necessary, oral hydration is preferred. The rehydration solution should contain glucose, electrolytes, and water. Use commercial sports drinks (e.g., Gatorade) or dextrose and electrolyte solutions available at pharmacies (e.g., Resol, Rehydralyte, Pedialyte). As an alternative, make a solution of ½ teaspoon salt, ½ teaspoon baking soda, and 4 tablespoons sugar in 1 liter of water (Carpenito, 2000). The World Health Organization's recommended rehydration solution is 2 g of salt plus 2 g of sugar in 1 liter of water. This can be flavored with lemon juice if desired (Waller & Caroline, 2000). Homemade solutions should be used within 24 hours of preparation. Intravenous or hypodermoclysis replacement may be required if the patient is unable to tolerate sufficient oral intake.

It is essential to provide good skin care. Keep the perianal area clean and protected. Avoid rubbing the area with wash clothes or towels. Use a pH-balanced cleanser or warm water applied using a squeeze bottle with gentle pressure. Sitz baths also help cleanse and promote comfort. Avoid soaps, since they are drying. After cleansing, apply a moisturizer followed by a barrier that contains zinc oxide, dimethicone, or silicone. Petrolatum-based products should be avoided, since they need to be reapplied frequently (Fleck, 2005). If the patient is experiencing massive amounts of diarrhea, consider the use of a fecal incontinence bag to protect skin, decrease caregiver burden, and help control odor.

Treat Cause of Diarrhea

- If the diarrhea is related to medications, stop the offending agents(s) when possible.
- If the diarrhea is due to fecal impaction, perform a manual disimpaction. Premedicate patients for this procedure. Waller and Caroline (2000) suggest sedation with midazolam, 1 mg intravenously, titrated up by 0.5-mg increments as needed, plus morphine. An oral benzodiazepine and opioid are also effective if the patient is premedicated 1 to 1½ hours before the procedure. Provide local anesthesia by applying lidocaine jelly onto the anus and then instilling 10 ml of 1% lidocaine jelly into the rectum. Wait 10 minutes before performing the digital removal of stool (Waller & Caroline, 2000). Following disimpaction, adjust laxatives to prevent future constipation.
- If the diarrhea is caused by infection, assess the potential of treating the infection. In acute, self-limited diarrhea, such as common viral-related diarrhea, no antiinfective treatment may be necessary. When pseudomembranous colitis is suspected, begin metronidazole, 500 mg orally every 8 hours for 10 days. Vancomycin, 125 to

250 mg orally every 6 hours for 10 days, should be reserved for second-line therapy (Hodgson & Kizior, 2004; Poutanen, 2004; Sykes, 2003).

■ For more prolonged infection-related diarrhea, which most often occurs in the AIDS population, the antiinfective is ideally selected based on the documented causative agent. Evaluation of the patient's physical status and preferences regarding treatment and the likelihood of disease response to treatment is essential in planning appropriate treatment. Doses of antiinfective treatments often need to be reduced in the presence of renal dysfunction. Consultation with an infectious disease specialist is recommended:

▶ AIDS patients with diarrhea respond better to antidiarrheal therapy and have fewer relapses of diarrhea when concurrently treated with antiretroviral therapy or protease inhibitors (Cohen et al., 2001; Maggi, Larocca, Quarto et al., 2000). Currently, there is debate on whether to continue an antiinfective at a maintenance dose after treatment of the acute infection in persons who are receiving highly active antiretroviral therapy (Aberg, Williams, Liu et al., 2003; Benson, Kaplan, Masur et al., 2004; Cohen et al., 2001).

▶ Cryptosporidiosis is best treated by effective antiretroviral therapy. Alternatively, nitazoxanide 500 mg orally every 12 hours for 3 days or paramomycin 25 to 35 mg/kg orally in three divided doses for 5 to 6 days (Benson et al., 2004) can be used.

▶ *Salmonella* spp. are usually treated with ciprofloxacin 500 to 750 mg orally twice daily. Duration of therapy for mild gastroenteritis is 7 to 14 days, and for advanced HIV therapy, it is continued for 4 to 6 weeks. Ciprofloxacin 500 mg orally twice daily may be continued for chronic suppression therapy (Benson et al., 2004).

▶ *Isospora belli* sp. are effectively treated with trimethoprim-sulfamethoxazole 80 to 160 mg/400 to 800 mg orally twice daily to four times daily for 10 days (Cohen et al., 2001; Verdier, Fitzgerald, Johnson et al, 2000; Woodruff & Glare, 2003).

▶ Cytomegalovirus often responds to treatment with ganciclovir or foscarnet intravenously for 21 to 28 days. The oral formulation of ganciclovir or valganciclovir may be used if symptoms are not severe enough to interfere with oral absorption (Benson et al., 2004). Ganciclovir is recommended for maintenance, since it is more cost effective and has fewer side effects (Somerville, 2003).

▶ A broad-spectrum antiinfective, such as ciprofloxacin or metronidazole, may be initiated if findings of studies are negative (Woodruff & Glare, 2003). Antiviral agents should also be considered when culture results are negative. However, remember that the protease inhibitors nelfinavir and ritonavir commonly cause diarrhea (Cohen et al., 2001).

▶ If diarrhea is caused by fat malabsorption, consider administering pancreatic enzymes. The starting dose of pancreatin or pancrelipase is two capsules or tablets orally with meals and one capsule or tablet with snacks. The dose can be increased to three capsules or tablets with meals, if needed (Hodgson & Kizior, 2004). Famotidine, an H_2 histamine receptor antagonist, has also been noted to increase fat absorption (Waller & Caroline, 2000). The recommended dose is 20 mg orally twice daily.

▶ If the diarrhea is due to bile salt malabsorption, administer cholestyramine. This medication absorbs and combines with bile acids to form an insoluble complex that is then eliminated in the feces. Administer 4 to 8 g orally three times daily (Hodgson & Kizior, 2004; Waller & Caroline, 2000).

Treat Discomfort

Discomfort associated with diarrhea includes gas pain and colicky pain. Simethicone is helpful for gas-related discomfort. Anticholinergic medications treat most colicky pain effectively. Examples of anticholinergic medications include propantheline (Pro-Banthine), 15 mg orally two or three times daily; hyoscyamine (Anaspaz, Levsin), 0.125 to 0.25 mg orally three or four times daily; and dicyclomine (Antispas, Bentyl), 20 mg orally three or four times daily (Hodgson & Kizior, 2004).

Control Diarrhea

Because diarrhea can be protective by flushing out irritative substances, avoid antidiarrheals for acute diarrhea. Adsorbent agents, such as attapulgite (Kaopectate), work by taking up substances nonspecifically, including bacteria, toxins, and water. They may be helpful for mild diarrhea in the healthy population. However, the large volumes required and their moderate effectiveness make them undesirable for palliative care (Sykes, 2003).

Mucosal prostaglandin inhibitors are helpful for acute diarrhea that requires an antidiarrheal for comfort and for those that involve an inflammatory process (e.g., radiation enteritis). Any nonsteroidal antiinflammatory drug (NSAID), except indomethacin, may be helpful (Sykes, 2003). Bismuth subsalicylate (Pepto-Bismol) is also a mucosal prostaglandin inhibitor. The recommended dosage is 30 ml or 2 tablets orally every 30 to 60 minutes, not to exceed eight doses per day for more than 2 days. Another GI antiinflammatory medication is mesalamine (Asacol). Administer 2400 mg/day orally in divided doses (Hodgson & Kizior, 2004). Psyllium-containing products such as Metamucil may also be useful for their ability to absorb excess fluid within the bowel (Montagnini, 2004).

Opioids are the mainstay of general antidiarrheal treatment in palliative settings (Sykes, 2003). They work by decreasing intestinal motility, leading to increased fluid absorption. Loperamide is the preferred opioid for diarrhea as it does not cross the blood-brain barrier and therefore has the highest antidiarrheal-to-analgesic ratio of the opioid-like agents (Mercadante, 2002). Loperamide is also about three times more potent than diphenoxylate and 50 times more potent than codeine. It is also long-acting, requiring only twice-daily dosing when long-term management of diarrhea is required. Tincture of opium (paregoric), which is sometimes used when diarrhea is refractory to loperamide, crosses the blood-brain barrier and thus causes systemic opioid effects. The bitter taste of tincture of opium may be nauseating to some persons. Dosages for all of these opioid antidiarrheals are as follows:

- Loperamide (Imodium): initial dose of 4 mg, followed by 2 mg after each loose stool. The generally accepted maximal dose is 16 mg/day (Hodgson & Kizior, 2004; Sykes, 2003; Waller & Caroline, 2000).
- Diphenoxylate (in Lomotil): initial dose of 5 mg, followed by 2.5 to 5 mg orally four times daily, titrated to patient response (Hodgson & Kizior, 2004; Sykes, 2003).
- Codeine phosphate: 10 to 60 mg orally four times daily. Codeine is usually avoided due to systemic opioid effects, but it is inexpensive (Skyes, 2003).
- 10% Tincture of opium: 0.3 to 1 ml orally four times daily (Waller & Caroline, 2000).

Octreotide, an analogue of the hormone somatostatin, inhibits GI motility, pancreatic secretion, and intestinal absorption. It has been demonstrated to be effective in the management of chemotherapy-induced diarrhea, diarrhea associated with dumping syndrome, and chronic diarrhea not responsive to specific antimicrobial therapy (Rosenoff, 2004; Sykes, 2003). It has also been shown to be helpful in controlling diarrhea due to secretory tumors and celiac plexus block (Mercadante, 2002; Sykes, 2003). Side effects include nausea, pain at the injection site, and headache. Because octreotide is expensive, this medication is generally reserved for those whose condition is refractory to other interventions. Dosages range from 150 to 600 mcg/day subcutaneously, either in divided doses or by continuous infusion. Waller and Caroline (2000) suggest the following:

- For chemotherapy or radiation therapy–induced diarrhea, administer 100 mcg subcutaneously twice daily.
- For postgastectomy dumping syndrome, administer 300 mcg/day by continuous infusion.
- For carcinoid syndrome, administer 150 to 300 mcg SC twice daily or 300 to 600 mcg/day by continuous infusion.

Clonidine may be helpful for some secretory diarrheas. This medication probably acts on enterocytes to suppress the release of secretory substances. The side effects of hypotension and sedation may limit its usefulness in palliative care (Mercadante, 2002).

PATIENT AND FAMILY EDUCATION

Detailed information from the patient and family is required in order to assess the potential causes of diarrhea and plan appropriate interventions. The clinician must teach the importance of prompt and detailed reporting of any changes in bowel patterns:

- Discuss the importance of reporting bowel functioning, including frequency, amount, color, and consistency of stools and any discomforts associated with bowel movements, to the health care team.
- Encourage adequate oral fluid intake to replace fluid losses due to diarrhea.
    - Provide instruction on the purchase or preparation of fluids with sugar and electrolytes.
    - If intravenous hydration is required at home, provide instruction on intravenous catheter site care and maintenance of the intravenous fluids.
- Teach the following dietary modifications to lessen diarrhea, taking into consideration the patient's desire and ability to eat.
    - Eat or provide small, frequent meals.
    - Avoid excessively hot, cold, or spicy foods.
    - Avoid caffeine.
    - Avoid milk products, fat, whole grains, and fresh fruits and vegetables.
    - Broaden the diet as tolerated, beginning with white bread, pasta, potatoes, rice, and fruits. The old mnemonic "BRAT" may be helpful in remembering acceptable foods: bananas, rice or rice cereals, applesauce, and toast.
    - In persons with a lactase deficiency, teach the use of lactose-free dairy products.
- Teach appropriate use of all medications, including antidiarrheals, anticholinergics, and antiinfective agents.
- Patients with prolonged diarrhea may require antidiarrheal medications on a schedule rather than as needed.

> As appropriate to the patient's condition and goals, teach patients with AIDS the importance of maintaining antiretroviral therapy during and after treatment for diarrhea.
> Instruction on giving subcutaneous injections or maintaining subcutaneous infusions is required for patients who are receiving octreotide.

■ Discuss the importance of perianal care:
> Teach the patient and family good, gentle cleansing techniques using a squeeze bottle of warm water.
> Teach how to monitor for skin breakdown.
> Teach appropriate use of skin barrier products.

EVALUATION AND PLAN FOR FOLLOW-UP

Frequently monitor the patient's bowel status, hydration status, and level of comfort. If diarrhea continues after instituting a treatment, appropriate changes must occur in the treatment plan. Determine if the cause was not correctly diagnosed or if a different treatment might be more effective. Encourage patients whose diarrhea continues for several days to keep intake and output records. This will assist in evaluating the need for supplemental oral or parenteral fluids.

At all times the patient is evaluated for comfort, including abdominal pain due to gas or GI spasm and discomfort associated with skin excoriation. Encourage the patient to describe the type of abdominal discomfort so that appropriate interventions are prescribed. Teach good skin care to prevent skin excoriation and instruct the patient and caregivers to report skin discomfort or any changes in the condition of the skin.

CASE STUDY The daughter of Mrs. A., an 82-year-old patient with advanced ovarian cancer, calls to report that her mother has had several bouts of diarrhea over the past 2 days. The daughter states that she gave her mother a few doses of loperamide (Imodium) both yesterday and today, but the diarrhea continues. She also reports that her mother is complaining of abdominal pain and cramping with the diarrhea. Mrs. A.'s medications include the following:

■ Sustained-release oxycodone, 40 mg orally twice daily, with a rescue dose of oxycodone, 10 mg orally every 1 to 2 hours as needed for pain
■ Docusate sodium–sennosides 50 mg/8.6 mg, 2 tablets orally at bedtime for constipation
■ Lorazepam, 1 mg orally every 6 hours as needed for anxiety
■ Digoxin, 0.125 mg orally daily for heart failure (well-controlled)

The clinician's questions elicit the following information. The diarrhea is dark and has the consistency of mucus. It occurred in small amounts, "maybe a quarter of a cup or so," five or six times over the past 24 hours. There is no pattern related to food intake. Mrs. A. is complaining of intermittent cramping pain in her lower abdomen and a sensation of rectal fullness: "like her bowels are still full even after the diarrhea." The patient's last regular bowel movement was 5 days ago.

The clinician suspects a fecal impaction with overflow diarrhea and instructs the family to give no additional loperamide and to give Mrs. A. a dose of her immediate-release oxycodone for the discomfort. The clinician schedules a home visit for later in the afternoon. Upon arrival the clinician notes that the patient's mucous membranes are dry and that she has poor skin turgor. The physical assessment reveals a distended abdomen with mild ascites. Bowel sounds are intermittent, high-pitched, and tinkling. There is dark liquid stool around the rectum, and a digital rectal examination reveals a large mass of hard, dry stool in the rectum.

The clinician tells the patient and family that the diarrhea is caused by a blockage of the bowel with hard stool. She explains the need for removal of the impaction, gives the patient an oil retention enema, and instructs the daughter to give Mrs. A. her lorazepam and immediate-release oxycodone. The clinician applies lidocaine jelly to the rectal area.

While waiting for the stool to soften as much as possible with the enema and for the medications to begin to work, the clinician explains that the combination of the pain medication and decreased fluid intake caused this blockage. The clinician discusses the following instructions with the patient and family:

- Increase the docusate sodium–sennosides 50 mg/8.6 mg to 2 tablets orally twice daily.
- Monitor bowel movements:
- If no bowel movement occurs in 2 days, give a 10-mg bisacodyl suppository. If there are no results, call the clinician.
- If diarrhea occurs, call the clinician.
- Increase fluid intake by mouth, as tolerated:
- Mix a solution of ½ teaspoon salt, ½ teaspoon baking soda, and 4 tablespoons sugar in 1 liter of water. Mrs. Anderson should sip the drink during the day, aiming to drink 1 liter of the fluid each day. Keep this solution refrigerated and discard any unused solution after 24 hours.
- If the patient is unable to drink at least 1 liter a day, contact the clinician.

The clinician also writes these instructions because the patient's discomfort and medications may interfere with her ability to understand and remember information at the present time.

Now that the local anesthetic and oil retention enema have had time to be effective, the clinician digitally removes the impaction and gives a cleansing enema. The nurse cleans the rectal area with a squeeze bottle of warm water and applies a silicone-based skin barrier cream to the reddened but intact skin. She reinforces the instructions and plans a follow-up telephone call in the morning.

REFERENCES

Aberg, J.A., Williams, P.L., Liu, T., et al; AIDS Clinical Trial Group 393 Study Team. (2003). A study of discontinuing maintenance therapy in human immunodeficiency virus-related subjects with disseminated *Mycobacterium avium* complex: AIDS Clinical Trial Group 393 Study Team. *J Infect Dis, 187(7)*, 1046-1052.

Anastasi, J.K. & Capili, B. (2000). HIV and diarrhea in the era of HAART: 1998 New York State hospitalizations. *Am J Infect Control, 28*, 262-266.

Benson, C.A., Kaplan, J.E., Masur, H., et al. (2004). *Treating opportunistic infections among HIV-infected adults and adolescents: Recommendations from CDC, the National Institutes of Health, and the HIV Medicine Association/Infectious Diseases of Society of America.* Retrieved November 15, 2005, from www.cdc.gov/mmwr/preview/mmwrhtml/rr5315a1.htm

Bickley, L.S. (2004). The abdomen. In L.S. Bickley (Ed.). *Bates' guide to physical examination and history taking* (8th ed., pp. 355-386). Philadelphia: Lippincott.

Carpenito, L.J. (2000). *Nursing diagnosis: Application to clinical practice* (8th ed.). Philadelphia: Lippincott.

Cohen, J., West, A.B., & Bini, E.J. (2001). Infectious diarrhea in human immunodeficiency virus. *Gastroenterol Clin North Am, 30(3)*, 637-664.

Fleck, C.A. (2005). Ethical wound management for the palliative patient. *Extended Care Product News, 100(4)*, 38-46.

Hodgson, B.B. & Kizior, R.J. (2004). *Saunders nursing drug handbook 2004.* St. Louis: Saunders.

Levy, M.H. (1991). Constipation and diarrhea in cancer patients. *Cancer Bull, 43*, 412-422.

Lingappa, V.R. (2003). Gastrointestinal disease. In S.J. McPhee, V.R. Lingappa, & W.F. Ganong (Eds.). *Pathophysiology of disease: An introduction to clinical medicine* (4th ed., pp. 340-379). New York: Lange Medical Books/McGraw-Hill.

Maggi, P., Larocca, A.M., Quarto, M., et al. (2000). Effect of antiretroviral therapy on cryptosporidiosis and microsporidiosis in patients infected with human immunodeficiency virus type 1. *Eur J Clin Microbiol Infect Dis, 19*, 213-217.

Mercadante, W. (2002). Diarrhea, malabsorption, and constipation. In A. Berger, R. Portenoy, & D. Weissman (Eds.). *Principles and practice of palliative and supportive oncology* (2nd ed., pp. 233-249). Philadelphia: Lippincott Williams & Wilkins.

Montagnini, M. (2004). Non-pain symptom management in palliative care. *Clin Fam Pract, 6(2)*, 395-422.

Poutanen, S.M. (2004). *Clostridium difficile*-associated diarrhea in adults. *Can Med Assoc J, 171(1)*, 51-58.

Rogers, H.M. (2005). Management of clients with intestinal disorders. In J.M. Black & J.H. Hawks (Eds.). *Medical-surgical nursing: Clinical management for positive outcomes* (7th ed., pp. 807-855). St. Louis: Elsevier Saunders.

Rosenoff, S.H. (2004). Octreotide LAR resolves severe chemotherapy-induced diarrhoea (CID) and allows continuation of full-dose therapy. *Eur J Cancer Care (Engl), 13(4)*, 380-383.

Sanchez, T.H., Brooks, J.T., Sullivan, P.S., et al; Adult/Adolescent Spectrum of HIV Disease Study Group. (2005). Bacterial diarrhea in persons with HIV disease, United States, 1992-2002. *Clin Infect Dis, 41(11)*, 1621-1627.

Somerville, K.T. (2003). Cost advantages of oral drug therapy for managing cytomegalovirus disease. *Am J Health-Sys Pharm, 60(23 Suppl 8)*, S9-S12.

Sykes, N. (2003). Constipation and diarrhoea. In D. Doyle, G. Hanks, N.I. Cherny, & K. Calman (Eds.). *Oxford textbook of palliative medicine* (3rd ed., pp. 483-496). New York: Oxford University Press.

Verdier, R., Fitzgerald, D., Johnson, W., et al. (2000). Trimethoprim-sulfamethoxazole compared with ciprofloxacin for treatment and prophylaxis of *Isospora belli* and *Cyclospora cayetanensis* infection in HIV-infected patients: A randomized controlled trial. *Ann Intern Med, 132*, 885-888.

Waller, A. & Caroline, N.L. (2000). *Handbook of palliative care in cancer* (2nd ed.). Boston: Butterworth-Heinemann.

Woodruff, R. & Glare, P. (2003). AIDS in adults. In D. Doyle, G. Hanks, N.I. Cherny, et al. (Eds.). *Oxford textbook of palliative medicine* (3rd ed., pp. 847-880). New York: Oxford University Press.

CHAPTER 27

DYSPNEA

Kim K. Kuebler, Jerald M. Andry, and Shawn Davis

■

The symptom of dyspnea, or breathlessness, has been defined as an uncomfortable awareness of breathing (Baines, 1978). The American Thoracic Society (ATS) defines *dyspnea* as "a subjective experience of breathing discomfort that consists of qualitatively distinct sensations that vary in intensity" (ATS, 1999). The experience is a combination of physiological, social, and environmental factors that potentiate physiological and behavioral response (ATS, 1999). Dyspnea not only is a common companion to pulmonary and cardiac diseases, but also often accompanies the dying process. The clinician providing management for the patient with dyspnea should always consider the underlying pathophysiology contributing to the patient's breathlessness. Having knowledge related to the cause of dyspnea will direct the clinician on how best to strategize his or her diagnostic evaluation and consideration for specific interventions.

The literature suggests that there is a large variation in the reported prevalence of dyspnea, which ranges from 21% to 79% (Bruera, Sweeney, & Ripamonti, 2002). "These variations are a result of the different natures of patient populations reported by different authors and the lack of a general consensus regarding the assessment and evaluation of dyspnea" (Bruera et al., p. 359, 2002). A number of authors have reported the incidence of dyspnea in different patient populations that include patients in the last month of life, patients with advanced cancer, and patients without intrathoracic malignancies, chronic congestive heart failure, and chronic obstructive pulmonary disease (COPD) (Bruera et al., 2002). Most cancer patients develop progressive dyspnea over days or weeks, yet for those patients who experience a sudden onset of dyspnea, a medical emergency should be considered (Bruera et al., 2002).

ETIOLOGY AND PATHOPHYSIOLOGY

Dyspnea encompasses complex interactions between peripheral and central sensory receptors and cognition, while the underlying causation remains unknown. Physiological, psychological, behavioral, social, and environmental factors play a role in the pathogenesis and perception of dyspnea (Rao & Gray, 2003). Although the underlying medical condition may not be treatable in the palliative care patient, dyspnea almost always responds to intervention or treatment.

Normal Control of Breathing

As simplistic as inhaling and exhaling seems, it is actually a complex of physiological mechanisms that are constantly adapting to a multitude of psychological, social, and environmental factors. The main function associated with the respiratory system is to obtain oxygen from the atmosphere to supply functioning cells and remove carbon dioxide (CO) produced by cellular metabolism (Levitzky, 2003). All respiratory processes are controlled by the central nervous system, which responds to stimuli in order to maintain homeostasis. The primary example is how the respiratory center in the medulla oblongata responds to stimuli from four primary sources (ATS, 1999; Guyton & Hall, 1996):

- Chemoreceptors in the aorta, carotid arteries, and medulla sense changes in Po_2, Pco_2, and pH and transmit signals back to the respiratory center to adjust breathing. The peripheral chemoreceptors (i.e., those in the aortic arch and carotid arteries) are most sensitive to changes in Po_2. When Po_2 decreases, ventilation increases. However, hypoxia must be fairly profound before this change in respiratory pattern is seen. The central chemoreceptors of the medulla are very sensitive to changes in pH. Changes in pH are closely related to Pco_2. Hypercapnia leads to a decrease in pH, which then stimulates ventilation.

- Mechanoreceptors in the diaphragm and chest wall sense changes in the work of breathing. When an increased workload is sensed, the respiratory center stimulates the diaphragm and respiratory muscles and attempts to expand the lungs.

- Vagal receptors in the airways and lungs also influence breathing. Afferent impulses are generated when (1) stretch receptors in the lungs are stimulated as the lungs expand, (2) irritant receptors in the bronchial walls are stimulated, or (3) C fibers in the interstitium of the lungs respond to increases in pulmonary interstitial or capillary pressure.

- Cortical areas of the brain affect breathing by allowing individuals to consciously increase or decrease their respiratory rate. It also appears that the chemoreceptors, mechanoreceptors, and respiratory center itself send messages to higher brain centers, leading to a cognitive awareness of the ventilatory demand.

Mechanisms Leading to Dyspnea

Patients may describe dyspnea by using several phrases such as "My breathing requires effort," "I feel a hunger for more air," or "I feel out of breath" (Harver, Mahler, Schwartzstein et al., 2000). In a palliative care patient, the perception of dyspnea includes several qualitatively distinct sensations that may be caused by one or more pathophysiological mechanisms (Manning & Schwartzstein, 1995). As described, receptors throughout the body will trigger the central nervous system when homeostasis is altered, which can ultimately lead to the feeling of dyspnea. However, specific data are not available to explain how dyspnea is processed by higher brain centers in humans (Guz, 1997). Research has shown that the known dyspnea pathways may be shared by painful stimuli such as heat, cold, and electrical stimulation (von Leupoldt & Dahme, 2005). Thus, there may be a common neural network explaining pain and dyspnea, which are common symptoms in the palliative care patient population. Before the brain can interpret changes and alter breathing patterns, peripheral stimuli must be gathered by various receptors.

Chemoreceptors found in the blood and brain detect blood-gas abnormalities. As stated, the central chemoreceptors of the medulla are particularly sensitive to fluctuations in pH. Any condition causing retention of CO_2, such as chronic obstructive pulmonary disease (COPD), leads to hypercapnia, which lowers blood pH. Thus, the respiratory system responds by increasing ventilation in order to "blow off" the excess CO_2. It is not known if the dyspnea caused by hypercapnia is a direct effect of chemoreceptor stimulation to higher brain centers or the cognitive perception of the increased ventilatory demand (ATS, 1999; von Leupoldt & Dahme, 2005).

Respiratory muscle abnormalities lead to a mismatch between the central respiratory motor output and the achieved ventilation. Respiratory muscle weakness, whether caused by generalized weakness or a neuromuscular disorder, is perceived as dyspnea. Many persons with advanced diseases experience anorexia, cachexia, and generalized weakness and are at risk for experiencing dyspnea. In diseases that cause hyperinflation of the lung and overexpansion of the thorax, the muscles of inspiration become weakened, leading to the sensation of dyspnea (ATS, 1999; Guyton & Hall, 1996). This dyspnea may be mediated via mechanoreceptor messages to the cortex.

Abnormal ventilatory impedance (e.g., narrow airways or increased airway resistance) leads to stimulation of increased central respiratory motor output. When the effort expended to breathe is not matched by the level of ventilation, dyspnea is perceived (ATS, 1999). This perception may result from vagal or mechanoreceptor stimulation of the cortex.

Cognitive factors also influence the perception of dyspnea (ATS, 1999; Guyton & Hall, 1996; Kuebler, Dahlin, Heidrich et al., 1996; Twycross, 1999). Although many physiological mechanisms lead to a perception of dyspnea, not all dyspnea is a direct result of pathological structural characteristics. Psychological states are interrelated to the dyspneic experience, which may be caused or exacerbated by anxiety, fear, hopelessness, and depression. Breathlessness precipitates anxiety, leading to increased breathlessness and even more anxiety; commonly called the "snowball effect." The patient's perception of dyspnea is decreased when he or she believes that the shortness of breath is treatable and that prompt access to treatment is available.

Dyspnea is predominantly experienced by persons with pulmonary, cardiac, and neuromuscular diseases (Ahmedzai, 1998; Carrieri-Kohlman & Janson-Bjerklie, 1993; Twycross, 1997). Table 27-1 summarizes many of the causes of dyspnea in the terminally ill. Note also that cognitive factors may contribute to all causes of dyspnea; thus, they are not included. Although respiratory muscle abnormality due to weakness may be present in almost all advanced diseases, Table 27-1 lists the diseases in which weakness is most profound.

ASSESSMENT AND MEASUREMENT

Patients who complain of being breathless will often seek some relief through position changes, pursed lip breathing, use of accessory muscles, and/or use of environmental aids such as a fan or sitting near an open window or refraining from being exposed to humidity. Breathlessness can be easily observed (objective evaluation) in the patient who is struggling to breathe—but is often considered a subjective experience. For the clinician, a simple approach used to assess and evaluate the patient's dyspnea would be

TABLE 27-1 ■ Causes of Dyspnea in Terminal Illness

Disease Process	Blood Gas Abnormalities	Increased Ventilatory Demand	Respiratory Muscle Abnormality	Ventilatory Impedence
Pulmonary Disease				
Chronic obstructive pulmonary disease	X	X	X	X
Asthma		X		X
Cystic fibrosis	X		X	X
Pneumonia	X			X
Pleural effusion	X	X		X
Malignancy	X	X	X	X
Radiation pneumonitis	X			X
Pulmonary embolism	X			X
Cardiovascular Disease				
Heart failure		X		X
Myopathies	X	X		
Anemia	X		X	
Superior vena cava syndrome	X			X
Neuromuscular Disease				
Muscular dystrophy		X	X	
Myasthenia gravis		X	X	
Amyotrophic lateral sclerosis		X	X	
Paralysis of diaphragm		X	X	

to ask the patient to quantify his or her difficulty in breathing from a numerical scale that is rated from 0 (no breathlessness) to 10 (severe breathlessness). A numerical value provides the clinician with an understanding of the patient's expression of his or her dyspnea intensity. The Edmonton Symptom Assessment System (ESAS) is an example of a numerical rating scale to evaluate the patient's intensity associated with multiple symptoms including dyspnea (Bruera, Kuehn, Miller et al.,1991).

There are several psychometrically valid and reliable dyspnea assessment tools that are used in clinical and research settings to assess and evaluate the symptom of dyspnea. The traditional approach to providing care for patients with chronic respiratory disease has primarily relied on pulmonary function tests (PFTs) to quantify the severity of the patient's disease and/or their response to therapy (Mahler, 2000). However, patients often present for medical attention as a result of their symptoms, particularly dyspnea and an impaired ability to perform activities of daily living, with both contributing to the interference of the patient's perceived quality of life (Mahler, 2000). The patient's perception of breathlessness that interferes with quality of life may not always be accurately reflected in the most recent spirometry evaluation (GOLD, 2003). As previously mentioned, simply asking the patient to rate his or her dyspnea or difficulty breathing from a numerical rating scale may serve as a useful indicator of the patient's self-description of his or her discomfort. Other examples of dyspnea evaluation tools will be briefly described below. The patient's physical status should be considered in instrument selection, since lengthy instruments are not generally appropriate in palliative care populations.

The St. George's Respiratory Questionnaire

The St. George's Respiratory Questionnaire (SGRQ) contains 76 items that are divided into three sections and include:

- Symptoms—affecting normal respirations to include the frequency and severity
- Activity—interference with the ability to engage in activities as a result of breathlessness
- Impact—influence that breathlessness has on a wide array of social and psychological difficulties:

Each of these sections is scored and then a final score is calculated to discern the severity of patient breathlessness (Jones, Quirk, & Baveystock, 1991). The SGRQ was developed to measure quality of life in patients with airway disease with the intent to exert greater sensitivity and be useful in patients with mild as well as severe disease (Jones et al., 1991).

Baseline and Transition Dyspnea Index

The Transition Dyspnea Index (TDI) was developed to provide a discriminative and evaluative assessment of dyspnea in pharmacotherapy trials for COPD (Witek & Mahler, 2003). This tool is divided into the Baseline Dyspnea Index (BDI) as a discriminative instrument to measure dyspnea at a single point in time (Mahler et al., 2004) and the TDI as an evaluative tool to assess changes in dyspnea from baseline. These tools consist of dyspnea indices that assess breathlessness in domains related to functional impairment, magnitude of task, and magnitude of effort (Mahler, Weinberg, Wells et al., 1998; Mahler, Ward, Fierro-Carrion et al., 2004).

The BDI/TDI evaluation tool has been proved useful in multiple clinical trials seeking to evaluate medication use to relieve dyspnea in patients with chronic lung disease. Successful demonstration of the relief of dyspnea with drug therapy depends on achieving consistent results using valid instruments (Witek & Mahler, 2003). The BDI/TDI, however, has received criticism from the interview process maintaining that the interpretation by the interviewer may introduce bias. Recently, the BDI/TDI was modified to allow patients to perform self-administration through a computerized venue. This has been further validated (Mahler et al., 2004).

Medical Research Council

The Medical Research Council Scale was developed in 1959 to provide patients an opportunity to grade their breathlessness based on a single dimension (i.e., daily tasks). This tool has been tested in patients with dyspnea from a variety of respiratory and cardiovascular origins (Fletcher, Elmes, & Wood, 1959).

HISTORY AND PHYSICAL EXAMINATION

Patients experiencing the sensation of dyspnea or breathlessness will often seek medical attention. The clinician encountering the dyspneic patient should consider asking the patient specifically about his or her shortness of breath. Because dyspnea is considered a subjective complaint, it is important to note that patients may often present with tachycardia and look in distress yet may not describe being dyspneic or distressed versus the patient who is not tachypneic or in apparent distress yet may describe having severe breathlessness (Pereira & Bruera, 2001).

The etiology of dyspnea may be easy to discern in most patients by taking a complete history and performing a physical examination. A detailed examination with a focus on the cardiac and respiratory systems is essential (Bruera et al., 2002). Simple measures such as a chest radiograph, digital oximetry, and a complete blood count and comprehensive metabolic profile tests can help in differentiating the cause of dyspnea (Bruera et al., 2002). Pulmonary function tests (PFTs) are useful for the patient with obstructive and restrictive pulmonary disease. These tests are easy to perform at the bedside and can also provide the clinician with valuable information on how the patient responds to specific interventions. If done appropriately, the patient will use a bronchodilator after the first evaluation and measurements are considered before and after bronchodilator use.

Differential diagnostics are important as dyspnea is a complex symptom that may arise from multiple insults. Common contributions to dyspnea can include the following (Bruera et al., 2002; Pereira & Bruera, 2001):

- Primary lung malignancy
- Pleural or pericardial effusion
- Carcinomatous lymphangitis
- Pulmonary embolism
- Chemotherapy-induced fibrosis
- Superior vena cava syndrome
- Depression and anxiety
- Pneumonia
- Muscle deconditioning (cachexia)
- COPD, neuromuscular disease
- Anemia
- Congestive heart failure (cor pulmonale)

DIAGNOSTICS

Diagnostic procedures can provide assistance in identifying the causes of dyspnea and monitoring the course of the illness, but the practitioner must evaluate the appropriateness of such diagnostic tests in palliative care. A diagnosis can sometimes be made based solely on the clinical presentation alone; thus, the burden and cost incurred by the patient must be considered. When a diagnosis is more complicated, a clinician may have a clinical history, physical examination, laboratory tests (complete blood cell count, metabolic panel), and possibly a chest radiograph as an initial work-up. Pulmonary diagnostics, such as spirometry and PFTs (outlined later), provide supporting information to help the clinician make the diagnosis (West, 2003). Additionally, spirometry and PFTs are valuable in following the progress of a patient's dyspnea over time. Other diagnostic tests that may not be used in palliative care include the following (Karnani, Reisfield, & Wilson, 2005; West, 2003):

- Pulse oximetry
- Echocardiography
- Brain natriuretic peptide
- Arterial blood gas
- Ventilation-perfusion ($\dot{V}/\dot{Q}$) scan

- Cardiopulmonary exercise testing
- Bronchoscopy
- Lung biopsy

Spirometry

Spirometry is a highly effort-dependent diagnostic test that measures the volume of air (liters) exhaled or inhaled by a patient as a function of time (Evans & Scanlon, 2003; Karnani et al., 2005). Spirometry allows clinicians to distinguish between obstructive (i.e., asthma and COPD) and restrictive (i.e., fibrosis, chest wall limitation, pleural diseases, neuromuscular disorders) diseases, in which patients experience dyspnea (Karnani et al., 2005; West, 2003). The typical end points measured via spirometry are the forced expiratory volume in 1 second (FEV_1), the forced vital capacity (FVC), and/or the forced expiratory volume in 6 seconds (FEV_6). FVC can be extremely challenging in older or impaired patients, so FEV_6 has been shown to be an acceptable surrogate alternative that is available in most newer spirometers. Spirometry has limitations because it does not allow clinicians to measure lung volumes; other PFTs are used to potentially identify the underlying cause of the patient's dyspnea (Karnani et al., 2005).

Pulmonary Function Tests

PFTs are used in addition to spirometry to determine the volume of air in the lungs at any given time. Such volumes include the total amount of air in the lungs at full inspiration (total lung capacity [TLC]), the amount of air left in the lungs at the end of normal expiration (functional residual capacity [FRC]), and the amount of air remaining after maximal expiration (residual volume [RV]) (Evans & Scanlon, 2003; Karnani et al., 2005). A clinician will may also order a diffusing capacity (DLCO) to estimate the patient's ability to absorb alveolar gases in the lung. The DLCO substitutes CO as a surrogate for oxygen in order to measure the amount of oxygen that is absorbed into the bloodstream (Evans & Scanlon, 2003). By knowing lung volumes and the amount of oxygen absorbed, clinicians are able to narrow the pathophysiology associated with dyspnea.

Radiography: Computed Tomography and Magnetic Resonance Imaging

Clinicians do not typically order radiographs, high-resolution computed tomography (CT) scans, and/or MRI for each patient who presents with dyspnea. However, such diagnostics are ordered to rule in and rule out underlying pathologies that are seen in palliative patients. High-resolution CT could be used to diagnose bronchiectasis and identify pulmonary embolism or idiopathic pulmonary fibrosis (Evans & Scanlon, 2003).

INTERVENTIONS AND TREATMENT

The treatment of dyspnea begins with determining and treating the underlying cause. This includes the appropriate selection of disease-specific and palliative therapies, taking into account prognosis, adverse events, costs, and potential outcomes to the patient. The most common reversible causes of dyspnea are bronchospasm, hypoxia, and anemia (Dudgeon & Lertzman, 1998). Appropriate management of dyspnea requires pharmacological and nonpharmacological treatments. Two types of drugs

TABLE 27-2 ■ Correctable Causes of Dyspnea/Breathlessness

Causes	Management
Respiratory infection	Antibiotics
	Expectorants
	Physiotherapy
Chronic obstructive pulmonary disease and asthma	Bronchodilators
	Corticosteroids
	Theophylline
	Physiotherapy
Hypoxia	Trial of oxygen
Bronchial obstruction and lung collapse	Corticosteroids
Mediastinal obstruction	Radiotherapy
	LASER therapy
	Stent
Lymphangitis carcinomatosa	Corticosteroids
	Diuretics
	Bronchodilators
Pleural effusion	Paracentesis
	Pleurodesis
Ascites	Diuretics
	Paracentesis
Pericardial effusion	Paracentesis
	Corticosteroids
Anemia	Blood transfusion
	Erythropoietin
Cardiac failure	Diuretics
	Digoxin
	Angiotensin-converting enzyme inhibitors
Pulmonary embolism	Anticoagulants (if appropriate)

From Twycross, R. (1999). Correctable causes of breathlessness. In R. Twycross. *Introducing palliative care* (p. 123). Oxon, UK: Radcliffe Medical Press.

that have proved useful in alleviating dyspnea in palliative care are opioids and drugs that decrease anxiety. Table 27-2 summarizes pharmacological options for the management of dyspnea based on cause. Many of the other medications described in this chapter concerning dyspnea relief have primarily been studied in other disease states such as asthma, COPD, and cancer.

Opioids

Opioids are commonly used medications to treat dyspnea in palliative care. The mechanisms of action by which opioids alleviate dyspnea are unclear but may include decreasing the central perception of dyspnea (similar to pain), decreasing anxiety, decreasing sensitivity to hypercapnia, reduction in oxygen consumption, and improved cardiovascular effects (Ahmedzai, 1998; Twycross, 1999; Vismara, Leaman, & Zelis, 1976). Because opioids are respiratory depressants, there are safety concerns. The risk of causing severe respiratory depression with opioid use depends on the prior exposure to opioids, route of administration, rate of titration, and underlying pathophysiology.

Data from several clinical studies reveal that 80% to 95% of terminal cancer patients achieved significant relief of dyspnea through the use of morphine (Bruera, Sala, Spruyt et al., 2005; Harwood, 1999; Mahler, 1990). A systematic review of 18 studies on the use of opioids in the management of dyspnea has been conducted (Jennings, Davies, Higgins et al., 2002). Most of the patients in the meta-analysis had COPD. The authors concluded that there is a significant positive effect of opioids in the treatment of breathlessness. In addition, oral or parenteral opioids showed a greater effect than nebulized formulations. Low-dose sustained-release oral morphine has been shown to provide significant improvements in refractory dyspnea in patients with COPD (Abernethy, Currow, Frith et al., 2003).

Nebulized formulations of opioids deliver medication directly to the airways and pulmonary circulation, avoiding first-pass metabolism by the liver. Studies evaluating the effectiveness of nebulized opioids have been inconclusive and predominantly negative; however, positive case reports have been published (Sarhill, Walsh, Khawam et al., 2000). Nebulized morphine was shown to be no more effective at reducing dyspnea than nebulized saline solution (Davis, 1996). Results of several small studies of nebulized morphine do not support its use to treat dyspnea (Brown, Eichner, & Jones, 2005). It has been suggested that nebulized opioids may not be delivered in a high enough concentration to affect dyspnea (Baydur, 2004). A recent preliminary study evaluating nebulized versus subcutaneous morphine to treat dyspnea in cancer patients showed that both routes of administration offered similar relief of dyspnea, but due to the low number of patients in the study, a difference between routes could not be determined (Bruera et al., 2005). Due to the number of conflicting studies and lack of large clinical trials, the utility of nebulized opioids to treat dyspnea remains controversial. They may be beneficial in some patient populations or when other therapies have failed.

The required dose of morphine to alleviate dyspnea is influenced by the patient's current opioid regimen. The opioid-naïve patient may begin with 5 to 6 mg of morphine every 4 hours as a starting dose. If a patient is receiving morphine for pain and remains dyspneic, increasing the dose by 25% to 50% is recommended (Thomas & von Gunten, 2003). The usual starting dose for nebulized morphine is 2 to 2.5 mg of preservative-free morphine in 3 ml of sterile saline solution. The dosage may be titrated up to 10 to 20 mg of morphine; however, a greater risk of bronchospasm is seen with higher doses. Once an effective dose is determined, both a sustained-release opioid for baseline control and an immediate release opioid for breakthrough can be used for chronic dyspnea.

Anxiolytics

Because fear and anxiety can be a large component of the sense of breathlessness, anxiolytics are often used to alleviate these causes. Benzodiazepines and phenothiazines have the ability to reduce respiratory drive, may reduce pulmonary ventilation, and may better control the emotional component of dyspnea.

Randomized controlled trials evaluating benzodiazepines versus placebo in COPD patients have yielded conflicting results regarding breathlessness and have shown that the medications are poorly tolerated in long-term studies (ATS, 1999; Mitchell-Heggs, Murphy, & Minty, 1980; Woodcock, Gross, & Geddes, 1981). In addition, alprazolam has been shown to be ineffective in treating dyspnea in COPD patients (Man, Hsu & Sproule, 1986). Despite the lack of evidence that anxiolytics reduce dyspnea, they are widely used. The use of these medications may be most beneficial when anxiety is prominent and when they are combined with an opioid (Thomas & von Gunten, 2003).

Phenothiazines have been poorly studied in dyspnea. Chlorpromazine has been shown to reduce breathlessness after exercise in healthy subjects (O'Neill, Morton, & Stark, 1985) and in COPD patients experiencing anxiety-associated dyspnea (McIver, Walsh, & Nelson, 1994). The combination of morphine with chlorpromazine or promethazine has been shown to be effective at reducing dyspnea (Dudgeon, 1997).

Various routes of administration of the anxiolytics are available, including oral, parenteral, and sublingual. Anxiolytics should be started at very low doses and titrated to dyspnea reduction. The following anxiolytics have been used to treat dyspnea (Thomas & von Gunten, 2003):

- Lorazepam, 0.5 to 1 mg every hour until dyspnea resides and then every 4 to 6 hours
- Diazepam, 5 to 10 mg every hour until dyspnea is settled and then every 6 to 8 hours; 2 to 5 mg in the elderly
- Clonazepam, 0.25 to 2 mg every 12 hours
- Midazolam, 0.5 mg intravenously every 15 minutes until dyspnea settles and then continuous subcutaneous or intravenous infusion
- Chlorpromazine (titrated to effect), 10 mg every 4 to 6 hours and as needed
- Promethazine (titrated to effect), 12.5 mg every 4 to 6 hours and as needed

Corticosteroids

In patients with advanced cancer, corticosteroids have been used to relieve dyspnea caused by superior vena cava syndrome and the inflammation induced by chemotherapy or radiation (LeGrand & Walsh, 1999; Wickham, 1998). The corticosteroids used are typically dexamethasone and prednisolone. Corticosteroids are used in the management of asthma, severe COPD, and fibrotic lung diseases as inhaled preparations, because these diseases have an inflammatory component in the lungs. Corticosteroids also cause bronchodilation, which may help relieve dyspnea (Barnes, 1995). This effect is enhanced when combined with a long-acting β_2 agonist, such as salmeterol or formoterol (Palmqvist, Arvidsson, Beckman et al., 2001). Possible side effects of corticosteroids include fluid retention, gastric toxicity, hyperglycemia, bruising, and decreased bone density (Calverley, 2005).

The following dosages are recommended for the treatment of dyspnea with corticosteroids (Ahmedzai, 1998; LeGrand & Walsh, 1999)

- Prednisolone, 30 to 60 mg/day
- Dexamethasone, 4 to 8 mg two to four times daily

Bronchodilators

Bronchodilators may significantly reduce the symptoms of dyspnea by treating reversible bronchospasm and decreasing important lung volumes (Barnes, 2000). Bronchodilators are standard therapy in asthma and COPD and have been used for symptomatic relief of dyspnea in cancer patients (Wickham, 1998). It is suggested that this class of medications is most beneficial for patients with cancer who also have obstructive lung disease and a history of smoking (Wickham, 1998).

The classes of medications that fall under bronchodilators include β agonists and anticholinergics. β Agonists are classified according to their receptor binding selectivity (α and β receptors) and their duration of action. They are termed sympathomimetics because they stimulate adrenergic receptors. Epinephrine and isoproterenol cause more cardiac stimulation (mediated by β_1 receptors) and are typically reserved for special circumstances. Short-acting β_2 agonists such as albuterol and the anticholinergic ipratropium are used for acute and maintenance therapy. Newer, long-acting bronchodilators are now available and include the β_2 agonists salmeterol and formoterol, used twice daily, and the anticholinergic tiotropium bromide, used once daily (Gross, 2004; Weder & Donohue, 2005). Tiotropium was found to decrease exertional dyspnea and enhance exercise endurance in COPD patients (O'Donnell, Fluge, Gerken et al., 2004). Table 27-3 highlights the most frequently used bronchodilators, with attention to usefulness, dose, and route.

Side effects of β_2 agonists include palpitations, tachycardia, tremor, and hypokalemia (Sears, 2002). Possible side effects of anticholinergics include dry mouth, urinary

TABLE 27-3 ■ Frequently Used Bronchodilators for Dyspnea or Breathlessness

Prototype	Clinical Usefulness	Dosage/Route
Nonselective Agonist		
Epinephrine	Acute Bronchospasm	Subcutaneous: titrate 0.2 to 1 mg as needed
	Sus-Phrine Longer-acting bronchodilation, acute asthma, anaphylaxis	Subcutaneous: titrate 0.5 to 1.5 mg every 6 hr as needed
	Epinephrine inhaler, Primatene, Vaponefrin Wheezing, broncho-constriction, asthma	Inhaler: 1 puff (200 mcg) every 3 to 4 hr as needed
Nonselective β Agonists		
Isoproterenol	Isuprel Intraoperative bronchospasm	Intravenous push: 0.2 mg (1 ml) in 10 ml of NaCl or 5% dextrose; titrate 0.01 to 0.02 mg
	Isuprel Chronic bronchoconstriction, asthma	SL: titrate 10- to 15-mg tablet as needed
	Isuprel inhaler Bronchoconstriction in asthma/COPD	Inhaler: 1 to 2 puffs (130 mcg each) up to five times daily as needed
Ethylnorepinephrine	Acute bronchospasm	Nebulizer: 5 to 15 deep inhalations of 10 mg/ml solution
		Subcutaneous, intramuscular: 1 to 2 mg (0.5 to 1 ml) as needed
Selective β₂ Agonists		
Albuterol sulfate	Proventil/Ventolin	Inhaler: 1 to 2 puffs (90 mcg each) every 4 to 6 hr
Salmeterol	Bronchodilation in asthma and COPD	Orally: 2 to 4 mg every 3 to 4 hr; maximum 8 mg qid
Xinofoate	Alupent	Inhaler: 3 to 4 puffs every 3 to 4 hr as needed; maximum 12 puffs daily
Formoterol	Bronchodilation for COPD	
Fumerate		Nebulizer: 10 deep inhalations of undiluted 5% solution every 4 hr as needed

Continued

TABLE 27-3 ■ Frequently Used Bronchodilators for Dyspnea or Breathlessness—cont'd

Prototype	Clinical Usefulness	Dose/Route
Selective β₂ Agonists—cont'd		
	Serevent Diskus	Orally: 10- to 20-mg tablets
	Maintenance of asthma/COPD	three to four times daily
	Foradil Aerolizer	Inhaler: 1 puff (50 mcg) twice daily
	Maintenance of asthma/COPD	Inhaler: 1 capsule inhaled
		twice daily
Anticholinergics		
Ipratropium	Atrovent	Inhaler: 2 puffs (18 mcg each)
bromide	Maintenance of COPD	four times daily
Tiotropium	Spiriva	Inhaler: 1 capsule inhaled daily
bromide	Maintenance of COPD	
Methylxanthines		
Theophylline	Elixophyllin, Slo-Phyllin, Uniphyl,	Orally: tablets (100, 200, 300, 400,
	Theo-Dur, Theo-24	and 450 mg), syrups, solutions
	Treat wheeze, shortness of	Initial dose 400 to 600 mg/day,
	breath from asthma and COPD	titrate to serum concentration
		of 10 to 20 mg/L
		Intravenous: infusion to serum
		concentration of 10 to 20 mg/L

Data from Katzung, B. (2001). *Basic and clinical pharmacology* (8th ed.). New York: McGraw-Hill; and Weder, M. & Donohue, J. (2005). Role of bronchodilators in chronic obstructive pulmonary disease. *Semin Respir Crit Care Med, 26(2),* 221-234.

retention, and glaucoma (Weder & Donohue, 2005). Side effects from inhaled anticholinergics are low because the molecules are positively charged and have little systemic absorption from the lungs (Gross, 2004). Their utility in palliative care must be weighed against potential side effects and practicality of use.

Theophylline

Theophylline is a methylxanthine that weakly inhibits the enzyme phosphodiesterase leading to bronchodilation, improved gas exchange, reduced inflammation, improved length-tension relationship of the diaphragm, and many other effects (Carrieri-Kohlman & Janson-Bjerklie, 1993; Hansel, Tennant, Tan et al., 2004). Theophylline is used as adjunct therapy in asthma and COPD, and most studies have included patients with nonmalignant disease. Therefore, similar to β₂ agonists and anticholinergics, theophylline is typically reserved for those patients with obstructive lung disease and those who smoke (Wickham, 1998).

The clinical use of theophylline is limited to its narrow therapeutic range and many drug-drug interactions (Hansel et al., 2004). Side effects of theophylline include nausea, headache, insomnia, palpitations, diuresis, and arrhythmias (Hansel et al., 2004). When used as a bronchodilator, doses that give a plasma concentration of 10 to 20 mg/L are optimal.

Oxygen

Oxygen therapy for the treatment of dyspnea in palliative patients is commonly performed by clinicians (Jantarakupt & Porock, 2005). In addition to the relief of breathlessness, therapeutic indications for oxygen use include hypoxemia or a tendency to develop pulmonary hypertension. If a patient's O_2 saturation falls below 90% at room air, the practitioner may consider starting oxygen by nasal cannula at 1 to 3 L/min, rechecking the patient's O_2 saturation in 20 to 30 minutes, and titrating up to 6 L/min if necessary (Ahmedzai, 1998; Luce & Luce, 2001, Pereira & Bruera, 1997). The results of O_2 titration are difficult to predict because neither the flow rate nor the route of administration has been shown to determine its effect on dyspnea in clinical trials. In fact, the published data are mixed regarding the use of oxygen for dyspnea. Oxygen was found to increase patients' oxygen saturation (SaO_2), thus reducing dyspnea, respiratory rate, and respiratory effort in patients with primary lung cancer and advanced disease (Bruera, de Stoutz, Velasco-Leiva et al., 1993; Swinburn, Mould, Stone et al., 1991). A separate controlled study by Davis (1999) showed no advantage of oxygen over compressed air in a separate controlled study. Due to inconclusive data, health care professionals should consider oxygen therapy on a case-by-case basis with the goal of making the patient as comfortable as possible.

Nonpharmacological Interventions

Palliative patients experiencing dyspnea typically have several comorbidities that may require numerous procedures and/or medications. Therefore, the clinician must use nonpharmacological interventions to maximize treatment benefit while trying to minimize potential side effects. Combined approaches (some discussed in depth later in the chapter) such as breathing retraining, exercise counseling, relaxation, and coping and adaptation strategies significantly improved breathlessness and the ability to perform activities of daily living in patients with advanced lung cancer (Dudgeon, 2005). Most of these and subsequent interventions can be taught and implemented easily into patients' daily activities by all levels of practitioners.

Clinician Demeanor

All clinicians who have interaction with the patient are instrumental therapeutic instruments, because patients react to the demeanor of the clinician. Thus, a calm, confident demeanor will reassure the patient and family and may diminish the anxiety associated with dyspnea and/or the underlying pathology (Thomas & von Gunten, 2003). As a patient's condition worsens, communication has been identified as a requirement for high-quality end-of-life care. Specifically, one group of patients surveyed would like to receive information regarding diagnosis and disease process, treatment, prognosis, advanced care planning, and what dying might be like (Curtis, Weinrich, Carline et al., 2002).

Breathing Techniques

Numerous dyspneic patients have experienced benefits from pursed-lip and diaphragmatic breathing techniques because they are able to decrease the air trapped in the lung (FRC), increase muscle productivity (recruitment) during inspiration and expiration, and increase the air consumed with each breath (tidal volume and alveolar ventilation), thus improving effective coughing and improving blood gases (Jantarakupt & Porock, 2005). Pursed-lip breathing (inhalation through the nose) allows for patients to slowly exhale through their lips, which allows for increased lung expansion and improved gas exchange by decreasing the time the airway is constricted (Jantarakupt & Porock, 2005).

Positioning

Several studies have shown that dyspneic patients with COPD have benefited by sitting in the "tripod" position. An example of the tripod is having sitting with feet wide apart and elbows resting on the knees (Jantarakupt & Porock, 2005). Such a position allows the abdominal wall to move outward, increasing transdiaphragmatic pressure, which provides more space for lung expansion and gas exchange (Sharp, Drutz, Moisan et al., 1980). Patients should learn numerous techniques that can improve patients' quality of life. Such positions include leaning on the banister when climbing stairs and leaning on a shopping cart while shopping. Patients should be encouraged to try various positions to determine which position works best for them (Sexton, 1990).

Exercise

The extent of exercise that palliative patients can tolerate will vary from patient to patient. However, practitioners should encourage patients to exercise leg and arm muscles using multiple techniques such as lifting weights, climbing small sets of stairs, walking on a treadmill, and using a cycle ergometer (Jantarakupt & Porock, 2005). Upper-extremity exercise is more beneficial to improving respiratory muscle strength and reducing dyspnea compared with lower-extremity exercise. Clinicians should consult with a physical therapist prior to beginning an exercise regimen. Additionally, patients should start with a low level of intensity, increase the level as the patient can tolerate, and maintain exercise for a minimum of 8 weeks (Jantarakupt & Porock, 2005).

Environmental Adjustments

Small, crucial changes to a patient's daily breathing technique can help improve a patient's dyspnea. Cold and dry air can stimulate the irritant receptors that provoke the cough reflex and allergic reactions, making dyspnea worse. Thus, patients should breathe through their mouth to warm and humidify the air before it passes the trachea. Additionally, patients should cover their mouth with a warm scarf when in cold conditions and use a humidifier when the air is extremely dry indoors. Dry air can impair cilia, which can lead to mucous plugging and dyspnea (Sexton, 1990). The ideal conditions for a dyspneic patient are a cool environment with gentle air movement. Dyspnea may be lessened by cool air from an open window or an oscillating fan set on low speed directed toward the patient's face (Jantarakupt & Porock, 2005; Manning & Schwartzstein, 1995). The cool air blown against the patient's cheek and nose is thought to affect the thermal and mechanical receptors in the distribution of the trigeminal nerve, resulting in a decreased perception of breathlessness (Dudgeon, 2005).

Relaxation Techniques

Complete muscle relaxation decreases oxygen consumption, decreases carbon dioxide production, and decreases the respiratory rate, which are all typically increased in a dyspneic patient (Sexton, 1990). Thus, relaxation techniques, such as Tai Chi, yoga, and/or controlled breathing techniques may help patients control dyspnea and decrease anxiety and possibly stop the vicious cycle of anxiety and dyspnea (Jantarakupt & Porock, 2005).

PATIENT AND FAMILY EDUCATION AND FOLLOW-UP

Dyspnea is a frightening experience for the patient and for those who observe the patient struggling to breathe. Once an etiology contributing to dyspnea has been established, it is important for the clinician to teach the patient and family how to utilize the appropriate interventions to manage this symptom. Patients may not always understand how to adequately navigate the medication delivery systems used in pulmonary medicine. Metered inhalers, dry powder inhalers, nebulized medications, and oral preparations may be overwhelming. Taking the time to evaluate how the patient demonstrates his or her use of these devices and learning the frequency of use will affect the compliance and adequate medication delivery to assist in symptom management. Exploring the emotional or psychological aspects associated with this symptom is also key as depression and anxiety may also require evaluation and management.

Asking the patient to record his or her incidence of dyspnea, the intensity of dyspnea that they experience, and the use of interventions and how these can interface with the dyspnea intensity score may also be useful when following up with the patient and evaluating the effectiveness of specific interventions.

CASE STUDY   M.W., a 58-year-old woman with an 8-month history of weight loss and increasing fatigue, recently noted severe shortness of breath and fever. She also has joint pain in her back, knees, and elbows. A chest radiograph and computed tomography scan reveal a central mass in the upper right lobe of her lung as well as mediastinal lymphadenopathy. Bronchoscopy washings and cytology are positive for stage IV metastatic squamous cell carcinoma of the right lung. Explorative thoracotomy reveals an unresectable tumor of the right lung with possible metastatic nodules in the left lung. M.W. is offered chemotherapy and radiation for treatment. M.W. decides not to pursue any aggressive therapies and enters a local hospice program. Initial medications include around-the-clock hydrocodone/APAP, which does not manage her pain or dyspnea appropriately. Pain is rated at a 9/10 and dyspnea is very severe, making it difficult to talk. Respiratory rate is currently 32, and M.W. is very anxious. She has discussed with the clinician the need to feel more comfortable at this stage of her life. After a complete physical examination, the clinician makes the following changes and interventions:

- Begin administration of equianalgesic sustained-release morphine and equivalent breakthrough dose. Pain should be adequately controlled 24 hours a day.
- Add prednisone, 20 mg/day, for both somatic pain and the inflammatory effects of dyspnea.
- Add chlorpromazine, up to 25 mg, three times daily for the relief of anxiety that M.W. is experiencing, which is having additional effects on her dyspnea— titrate as indicated.

- Instruct M.W. in the use of pursed-lip breathing, relaxation techniques, and position changing, and reporting changes in symptoms.
- Consult the interdisciplinary team to support recent diagnosis and functional limitations.
- Provide oxygen therapy for palliation of breathlessness as needed.

REFERENCES

Abernethy, A., Currow, D., Frith, P., et al. (2003). Randomised, double blind, placebo controlled crossover trial of sustained release morphine for the management of refractory dyspnea. *BMJ, 327,* 523-529.

Ahmedzai, S. (1998). Palliation of respiratory symptoms. In D. Doyle, G.W.C. Hanks, & N. MacDonald (Eds.). *Oxford textbook of palliative medicine* (2nd ed., pp. 583-616). New York: Oxford University Press.

American Thoracic Society (ATS). (1999). Dyspnea mechanisms, assessment and management: A consensus statement. *Am J Respir Crit Care Med 159,* 321-340.

Baines, M. (1978). Control of other symptoms. In C. Saunders (Ed.). *The management of terminal disease.* Chicago: Year–Book.

Barnes, P. (1995). Inhaled glucocorticosteroids for asthma. *N Engl J Med, 332,* 868-875.

Barnes, P. (2000). Chronic obstructive pulmonary disease. *N Engl J Med, 343,* 269-280.

Baydur, A. (2004). Nebulized morphine: A convenient and safe alternative to dyspnea relief? *Chest, 123,* 363-365.

Brown, S., Eichner, S., & Jones, J. (2005). Nebulized morphine for relief of dyspnea due to chronic lung disease. *Ann Pharmacother, 39(6),* 1088-1092.

Bruera, E., de Stoutz, N., Velasco-Leiva, A., et al. (1993). Effects of oxygen on dyspnea in hypoxemic terminal-cancer patients. *Lancet, 342,* 13-14.

Bruera, E., Kuehn, N., Miller, M., et al. (1991). The Edmonton Symptom Assessment Scale (ESAS): A simple method for the assessment of palliative care patients. *J Palliat Care, 7(2),* 6-9.

Bruera, E., MacEachern, T., Ripamonti, C., et al. (1993). Subcutaneous morphine on the dyspnea of terminal cancer patients. *Ann Intern Med, 119(9),* 906-907.

Bruera, E., Sala, R., Spruyt, O., et al. (2005). Nebulized versus subcutaneous morphine for patients with cancer dyspnea: A preliminary study. *J Pain Symptom Manage, 29(6),* 613-618.

Bruera, E., Sweeney, C., & Ripamonti, C. (2002). Management of dyspnea. In A. Berger, R. Portenoy, & D. Weissman (Eds.). *Palliative care and supportive oncology* (pp. 357-371). Philadelphia: Lippincott Williams & Wilkins.

Calverley, P.M. (2005). The role of corticosteroids in chronic obstructive pulmonary disease. *Semin Respir Crit Care Med, 26(2),* 235-245.

Carrieri-Kohlman, V. & Janson-Bjerklie, S. (1993). Dyspnea. In Carrieri-Kohlman, V., Lindsey, M., & West, C. (Eds.). *Pathophysiological phenomena in nursing* (2nd ed., pp. 247-278). Philadelphia: Saunders.

Curtis, J., Wenrich, M., Carline, J., et al. (2002). Patients' perspectives on physician skill in end-of-life care. Differences between patients with COPD, cancer, and AIDS. *Chest, 122,* 356-362.

Davis, C. (1996). Single-dose, randomized, controlled trial of nebulized morphine in patients with cancer-related breathlessness. *Palliat Med, 10,* 64-65.

Davis C. (1999). Palliation of breathlessness. In C. von Gunten (Ed.). *Palliative care and rehabilitation of cancer patients* (pp. 59-74). Boston: Kluwer Academic Publishers.

Dudgeon, D. (1997). Dyspnea clinical perspectives. In *Symptoms in terminal illness: A research workshop, treating symptoms at the end-of-life* (pp. 1-22). Rockville, Md.: National Institutes of Health.

Dudgeon, D. (2005). Management of dyspnea at the end of life. In D. Mahler & D. O'Donnell (Eds.). *Dyspnea: Mechanisms, measurement and management* (2nd ed., pp. 429-461). Boca Raton, Fla.: Taylor & Francis.

Dudgeon, D. & Lertzman, M. (1998). Dyspnea in the advanced cancer patient. *J Pain Symptom Manage, 16,* 212-219.

Evans, S. & Scanlon, P. (2003). Current practice in pulmonary function testing. *Mayo Clin Proc, 78,* 758-763.

Fletcher, C., Elmes, P., & Wood, C. (1959). The significance of respiratory symptoms and the diagnosis of chronic bronchitis in a working population. *BMJ, 1*, 257-266.

GOLD. (2003). *Global initiative for chronic obstructive lung disease: Global strategy for the diagnosis, management, and prevention of chronic obstructive pulmonary disease.* Bethesda, Md.: U.S. Department of Health and Human Services, Public Health Service, National Institutes of Health.

Gross, N. (2004). Tiotropium bromide. *Chest, 126(6),* 1946-1953.

Guyton, A.C. & Hall, J.E. (1996). *Textbook of medical physiology* (9th ed.). Philadelphia: Saunders.

Guz, B. (1997). Breathing and breathlessness. *Respir Physiol, 109,* 197-204.

Hansel, T., Tennant, R., Tan, A., et al. (2004). Theophylline: Mechanism of action and use in asthma and chronic obstructive pulmonary disease. *Drugs of Today, 40(1),* 55-69.

Harver, A., Mahler, D., Schwartzstein R., et al. (2000). Descriptors of breathlessness in health individuals: distinct and separable constructs. *Chest, 118,* 679-690.

Harwood, K. (1999). Dyspnea. In C. Yarbro, M. Frogge, & M. Goodman (Eds.). *Cancer symptom management* (pp. 45-55). Sudbury, Mass.: Jones & Bartlett.

Jantarakupt, P. & Porock, D. (2005). Dyspnea management in lung cancer: Applying the evidence from chronic obstructive pulmonary disease. *Oncol Nurs Forum, 32(4),* 785-795.

Jennings, A., Davies, A., Higgins, P., et al. (2002). A systematic review of the use of opioids in the management of dyspnea. *Thorax, 57,* 939-944.

Jones, P., Quirk, F., & Baveystock, C. (1991). The St George's Respiratory Questionnaire. *Respir Med, 85(Suppl B),* 25-31.

Karnani, N., Reisfield, G.M., & Wilson, G.R. (2005). Evaluation of chronic dyspnea. *Am Fam Physician, 71(8),* 1529-1537, 1538.

Kuebler, K, Dahlin, C.M., Heidrich, D.E., et al. (1996). *Hospice and palliative care clinical practice protocol: Dyspnea.* Pittsburgh, Pa.: Hospice Nurses Association.

LeGrand, S. & Walsh, D. (1999). Palliative management of dyspnea in advanced cancer. *Curr Opin Oncol, 11,* 250-254.

Levitzky, M. (2003). Function and structure of the respiratory system. In *Pulmonary physiology* (6th ed., pp. 1-10). New York: McGraw-Hill.

Luce, J. & Luce J. (2001). Management of dyspnea in patients with far-advanced lung disease. *JAMA 285(10),* 1331-1337.

Mahler, D. (1990). Acute dyspnea. In D. Mahler (Ed.). *Dyspnea* (pp. 127-144). Mt. Kisco, N.Y.: Futura.

Mahler, D. (2000). How should health-related quality of life be assessed in patients with COPD? *Chest, 117,* 54S-57S.

Mahler, D., Ward, J., Fierro-Carrion, G., et al. (2004). Development of self-administered versions of modified baseline and transition dyspnea indexes in COPD. *J Chron Obstructive Pulm Dis 1(2),* 165-172.

Mahler, D., Weinberg, D., Wells, C., et al. (1998). The measurement of dyspnea. In: D. Mahler (Ed.). *Dyspnea* (pp. 149-198). New York: Marcel Dekker.

Man, G., Hsu, K., & Sproule, B. (1986). Effect of alprazolam on exercise and dyspnea in patients with chronic obstructive pulmonary disease. *Chest, 90,* 832-836.

Manning, H. & Schwartzstein, R. (1995). Mechanisms of disease: pathophysiology of dyspnea. *N Engl J Med, 333(23),* 1547-1553.

McIver, B., Walsh, D., & Nelson, K. (1994). The use of chlorpromazine for symptom control in dying cancer patients. *J Pain Symptom Manage,* 9(5), 341-345.

Mitchell-Heggs, P., Murphy, K., & Minty, K. (1980). Diazepam in the treatment of dyspnea in the pink puffer syndrome. *Q J Med, 193,* 9-20.

O'Donnell, D., Fluge, T., Gerken, F., et al. (2004). Effects of tiotropium on lung hyperinflation, dyspnoea and exercise tolerance in COPD. *Eur Respir J, 23(6),* 832-840.

O'Neill, P., Morton, P., & Stark, R. (1985). Chlorpromazine: A specific effect on breathlessness? *Br J Clin Pharmacol, 19,* 793-797.

Palmqvist, M., Arvidsson, P., Beckman, O., et al. (2001). Onset of bronchodilation of budesonide/formoterol vs. salmeterol/fluticasone in single inhalers. *Pulm Pharmacol Ther, 14,* 29–34.

Pereira, J. & Bruera, E. (1997). Dyspnea. In *The Edmonton aid to palliative care* (pp. 62-63). Edmonton, Canada: Division of Palliative Care, University of Alberta.

Pereira, J. & Bruera, E. (2001). Dyspnea. In: J. Pereira & E. Bruera (Eds). *Alberta palliative care resource* (pp. 65-68). Edmonton, Alberta: Alberta Cancer Board.

Rao, A. & Gray, D. (2003). Breathlessness in hospitalised adult patients. *Postgrad Med J, 79,* 681-685.

Sarhill, N., Walsh, D., Khawam, E., et al. (2000). Nebulized hydromorphone for dyspnea in hospice care of advanced cancer. *Am J Hospice Palliat Care, 17(6),* 389-391.

Sears, M. (2002). Adverse effects of beta-agonists. *J Allergy Clin Immunol, 110(6),* S322-S328.

Sexton D. (1990). *Nursing care of the respiratory patient.* Norwalk, Conn.: Appleton and Lange.

Sharp, J., Drutz, W., Moisan, T., et al. (1980). Postural relief of dyspnea in severe chronic pulmonary disease. *Am Rev Respir Dis, 122,* 201-211.

Swinburn, C., Mould, H., Stone, T., et al. (1991). Symptomatic benefit of supplemental oxygen in hypoxemic patients with chronic lung disease. *Am Rev Respir Dis, 143,* 913-915.

Thomas, J. & von Gunten, C. (2003). Management of dyspnea. *J Support Oncol, 1,* 23-34.

Twycross, R. (1999). Correctable causes of breathlessness. In R. Twycross. *Introducing palliative care* (p. 123). Oxon, UK: Radcliffe Medical Press.

Twycross, R.G. (1997). *Symptom management in advanced cancer* (2nd ed.). New York: Radcliffe Medical Press.

Vismara, L., Leaman, D., & Zelis, R. (1976). The effects of morphine on venous tone in patients with acute pulmonary edema. *Circulation, 54,* 335–337.

von Leupoldt, A. & Dahme, B. (2005). Cortical substrates for the perception of dyspnea. *Chest, 128,* 345-354.

Weder, M. & Donohue, J. (2005). Role of bronchodilators in chronic obstructive pulmonary disease. *Semin Respir Crit Care Med, 26(2),* 221-234.

West, J. (2003). Obstructive diseases and restrictive diseases. In B. Sun (Ed.). *Pulmonary pathophysiology, The essentials* (6th ed.). Philadelphia: Lippincott Williams & Wilkins, pp. 51-99.

Wickham, R. (1998). Managing dyspnea in cancer patients. *Development in Supportive Cancer Care,* 2(2), 33-40.

Witek, T. & Mahler, D. (2003). Minimal important difference of the transition dyspnoea index in a multinational clinical trial. *Eur Respir J, 21,* 267-272.

Woodcock, A., Gross, E., & Geddes, D. (1981). Oxygen relieves breathlessness in "pink puffers." *Lancet, 1,* 907-909.

CHAPTER 28

FATIGUE

Louise P. Meyer

■

DEFINITION AND INCIDENCE

The experience of fatigue is considered subjective and, not unlike pain and anxiety, remains a challenge to define. There has been a heightened awareness during the past 20 years that the incidence of fatigue is extremely high among all patients. Current research demonstrates that it is highly prevalent throughout all stages of cancer, affects both genders, and crosses all age groups (Burks, 2001; Curt, Breitbart, Cella et al., 2000; Nail, 2002). Although several authors, as well as the National Comprehensive Cancer Network (NCCN), offer definitions that highlight various aspects of the experience of extreme tiredness, there is as yet no universal or "gold standard" definition of fatigue in the context of health and disease (Glaus, 1998; NCCN, 2005; Neuenschwander & Bruera, 1998; Portenoy & Miaskowski, 1998). Fatigue remains the symptom reported most consistently by patients with a cancer diagnosis; it is considered the one symptom that is the most distressing. It interferes with daily activities of living and results in a decrease in quality of life (Glaus, Crow, & Hammond, 1994; Richardson, 1995).

With a growing interest in the treatment and study of fatigue, there is a heightened need for a common definition that would provide a better understanding of this symptom. Glaus (1998) notes that defining *fatigue* remains difficult in part because there are so many unanswered questions: It is not clear whether fatigue is a single entity or involves various related phenomena. What is generally agreed upon is that cancer-related fatigue is subjective and multidimensional and that it should be measured by self-assessment and self-report. It is not yet understood what causes extreme tiredness in patients with advanced illness, nor is it understood why at least 10% to 30% of patients experience fatigue that persists for months to years after the completion of treatment (Bower, Ganz, Aziz et al., 2002; Nail, 2004). The fact that there is still not an agreed-upon definition remains the greatest challenge. As early as 1987, Piper, Lindsey, and Dodd defined *cancer-related fatigue* as a "persistent feeling of exhaustion and decreased physical and mental capacity unrelieved by rest or sleep." A later definition proposed by Cella, Peterman, Passik et al. (1998) defined *fatigue* as "a subjective state of overwhelming and sustained exhaustion and decreased capacity for physical and mental work that is not relieved by rest." The most recent definition put forth as a result of the work of the NCCN defines *fatigue* as "a persistent, subjective sense of tiredness related to cancer or cancer treatment that interferes with usual functioning" (Mock, Atkinson, Barsevick et al., 2003; NCCN, 2005).

The author would like to acknowledge Sandy McKinnon for her contributions that remain unchanged from the first edition of this textbook.

This definition leaves out the important fact that the main difference between cancer-related fatigue and non–cancer-related fatigue is that it is unrelieved by rest (Mock, 2003). A comprehensive definition should include specific criteria such as severity, duration, and effect as well as the fact that it is not relieved by rest. It should also include the effect on quality of life and functional ability. This would increase the visibility of this problem and provide a real focus for research (Morrow, Abhay, Roscoe et al., 2005; Portenoy & Miaskowski, 1998; Winningham, Nail, Burke et al., 1994).

Fatigue may include symptoms similar to malaise, weakness, asthenia, lassitude, and loss of strength, as well as difficulty in concentrating and decreased energy (Iop, Manfredi, & Bonura, 2004). Some authors use the terms "fatigue" and "asthenia" interchangeably (Neuenschwander & Bruera, 1998). Cella and colleagues (1998) conceptualize fatigue as a multidimensional phenomenon that includes physical, emotional, and cognitive components. Ferrell, Grant, Dean et al. (1996) note that fatigue has a significant effect on all dimensions of quality of life including physical, spiritual, psychological, and social. Aaronson, Teel, Cassmeyer et al. (1999) define *fatigue* as the awareness of a decreased capacity for physical and/or mental activity due to an imbalance in the availability, utilization, and/or restoration of resources needed to perform activity.

Most researchers agree that cancer-related fatigue is a multicausal, multidimensional symptom (Cella et al., 1998; Glaus, 1998; Neuenschwander & Bruera, 1998; Piper, Dibble, Dodd et al., 1998; Portenoy & Miaskowski, 1998; Winningham et al., 1994). Although sparse, most reports place the incidence of fatigue in the terminally ill between 75% and 100% (Lawrence, Kupelnick, Miller et al., 2004; Maughan, James, Kerr et al., 2002; Wolfe, Grier, Klar et al., 2000). It is one of the most common symptoms reported by patients with cancer and clearly can be both extremely distressing and debilitating (Clark & Lacasse, 1998; Glaus, 1998; Portenoy & Miaskowski, 1998). High levels of fatigue may be experienced by patients receiving treatment as well as those with advanced disease. This may result in a permanent decrease in level of functioning (Given, Given, Azzouz et al., 2001; Mock, McCorkle, Ropka et al., 2002). There needs to be more research in this area. Fatigue is also a common symptom in many chronic diseases such as rheumatoid arthritis, diabetes, multiple sclerosis, and acquired immunodeficiency syndrome (AIDS), as well as the poorly understood chronic fatigue syndrome (Aaronson et al., 1999). Fatigue may precede a diagnosis of cancer and may be debilitating enough to lead patients to refuse further anticancer treatment (Neuenschwander & Bruera, 1998).

Most research into cancer-related fatigue has focused on the period surrounding treatment, and there is much work to be done to further understanding of fatigue in cancer survivors, patients with terminal disease, and adolescents. Research has just started to extend beyond the adult population (Erickson, 2003). Fatigue in cancer patients may be perceived as inevitable by care providers, family, and patients themselves (Neuenschwander & Bruera, 1998), and complaints may not be taken seriously (Clark & Lacasse, 1998). Fatigue-related problems often emerge after the more distressing symptoms such as pain or nausea have been relieved.

ETIOLOGY AND PATHOPHYSIOLOGY

Fatigue is reported to affect 70% to 100% of patients regardless of age. It can be an effect of therapy or the cancer itself or both (Curt et al., 2000; Erickson, 2003; Jacobsen,

Hann, Azzarello et al., 1999; Malik, Makower, & Wadler, 2001). It can be a presenting symptom as well as a symptom seen in advanced cancer and palliative care. Better management of other symptoms such as nausea, vomiting, and pain has made fatigue a more distressing symptom than it has been in the past. Fatigue as a physiological phenomenon may be a beneficial and protective symptom against overexertion during both prolonged physical and intellectual efforts (Aaronson et al., 1999). The feeling of being tired after a good exercise session or a hard day's work can even be pleasant (Clark & Lacasse, 1998; Glaus, 1998). This phenomenon is to be distinguished from fatigue as a pathological finding that is distressing and serves no beneficial function. Mock (2003) believes that cancer patients may need to repair additional cells as a result of treatment with chemotherapy or radiation therapy. At the same time, the body has less reserve energy to perform this task as a result of anorexia, cachexia, nausea, and diarrhea. Fatigue associated with cancer has been found to be more persistent and more emotionally overwhelming and lacks the normal circadian rhythm (Glaus, 1998). It is not relieved by a good sleep and paradoxically may contribute to sleep difficulties (Engstrom, Strohl, Rose et al., 1999).

Fatigue has been associated with most severe and chronic illnesses, including cancer, end-stage organ failure, neuromuscular disorders, and major depression. However, the pathogenesis of fatigue is not yet well understood and is the subject of much speculation, conjecture, and research. Cella and associates (1998) list several factors that may contribute to cancer-related fatigue:

- Preexisting conditions (e.g., congestive heart failure, fibromyalgia)
- Direct effects of cancer ("tumor burden")
- Cancer treatment effects
- Surgery
- Chemotherapy
- Radiation therapy
- Biologic response modifiers
- Conditions related to cancer or its treatment:
  - Anemia
  - Dehydration
  - Malnutrition
  - Infection
- Cytokine production
- Altered muscle metabolism (e.g., decreased protein synthesis or accumulation of metabolites)
- Symptoms of cancer or its treatment (e.g., pain, nausea)
- Disruption of sleep-rest cycle
- Immobility
- Emotional demands of dealing with cancer
- Stress
- Anxiety
- Depression

Most often, fatigue is the result of multiple factors, each requiring individual attention and treatment, if possible (Cella et al., 1998). Some of the potential causes listed are considered in more detail in the discussion that follows.

Anemia

Anemia is one of the few conditions with a direct causal relationship to fatigue. In general, patients who have a hemoglobin (Hb) level of less than 12 g/dL are considered anemic (Mercandante, Gebbia, Marrazzo et al., 2000). However, this does not mean that the clinician can state with certainty that there is threshold Hb level below which a person experiences fatigue (Morrow et al., 2005). The factors that contribute to anemia are both extrinsic and intrinsic. The extrinsic factors are radiotherapy and chemotherapy. The intrinsic factors are bone marrow involvement, blood loss, and nutritional deficiencies (Dicato, 2003). Transfusions of packed red blood cells in patients with low Hb levels may or may not provide relief from distressing fatigue. Many patients have anemia of chronic disease that is due to the cancer itself. This will cause a blunting effect on erythropoietin and a lack of normal response to erythropoietin (Glaspy, 2001). It appears that persons with slowly decreasing Hb levels may have less severe symptoms than those whose Hb level drops rapidly. Thus, some persons with terminal illnesses may have significant anemia but few physical signs and symptoms. Interestingly, although most anemic patients report high levels of fatigue, the majority of fatigued patients are not anemic (Irvine, Vincent, Graydon et al., 1994).

Medications

Many medications used to treat cancer symptoms also cause drowsiness or fatigue, including opioids, hypnotics, benzodiazepines, tricyclic antidepressants, and dopamine antagonists. Many persons with terminal illnesses are taking one or more of these medications to treat other uncomfortable symptoms. Careful titration of medications to their lowest effective dose may assist in minimizing this effect. It is also important to determine which medications can be eliminated completely, thus minimizing the deleterious effects of medications.

Cytokines

Cells within the body's immune system, and possibly within the tumor itself, produce proteins called cytokines (e.g., interleukins, interferons, and tumor necrosis factor). It is theorized that cytokines play a role in producing fatigue in illnesses such as cancer, infections, and chronic fatigue syndrome, but the exact mechanism is not yet known (Cleeland, Bennett, Dantzer et al., 2003; Gutstein, 2001). Nor is the mechanism for the persistence of fatigue known (Andrews & Morrow, 2001). Some of the cytokines that have been implicated in the development of cancer-related fatigue include the proinflammatory cytokines such as interleukin (IL)-1 beta, IL-6, and tumor necrosis factor (Bower et al., 2002), as well as the antiinflammatory cytokines such as IL-10 (Cleeland et al., 2003). There needs to be further research in this area to see if there is a relationship between cytokines and fatigue.

Malnutrition and Cachexia

The profound fatigue or asthenia associated with advanced cancer was once thought to be the result of malnutrition and cachexia (Neuenschwander & Bruera, 1998). It is now believed to be more complex than insufficient caloric intake. Cytokine production may be the underlying mechanism for the anorexia-cachexia syndrome and may also cause the symptom of fatigue. Several cytokines, including IL-1, IL-6, and tumor necrosis factor, as well as interferon-gamma, have been implicated as possible mediators of the cachectic syndrome. There also seems to be an inverse relationship between IL-6 and serum albumin. Neuropeptides also seem to play a role in cachexia (Kuzrock, 2001). Similarly, cytokines may contribute to the fatigue associated with some infections (Walker, Schleinich, & Bruera, 1998).

Neurological Dysfunction

Autonomic dysfunction associated with malignancy may cause postural hypotension, occasional syncope, fixed heart rate, and nausea (Neuenschwander & Bruera, 1998). However, almost all the work has been done with patients who have chronic fatigue syndrome and fibromyalgia. There has been no research done in this area with cancer patients, but one in which cancer related research is warranted.

Metabolic and Endocrine Disorders

Preexisting illnesses and secondary conditions such as diabetes mellitus; Addison's disease; electrolyte imbalances such as low sodium, potassium, and magnesium levels; and hypercalcemia may produce fatigue (Neuenschwander & Bruera, 1998; Portenoy & Miaskowski, 1998).

Overexertion

Trying to keep up with a pre-illness lifestyle may contribute to exhaustion (Neuenschwander & Bruera, 1998). Having unrealistic expectations about physical capacities should trigger further emotional evaluation.

Sleep Disruption

Lack of sleep may be related to several concerns, including symptom distress (pain, dyspnea), waking for care needs (medication, repositioning), side effects of medication (steroids, methylphenidate, opioids), and daily inactivity (Engstrom et al., 1999). Rest and immobility may have the paradoxical effect of increasing fatigue and decreasing the efficiency of neuromuscular functioning (Cella et al., 1998). Ancoli-Israel, Moore, and Jones (2001) reported that patients with a poorer quality of sleep had more severe fatigue. It is related to the sleep-wake cycles as well as the quality and quantity of sleep at night. The dimensions of fatigue such as physical, attentional, and cognitive are related in some way to the desynchronized sleep-wake cycles and disrupted sleep. There is also mounting evidence that altered circadian rhythms contribute to fatigue. Roscoe, Morrow, Hickok et al. (2002) demonstrated that there is a positive relationship between interrupted circadian rhythm and measurement of fatigue and depression. Carpenter, Gautam, Freedman et al. (2001) looked at breast cancer patients and healthy participants. The breast cancer group did not have the same circadian pattern as the healthy group.

Depression

Fatigue may be the physical expression of feelings of hopelessness and demoralization as the illness progresses. In addition, depression may be masked. Treatments for major depression may involve medications that exacerbate fatigue (Cella et al., 1998). Fatigue and depression frequently coexist in patients with cancer. There have been few studies that have looked at the relationship between fatigue and depression. Morrow, Hickok, Roscoe et al. (2003) looked at whether there was a causal relationship between them and whether a selective serotonin reuptake inhibitor antidepressant would have any effect on fatigue while reducing depression. The conclusion of the study was that it did not have any effect on fatigue although it did reduce the level of depression. It would appear that there is another mechanism causing the fatigue that does not involve this pathway.

ASSESSMENT AND MEASUREMENT

Researchers and clinicians agree that accurate assessment and measurement of fatigue are critical to advancing the knowledge and ability to treat effectively. There are a number of appropriate and validated tools in existence with which to assess and measure fatigue. They include the Brief Fatigue Inventory, the Revised Piper Fatigue Scale, the Cancer Fatigue Scale, the Revised Schwartz Cancer Fatigue Scale, and the Multidimensional Fatigue Inventory (Mendoza, Wang, Cleeland et al., 1999; Okuyama, Akechi, Kugaya et al., 2000; Piper et al., 1998; Schwartz & Meek, 1999; Smets, Garssen, Bonke et al., 1995). Piper and coworkers (1998) suggest that a simple rating of fatigue intensity from 0 to 10 is reasonable in many circumstances (Table 28-1). The authors add that patients should be asked the following as well:

- How has fatigue affected activities of daily living?
- Has the ability to concentrate or remember been affected?
- How has fatigue affected mood?

These screening questions are helpful in determining the need for further assessment, referrals, and supportive therapies such as home care, occupational therapy, or assistive equipment (Piper et al., 1998). The symptoms of fatigue must be viewed in the context of the person's life, level of distress, and overall treatment goals, recognizing that these goals may change over time (Portenoy & Miaskowski, 1998).

Initial assessment includes identifying temporal features, such as onset and daily patterns, determining any relationship between the fatigue and events such as

TABLE 28-1 ■ **Multidimensional Measures of Fatigue**

Measure	First Author, Year	Dimensions Measured
Brief Fatigue Inventory	Mendoza, 1999	Severity, interference
Cancer Fatigue Scale	Okuyama, 2000	Physical, cognitive, affective
Fatigue Symptom Inventory	Hann, 1998	Severity, frequency, diurnal variation, interference
Multidimensional Fatigue Inventory	Smets, 1995	General, physical, mental, reduced activity, reduced motivation
Multidimensional Fatigue Symptom Inventory	Stein, 1998	General, physical, emotional, mental, vigor
Revised Piper Fatigue Scale	Piper, 1998	Behavioral/severity, affective meaning, sensory, cognitive/mood
Revised Schwartz Cancer Fatigue Scale	Schwartz, 1999	Physical, perceptual

Adapted with permission from Jacobsen, P. (2004). Assessment of fatigue in cancer patients. *J Natl Cancer Inst Monogr, 32,* 94, Table 1.

chemotherapy, and assessing factors that relieve and exacerbate the fatigue. Screening laboratory tests may include complete blood cell count; electrolyte, serum calcium, creatinine, glucose, and transaminase levels; and possibly a thyrotropin (thyroid-stimulating hormone) evaluation if hypothyroidism is suspected (Walker et al., 1998).

There are several unresolved issues related to the assessment of fatigue. The first is the ability to distinguish between fatigue and depression. Fatigue and depression have common symptoms such as loss of concentration. The second issue is the use of self-reports of fatigue as a basis for clinical decision making. The third issue was the ability to detect temporal changes in fatigue. There is a lot of variability in the level of fatigue in patients receiving chemotherapy or radiation therapy. Depending on how the measurement tool is worded, it may be difficult to capture the changes over the course of the day or week (Jacobsen, 2004).

Fatigue is a multidimensional problem, and more sophisticated assessment may be helpful in some cases (Piper et al., 1998; Portenoy & Miaskowski, 1998). Although most fatigue assessment instruments have been developed for research, they may be helpful in clinical practice if they are easy to use. Multidimensional tools such as the Piper Fatigue Self-Report Scale, which looks at severity, distress, and effect of fatigue, are available for use in clinical situations and can aid in the evaluation of intervention strategies (Piper et al., 1998).

HISTORY AND PHYSICAL EXAMINATION

It is important to ask about fatigue during an initial history and follow-up visits with patients. As previously noted, fatigue may be viewed as inevitable by patients and families or may not be noticed until more distressing symptoms have been relieved (Neuenschwander & Bruera, 1998). It is important to ask about the five primary factors associated with fatigue: pain, emotional distress, sleep disturbance, anemia, and hypothyroidism (Patarca-Montero, 2004).

The clinician must look for potential causes and associations for fatigue. For example, questioning about nighttime medications may uncover the cause of morning fatigue (Portenoy & Miaskowski, 1998). A review of all medications is essential in order to ascertain which may be contributing to drowsiness or fatigue. In addition, a comprehensive review of systems, assessment of activity level, and nutritional and metabolic assessment needs to be done. All treatable causes of fatigue need to be assessed and treated or ruled out.

Patients with moderate and severe levels of fatigue need a complete assessment. A comprehensive history should be taken. Factors such as disease type, response to treatment, and the treatment itself should be considered when assessing possible contributing factors of fatigue (Escalante, 2003).

DIAGNOSTICS

The extent of laboratory or radiological investigations must be decided on a case-by-case basis. Tests may be costly and burdensome and should be pursued only when the cause is uncertain and there is a potential to make a change in treatment (Patarca-Montero, 2004; Portenoy & Miaskowski, 1998). It is necessary to have a good understanding of the patient's goals and degree of distress caused by the fatigue. Laboratory tests for possible hematological or metabolic problems are helpful and have previously been identified in this chapter.

INTERVENTION AND TREATMENT

Patients may not report fatigue, believing it to be inevitable and untreatable. Passik, Kirsh, Donaghy et al. (2002) conducted a survey of 200 cancer patients. More than two thirds of the patients never told their clinician that they felt fatigued. The most common reasons given were the clinician's failure to offer interventions, the patient's lack of awareness of possible effective interventions, and the patient's not wanting to complain. Clinicians may not be asked about fatigue during visits, and its effect may be underestimated or ignored completely (Cella et al., 1998). Patients fear that increased levels of fatigue mean that their disease is progressing, when in fact it may be an effect of the treatment. Expectations for improvement should be discussed. Fatigue may not be reversible, and this possibility should be compassionately communicated. On the other hand, knowing that chemotherapy-related fatigue is short term can in itself be therapeutic (Portenoy & Miaskowski, 1998).

The goal of care is to "reverse the reversible." Reversible causes of fatigue may coexist with irreversible causes, and the goal of care may be to improve function and minimize fatigue rather than to eliminate it (Cella et al., 1998; Neuenschwander & Bruera, 1998). Determining goals should be a collaborative process for the patient and practitioner. Many possible treatments for fatigue can be tiring, and a trial-and-error process can be frustrating (Portenoy & Miaskowski, 1998). Often, several treatment options will be used at the same time to develop an effective treatment plan that works for the patient (Escalante, 2003).

The following interventions may be helpful:

- Treat underlying problems such as dehydration, hypercalcemia, hypothyroidism, hypokalemia, and hypoxia (Cella et al., 1998, Escalante, 2003).
- Suggest keeping a diary to record actions and activities that increase or decrease fatigue, as an aid in planning daily and weekly activities (Clark & Lacasse, 1998).
- Teach energy conservation techniques, such as sitting instead of standing and using assistive devices such as bath chairs, raised toilet seats, or wheelchairs. Consider consultations with physical or occupational therapists.
- Teach patients and caregivers ways to reduce stress. For some patients, participation in support groups is helpful. Use of yoga, meditation, massage, and visual imagery is also helpful in reducing stress (Escalante, 2003).
- Encourage a balance between rest and exercise. Further research is still needed to determine the role of exercise in cases of pathologic fatigue, but it is clear that excessive rest may be as fatigue inducing as excessive exercise (Neuenschwander & Bruera, 1998; Portenoy & Miaskowski, 1998). Eight randomized controlled trials were reviewed by Watson and Mock (2004) using exercise as an intervention. It is clear that physical therapy as well as a rehabilitation specialist needs to be involved in the development of an exercise program. The following recommendations are made, based on the results of these trials:
  - The exercise program should begin at the start of treatment.
  - It should be of low to moderate intensity.

- It should be progressive, starting with 15 minutes of exercise and progressing to 30 minutes, 3 to 5 days a week.
- It should be mainly aerobic in nature.
- An exercise diary should be kept to document exercise and encourage adherence to the program (Watson and Mock, 2004).
- When developing an exercise program, take into account contraindications to exercise, including cardiac abnormalities, recurrent unexplained pain or nausea, extreme fatigue, and cyanosis (Escalante, 2003; Portenoy & Miaskowski, 1998; Watson & Mock, 2004).
- Encourage good sleep habits such as napping earlier in the day for a brief period of time (not more than 30 minutes), not napping in the evening, establishing a bedtime routine, using relaxation exercises, and avoiding stimulants (Portenoy & Miaskowski, 1998). A pilot study of a sleep program by Davidson, Waisberg, Brundage et al. (2001) in a small group of patients included: stimulus control therapy, relaxation training, and consolidation of sleep and reduction of cognitive-emotional arousal. This small program demonstrated that total good sleep time and fatigue were improved. More studies need to be done investigating sleep therapy as a treatment for fatigue.

Pharmacology

To avoid unnecessary medications and polypharmacy, Portenoy and Miaskowski (1998) offer the following suggestions:

- Reduce or discontinue medications known to cause fatigue:
  - Antiemetics
  - Hypnotics (sleeping pills may increase sleep while compounding the problem of daytime fatigue [hangover effect]; assess whether sleep is restorative or non-restorative)
  - Anxiolytics
  - Antihistamines (H_1 or H_2 blockers)
  - Analgesics (in the presence of distressing fatigue, try reducing the daily dose by 25%)
- Use antidepressants for patients with major depression who are experiencing fatigue. Consider using one of the selective serotonin reuptake inhibitors that is less sedating than other classes of antidepressants.
- Psychostimulants may be helpful in treating opioid-related fatigue and depression in elderly and medically ill patients. However, these medications may also cause insomnia, anxiety, anorexia, confusion, and tachycardia.
  - Methylphenidate (Ritalin): Walker and colleagues (1998) first suggested starting with a morning trial dose of 5 to 10 mg orally; because this medication has a short half-life, beneficial effects are apparent within 24 hours; if the patient shows improvement, suggest 10 mg with breakfast and 5 mg with lunch; avoid doses after noon to prevent sleeplessness at night. These recommendations are for immediate-release medication; for sustained-release, 5 to 10 mg daily is recommended. Sarhill, Walsh, Nelson et al. (2001), Breitbart, Rosenfeld, Kaim et al. (2001), and Homsi, Nelson, Sarhill et al. (2001) all have done small studies in patients with advanced cancer using Ritalin with

positive results. Despite these studies, there is no consensus regarding the use of psychostimulants in this patient population.

▶ Modafinil is a wake-promoting agent that has been shown to improve wakefulness. It is not a dopamine antagonist; it has a low abuse potential and fewer side effects than psychostimulants. In clinical studies with multiple sclerosis patients by Rammohan, Rosenberg, Lynn et al. (2002) and Zifko, Rupp, Schwartz et al. (2002), patients experienced decreased fatigue and increased levels of alertness. A dosage of 100 to 200 mg/day has been shown to be effective in this patient group. No data are yet available in patients with cancer.

▶ Pemoline (Cylert) is helpful in treating fatigue related to multiple sclerosis, but is also associated with liver toxicity; consider using pemoline only if treatment with methylphenidate is unsuccessful.

■ Erythropoietin: Research supports that erythropoietin increases hematocrit and improves energy and quality of life. Poor performance status, often seen in patients with advanced cancer, is linked to high levels of fatigue (Pater, Zee, Palmer et al., 1997). A study of more than 2000 patients, including those with advanced cancer, demonstrated that cancer patients experienced increased energy levels, which were positively correlated with quality of life (Glaspy, Bukowski, Steinberg et al., 1997). In a review by Crawford (2002), a number of trials in the 1990s demonstrated that recombinant human erythropoietin improved hemoglobin and decreased the need for transfusions. It was not put into clinical practice because of a common misperception by clinicians that mild to moderate anemia in cancer patients was asymptomatic and thus did not warrant any intervention. Balducci and Extermann (2000) recommend that patients with advanced cancer have their symptoms aggressively treated, including fatigue. Fatigue was reported as the most prevalent symptom in a study of hospice patients by Henriksen, Riis, Christophersen et al. (1997).

■ Corticosteroids: The stimulant effect of corticosteroids is often helpful for persons with advanced disease and multiple symptoms. Dexamethasone, 1 to 2 mg twice daily, or prednisone, 5 to 10 mg twice daily, may be used. Rousseau (2001) recommends the use of high-dose corticosteroids in the terminally ill to provide symptomatic relief of symptoms, including fatigue.

Complementary Therapies

There are several other interventions that may assist in alleviating fatigue or coping with the distress of fatigue. These include but are not limited to the following:

■ Stress management
■ Visual imagery
■ Distraction to reduce boredom (e.g., hobbies, gardening, music)
■ Hot baths
■ Cognitive-behavioral therapy: Counseling of patients and families has been shown to have a positive effect. Not enough attention is paid to providing counseling early on, and both patients and families have a need for information and support throughout the illness. Studies by Elmberger, Bolund, and Lutzen (2000) and Singer and Schwarz (2002) demonstrate that counseling reduces anxiety and increases well-being. A social worker should be involved in the care of cancer patients

throughout their illness. Ream, Richardson, and Alexander-Dann (2002) developed a four-part educational program that provided patients with education and the opportunity to discuss their fatigue with someone. Although this was just a pilot study, there was evidence that the program helped to lessen fatigue and improve well-being.

PATIENT AND FAMILY EDUCATION

Patients and families may need coaching and support to let go of certain activities in order to save energy for whatever is most important. Delegation is a difficult task for many people, especially women and mothers, to learn. There may be a need to set limits on visitors and some social activities. Fatigue is not usually influenced quickly (Clark & Lacasse, 1998). Despite these potential losses, acceptance of limitations can lead to adaptation (Walker et al., 1998).

Patients and families may associate fatigue with a worsening of the disease and may be reassured by alternative explanations for this symptom and encouraged by the possibilities for improvement. They should have an understanding of the nature of the symptom, options for therapy, and expected outcomes (Portenoy & Miaskowski, 1998).

EVALUATION AND PLAN FOR FOLLOW-UP

The effect of fatigue and the goals of care change over time (Portenoy & Miaskowski, 1998). Treatment of fatigue requires early identification, careful assessment, and close follow-up. Success in the management of fatigue is highly individualized and correlated with each person's goals (Clark & Lacasse, 1998).

CASE STUDY   J. is a 34-year-old mother of two children: a 10-year-old and a lively 6-year-old. Her husband is very supportive. J. was diagnosed with colon cancer 4 years ago and was treated with resection, colostomy, and radiation treatments. Unfortunately an abdominal CT scan performed 1 year ago revealed liver metastases. Chemotherapy failed to help, and J. knows that her time is limited. She is determined to be at home for as long as possible. Problems with pain and nausea are under reasonable control. The clinician visits J. at home one afternoon. Her husband has taken the children out to a movie and J. begins by saying that she is feeling "exhausted." She adds that she has not been sleeping at night or, rather, has to wake up to take her pain medication every 4 hours. The clinician identifies the following contributing factors to J.'s fatigue and initiates corrective actions:

- She is on a short-acting pain medication with a stable pain problem.
  - Switch to a long-acting preparation to facilitate sleep at night and provide more complete pain relief while using the short-acting medication for breakthrough pain.

- She has been trying to keep the environment as "normal" as possible for the children by trying to do all the cooking and cleaning herself.
  - Encourage J. to consider hiring a housekeeper or asking for more help from family and friends. Involve children in some simple household tasks with Mom supervising. It will provide an opportunity for them to spend time together.
  - Review energy conservation techniques with J.
  - Consult an occupational therapist for additional instruction in tools and techniques for energy conservation in daily activities.
- J. has been "too tired to eat."
  - She should consider help with cooking so that she will have enough energy to eat with her family.
  - Review nutritional intake. It is important that her diet contain foods that are high in energy.
  - Consider liquid supplements.
- J. is concerned about her fatigue and her ability to continue fulfilling her role as mother and wife.
  - Discuss J.'s goals and expectations.
  - Consider use of erythropoietin if appropriate. Also consider use of modafinil and methylphenidate to help improve her energy level. And consider the possibility of J. taking short walks with her family as an opportunity to spend time together and improve her energy level. If she is able, an exercise program should be developed by a physical therapist to help her increase her endurance and energy.
  - Help J. adjust to her limitations.
  - Assist J. to identify the underlying meaning of her "chores" as mother and wife and other ways to fulfill these roles.
  - Consult a counselor or social worker to provide additional counseling and support.

REFERENCES

Aaronson, L.S., Teel, C.S., Cassmeyer, V., et al. (1999). Defining and measuring fatigue. *Image—J Nurs Scholar, 31(1)*, 45-50.

Ancoli-Israel, S., Moore, P., & Jones, V. (2001). The relationship between fatigue and sleep in cancer patients: a review. *Eur J Cancer Care, 10(4)*, 245-255.

Andrews, P. & Morrow, G. (2001). Approaches to understanding the mechanisms involved in fatigue associated with cancer and its treatments: a speculative review. *ESO Sci Updates, 5*, 79-93.

Balducci, L. & Extermann, M. (2000). Management of the frail person with advanced cancer. *Crit Rev Oncol/Hematol, 33(2)*, 143-148.

Bower, J., Ganz, P., Aziz, N., et al. (2002). Fatigue and proinflammatory cytokine activity in breast cancer survivors. *Psychosom Med, 64*, 604-611.

Breitbart, W., Rosenfeld, B., Kaim, M., et al. (2001). A randomized, double-blind, placebo-controlled trial of psychostimulants for the treatment of fatigue in ambulatory patients with human immunodeficiency virus disease. *Arch Intern Med, 161(3)*, 411-420.

Burks, T. (2001). New agents for the treatment of cancer-related fatigue. *Cancer, 92(9 Suppl)*, 1714-1718.

Carpenter, J., Gautam, S., Freedman, R., et al. (2001). Circadian rhythm of objectively recorded not flashes in postmenopausal breast cancer survivors. *Menopause, 8(3)*, 181-188.

Cella, D., Peterman, A., Passik, S., et al. (1998). Progress toward guidelines for the management of fatigue. *Oncology, 12(11A, NCCN Proceedings),* 369-377.

Clark, P.M. & Lacasse, C. (1998). Cancer-related fatigue: Clinical practice issues. *Clinl J Oncol Nurs, 2(2),* 45-53.

Cleeland, C., Bennett, G., Dantzer, R., et al. (2003). Are the symptoms of cancer and cancer treatment due to a shared biologic mechanism? *Cancer, 97(11),* 2919-2925.

Crawford, J. (2002). Recombinant human erythropoietin in cancer-related anemia: review of the clinical evidence. *Oncology, 16(9 Suppl 10),* 41-53.

Curt, D., Breitbart, W., Cella, D., et al. (2000). Impact of cancer-related fatigue on the lives of patients: new findings from the Fatigue Coalition. *Oncologist, 5,* 353-360.

Davidson, J., Waisberg, J., Brundage, M., et al. (2001). Non-pharmacologic group treatment of insomnia: a preliminary study with cancer survivors. *Psycho-oncology 10(5),* 389-397.

Dicato, M. (2003). Anemia in cancer: some pathophysiological aspects. *Oncologist, 8,* 19-21.

Elmberger, E., Bolund, C., & Lutzen, K. (2000). Transforming the exhausting to energizing process of being a good parent in the face of cancer. *Health Care for Women International, 21(6),* 485-499.

Engstrom, C.A., Strohl, R.A., Rose, L., et al. (1999). Sleep alterations in cancer patients. *Cancer Nurs, 22(2),* 143-148.

Erickson, J. (2003). Fatigue in adolescents with cancer: a review of the literature. *Clinl J Oncol Nurs, 8(2),* 139-145.

Escalante, C. (2003). Treatment of cancer-related fatigue: an update. *Support Care Cancer, 11,* 79-83.

Ferrell, B.R., Grant, M., Dean, G.E., et al. (1996). "Bone tired": The experience of fatigue and its impact on quality of life. *Oncol Nurs Forum, 23,* 1539-1549.

Given, B., Given, C., Azzouz, F., et al. (2001). Physical functioning of elderly cancer patients prior to diagnosis and following initial treatment. *Nurs Res, 50,* 222-232.

Glaspy, J. (2001). Anemia and fatigue in cancer patients. *Cancer, 92(6 Suppl),* 1719-1724.

Glaspy, J., Bukowski, R., Steinberg, D., et al. (1997). Impact of therapy with epoetin alfa on clinical outcomes in patients with nonmyeloid malignancies during cancer chemotherapy in community oncology practice. Procrit Study Group. *J Clin Oncol, 15(3),* 1218-1224.

Glaus, A. (1998). *Fatigue in patients with cancer: Analysis and assessment.* New York: Springer.

Glaus, A., Crow, R., & Hammond, S. (1994). A qualitative study to explore the concept of fatigue/tiredness in cancer patients and in healthy individuals. *Support Cancer Care, 5,* 82-96.

Gutstein, H. (2001). The biologic basis of fatigue. *Cancer, 92(6 Suppl),* 1678-1683.

Henriksen, H., Riis, J., Christophersen, B., et al. (1997). Distress symptoms in hospice patients [in Danish]. *Ugeskr Laeger, 159(47),* 6992-6996.

Homsi, J., Nelson, K., Sarhill, N., et al. (2001). A phase II study of methylphenidate for depression in advanced cancer. *Am J Hospice Palliat Care, 8(6),* 403-407.

Iop, A., Manfredi, A., & Bonura, S. (2004). Fatigue in cancer patients receiving chemotherapy: an analysis of published studies. *Ann Oncol, 15,* 712-720.

Irvine, D., Vincent, L., Graydon, J., et al. (1994). The prevalence and correlates of fatigue in patients receiving treatment with chemotherapy and radiotherapy: a comparison with the fatigue experience by healthy individuals. *Cancer Nurs, 17,* 367-378.

Jacobsen, P. (2004). Assessment of fatigue in cancer patients. *J Natl Cancer Inst Monogr, 32,* 92-97.

Jacobsen, P., Hann, D., Azzarello, L., et al. (1999). Fatigue in women receiving adjuvant chemotherapy for breast cancer: characteristics course and correlate. *J Pain Symptom Manage, 18(4),* 233-242.

Kuzrock, R. (2001). The role of cytokines in cancer-related fatigue. *Cancer, 92(6 Suppl),* 1684-1688.

Lawrence, D., Kupelnick, B., Miller, K., et al. (2004). Evidence report on the occurrence, assessment, and treatment of fatigue in cancer patients. *J Natl Cancer Inst Monogr, 32,* 40-50.

Malik, U., Makower, D., & Wadler, S. (2001). Interferon-mediated fatigue. *Cancer, 92(6 Suppl),* 1664-1668.

Maughan, T., James, R., Kerr, D., et al.; British MRC Colorectal Cancer Working Party. (2002). Comparison of survival, palliation, and quality of life with three chemotherapy regimens in metastatic colorectal cancer: a multicentre randomized trial. *Lancet, 359,* 1555-1563.

Mendoza, T., Wang, X., Cleeland, C., et al. (1999). The rapid assessment of fatigue severity in cancer patients: use of the Brief Fatigue Inventory. *Cancer, 85,* 1186-1196.

Mercadante, S., Gebbia, V., Marrazzo, A., et al. (2000). Anemia in cancer: pathophysiology and treatment. *Cancer Treat Rev, 26,* 303-311.

Mock, V. (2003). Clinical excellence through evidence-based practice: fatigue management as a model. *Oncol Nurs Forum, 30(5)*, 790-796.

Mock, V., Atkinson, A., Barsevick, A., et al. (2003). Cancer-related fatigue clinical practice guidelines in oncology. *J Natl Comprehen Cancer Network, 1,* 308-331.

Mock, V., McCorkle, R., Ropka, M., et al. (2002). Fatigue and physical functioning during breast cancer treatment [abstract]. *Oncol Nurs Forum, 29,* 338.

Morrow, G., Abhay, R., Roscoe, J., et al. (2005). Management of cancer-related fatigue. *Cancer Investigations, 23,* 229-239.

Morrow, G., Hickok, J., Roscoe, J., et al.; University of Rochester Cancer Center Community Clinical Oncology Program. (2003). Differential effects of paroxetine on fatigue and depression: a randomized double-blind trial from the University of Rochester Cancer Center Community Clinical Oncology Program. *J Clin Oncol, 21(24),* 4635-4641.

Nail, L. (2002). Fatigue in patients with cancer. *Oncol Nurs Forum, 29,* 537-553.

Nail, L. (2004). My get up and go got up and went: fatigue in people with cancer. *J Natl Cancer Inst Monogr, 32,* 72-75.

National Comprehensive Cancer Network (NCCN). (2005). Practice Guidelines. Cancer related fatigue panel 2005 guidelines, version 1, 2005, March. Rockledge, Pa.: National Comprehensive Cancer Network (www.nccn.org).

Neuenschwander, H. & Bruera, E. (1998). Asthenia. In D. Doyle, G.W.C. Hanks, & N. MacDonald (Eds.), *Oxford textbook of palliative medicine* (2nd ed., pp. 573-581). New York: Oxford University Press.

Okuyama, T., Akechi, T., Kugaya, A., et al. (2000). Development and validation of the cancer fatigue scale: a brief three-dimensional, self-rating scale for the assessment of fatigue in cancer patients. *J Pain Symptom Manage, 19,* 5-14.

Passik, S., Kirsh, K., Donaghy, K., et al.; Fatigue Coalition. Fatigue Coalition. (2002). Patient-related barriers to fatigue communication: initial validation of the fatigue management barriers questionnaire. *J Pain Symptom Manage, 24(5),* 481-493.

Patarca-Montero, P. (2004).Treatment of cancer-related fatigue. In *Handbook of cancer-related fatigue* (pp. 173-248). New York: Haworth Medical Press.

Pater, J., Zee, B., Palmer, M., et al. (1997). Fatigue in patients with cancer: results with National Cancer Institute of Canada Clinical Trials Group studies employing the EORTC QLQ-C30. *Support Care Cancer, 5(5),* 410-413.

Piper, B., Lindsey, A., & Dodd, M. (1987). Fatigue mechanisms in cancer patients: developing nursing theory. *Oncol Nurs Forum 14(6),* 17-23.

Piper, B.F., Dibble, S.L., Dodd, M.J., et al. (1998). The revised Piper Fatigue Scale: Psychometric evaluation in women with breast cancer. *Oncol Nurs Forum, 25,* 677-684.

Portenoy, R.K. & Miaskowski, C. (1998). Assessment and management of cancer-related fatigue. In Berger, A., Weissman, D., & Portenoy, R.K. (Eds.). Principles and Practice of Supportive Oncology (pp. 109-118). Philadelphia: Lippincott.

Rammohan, K.W., Rosenberg, J.H., Lynn, D.J., et al. (2002). Efficacy and safety of modafinil (Provigil) for the treatment of fatigue in multiple sclerosis: a two centre phase 2 study. *J Neurol Neurosurg Psychiatr, 72(2),* 179-183.

Ream, E., Richardson, A., & Alexander-Dann, C. (2002). Facilitating patients' coping with fatigue during chemotherapy-pilot outcomes. *Cancer Nurs 25(4),* 300-308.

Richardson, A. (1995). Fatigue in cancer patients: a review of the literature. *Eur J Cancer Care, 4(1),* 20-32.

Roscoe, J., Morrow, G., Hickok, J., et al. (2002). Temporal interrelationships among fatigue, circadian rhythm and depression in breast cancer patients undergoing chemotherapy treatment. *Support Care Cancer, 10,* 329-336.

Rousseau, P. (2001). The palliative use of high-dose corticosteroids in three terminally ill patients with pain. *Am J Hospice Palliat Care, 18(5),* 343-346.

Sarhill, N., Walsh, D., Nelson, K., et al. (2001). Methylphenidate for fatigue in advanced cancer: a prospective open label pilot study. *Am J Hospice Palliat Care, 18(3),* 187-192.

Schwartz, A. & Meek, P. (1999). Additional construct validity of the Schwartz Cancer Fatigue Scale. *J Nurs Measure, 7,* 35-45.

Singer, S. & Schwarz, R. (2002). Psychosocial aftercare of patients with endometrial or cervical cancer. *Zentralblatt Gynakologie, 124(1),* 64-70.

Smets, E., Garssen, B., Bonke, B., et al. (1995). The Multidimensional Fatigue Inventory (MFI) psychometric properties of an instrument to assess fatigue. *J Psychosomat Res, 39,* 315-325.

Walker, P., Schleinich, M.A. & Bruera, E. (1998). Asthenia. In N. MacDonald (Ed.), *Palliative medicine: A case-based manual* (pp. 29-33). Toronto: Oxford University Press.

Watson, T. & Mock, V. (2004). Exercise as an intervention for cancer-related fatigue. *Physical Ther, 84(8),* 736-743.

Winningham, M.L., Nail, L.M., Burke, M.B., et al. (1994). Fatigue and the cancer patient: The state of the knowledge. *Oncol Nurs Forum, 21,* 23-36.

Wolfe, J., Grier, H., Klar, N., et al. (2000). Symptoms and suffering at the end of life in children with cancer. *N Engl J Med, 342,* 326-333.

Zifko, U.A., Rupp, M., Schwarz, S., et al. (2002). Modafinil in treatment of fatigue in multiple sclerosis: Results of an open-label study. *J Neurol, 249,* 983-987.

CHAPTER 29

HICCUPS

Peg Esper

■

DEFINITION AND INCIDENCE

The term "hiccups" describes the spasmodic movement of the diaphragm that is followed by a rapid closure of the glottis. Men are more likely to experience episodes of hiccups, which can occur between 2 and 60 times per minute (Ripamonti & Fusco, 2002). The medical term for "hiccup" is derived from the Latin word *singultus*, which means "a gasp or sigh" (Krakauer, Zhu, Bounds et al., 2005).

Hiccups have been classified in the literature as being episodic (or a "bout" of hiccups); protracted, which last over 48 hours; or intractable, lasting longer than 1 month (Waller & Caroline, 2000). These classifications appear to be more arbitrarily than scientifically based, and most individuals would probably agree that hiccups lasting more than a few hours is likely to be personally defined as intractable.

Hiccups can be experienced by individuals with and without a documented illness. The benign occurrence of hiccups is generally limited. Healthy individuals rarely require intervention beyond self-help measures. Individuals with advanced illness, however, may develop an intractable form of hiccups that can become debilitating and lead to such symptoms as anxiety, depression, dyspnea, nausea, pain, and fatigue. The actual incidence of hiccups in individuals with cancer and other chronic illnesses has not been well documented, but the occurrence of idiopathic singultus is reported to be 1:100,000 people in the general population (Petroianu, 2005).

ETIOLOGY AND PATHOPHYSIOLOGY

Hiccups are attributed to a variety of causes but generally can be placed into one of the six following categories (Krakauer et al., 2005; Ripamonti & Fusco, 2002):

- Conditions that cause inflammation of the peripheral branches of the phrenic and vagal nerves, such as gastric and abdominal distention (having a variety of causes, including bowel obstruction and intraabdominal hemorrhage), excessive ingestion of food, sudden changes in the gastric temperature, esophageal reflux or obstruction, pleuritis, pericarditis, pulmonary edema, pneumonia, and mediastinal or cervical tumors
- Central nervous system disorders, such as intracranial tumors, head injury, and stroke

The author wishes to acknowledge Patricia H. Berry for her contributions that remain unchanged from the first edition.

- Metabolic and toxic causes, such as renal failure or insufficiency, hypocalcemia, hyponatremia, alcohol abuse, chemotherapeutic agents, barbiturates, benzodiazepines, and parenteral corticosteroids
- Infectious disorders (infrequent), including meningitis, abscess, tuberculosis, and influenza
- Psychogenic disturbances, such as anxiety, emotional stress, and excitement
- Idiopathic causes, when a causative factor is not identified; because extensive evaluation is often unwarranted in a terminally ill patient

Hiccups generally involve the left diaphragm but have a minimal effect on ventilation. An increase in P_{CO_2} decreases the frequency of hiccups (Waller & Caroline, 2000).

In patients near death, gastric distension is most likely the underlying cause of hiccups, accounting for 95% of cases (Twycross, 1997).

ASSESSMENT AND MEASUREMENT

A complete evaluation for hiccups includes identification of possible contributing etiologies. The ability to intervene and the methods of intervention will be based on the patient's current stage of illness.

HISTORY AND PHYSICAL EXAMINATION

Underlying medical diagnoses often suggest the cause of hiccups. The history and physical examination should be directed to rule out the causes discussed. In addition, the following aspects of the history and physical examination should be considered:

- Length of the episode and its effect on the patient's quality of life
- Review of medications (renal hemodialysis patients have been reported to have hiccups following ingestion of "star fruit") (Noble & Green, 2001)
- Comprehensive medical history to evaluate for history of any recent surgery, stroke, or renal dialysis
- Measures, if any, the patient has used in an attempt to relieve the hiccups (a patient who indicates that inducing emesis relieved hiccups may have increased acidity causing the hiccup problem)
- Check for foreign bodies in the ear canal, since they can stimulate hiccups
- Examination of the body for possible sources of irritation to the diaphragm, vagus, and phrenic nerves (Petroianu, 2005)
- Evaluation for neurological findings that may be associated with hiccups such as multiple sclerosis and increased intracranial pressure (Petroianu, 2005)

DIAGNOSTICS

Diagnostic tests will generally not yield a cause for hiccups. However, a radiographic study may be beneficial in patients with an optimal performance status.

Laboratory studies may be used to evaluate for electrolyte disturbances that may be related.

INTERVENTION AND TREATMENT

Treatment for hiccups in end-stage illness is often questionable. However, if an underlying cause is identified and the treatment is consistent with the goals of care and desires of the patient and family, treatment is appropriate. For example, if the underlying cause is related to pneumonia, treating the pneumonia with the intent of providing comfort—in this case, relief of distressing hiccups—is entirely appropriate. In addition, if medications are identified as a possible cause, discontinuing the offending medication and substituting another may also be appropriate.

Pharmacological Interventions

The pharmacological approaches to hiccups can be organized into several categories: phrenic and/or vagal stimulation, reduction of gastric distention, muscle relaxation, and central suppression of the hiccup reflex. Table 29-1 summarizes a number of possible pharmacological interventions.

Complementary and Nonpharmacological Interventions

Nonpharmacological interventions for hiccups are numerous. Most patients and families have attempted these before contacting a clinician. It is still appropriate to try these approaches if they have not been attempted but to consider the degree of distress related to hiccups and add pharmacological approaches as appropriate. The use of Aschner's oculocardiac reflex (compression of the eyeball) has been identified as one means of terminating hiccups (Petroianu, 2005). Table 29-1 lists a variety of other nonpharmacological methods to control hiccups.

Intensive Measures

Consideration of invasive and more intensive physical measures must be carefully evaluated for use in the palliative care setting. Such measures may include nasogastric tube insertion, transesophageal diaphragmatic pacing, and vagus nerve stimulation (Andres, 2005; Payne, Tiel, Payne et al., 2005; Petroianu, 2005).

PATIENT AND FAMILY EDUCATION

Hiccups can be a distressing symptom for both patient and family. As with all symptoms, patients and families should be taught about the probable underlying cause and proposed treatment plan(s) and urged to contact their clinician if the planned interventions are not effective. They also need to be reassured that control of distressing symptoms is the highest priority in their plan of care, in keeping of course with the wishes and goals of the patient and family. The consequences of no treatment should be part of the overall goal-setting discussion.

TABLE 29-1 ■ Interventions for Hiccup Management

Agent	Suggested Dosing
Pharmacological Approaches	
Baclofen	5 to 20 mg orally twice or three times daily
Carbamazepine	200 mg orally three or four times daily
Chlorpromazine	25 to 50 mg intramuscularly initially, followed by 25 to 50 mg orally three times daily
Gabapentin	300 to 400 mg orally three times daily
Haloperidol	5 mg intravenously every 6 hr initially and/or 1 to 4 mg subcutaneously three times daily
Methylphenidate	5 mg orally twice daily
Metoclopramide	10 mg intravenously over 2 min, followed by 10 orally three to four times daily
Simethicone-containing antacids	Four times a day (before meals and at bedtime)
Nonpharmacological Approaches	
Acupuncture	
Biting a lemon	
Breathing into a paper bag	
Drinking peppermint water (do not combine with metoclopramide)	
Dropping a cold key down the back of the shirt	
Holding breath	
Repeated tapping over C5 dermatome	
Supra-supramaximal inspiration	
Swallowing a teaspoon of dry sugar	
Swallowing dry bread	

Data from Hernandez, J.L., Pajaron, M., Garcia-Regata, O., et al. (2004). Gabapentin for intractable hiccup. *Am J Med, 117*(4), 279-281; Krakauer, E.L., Zhu, A.X., Bounds, B.C., et al. (2005). Case records of the Massachusetts general hospital. Weekly clinicopathological exercises. Case 6-2005. A 58-year-old man with esophageal cancer and nausea, vomiting, and intractable hiccups. *N Engl J Med, 352*(8), 817-825; Marechal, R., Berghmans, T., & Sculier, P. (2003). Successful treatment of intractable hiccup with methylphenidate in a lung cancer patient. *Support Care Cancer, 11*(2), 126-128; Moro, C., Sironi, P., Berardi, E., et al. (2005). Midazolam for long-term treatment of intractable hiccup. *J Pain Symptom Manage, 29*(3), 221-223; Morris, L.G., Marti, J.L., & Ziff, D.J. (2004). Termination of idiopathic persistent singultus (hiccup) with supra-supramaximal inspiration. *J Emerg Med, 27*(4), 416-417; Sanchack, K.E. (2004). Hiccups: When the diaphragm attacks. *J Palliat Med, 7*(6), 870-873; and Smith, H.S., & Busracamwongs, A. (2003). Management of hiccups in the palliative care population. *Am J Hospice Palliat Care, 20*(2), 149-154.

EVALUATION AND PLAN FOR FOLLOW-UP

Treatment is judged successful when the hiccups are resolved (in terms of patient-determined goals) or do not recur. In some cases, several trials and combinations of different interventions may occur before the symptom is resolved to the patient's and family's satisfaction. Although there is little in the literature regarding hiccups in end-of-life care, it is reasonable to expect them to occur as the patient status changes. Continual patient evaluation and inquiries about new or recurrent symptoms and their management are important factors.

CASE STUDY   Mrs. C. is a 36-year-old woman with metastatic breast cancer. She has known bone and liver involvement. Her pain has been under adequate control until she started experiencing intractable hiccups during the past 4 days. She reports trying a variety of "home remedies," which included holding her breath, breathing into a paper bag, and biting into a lemon. She obtains occasional relief of symptoms but only for a short duration, and they are back again.

Her current medications include a 50-mg fentanyl patch that is changed every 72 hours, 10 to 20 mg of immediate-release morphine for breakthrough pain every 2 to 3 hours as needed, senna 2 tablets three times daily, prednisolone 20 mg daily, and lorazepam 1 mg orally every 8 hours as needed for anxiety.

The ongoing hiccups have increased her pain level to the point where she has increased the frequency of her breakthrough medication. As a result, she is also starting to have more problems with constipation. She is starting to feel nauseated from the hiccups as well as experiencing increased agitation, anxiety, and frustration.

The physical examination revealed a mildly distended abdomen and slightly diminished bowel sounds. The liver was moderately enlarged, crossing the midline, and increased in size from her last examination. The clinician believes the etiology of her hiccups to likely be related to increased compression of the diaphragm and stomach from progressive hepatic metastasis but also multifactorial.

A trial of methylphenidate 10 mg orally every 6 hours is initiated. This relieved Mrs. C.'s nausea and her constipation has improved, but her hiccups have not resolved completely. A trial dose of chlorpromazine 25 mg is given and effectively stops the hiccups, but the patient experienced mild delirium with it. This led to the initiation of baclofen 5 mg three times daily. Within 24 hours, the patient had no further complaints of hiccups. She started to experience loose stools, which was believed to possibly be related to the methylphenidate, which had not been discontinued. The dosage of this was decreased to 10 mg orally twice daily, and the patient had no further problems with diarrhea but has maintained improved bowel function and has no nausea.

REFERENCES

Andres, D.W. (2005). Transesophageal diaphragmatic pacing for treatment of persistent hiccups. *Anesthesiology, 102(2)*, 483.

Krakauer, E.L., Zhu, A.X., Bounds, B.C., et al. (2005). Case records of the Massachusetts General Hospital. Weekly clinicopathological exercises. Case 6-2005. A 58-year-old man with esophageal cancer and nausea, vomiting, and intractable hiccups. *N Engl J Med, 352(8)*, 817-825.

Noble, J. & Green, H.L. (2001). *Textbook of primary care medicine* (3rd ed., pp. 187-189). St. Louis: Mosby.

Payne, B.R., Tiel, R.L., Payne, M.S., et al. (2005). Vagus nerve stimulation for chronic intractable hiccups. Case report. *J Neurosurg, 102(5)*, 935-937.

Petroianu, G.A. (2005). Hiccups. In R.E. Rakel & E.T. Bope (Eds.). *Conn's current therapy 2005* (57th ed., pp. 12-16). Philadelphia: Saunders. Retrieved January 21, 2005, from MDConsult online database at www.mdconsult.com

Ripamonti, C. & Fusco, F. (2002). Respiratory problems in advanced cancer. *Support Care Cancer, 10(3)*, 204-216.

Twycross R. (1997). *Symptom management in advanced cancer* (2nd ed.). Oxon, UK: Radcliffe Medical Press.

Waller, A. & Caroline, N. (2000). *Handbook of palliative care in cancer* (2nd ed.). Boston: Butterworth-Heinemann.

CHAPTER 30

LYMPHEDEMA

Jane M. Armer and Sheila H. Ridner

■

Although it is hoped that lymphedema may decrease in incidence due to improved surgical techniques and procedures, lymphedema still occurs in a significant percentage of individuals and may be of sufficient degree to increase patient's risk for infection, affect mobility, and cause a decline in overall quality of life (Muscari, 2004). It is important for the advanced practice nurse (APN) and all other palliative care health professionals to understand how to manage a patient with lymphedema.

DEFINITION AND INCIDENCE

Lymphedema is a condition in which excessive fluid and protein accumulate in the extravascular and interstitial space. This occurs when the lymphatic system cannot either accept or transport lymph (the colorless fluid that bathes the cells of the body, carrying away byproducts of metabolism and helping to fight infection) into the circulatory system (Browse, Burnand, & Mortimer, 2003; Rockson, 2001). Primary lymphedema due to genetic and familial abnormalities in the lymphatic structure or function may occur in 1 of every 10,000 individuals (Townsend, Beauchamp, Evers et al., 2001). Incidence of secondary lymphedema varies depending on the cause. For example, 15% to 20% of breast cancer survivors in the United States may develop lymphedema, and approximately 90 million individuals worldwide may have secondary lymphedema caused by filarial (parasitic) infections (Petrek, Pressman, & Smith, 2000; Townsend et al., 2001). Although the occurrence of lymphedema in palliative care settings is unknown, one lymphedema clinic reported that approximately 30% of their clients were advanced cancer patients with lower limb swelling (Logan, 1995), and lymphedema is cited in the literature as a distressful symptom experienced by patients in palliative care settings (Winn & Dentino, 2004).

Lymphedema is a chronic medical condition requiring careful management. Because lymphedema can develop at any time throughout life (Browse et al., 2003; Foldi, Foldi, & Kubik, 2003), the clinician may have to address both recent-onset (acute) and long-existing (chronic) lymphedema in patients receiving palliative care.

ETIOLOGY AND PATHOPHYSIOLOGY

In healthy individuals, blood capillaries and lymphatic structures support fluid exchange at the blood capillary–interstitial–lymphatic interface. Capillary pressure, negative interstitial pressure, and interstitial fluid colloid osmotic pressure collectively exert approximately 41 mm Hg outward pressure, and plasma colloid osmotic pressure exerts 28 mm Hg inward pressure, resulting in a net filtration pressure of 13 mm Hg from the arterial side of capillaries into the interstitial space (Guyton & Hall, 2000). Approximately 90% of this fluid reenters the blood circulatory system through venous ends of capillaries, and the remaining 10% enters lymphatic collectors. Fluid return to the venous end of the capillary is facilitated by the net venous reabsorption pressure of 7 mm Hg created by the imbalance between capillary, negative interstitial, and interstitial fluid colloid pressure of 21 mm Hg outward pressure and the inward plasma colloid osmotic pressure of 28 mm Hg (Guyton & Hall, 2000). Fluid and the larger protein molecules enter the lymphatic system through small one-way valves and are moved by contraction of lymphangions (segments of vessels), contraction of surrounding muscles, and contractile filaments in the endothelial cells through the lymphatic vessels into the blood circulatory system (Ridner, 2002).

When the lymphatic system can no longer transport the normal fluid and protein load or when there is reduced lymphatic transport capacity coupled with increased lymph, lymphedema develops (Browse et al., 2003; Foldi et al., 2003). Lymphedema can arise from either primary (idiopathic) or secondary (acquired) conditions. Primary lymphedema occurs in the presence of malformation of lymph vessels and/or lymph nodes and is associated with many medical conditions (Table 30-1). Primary lymphedema is classified based on timing of first noted swelling (Foldi et al., 2003):

- Congenital lymphedema, present at birth
- Lymphedema praecox, develops after birth but before age 35
- Lymphedema tarda, develops after age 35

TABLE 30-1 ■ Lymphedema: Etiologies and Causes

Primary Lymphedema: Associated Diseases

Nonne-Milroy syndrome	Hennekam syndrome
Turner syndrome	Mixed vascular and lymphatic disorders
Noonan syndrome	Milroy syndrome
Fibrosis of inguinal nodes	Meige syndrome
Yellow nail syndrome	Lymphedema and distichiasis
Adams-Olivier syndrome	Neurofibromatosis
Proteus syndrome	Aagenaes syndrome
Klippel-Trenaunay syndrome	Prader-Willi syndrome

Secondary Lymphedema: Selected Causes

Category	Examples
Infection	Filariasis, tuberculosis, toxoplasmosis, postsurgical infection
Trauma	Surgery, automobile accident, crush injuries, burns, vein removal, self-inflicted injury
Cancer and cancer treatment	Tumor occluding lymphatic structures (new or recurrent), lymphatic-infiltrating metastatic disease, Kaposi's sarcoma, surgery, radiation, and postsurgical infection
Venous disease	Postthrombic conditions, venous ulcerations, intravenous drug abuse causing venous thrombosis and/or abscesses
Immobility	Paralysis, extreme fatigue, venous stasis
Inflammation	Rheumatoid arthritis, dermatitis, psoriasis

Secondary lymphedema, lymphedema with a known cause, is the most common lymphedema in developed countries (see Table 30-1). It can occur immediately after the known insult to the lymphatic system or have a latency stage and appear many years later (Foldi et al., 2003). Any patient who has had a lymph node dissection or a tumor that impedes lymphatic circulation is at risk for developing lymphedema.

Both primary and secondary lymphedema may appear first as acute and then chronic disease (lasting longer than 6 months) that can progress over time through three stages of severity. Physical presentation of swelling is the same regardless of cause. Initially, in grade I, the limb will swell and pit with pressure, and elevation will relieve the swelling. In grade II, the limb will become firmer, not pit with pressure, and skin changes, hair loss, and alteration in nails may be noted. In grade III, elephantiasis results with very thick skin and large skin folds (Pain & Purushotham, 2000).

ASSESSMENT AND MEASUREMENT

Lymphedema assessment may entail evaluation of new-onset acute swelling or preexisting lymphedema. In both cases, it is imperative to assess immediately for infection and, if present, initiate treatment (Feldman, 2005; Olszewski, 2005; Weissleder & Schuchhardt, 2001) (Table 30-2). Awakening with a hot, painful, swollen limb may be the first sign or symptom of lymphedema onset. Likewise, individuals with chronic lymphedema can rapidly develop cellulitis or lymphangitis. Infections can quickly escalate into emergency situations such as life-threatening septicemia. When assessing infection, look for redness, spreading either locally or in a distinct red line. Touch the area to determine if it is warm and/or painful. Observe for oozing or drainage in the area. Check the patient's temperature. Palpate for enlarged nodes. Many patients

TABLE 30-2 ■ Lymphedema: Assessment Checklist

Symptom	Yes	No
Bruising		
Rash		
Blistering		
Dusky in color		
Unusual hair loss		
Swelling		
Enlarged lymph node		
Oozing fluid		
Pitting with pressure		
Hard, nonpitting		
Dry and/or flaky		
Hard, nonpitting		
Raised lumps		
Cracking		
Warm to touch		
Cool to touch		

report feeling flu-like symptoms both before and after immediate signs of infection, so inquire about aching, fatigue, nausea, vomiting, weakness, dizziness, chills, or sweating. Any of these signs or symptoms requires immediate antibiotic treatment, and, in the case of a patient near end-of-life, hospitalization may be considered.

When an infection is present and appropriately treated and if no signs or symptoms of infection are noted, both subjective and objective manifestations of lymphedema and associated psychological sequelae should be assessed.

Subjective Symptoms

Subjective indicators may include patient-reported swelling, jewelry or clothing feeling tight, and feeling of heaviness in limbs (Armer, Radina, Porock et al., 2003). For patients with chronic lymphedema, alteration in limb sensation (heaviness, tightness, aching, burning, swelling, hardness, stabbing, pins and needles, and numbness) and fatigue may be reported (Armer & Porock, 2001; Ridner, 2005). Patients may also report a decrease or change in physical activity and demonstrate signs of psychological distress, such as depressed mood, frustration, anger about the swelling, and feeling helpless to manage their condition (Ridner, 2005). These subtle or overt changes in sensation may be the first indicators of lymphedema, lymphedema progression, or complications such as infection prior to objective changes.

Objective Signs

Currently, there is no accepted "gold standard" for objective measurement of limb swelling associated with lymphedema. However, multiple methods can be used to measure swelling in affected limbs: (1) water displacement, (2) limb girth measured in cm with a tape measure, (3) infrared laser scanning, and (4) bioelectrical impedance. It is notable that swelling associated with truncal, breast, genital, and head and neck lymphedema may be best assessed with subjective symptom report and observation, as objective fluid assessment measurements are, at best, limited.

Water displacement: Patients are required to remove clothing covering the swollen limb and then to place the uncovered limb in a cylinder of water. The amount of water displaced by the limb estimates the limb volume (Megens, Harris, Kim-Sing et al., 2001). Limbs with wounds cannot be assessed with water displacement. End-of-life patients may be too frail, weak, and fatigued to extend the limb vertically into the water displacement volumeter until overflow dripping stops.

Circumferential measurement: Patients must remove all limb coverings and sit, extending limbs horizontally while measurement increments are marked on their skin or on a strip of adhesive tape attached to the skin. A nonstretch tape is then placed around the limb at intervals of 10, 5, or 4 cm from wrist to axilla or ankle to groin. Both limbs are measured for comparison at similar anatomic or centimeter locations, or total bilateral limb volume is calculated for comparison. This is the most commonly used method of limb volume measurement in clinical settings; however, measurement error may potentially mask lymphedema occurrence or progression or falsely implied lymphedema (Armer, 2005).

Perometer: This optoelectronic volumetry device (Juzo, Cuyahoga Falls, OH) uses infrared laser technology (Petlund, 1991). The perometer estimates total limb volume and records limb shape, using PeroPlus computer software (Juzo, 2002).

Clothing must be removed from the limb before measurement. The size and nonportable nature of the machine require that patients come into the clinic for limb measurement.

Bioelectrical impedance: A bioelectrical impedance device known as the Lymphometer (ImpediMed, Queensland, Australia) is being used in research settings to estimate limb volume and assess presence of lymphedema. This device uses low-voltage electric current to determine extracellular fluid (lymph) (Cornish, Chapman, Thomas et al., 2000). Clothing remains on, the procedure is quick and painless, and the device is portable.

Varying standards are used to diagnose lymphedema. For example, a 2- to 10-cm increase in circumference, 200-ml limb volume increase, or a 5% to 10% limb volume increase, compared with prior measurements in the same area or to the contralateral limb, is a standard for the definition of lymphedema as cited in the literature (Bland, Perczyk, Du et al., 2003). Thus, measurements falling within these ranges may indicate lymphedema. When using bioelectrical impedance, ratios of affected to unaffected limb volumes are calculated; manufacturer-suggested cut points for possible lymphedema have been established.

In addition to actual volume measurement, asymmetry in limbs, head and neck, trunk, or genital areas due to swelling secondary to lymph fluid accumulation may be observed. In some cases, Stemmer's sign may be present. This skinfold sign is typically assessed by placing a finger on each side of the base of a toe or finger and squeezing gently; in addition, use of this technique in other body segments, such as limbs and trunk, has been documented (Weissleder & Schuchhardt, 2001). When lymphedema is present, a thickening of this fold is noted when compared to a nonlymphedematous digit. However, the absence of Stemmer's sign does not rule out lymphedema.

HISTORY AND PHYSICAL EXAMINATION

When conducting a history and physical examination of a patient with lymphedema, it is important to keep in mind possible differential (or comorbid) diagnoses, such as myxedema, lipidema, deep vein thrombosis, cancer recurrence, chronic venous insufficiency, cellulitis, or other infections (Rockson, 2001).

History should include the following:
- Review of all current and prior medical diagnoses including infections
- Course of current illness including onset (new or preexisting) of swelling, location of swelling, and exacerbation and remission of symptoms
- Review of current medications and medical treatment (e.g., radiation, surgery, antibiotic therapy, etc.)
- Review of possible causes (surgery, tumor, previous trauma)
- Family history of lymphedema or possibly undiagnosed chronic limb and/or body swelling
- Symptom review: heaviness or other sensations in affected area, skin crease depth in limb, perceived swelling, tighter-fitting clothing or jewelry on the affected side, pain, decrease or difficulty in mobility

Physical examination should include the following:
- Location and spread of swelling

- Stemmer's sign test
- Signs of infection as previously discussed
- Volume measurement if possible
- Determination of stage of lymphedema
- Skin assessment (see Table 30-2)

DIAGNOSTICS

Lymphedema onset is often multifactorial and challenging to diagnose in palliative care settings (Cheville, 2002). For this reason, it is helpful to distinguish between the progression of established lymphedema due to diminished efficacy of treatment and edema related to direct tumor spread and/or other systemic factors (Cheville, 2002). Many cancer patients with secondary lymphedema experience progression of previously controlled lymphedema with advancing disease, largely due to reduced ability to adhere to the rigorous complete decongestive therapy (CDT) maintenance regimen (Cheville, 2002). Further, lymphedema may develop or progress secondary to direct tumor spread, independently of the adequacy of a CDT program (Cheville, 2002). For example, new-onset edema in the legs, genitalia, and/or lower trunk may reflect tumor recurrence, particularly in cancers such as cervical, uterine, ovarian, prostate, and lymphomas. Palliative radiation therapy to reduce tumor bulk or slow disease progression may also cause lymphedema. Additionally, certain systemic conditions associated with advancing illness may produce or exacerbate lymphedema (e.g., fluid and electrolyte imbalances, reduced protein synthesis, renal failure, and compromised cardiac function) (Cheville, 2002).

If, after completion of the history and physical examination, additional information is needed to make a differential diagnosis and/or to determine type of treatment, additional diagnostic testing can be done. Potential risks, possible discomfort, and cost must be balanced with potential benefits, including whether the overall plan of care and, specifically, care for the swollen limb, will be affected by the findings.

Magnetic resonance imaging (MRI), duplex scanning, or phlebography can be used to rule out deep vein thrombosis (Townsend et al., 2001). MRI, ultrasonography, or phlebography can be used to rule out chronic deep venous insufficiency. Computed tomography scans can help identify lymphatic obstructions and guide lymphedema therapists to potentially unobstructed drainage pathways that can be used during treatment (Cheville, 2002).

Lymphoscintigraphy, the primary diagnostic method used to visualize the lymphatics (Williams, Witte, Witte et al., 2000), must be done in a nuclear medicine setting by an experienced clinician. This procedure involves injection of a radioactively tagged tracer and scanning to evaluate lymph flow and lymphatic structure. It is used frequently to determine the structural cause of lymphedema and, in some situations, to monitor the effectiveness of treatment (Szuba, Strauss, Sirsikar et al., 2002).

INTERVENTION AND TREATMENT

Clinician collaboration with certified lymphedema therapists, the patient, and caregiver(s) is needed to determine if the risks and discomforts associated with the treatment

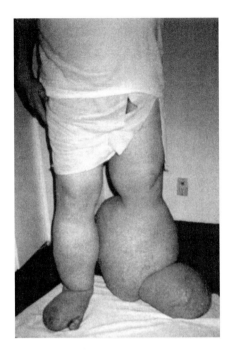

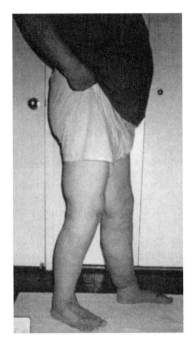

Figure 30-1 Below-knee lymphedema before treatment. (From www. nortonschool.com/aboutlymphedema.html.)

Figure 30-2 Below-knee lymphedema after treatment. (From www.nortonschool.com/aboutlymphedema.html.)

outweigh potential benefits. In patients nearing death, no treatment may be needed, unless infection is present. Successful treatment of lymphedema is directly related to understanding the underlying pathological condition(s) causing the problem and its accompanying symptoms. Sometimes it may not be possible to control worsening lymphedema. Thus, it is imperative that in addition to initiating treatment for the swelling, the clinician must also intervene as needed for symptoms such as pain, depressed mood, increased fatigue, difficulties in carrying out activities of daily living, and decreased self-esteem (Geller, Vacek, O'Brien et al., 2003; Ridner, 2005). If generalized infection is present, the use of compression bandages, manual lymph drainage, and exercises should be stopped until the patient is afebrile, skin temperature returns to normal, and erythema is receding (Feldman, 2005). If there is an open wound, it must be addressed immediately.

Infection Management

Because microorganisms penetrating the skin may trigger infections, meticulous skin care among patients with lymphedema is a necessary preventative measure. When infection occurs, Olszewski (1996, 2005) recommends skin bacteriological cultures for patients experiencing frequently recurring episodes of dermatitis, lymphangitis, and lymphadenitis and treatment with effective antibiotics such as penicillin or erythromycin.

Dermatolymphangioadenitis (DLA) may occur in persons with chronic lymphedema and is followed by an increase in swelling in the affected area (Olszewski, 2005). Episodes of DLA are most frequently observed in the postsurgical, posttraumatic, and postdermatitis types of secondary lymphedema, as well as in the late and advanced stages of primary forms (Olszewski, 2005). Among the bacterial strains most commonly isolated are *Staphylococcus epidermidis* and other coagulase-negative staphylococci, micrococci, and *Acinetobacter* but not streptococci. Antibiotics for acute episodes should be prescribed based on the causative agent. Once a patient has had DLA, it frequently recurs. To prevent DLA recurrence, Olszewski (2005) recommends administration of long-term (minimally over 3 months and up to 12 months)intramuscular penicillin accompanied by local anesthetic. Oral penicillin may be considered for those able to swallow. For patients with penicillin allergy, erythromycin is given orally for an extended period of time (3 to 12 months).

Lymphedema Management

When treating lymphedema, the current "gold standard" treatment is CDT, a two-phase treatment protocol for both primary and secondary lymphedema (Badger, Preston, Seers et al., 2004; Harris, Hugi, Olivotto et al., 2001; Rockson, 2001). Phase 1 consists of intensive, manual lymphatic drainage (MLD), a specialized massage; around-the-clock two-way short-stretch compression bandaging; a program of exercises; and meticulous skin care. Phase 2, the maintenance phase, includes life-long wearing of daytime elastic sleeves or stockings, nighttime compression wrapping, exercises, and skin care. To work consistently in palliative care, conventional approaches to lymphedema management such as CDT may need to be modified substantially (Cheville, 2002). For example, compressive bandaging may need to be modified due to skin metastases, painful areas, radiation burns, pathological fractures, and other adverse conditions. Further, if lymphatic obstruction is undetectable with conventional imaging, the therapist may have to rely on anatomic understanding of the lymphatic system to identify patient drainage pathways (Cheville, 2002). Thus, lymphedema therapists and clinicians must work together and recognize that their attention, acceptance of the patient, and willingness to adapt and persevere may be, in and of themselves, therapeutic independent of objective improvement (Cheville, 2002). Table 30-3 discusses adaptations of CDT for palliative care needs.

Sequential pneumatic compression pumps, single or multicompartmentalized compression devices consisting of cells that deflate and inflate, are sometimes used as an alternative to CDT when access to lymphedema therapists or caregivers is limited and the patient has limited mobility or energy. When properly applied, these pumps move fluid proximally within the limb but cannot move fluid from the limb into the trunk as does CDT (Rockson, 2001). When the patient or caregiver has limited energy or mobility for completion of the full range of CDT, the pump may also be used in conjunction with modified CDT techniques to aid movement of fluid from the limb into the trunk. Caution must be taken to prevent tissue injury and worsening of lymphedema and related symptoms due to inappropriate placement and pressures greater than sustainable by the fragile lymphatic collectors (Boris, Weindorf, & Lasinski, 1998; Eliska & Eliskova, 1995).

TABLE 30-3 ■ Lymphedema Treatment: Adapting Complete Decongestive Therapy (CDT) for Palliative Care

Key Considerations	Description
Skin breakdown	Compression will limit edema and facilitate diffusion of oxygen and nutrients. Place compressive bandages over painless areas of skin breakdown that are free of infection. Dressings should not adhere to the wound. Use petroleum jelly–impregnated or other nonadherent gauze to avoid discomfort during dressing changes. Adhering bandages or dressing materials can be "soaked off" to prevent ripping the skin. Change bandages BID if skin breakdown occurs within the area of CDT treatment. Instruct patient and caregivers on safe and effective bandaging.
Bandaging materials	Tailor palliative CDT program for each patient. Use Artiflex or extra foam padding to protect bony prominences. Use fewer than normal bandages for patients whose additional care is demanding and when maintenance rather than reduction of limb volume is goal. Protect skin adjacent to wrapped areas if taut, irritated, or friable. Cut Tubigrip and sew to protect surrounding skin from abrasive short-stretch bandages. If lymphorrhea is present, to absorb moisture, use calcium alginate padding next to the skin. Apply impermeable membrane just outside the alginate to avoid wet bandages.
Anticipate progression	Phase II (maintenance) CDT program must consider future functional deterioration. Educate patient and caretakers in strategies to adapt and modify their phase II program. Consider use of a Mediassist device, Legacy or Tribute garment, or Reid Sleeve to increase the probability of success. Donning garments is difficult for weak patients. Layer two compressive garments of a lower class or use a zippered garment.
Remedial exercise	Consider progressive weakness. Exercise performance with gravity eliminated may extend the utility of the program. Modify exercises in consideration of plegic or painful structures. Do not stress skeletal structures with potential bone metastases. Obtain a report of most recent bone scan or skeletal survey to use in devising a safe and humane exercise program.
Manual lymphatic drainage	Clinician and therapist must work closely with the interdisciplinary palliative care team and familiarize themselves with malignant sources of lymphatic obstruction. Lymphatic obstruction may be undetectable by conventional imaging. In such cases, anatomic understanding of the lymphatic system is critical to identify patent drainage pathways.

Data with permission from Cheville, A.J. (2002). *Lymphedema and palliative care. National Lymphedema Network. LymphLink, 14,* 3-4 (reprint). Retrieved from www.lymphnet.org/newsletter/newsletter.htm.

Although careful monitoring and frequent revision to lymphedema treatment modalities are required in palliative care settings, the therapeutic benefits of treatment, such as reestablishing the patient's perception of control, empowerment of caregivers, reducing infection risk, improving mobility, and decreasing risk of skin breakdown, make such treatment an important component of palliative care for individuals with lymphedema (Cheville, 2002).

EVALUATION AND FOLLOW-UP

Volume reduction treatment in the initial intensive phase (and in regular lymphatic follow-up sessions after intensive therapy) usually continues until limb volume plateaus. At that point, patients are transitioned to at-home self-care techniques. Once a

TABLE 30-4 ■ Lymphedema Management: Guide for Chronic Edema

Category	Patient Status	Intervention
Mild and uncomplicated edema	■ Excess limb volume < 20% ■ No trunk, head, or genital swelling ■ No arterial insufficiency or malignancy	■ Education, information, and advice ■ Daily: skin care, exercise, simple lymphatic drainage, and compression ■ Monitoring and referral if required
Moderate to severe, complicated edema	■ Excess limb volume >20% with trunk, head, or genital edema ■ Distorted limb shape ■ Skin problems ■ Evidence of active controlled malignancy, arterial and/or venous insufficiency, current acute inflammatory episode, and/or lymphorrhea	■ Education, information, and advice ■ Multilayer LE bandaging, manual lymph drainage, isotonic exercises, skin care, compression garments ■ Referral to other members of the health care team ■ Transfer to maintenance program as required
Edema and advanced disease	■ Edema associated with advanced disease ■ Trunk and/or midline edema, lymphorrhea, tension in the tissues, impaired mobility and function, pain, infection	■ Education, information, and advice ■ Emphasis on quality of life ■ Daily skin care, support and positioning of the limb, exercises, lymphatic drainage ■ Specialist interventions such as manual lymphatic drainage, modified multilayer bandaging, compression garments, appliance to aid mobility and function

Data from the British Lymphology Society. (2006). *Chronic oedema population and need.* Retrieved March 22, 2006, from www.lymphoedema.org/bls/membership/definitions.htm; and Williams, A. (2004). *An overview of non-cancer related chronic oedema—A UK perspective.* Retrieved December 12, 2004, from www.worldwidewounds.com/2003/april/Williams/Chronic-Oedema.html.

patient has been diagnosed with lymphedema, the clinician will need to observe for any change in the lymphedematous area at each patient visit. This evaluation should include assessment for signs and symptoms of infection, increased swelling, pain, and emotional distress. Table 30-4 details situations requiring referral to specialists in lymphedema management.

PATIENT AND FAMILY EDUCATION

Clinicians and lymphedema therapists caring for the patient must communicate clearly with each other and with the patient and caregivers. Issues such as how and who will provide the self-care required after hands-on, phase I intensive professional therapy is completed must be clearly understood. Information about restrictions on activity must also be provided and instructions on how to assist the patient during movement given. Self-care will include daily cleaning of the skin in the swollen area with nonsoap or mild soap or cleansers, drying the area thoroughly, and applying oil-based pH-neutral creams or lotions to maintain hydration. Unscented products are recommended (Mortimer & Badger, 2004). Patients and caregivers should be taught signs or symptoms of infection and to examine the patient for such signs or symptoms during each cleaning and instructed to contact the clinician immediately if any are noted. Prescribed garments or bandages should be applied and patients and caregivers warned to never use nonprescribed alternatives such as Ace bandages. Patients and caregivers need to be encouraged to tell the clinician when the burdens of lymphedema or its treatment become overwhelming.

CONCLUSION

Lymphedema is a distressing problem for the palliative care patient and his or her family. Timely assessment for the presence and/or worsening of lymphedema and quick intervention are necessary to provide patient comfort. Management of any developing infection in the swollen area is imperative. If treatment becomes too burdensome for the patient, the clinician should reevaluate and modify treatment goals accordingly.

CASE STUDY

H., age 79, is a widowed, intermediate-level nursing care facility resident. She is alert and articulate and has a keen interest in the bustling activity around her. She is a 26-year breast cancer survivor who underwent a radical mastectomy. Three months ago, H. was told the pain in her back and ribs was due to metastasis of her breast cancer. Although the prognosis is uncertain, palliative care is planned. H. has had grade II lymphedema of the left arm for 10 years. The arm is approximately one-and-a-half times larger than the other arm; by circumferential assessment, limb volume is 1000 ml greater on the affected side. The arm is brawny, nonpitting, and firm to palpation. When she is in a wheelchair, she wears a hemiplegic-style sling due to heaviness of the limb and her inability to bear the weight of the limb without assistance. She cannot manage her four-legged walker because of weakness and heaviness of the limb. She has weeping (lymphorrhea) and occasional "shooting" pains in the arm and has had six episodes of cellulitis over the past 18 months, with each episode treated with oral antibiotics. H. takes oral medication for hypertension and diabetes, has stress incontinence due to a "fallen" uterus (treated palliatively with a pessary, which is managed with nursing assistance), and takes an antiinflammatory medication as needed for arthritis pain. She limits her fluids through the day and especially at bedtime due to worry about "accidents" from stress incontinence.

H. says she has a "fat arm" that she knows "no one wants to look at." She has not been fitted for a compression sleeve for many years and does not regularly wear a sleeve in the daytime or a bandage at night. She has never had CDT, as her doctor once told her there was no effective treatment to "cure" the lymphedema. Over the years, her only treatment has been the occasional wearing of a heavy flesh-colored sleeve that was "too hot" in warm weather, "bothersome" in doing her gardening and housework, and "not very pretty" to wear in public.

The clinician is asked to see H. today because a 4-day wound has failed to heal after her forearm on the affected side was injured during a wheelchair transfer.

The wound has a border of a 0.5-cm ring of erythema and produces a colorless exudate. The surrounding area is warm to the touch and the forearm is tender. No elevation of temperature is noted.

Plan of care to manage the wound on the affected arm and the lymphedema:

- Discuss goals in managing her lymphedema. Incorporate her goals and priorities for herself and her health in the plan of care in view of the recent evidence of breast cancer progression.
- Clean and dress wound with petroleum jelly impregnated gauze over antibiotic cream (e.g., Bactroban) twice daily.
- Administer oral antibiotics (erythromycin because of a history of penicillin allergy) for 14 days.
- Monitor hydration and nutrition, including adequate dietary protein. Explain to H. that adequate fluid intake is necessary for healing and maintaining health and comfort, and that concentrated urine is associated with more frequent urination and increased risk of a urinary tract infection.
- Refer to a therapist(s) with special training in lymphedema management to assess eligibility and readiness for a course of intensive CDT therapy. Assess H.'s openness to CDT for comfort, as well as for reduction of limb volume.
- Determine alternative strategies for reducing limb volume and weeping to promote comfort and healing and to reduce risk of future infection. Explore use of a washable, custom-fit, foam-filled compression garment (e.g., Legacy, Tribute) to facilitate healing, reduce limb volume, and improve comfort.
- Evaluate need for pain medication. Encourage elevation of the affected arm on a soft pillow to reduce fluid accumulation as a result of being in a dependent position.
- Educate patient, family, and staff on how to care for limb: keep area clean, elevate swollen arm, observe for redness, heat, or foul odor.

With the complexities and stressors of advanced disease, the posttreatment consequence of lymphedema, and other comorbidities, H.'s case is challenging—and not so unusual in the world of chronic illness and palliative care. As in this case study, individualized, holistic, and multidisciplinary patient care partnered with ongoing education of patients and staff are key ingredients in treatment plans that can improve quality of life.

REFERENCES

Armer, J.M. (2005). The problem of post-breast cancer lymphedema: Impact and measurement issues. *Cancer Investigation, 1,* 71-77.

Armer, J. & Porock, D. (2001). Self-reported fatigue in women with lymphedema. *LymphLink, 13(3),* 1-4.

Armer, J.M., Radina, M.E., Porock, D., et al. (2003). Predicting breast cancer-related lymphedema using self-reported symptoms. *Nurs Res, 52,* 370-379.

Badger, C., Preston, N., Seers, K., et al. (2004). Physical therapies for reducing and controlling lymphedema of the limbs. Cochrane Breast Cancer Group. *Cochrane Database of Systematic Reviews, 4,* CD003141.

Bland, K.L., Perczyk, R., Du, W., et al. (2003). Can a practicing surgeon detect early lymphedema? *Am J Surg, 186,* 509-513.

Boris, M., Weindorf, S., & Lasinski, B. (1998). The risk of genital edema after external pump compression for lower limb lymphedema. *Lymphology, 31,* 15-20.

British Lymphology Society. (2006). *Chronic oedema population and need.* Retrieved March 22, 2006, from www.lymphoedema.org/bls/membership/definitions.htm.

Browse, N., Burnand, K.G., & Mortimer, P.S. (2003). *Diseases of the lymphatics.* London, England: Arnold.

Cheville, A.J. (2002). *Lymphedema and palliative care. National Lymphedema Network. LymphLink, 14,* 1-4 (reprint). Retrieved from www.lymphnet.org/newsletter/newsletter.htm.

Cornish, B.H., Chapman, M., Thomas, B.J., et al. (2000). Early diagnosis of lymphedema in post-surgery breast cancer patients. *Ann N Y Acad Sci, 904,* 571-575.

Eliska, O. & Eliskova, M. (1995). Are peripheral lymphatics damaged by high pressure manual massage? *Lymphology, 28,* 21-30.

Feldman, J.L. (2005 October). The challenge of infection in lymphedema. National Lymphedema Network. *LymphLink.*

Foldi, M., Foldi, E., & Kubik, S. (Eds.). (2003). *Textbook of lymphology for physicians and lymphedema therapists.* Munchen, Germany: Urban & Fischer.

Geller, B.M., Vacek, P.M., O'Brien, P., et al. (2003). Factors associated with arm swelling after breast cancer surgery. *J Women Health, 12,* 921-930.

Guyton, A.C. & Hall, J.E. (2000). *Textbook of medical physiology* (10th ed.). Philadelphia: Saunders.

Harris, S.R., Hugi, M.R., Olivotto, I.A., et al. (2001). Clinical practice guidelines for the care and treatment of breast cancer lymphedema. *Can Med Assoc J, 164,* 191-199.

Juzo Compression Therapy Garments. (2002). *Perometer Plus: A complete compression garment measurement system.* Cuyahoga Falls, Ohio: Author.

Logan, V.B. (1995). Incidence and prevalence of lymphedema: a literature review. *J Clin Nurs, 4,* 213-219.

Megens, A.M., Harris, S.R., Kim-Sing, C., et al. (2001). Measurement of upper extremity volume in women after axillary dissection for breast cancer. *Arch Phys Med Rehabil, 82,* 1639-1644.

Mortimer, P.S. & Badger, C. (2004). Lymphoedema. In D. Doyle, G. Hanks, N.I. Cherney, & K. Calmans (Eds.). *Oxford textbook of palliative medicine* (3rd ed.). Oxford: Oxford University Press.

Muscari, E. (2004). Lymphedema: Responding to our patients' needs. *Oncol Nurs Forum, 31,* 905-912.

Olszewski, W.L. (1996). Inflammatory changes of skin in lymphedema of extremities and efficacy of benzathine penicillin administration. National Lymphedema Network. *LymphLink, 8,* 1-2.

Olszewski, W.L. (2005 October). *An alternative viewpoint from across the world on the management of infections in LE. National Lymphedema Network LymphLink.* Retrieved from www.lymphnet.org/newsletter/newsletter.htm.

Pain, S.J. & Purushotham, A.D. (2000). Lymphedema following surgery for breast cancer. *Br J Surg, 87,* 1128-1141.

Petlund, C.F. (1991). Volumetry of limbs. In W.L. Olszewski (Ed.). *Lymph stasis: Pathophysiology, diagnosis and treatment* (pp. 444-451). Boston: CRC Press.

Petrek, J.A., Pressman, P.I., & Smith, R.A. (2000). Lymphedema: Current issues in research and management. *CA Cancer J Clin, 50,* 292-307.

Ridner, S.H. (2002). Breast cancer lymphedema: Pathophysiology and risk reduction guidelines. *Oncol Nurs Forum, 29,* 1285-1293.

Ridner, S.H. (2005). Quality of life and a symptom cluster associated with breast cancer treatment-related lymphedema. *Support Care Cancer, 13,* 904-911.

Rockson, S.G. (2001). Lymphedema. *Am J Med, 110,* 288-295.

Szuba, A., Strauss, W., Sirsikar, S.P., et al. (2002). Quantitative radionuclide lymphoscintigraphy predicts outcome of manual lymphatic therapy in breast cancer-related lymphedema of the upper extremity. *Nucl Med Commun, 23,* 1171-1175.

Townsend, C.M., Jr., Beauchamp, R.D., Evers, B.M., et al. (2001). *Sabiston textbook of surgery: The biological basis of modern surgical practice* (16th ed.). Philadelphia: Saunders.

Weissleder, H., & Schuchhardt, C. (Eds.) (2001). *Lymphedema diagnosis and therapy.* Köln [Cologne]: Germany: Viavital Verlag GmbH.

Williams, A. (2004). *An overview of non-cancer related chronic oedema—A UK perspective.* Retrieved December 12, 2004, from www.worldwidewounds.com/2003/april/Williams/Chronic-Oedema.html.

Williams, W.H., Witte, C.L., Witte, M.H., et al. (2000). Radionuclide lymphangioscintigraphy in the evaluation of peripheral lymphedema. *Clin Nucl Med, 25,* 451-464.

Winn, P.A. & Dentino, A.N. (2004). Quality palliative care in long-term care settings. *J Am Med Dir Assoc, 5,* 197-206.

CHAPTER 31

NAUSEA AND VOMITING

Valarie A. Pompey

■

DEFINITION AND INCIDENCE

Nausea is a subjective feeling that usually, but not always, precludes vomiting. Descriptors include "queasy," "butterflies," and "sick to stomach."

Retching, an involuntary attempt to vomit, consists of rhythmic, labored spasmodic movement of the diaphragm and abdominal muscles causing regurgitation into the esophagus (Woodruff, 2004). Retching often follows nausea and precedes vomiting. Descriptors include "dry heaves."

Vomiting, often confused with nausea, is the forceful contraction of the abdominal muscles (stomach), to cause the expulsion of stomach contents through the mouth (National Comprehensive Cancer Network [NCCN], 2005). Common descriptors include "throwing up."

Nausea and vomiting (N/V) are two of the most frequently reported and feared side effects experienced by patients throughout their cancer experience. N/V affects 60% to 80% of cancer patients undergoing active treatment (Cunningham, 2005), 50% to 60% of patients with advanced disease (Herndon, Jackson, & Hallin, 2002), and as many as 40% of terminally ill patients within in their last week of life (Kazanowski, 2001). If untreated, complications can lead to unnecessary hospitalizations and diminished quality of life (Figure 31-1). N/V is particularly prevalent in persons with breast, stomach, and gynecological cancers, as well as persons with AIDS (Kazanowski, 2001). At end-of-life, N/V is commonly seen as a result of certain conditions such as bowel obstruction, hypercalcemia, constipation or impaction, use of opioids, uremia, and increased intracranial pressure secondary to metastatic disease in the brain. Effective management of these individual symptoms during initial and continued therapy profoundly influences symptom response throughout the cancer trajectory (Rhodes & McDaniel, 2001).

ETIOLOGY AND PATHOPHYSIOLOGY

Still not well defined, the physiological mechanisms for N/V are complex and may involve one or more mechanisms and can occur from one or more neurotransmitters (Wickham, 2005). The vomiting center (VC), located in the brainstem along with the chemoreceptor trigger zone (CTZ), located in the area postrema of the fourth ventricle

The author would like to acknowledge Julie Griffie and Sandy McKinnon for their contributions that remain unchanged from the first edition of this book.

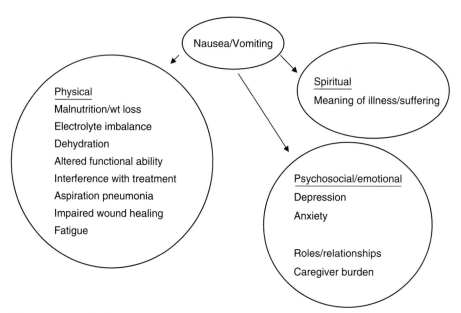

Figure 31-1 Multidimensional effects of nausea and vomiting. Data from Woodruff, R. (2004). Nausea and vomiting. In *Palliative medicine* (4th ed., pp. 223-237). New York: Oxford University Press; and King, C.R. (2001). Nausea and vomiting. In B.R. Ferrell & N. Coyle (Eds.). *Palliative nursing* (pp. 107-121). New York: Oxford University Press.

of the brain, coordinate the processes involved in N/V. The CTZ is stimulated by chemicals and neurotransmitters found in the cerebrospinal fluid and blood. The CTZ, the VC, and the gastrointestinal tract have many neurotransmitter receptors. Activation of these receptors by noxious stimuli results in the symptoms of N/V. The principal neuroreceptors involved in the emetic response include dopamine and serotonin (5-hydroxytryptamine$_3$ [5-HT$_3$]) receptors. Other receptors involved in signal transmission include acetylcholine, corticosteroid, histamine, cannabinoid, opiate, and neurokinin-1 (NK-1), which are located in the VC and vestibular center of the brain (NCCN, 2005) (Table 31-1).

The VC is located in the lateral reticular formation of the medulla oblongata and is situated close to areas in the brain responsible for respiration, salivation, vasomotor processes, and vestibular apparatus (Ezzone, 2000). The VC, which coordinates the process of N/V, receives signals from the cerebral cortex and higher brainstem, thalamus, hypothalamus, and the vestibular system. It also receives emetic impulses via the vagus and splanchnic nerves from the pharynx and gastrointestinal tract when enterochromaffin cells in the upper gastrointestinal tract are stimulated (Figure 31-2). The VC also receives signals from the CTZ, which can initiate vomiting only via the VC (Mannix, 1999).

Vomiting occurs when efferent impulses are sent from the VC to the salivation center, abdominal muscles, respiratory center, and cranial nerves. Box 31-1 lists common causes of N/V in the palliative care setting; the causes most frequently identified in persons with end-stage disease are identified by an asterisk.

TABLE 31-1 ■ Mechanisms and Neuroreceptors of Nausea and Vomiting

Receptors and Neurotransmitters	Trigger	Antiemetic Class
Gastrointestinal Tract		
Serotonin (5-HT$_3$)	Irritation	Antihistamine
	Gastric stasis	5-HT$_3$ antagonist
	Hepatomegaly	Anticholinergic
	Radiation therapy	
	Chemotherapy	
	Obstruction	
Vestibular Apparatus		
Histamine (H$_1$)	Motion	Antihistamine
Acetylcholine		Anticholinergic
Chemoreceptor Trigger Zone		
Substance P	Chemicals	NK-1 antagonist
Dopamine (D$_2$)	Electrolyte imbalance	Antidopaminergic
Serotonin (5-HT$_3$)	Drugs	5-HT$_3$ antagonist
Cortex		
Pressure receptors	Anxiety, stress	
	Raised intracranial pressure	
	Sights, smells, taste	
Vomiting Center		
Acetylcholine	Gastrointestinal tract	
Histamine receptor (H$_1$)	Vestibular apparatus	
Serotonin (5-HT$_2$)	Cortex	
	Chemoreceptor trigger zone	

ASSESSMENT AND MEASUREMENT

Identification of the possible cause(s) of N/V begins with a detailed history and physical examination. In patients with advanced cancer, N/V is frequently due to multiple causes (Woodruff, 2004). Questions about onset, precipitating and aggravating factors, quality (duration, frequency, and severity), and relieving factors should be documented so that an individualized approach to management can be implemented. Assessment of the gastrointestinal status, that is, abdominal distention, presence of bowel sounds, and presence of other associated symptoms such as constipation, should be part of the total process. It is also very important to remember that the most reliable way to assess nausea is through the patient's report.

Temporal Characteristics
- Onset: When did it start?
- Pattern: Specific times of the day? Continuous or intermittent?
  - If it is intermittent, what are the frequency and length of episodes?
  - Does nausea precede vomiting, or does vomiting come without warning?
- Relieving and aggravating factors: What makes it better or worse?
  - Affected by movement?
  - Better or worse with eating?

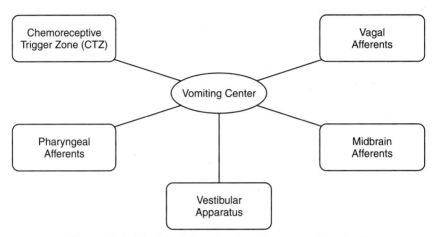

Figure 31-2 Physiological mechanism of nausea and vomiting.

- ❱ After certain drugs?
- ❱ In certain situations?
- ❱ With certain smells?

Risk Factors

Disease Related

- Primary or metastatic tumor of the central nervous system that includes the VC or increased intracranial pressure
- Obstruction of a portion of the gastrointestinal tract
- Food toxins, infection, or motion sickness
- Metabolic abnormalities, such as hyperglycemia, hyponatremia, hypercalcemia, and renal or hepatic dysfunction
- Advanced stomach and breast cancers, any cancer at end-stage
- Pharyngeal irritation from tenacious sputum, candidiasis
- Hepatomegaly

Treatment Related

- Stimulation of receptors of the labyrinth of the inner ear
- Obstruction, irritation, inflammation, and delayed gastric emptying stimulating the gastrointestinal tract through the vagal visceral afferent pathway
- Stimulation of the VC through cellular by-products associated with cancer treatments. Chemotherapy drugs are classified by their potential to cause chemotherapy-induced nausea and vomiting (CINV) within the first 24 hours of drug administration. N/V occurring within the first 24 hours of chemotherapy drug administration is called *acute*. N/V that persists for several hours or days 24 hours or more after treatment is termed *delayed*. *Anticipatory* N/V can develop depending on how successful prior experiences at control have been and is usually triggered by cues linked to prior treatments such as smells, sounds, etc.

Box 31-1	**Common Causes of Nausea and Vomiting in Palliative Care**

GASTROINTESTINAL

Gastrointestinal obstruction*
Constipation*
Gastritis*
Gastric stasis*
Squashed stomach syndrome
Gastrointestinal infection
Carcinomatosis
Extensive liver metastasis

PHARYNGEAL IRRITATION

Candida spp. infection
Thick sputum
Cough

CENTRAL NERVOUS SYSTEM

Increased intracranial pressure*
Posterior fossa tumors or bleeding
Meningitis, infectious or neoplastic

MEDICATIONS

Opioids*
Antibiotics
Chemotherapy
Corticosteroids
Digoxin
Nonsteroidal anti-inflammatory drugs (NSAIDs)
Iron

METABOLIC*

Hypercalcemia
Liver failure
Renal failure

PSYCHOLOGICAL AND EMOTIONAL

Anxiety
Pain
Conditioned response (anticipatory nausea)

SITUATIONAL

Odors
Inadequate mouth care

*Indicates the causes most frequently identified in persons with end-stage diseases.

- Stimulation of the VC through afferent pathways from radiation therapy of the gastrointestinal tract. Radiation-induced nausea and vomiting (RINV) depends on the site of treatment, size of treatment field, and radiation dose. Patients at highest risk have received a large volume of radiation to the upper abdominal tissues. Time to onset of radiation is related to the dose fraction: 10 to 15 minutes after total body irradiation or hemibody irradiation to as much as 1 to 2 hours after smaller doses of radiation to a specific site (i.e., upper abdomen). RINV may persist for several hours (Wickham, 2005).
- Side effects of medications such as digitalis, morphine, antibiotics, iron, vitamins, and chemotherapy agents. Emetogenicity of various chemotherapy agents is given in Box 31-2.
- Side effects of concentrated nutritional supplements
- Postoperative nausea and vomiting (PONV) is related to the anesthesia rather than the surgical procedure itself. PONV is more likely to occur after certain surgeries, such as craniotomy, laparotomy, and major breast surgery. N/V potentiates patient discomfort and increases the risk for postoperative complications, such as wound dehiscence, bleeding, dehydration, and electrolyte imbalance (Wickham, 2005).

Patient Related

- Previous experience with N/V
- Alcohol use (chronic or heavy drinkers experience less N/V than do nondrinkers).
- Gender: Women are at greater risk for CINV, PONV, and N/V from other causes.

Situational

- Increased levels of tension, stress, emotions, and anxiety
- Noxious odors or visual stimuli
- Conditioned (anticipatory) responses to previous cancer and other stressful experiences. History of motion sickness increases risk. This occurs in 25% of chemotherapy patients.

Treatment Options

Ask what has been tried to treat the nausea.

- Pharmacological interventions, including prescription medications, over-the-counter medications, and home, herbal, and natural remedies
- Nonpharmacological interventions such as alternative and complementary therapies

Additional symptoms (sequelae) (Berendt, 1998; Griffie & McKinnon, 2002) should be sought.

- Change in bowel pattern? Have bowels moved in the last 24 hours? When was the last bowel movement?
- What medications have been tried in the last 24 hours?
- What other medications have been tried for this episode of the nausea?
- What does the patient feel is the cause of the nausea?
- What is the content of the vomitus: food, bile, presence of blood or feces?
- What is the volume of the emesis (large volume suggests gastric stasis)?
- Heartburn or reflux symptoms?

| Box 31-2 | Therapy-Related Risk Factors for Nausea and Vomiting |

CHEMOTHERAPY

Emetic Risk of Chemotherapy (Generic Names)

High (>90%)

Carmustine (>250 mg/m^2)
Cisplatin (>50 mg/m^2)
Cyclophosphamide (>1500 mg/m^2)
Dacarbazine (>500 mg/m^2)
Mechlorethamine
Procarbazine (orally)
Streptozocin

Moderate (30% to 90%)

Aldesleukin (IL-2)
Cyclophosphamide (<1500 mg/m^2)
Carmustine (<250 mg/m^2)
Doxorubicin
Cisplatin (<50 mg/m^2)
Epirubicin
Cytarabine (>1 g/m^2)
Idarubicin
Irinotecan
Ifosfamide
Melphalan (<50 mg/m^2)
Methotrexate (250 to 1000 mg/m^2)
Carboplatin
Cyclophosphamide (orally)

Low (10% to 30%)

Doxorubicin (liposomal)
5-Fluorouracil
Mitoxantrone (<12 mg/m^2)
Gemcitabine
Temozolomide
Mitomycin
Etoposide (orally)
Paclitaxel
Cytarabine (100-200 mg/m^2)
Topotecan
Docetaxel
Trastuzumab

Minimal (<10%)

Asparaginase
Methotrexate (<50 mg/m^2)
Bleomycin
Capecitabine
Rituximab
Bevacizumab
Vincristine
Vinblastine
Vinorelbine (intravenously)

Continued

Box 31-2	Therapy-Related Risk Factors for Nausea and Vomiting—cont'd

RADIATION THERAPY

Low Risk (0 to 10%)	Moderate Risk (10% to 55%)	High Risk (55% to 90%)
Head and neck	Hemibody to lower body	Total body irradiation
Extremities	Thorax	Hemibody to upper body
	Pelvis	Entire abdomen
		Upper abdomen

SURGERY POSTANESTHESIA

Low Risk (0 to 10%)	Moderate Risk (10% to 55%)	High Risk (55% to 90%)
Craniotomy	Ear, nose, throat	Major breast surgery
Laparotomy	Laparoscopy	Strabismus surgery

Data from Wickham, R. (2005). Nausea and vomiting: Palliative care issues across the cancer experience. *Oncol Support Care Q, 1(4)*, 44-57; and Cunningham, R.S. (2005). Using clinical practice guidelines to improve clinical outcomes in patients receiving emetogenic chemotherapy. *Oncol Support Care Q, 3(1)*, 4-10. Pittsburgh: Oncology Education Services (OES).

- How distressing is the nausea to the patient on a visual analog scale of 0 to 10?
- What are the patient goals for comfort?
- Are there any associated symptoms such as anxiety, pain, odynophagia or dysphagia, or cough that may require simultaneous intervention?

HISTORY AND PHYSICAL EXAMINATION

Physical examination is considered an essential and complementary element to collection of the patient's history during the assessment process. Often, information gathered from the physical examination helps determine the cause of N/V and guides the practitioner in selecting the appropriate treatment.

- Conduct a general physical examination (Berendt, 1998; Griffie & McKinnon, 2002).
  - Note any recent weight change.
  - Check for fever to rule out infection.
  - Assess for signs of dehydration.
  - Assess intake versus output.
  - Assess mental status changes and orientation or level of consciousness.
  - Conduct a psychosocial assessment: Explore anxiety-producing events and coping abilities.
  - Fundi of eyes should be examined for papilledema if cerebral metastasis is suspected, although increased intracranial pressure should not be excluded in its absence.

- Oropharynx should be checked for infection (stomatitis or thrush), dryness of mucous membranes (dehydration), and presence of tenacious sputum.
- Cardiovascular status (pulse, tachycardia; blood pressure, check for postural hypotension) should be determined.
- Abdomen should be checked for ascites, hepatomegaly, abdominal distention, tenderness or pain, masses, and presence and character of bowel sounds.
- Rectal examination should be conducted for tenderness, constipation, impaction, and masses, and a stool examination should be conducted for occult blood.
- Skin assessment should be performed for jaundice, uremic frost, pruritus, and turgor.
- Consider medical diagnosis, especially disease processes with a potential to cause N/V, such as gastrointestinal or genitourinary malignancies, primary or metastatic brain tumors, liver failure, and renal failure.
    - Bowel obstruction is relatively common in patients with abdominal tumors, especially those with colorectal and ovarian cancers.
    - Increased intracranial pressure is usually due to primary or secondary brain tumors or metastasis and/or to accompanying cerebral edema.
    - Uremia is usually caused by primary or secondary breast or bladder tumors (C. Poe, 2005, personal communication).
    - Determine treatment history: Is the patient undergoing active treatment with chemotherapy or radiation therapy? Has there been recent or past treatment with chemotherapy or radiation?
    - Review the surgical history. Have there been any recent gastrointestinal surgeries or procedures?
    - Review current medications that may contribute to nausea (e.g., opioids, steroids, digoxin).
    - Evaluate the patient's past experiences with N/V and the effectiveness of interventions used in prior experiences.
    - Investigate other possible etiologies such as uncontrolled pain, pancreatic disease, psychological distress, gastric irritation, hypercalcemia, or acute gastrointestinal infection unrelated to the disease (C. Poe, 2005, personal communication).

DIAGNOSTICS

The following tests may be necessary and appropriate if other forms of assessment fail to identify the cause(s) of N/V (Campbell & Hately, 2000). Possible causes include disease recurrence or progression, central nervous system metastases, abdominal abnormalities, infection, metabolic abnormalities, and obstruction by tumor or stool.

- Laboratory studies
    - Blood urea nitrogen, creatinine
    - Ionized calcium
    - Liver function tests
    - Serum drug levels
    - Complete blood cell count with differential
    - Serum sodium to identify dehydration

- Radiographic studies
  - Computed tomography scanning
  - Magnetic resonance imaging
  - Abdominal flat plate
  - Endoscopy

INTERVENTION AND TREATMENT

Interventions to eliminate causes of N/V are the first step to its management (Gullatte, Kaplow, & Heidrich, 2005). When that is not possible, antiemetics are the mainstay to management of N/V in any setting. Understanding the underlying cause and using an individualized approach to care are key in selecting the most appropriate agent for successful management. Nurses working in palliative care have the challenge of providing care to patients with several comorbidities, resulting in multiple symptoms requiring simultaneous intervention (Campbell & Hately, 2000). Because of this unique challenge, multiple drugs in conjunction with nonpharmacological approaches and utilization of the interdisciplinary team may be needed to control symptoms. Successful management of N/V with multifactorial causes is dependent on the following (Campbell & Hately, 2000; King, 2001):

- Assessment
- Accurate diagnosis and identification of cause(s) and identification of emetic pathway
- Choice of the correct antiemetic
- Choice of the most efficacious route that ensures delivery of the antiemetic to the site of action
- Effective titration of dose and regular administration of the antiemetic
- Treatment of reversible causes
- Change to and adjustment of the protocol if it is not working
- Appropriate adjuvant medications and nonpharmacological interventions
- Individualized and holistic nursing care (remember that anxiety or psychological stress can cause nausea)
- Consideration and evaluation of the potential adverse or opposing effects of drug(s) used to treat N/V

Pharmacological Interventions

Antiemetics are considered the drug of choice, yet they often prove to be ineffective when used alone. This is most likely due to inadequate dose, incomplete diagnosis, or incorrect diagnosis. If the cause is multifactorial, select the most potent antiemetic for the probable cause, rather than one multipurpose agent. Most palliative care programs have available a compounding pharmacist who can prepare a combination of antiemetics in convenient vehicles for administration, such as suppository, oral suspension, topical, or transdermal forms. Common combinations in the palliative setting include the following (Griffie & McKinnon, 2002):

- Diphenhydramine, dexamethasone, and metoclopramide
- Diphenhydramine, lorazepam, and haloperidol
- Haloperidol, lorazepam, metoclopramide, and diphenhydramine

Table 31-2 outlines medications used to treat nausea and vomiting in the palliative care setting.

Nonpharmacological Interventions

Use of the interdisciplinary team for management of symptoms is unique to palliative care. Psychological interventions to control physiological responses (King, 2001) are a common and quite successful approach in the palliative care setting. The intent of these interventions is to focus attention on other stimuli rather than on the symptoms of N/V.

TABLE 31-2 ■ Medications for the Treatment of Nausea and Vomiting

Specific Medication	Recommended Dosing Schedule
Dopamine Antagonists	
Prochlorperazine (Compazine)	Orally, intravenously, intramuscularly 10 mg every 6 hr; per rectum 25-mg suppository every 12 hr
Chlorpromazine (Thorazine)	Orally, intravenously, intramuscularly 25 to 50 mg every 6 hr; per rectum 25-mg suppository every 6 hr
Haloperidol (Haldol)	Orally, intravenously, subcutaneously, intramuscularly 0.5 to 2 mg every 6 hr
Thiethylperazine (Torcan)	Intravenously, orally 10 mg every 8 hr
Promethazine (Phenergan)	Intravenously, orally 25 mg every 6 hr; per rectum 12.5- to 50-mg suppository every 6 hr
Metoclopramide HCl (Reglan)	Orally 10 mg $\frac{1}{2}$ hr before meals and at bedtime
Serotonin Antagonists	
Ondanstron (Zofran)	Intravenously 32 mg or orally 24 mg prior to treatment; orally 4 to 8 mg every 8 hr
Granisetron (Kytril)	Intravenously or orally 1 to 2 mg daily
Dolasetron mesylate (Anzemet)	Intravenously or orally 100 mg intravenously or orally daily
Palonosetron (Aloxi)	Intravenously 0.25 mg 30 min before chemotherapy.
Prokinetic Drugs	
Metoclopramide HCl (Reglan)	Orally 10 mg $\frac{1}{2}$ hr before meals and at bedtime
Corticosteroids	
Dexamethasone (Decadron)	Dose and schedule are empiric; orally or intravenously 4 to 10 mg every 6 hr
Benzodiazepines	
Lorazepam (Ativan)	Orally or intravenously 0.5 to 2.0 mg every 6 hr
Cannabinoids	
Dronabinol (Marinol)	Orally 2.5 to 10 mg every 6 hr
Antihistamines	
Diphenhydramine (Benadryl)	Orally or intravenously 25 to 50 mg every 6 hr
Hydroxyzine (Vistaril)	Orally or intramuscularly 25 to 50 mg every 6 hr
Antisecretory Agents	
Octreotide acetate (Sandostatin)	Subcutaneously 100 to 600 mcg/24 hr; used in intestinal obstruction to reduce gastrointestinal secretions and motility
Substance P/Neurokinin-1 Antagonist	
Aprepitant (Emend)	Orally 125 mg day 1, 80 mg days 2 and 3, day 1 at 1 hr before chemotherapy, days 2 and 3 in morning
Scopolamine hydrobromide (Transderm-Scop)	1.5-mg patch every 72 hr

Most interventions are based on behavioral therapies such as relaxation techniques, guided imagery, distraction, systemic desensitization, massage and music therapy, self-hypnosis, acupuncture, acupressure, and biofeedback (Ezzone, 2000; King, 2001). Patient and family involvement is the mainstay of successful symptom management. Box 31-3 outlines some self-care activities that patients and their caregivers can implement independently and as an adjunct to nursing interventions to control N/V.

PATIENT AND FAMILY EDUCATION

Working closely with patients and their caregivers to prevent the causes of N/V or to aggressively managing existing symptoms requires teaching patients and/or families interventions for independent management. If those interventions do not prove successful, the importance of prompt notification of the clinician regarding refractory symptoms is paramount to prevent complications. Educational materials on disease states, effects of cancer treatment, and written information on how to manage side effects are invaluable resources to refer to when away from the clinical setting. Reliable and consistent information is important to assist patients in coping with the cancer treatment process (Berendt, 1998; Ezzone, 2000; Griffie & McKinnon, 2002).

■ Encourage use of self-care diaries and logs to record the frequency of N/V.
■ Instruct patient to notify clinician when
  ▶ More than three episodes of vomiting occur in a day or 2 consecutive days of vomiting.
  ▶ Vomiting occurs soon after oral administration of antiemetics.
  ▶ Fever develops.
  ▶ There is increased or escalating pain or weakness.
  ▶ There are signs and symptoms of dehydration and aspiration.
  ▶ There is weight loss.

Box 31-3	Self-Care Activities for the Management of Nausea and Vomiting

Oral care should be provided after each episode of nausea and vomiting.
Apply cool, damp cloth to forehead, neck, and wrists.
Decrease noxious stimuli like odors and pain.
Restrict fluids with meals.
Eat frequent small meals.
Eat bland, cool, or room-temperature food.
Provide clear liquids, Popsicles, and/or Gatorade for 24 hours following acute nausea and vomiting episodes.
Have patient wear loose-fitting clothes.
Provide fresh air with fan, open windows.
Have patient avoid sweet, salty, fatty, and spicy foods.
Limit sounds, sights, and smells that precipitate nausea and vomiting.
Patient should avoid moving and reclining for 30 min after eating.

Data from King, C.R. (2001). Nausea and vomiting. In B.R. Ferrell & N. Coyle (Eds.). *Palliative nursing* (pp. 107-121). New York: Oxford University Press; and Rhodes, V. & McDaniel, R. (2001). Nausea, vomiting and retching: Complex problems in palliative care. *CA Cancer J Clin, 51(4)*, 232-248.

- There is blood or feces in vomit.
- Instruct patient about correct dose and administration of medication.
- Teach patient to avoid eating or drinking for 1 to 2 hours after vomiting and encourage fluid intake. Clear liquid diet for 24 hours may allow the gastrointestinal tract to rest and give the antiemetics time to work.
- Instruct patients and caregivers that the patient should be allowed to eat when and what he or she chooses.
- Suggest that eating smaller meals throughout the day is more tolerable.
- Provide effective management of symptoms such as pain, anxiety, and cough to prevent breakthrough nausea.
- Suggest environmental modification—cool, well-ventilated, lowered lighting and noise levels, and absence of noxious sights and smells.
- Teach nonpharmacological relaxation and distraction activities.
- Inform patient that treatment of any symptom including N/V is a patient choice; instruct patient about consequences of no treatment as part of overall goal setting when developing a plan of care.
- Instruct on positioning techniques to decrease risk of aspiration.

EVALUATION AND FOLLOW-UP

Effective management of any symptom involves the evaluation of patient response to mutually identified goals through routine follow-up. As with pain, when there is a new intervention initiated or dose change, patient contact should occur within 24 hours. In the home care setting, if a return visit is not feasible, a skilled clinician can accomplish this follow-up with a telephone call followed by face-to-face contact as soon as possible.

CASE STUDY

Mr. B. is a 78-year-old man who has advanced prostate cancer. He enters the clinic for control of nausea. He has been under treatment for the past 7 years and now has uncontrolled disease with widespread metastatic sites of cancer, including the bladder. He has nephrostomy tubes in place. Three months ago, he underwent a colostomy for blockage of his lower bowel. Mr. B. is receiving leuprolide acetate injections every 3 months. He has not had radiation therapy in the past year. He reports a weight loss of 30 pounds over the last 4 months. When asked what the physicians told him about his disease status, he states, "They told me 6 to 9 months, 6 months ago."

The clinician obtains the following assessment data regarding Mr. B.'s nausea: The nausea is constant and began after the colostomy was placed. It has gradually increased in intensity and now has accompanying episodes of emesis, about every third day. His emesis consists of small amounts of digested food. He reports that eating large amounts of food makes it worse. He cannot name anything that he has tried that makes it worse or makes it better. The colostomy is functioning. Bowel sounds are normal and laboratory values are normal.

Mr. B. has not taken anything for the nausea. He reports trying to avoid any extra pills but now feels he no longer can avoid medications. His only medication, besides the every-3-month leuprolide acetate injection, is clonidine (Catapres) daily. He does not take any over-the-counter medications. Mr. B. states that he does not want to undergo any further evaluation tests if they can be avoided.

In determining the best pharmacological choices, the clinician considers that the nausea is constant, the cause is not known, and there are no signs or symptoms of intestinal obstruction. A dopamine antagonist is perhaps the best beginning point to provide broadest coverage of possible causes. Prochlorperazine, 10 mg orally every 6 hours around the clock, is an appropriate starting regimen.

This patient will likely benefit from nonpharmacological interventions as well. Suggest small meals. Assure Mr. B. that there are a number of approaches to therapy and that any medications are easily adjusted to find the best medication and dose for him. Allow time for Mr. B. to talk about his statement, "They told me 6 to 9 months, 6 months ago," as this may open a wide variety of emotional concerns that need to be addressed.

Mr. B. and his family are given the following instructions:

- Start the prochlorperazine, 10 mg orally every 6 hours around the clock.
- Keep a record of episodes of nausea and emesis and note any relationship to time of last meal.
- Contact clinician if no relief in intensity of nausea occurs in 3 days (mutually agreed-upon goal).

REFERENCES

Berendt, M.C. (1998). Alterations in nutrition: Nausea and vomiting. In J.K. Itano & K.N. Taoka (Eds.). *Core curriculum for oncology nursing* (pp. 238-243). Pittsburgh: Oncology Nursing Society.

Campbell, T. & Hately, J. (2000). The management of nausea and vomiting in advanced cancer. *Int J Palliat Nurs, 6(1),* 18-25.

Cunningham, R.S. (2005). Using clinical practice guidelines to improve clinical outcomes in patients receiving emetogenic chemotherapy. *Oncol Support Care Q, 3(1),* 4-10. Pittsburgh: Oncology Education Services (OES).

Ezzone, S.A. (2000). Nausea and vomiting. In B.M. Nevidjon & K.W. Sowers (Eds.). *A nurse's guide to cancer care* (pp. 295-310). Philadelphia: Lippincott.

Griffie, J. & McKinnon, S. (2002). Nausea and vomiting. In K.K. Kuebler, P. Berry, & D.E. Heidrich (Eds.). *End of life care: Clinical practice guidelines* (pp. 333-343). Philadelphia: Saunders.

Gullatte, M.M., Kaplow, R., & Heidrich, D.E. (2005). Nausea and vomiting. In K.K. Kuebler, M.P. Davis, & C.D. Moore (Eds). *Palliative practices: An interdisciplinary approach* (pp. 229-231). St. Louis: Elsevier/Mosby.

Herndon, C.M., Jackson, K.C., & Hallin, P.A. (2002). Management of opioid-induced gastrointestinal effects in patients receiving palliative care. *Pharmacotherapy, 22(2),* 240-250.

Kazanowski, M.K. (2001). Nausea and vomiting near end of life. In M.L. Matzo & D.W. Sherman (Eds.). *Palliat care nursing* (pp. 340-342). New York: Springer.

King, C.R. (2001). Nausea and vomiting. In B.R. Ferrell & N. Coyle (Eds.). *Palliative nursing* (pp. 107-121). New York: Oxford University Press.

Mannix, K.A. (1999). Palliation of nausea and vomiting. In D. Doyle, G. Hanks, & N. MacDonald (Eds.). *Oxford textbook of palliative medicine* (2nd ed., pp. 489-498). New York: Oxford University Press.

National Comprehensive Cancer Network. (2005). *Antiemesis guidelines. NCCN Clinical Practice Guidelines in Oncology.* Retrieved from www.nccn.org.

Rhodes, V. & McDaniel, R. (2001). Nausea vomiting and retching: Complex problems in palliative care. *CA Cancer J Clin, 51(4),* 232-248.

Wickham, R. (2005). Nausea and vomiting: Palliative care issues across the cancer experience. *Oncol Support Care Q 1(4),* 44-57.

Woodruff, R. (2004). Nausea and vomiting. In *Palliative medicine,* (4th ed., pp. 223-237). New York: Oxford University Press.

CHAPTER 32

PAIN

Debra E. Heidrich and Peg Esper

■

DEFINITION AND INCIDENCE

The International Association for the Study of Pain (IASP) defines *pain* as an unpleasant sensory and emotional experience associated with actual or potential tissue damage or described in terms of such damage (IASP, 1979). Pain, however, is a highly personal and subjective experience. McCaffery (1968) proposed the definition most applicable to clinical practice: "Pain is whatever the experiencing person says it is, existing whenever he/she says it does." The patient's self-report of pain is its single most reliable indicator. In other words, the patient's report must be accepted at face value (American Pain Society, 2003).

Pain may be classified based on duration or by inferred pathophysiology. The interventions selected to treat pain will be influenced by both of these types of classification (McCaffery & Pasero, 1999). These classifications are as follows:

Types of Pain Based on Duration

- Acute pain is relatively brief in duration. There is a recognized cause of the pain, and the pain diminishes as healing takes place. With acute pain, there may or may not be observable autonomic signs of discomfort (e.g., increased pulse rate and blood pressure) and nonverbal signs (e.g., tense muscles, facial grimace).
- Chronic pain is described as pain that persists after the resolution of the initial injury. It is perceived as irreversible and meaningless. Due to physiologic and behavioral adaptation, there are few or no autonomic or nonverbal signs of discomfort.
- Breakthrough pain (also called episodic pain) is defined by Portenoy and Hagen (1990) as a "transitory exacerbation of pain that occurs on a background of otherwise stable pain in a patient receiving chronic opioid therapy" (p. 273). Breakthrough pain tends to occur in persons with higher pain severity and is associated with distress and disability (Caraceni, Martini, Zecca et al., 2004; Zeppetella, O'Doherty, & Collins, 2000). The three subtypes of breakthrough pain are listed next (Mercadante & Portenoy, 2001; Portenoy & Hagen, 1990). Assessment of the onset, duration, frequency, and precipitating factors assists in determining the type and guides the treatment.
  - ▶ End-of-dose failure occurs when the blood levels of analgesics are declining. This indicates a need to increase the dose or the frequency of administration of the analgesic.

The author would like to acknowledge Julie Griffie, Sandy McKinnon, and Patricia H. Berry for their contributions that remain unchanged from the first edition of this book.

> Incident pain occurs due to movement, such as position changes in bed, standing, walking, and coughing. It also includes discomfort from involuntary activities, such as pain due to bowel or bladder distention.

> Nonincident breakthrough pain has no identified precipitant.

Types of Pain Based on Inferred Pathophysiology

- Nociceptive pain arises from direct stimulation of the afferent nerves in the skin, soft tissue, or viscera. This type of pain may be further classified as somatic pain, caused by stimulation of nociceptors in the skin, joints, muscle, bone, or connective tissue; or visceral pain, caused by stimulation of nociceptors in the visceral organs (Figure 32-1).

- Neuropathic pain results from abnormal processing of sensory input due to nerve damage. This type of pain may be further classified as centrally generated pain or peripherally generated pain.

Patients may experience several different types of pain at the same time; some of these pains may be somatic, some visceral, some neuropathic, and some mixed. Because interventions are based on the type and severity of pain, thorough assessment of each site of pain is critical to appropriate pain management.

Pain is a common symptom with advanced diseases, affecting at least up to 90% of people with metastatic cancer, 90% of those with acquired immunodeficiency syndrome (AIDS), 65% of people with multiple sclerosis, 78% of people with cardiac disease, 8% of people with cerebrovascular disease, and 20% of people with diabetes (Anderson, Vestergaard, Ingeman-Nielsen et al., 1995; Biovie, 1999; Breitbart, Passik, & Rosenfeld, 1999; Corbett, 2005; Levenson, McCarthy, Lynn et al., 2000; McCarthy, Lay, & Addington-Hall, 1996; Ogle & Hopper, 2005). Breakthrough pain occurs in up to 89% of persons with advanced cancer (Zeppetella et al., 2000). The incidence of breakthrough pain in nonmalignant diseases is not investigated as extensively but is reported with many different disease processes (Svendsen, Andersen, Arnason et al., 2005). Zeppetella, O'Doherty, & Collins (2001) reported breakthrough pain in 63% of persons admitted to a hospice with noncancer diagnoses. Important to note and just as significant is the fact that many persons also experience pains unrelated to their primary diagnosis, such as arthritis and chronic low back pain.

Pain control at the end-of-life remains an important, yet often neglected, issue. Data from the SUPPORT study showed a high incidence of uncontrolled pain (from 74% to 95%) in very ill and dying hospitalized adults despite planned interventions from

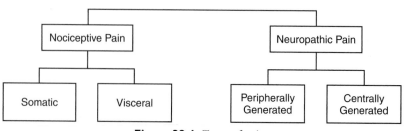

Figure 32-1 Types of pain.

nurses encouraging physicians to attend to pain control (SUPPORT Study Principal Investigators, 1995). A recent study shows that patient satisfaction with pain control has improved only slightly since the implementation of pain standards by the Joint Commission on the Accreditation of Healthcare Organizations in 2001 (Leddy & Wolosin, 2005).

Uncontrolled pain causes physical, psychosocial, emotional, spiritual, and financial burdens and decreases quality of life. Pain interferes with activities of daily living, decreases strength and endurance, stimulates nausea, impairs appetite, interferes with sleep, and impairs immune response (Page, 2005); it interferes with social and intimate relations, contributing to isolation. Pain is also associated with high emotional distress (Vachon, 2004). A study by Sela, Bruera, Conner-Spady et al. (2002) showed gender differences in the affective responses to cancer pain: men most often reported frustration, anger, and exhaustion due to pain, and women described exhaustion, helplessness, frustration, hopelessness, and anger as their top concerns. Spiritual distress may be a cause or an effect of pain (Georgesen & Dungan, 1996). In addition, pain increases caregiver burden and diminishes important social supports for both the patient and the family. Finally, some pain medications and other treatment regimens are expensive, causing economic stress at a particularly vulnerable time.

ETIOLOGY AND PATHOPHYSIOLOGY

Nociceptive pain occurs when a pain stimulus is generated from either somatic or visceral structures. Pain from somatic structures, including bone, joints, muscle, skin, and connective tissue, is usually described as "aching" or "throbbing," and the patient can often point to the exact area where the painful stimulus is occurring (i.e., it is well localized). Stimuli from visceral tissues (mainly thoracic, abdominal, and pelvic organs) cause pain that is described as gnawing and aching. Visceral pain may or may not be well localized. In fact, visceral pain may be felt in areas other than the original site, a phenomenon known as *referred pain* (Hudspith, Siddall, & Munglani, 2006). Figure 32-2 illustrates some commonly reported sites where pain may be referred from visceral organs.

Neuropathic pain is not as clearly understood as nociceptive pain. Peripherally generated neuropathic pains involve abnormal processing of sensory input from the peripheral nerves and may be described as "aching," "burning," "tingling," or "shocklike." Centrally generated neuropathic pains involve abnormal processing of sensory input at the spinal cord level, leading to hyperexcitability. This causes an abnormal continuation of pain impulses, even in the absence of further pain stimuli, or an abnormal processing of stimuli such that normally nonpainful stimuli are perceived as painful (allodynia). Neuropathic pain syndromes can be difficult to treat. The words used to describe an individual's pain assist in determining the type of pain and inferring a cause (Table 32-1).

Nociceptive Pain Processes

There are four processes involved in nociceptive pain: transduction, transmission, perception, and modulation. Transduction begins when mechanical, thermal, or chemical stimuli cause tissue damage. The damage itself and the inflammatory response to the

POSTERIOR   ANTERIOR

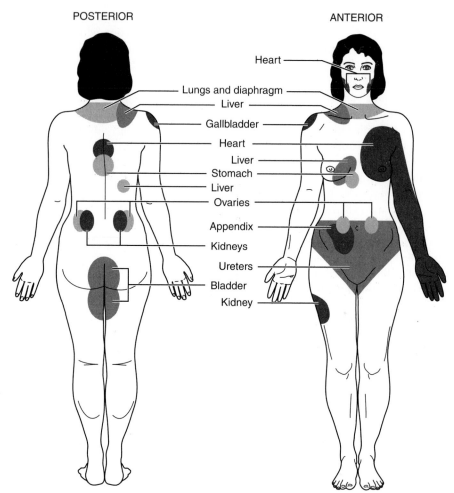

Figure 32-2 Commonly reported sites where pain may be referred from visceral organs. (From Brockrath, M. [1985]. *Fundamentals. Nursing Now* [p. 18]. Springhouse, Pa.: Springhouse.)

damage release substances that stimulate or sensitize the pain fibers (Figure 32-3). In the presence of sufficient stimulation, the nerve membrane becomes permeable to sodium, leading to depolarization. An efflux of potassium causes repolarization. Repeated depolarization and repolarization generate an impulse and transduction is complete (Hudspith et al., 2006; McCaffery & Pasero, 1999; Wilke, 1995). In addition to transduction, peripheral pain fibers have the ability to release substances in response to injury (including substance P) that contribute to the inflammatory process and further increase the sensitization of the pain fibers (Hudspith et al., 2006). This explains why light touch of an inflamed area is perceived as painful.

The second phase of nociception is transmission of the impulse from the site of injury to the dorsal horn of the spinal cord, up to the brainstem, and out to the thalamus and cortex. Nociceptive fibers carry the impulse to the dorsal horn of the spinal cord, where

TABLE 32-1 ■ Classifications and Examples of Pain

Pain Type	Subtype	Descriptors	Examples

Nociceptive	Somatic	Aching
		Throbbing
		Well-localized
			Acute somatic pain:
			  Surgical incisions
			  Muscle or joint sprain
			Chronic somatic pain:
			  Arthritis
			  Metastatic cancer to the
			    bone

Nociceptive	Visceral	Aching
		Gnawing
		Deep and squeezing
		Intermittent cramping
		Poorly localized; referred
			Acute visceral pain:
			  Angina
			  Bladder irritation (e.g.,
			    infection)
			  Acute bowel obstruction
			Chronic visceral pain:
			  Pancreatic cancer
			  Metastatic cancer to the liver

Neuropathic:
  centrally
  generated
	Deafferentation	Burning
		Aching
		Lancinating
		Pricking
		Lacerating
		Pressing
			Phantom limb pain (may
			  have both central and
			  peripheral mechanisms)
			Spinal cord injury
			Stroke
			PHN

	Sympathetically
	  maintained
		Burning
		Hyperalgesia
		Allodynia
		Accompanied by excessive
		  sweating and vasomotor
		  changes
			Complex regional pain
			  syndrome types I and II

Neuropathic:
  peripherally
  generated
	Polyneuropathies	Deep aching
		Superficial burning, stinging,
		  or prickling
		Shocklike; lancinating
		Pain felt along distribution of
		  many peripheral nerves
			Diabetic neuropathy
			Drug-induced neuropathy
			  (e.g., due to vinca alkaloid
			  chemotherapy)

	Mononeuropathies	Burning
		Severe aching
		Intermittent stinging or
		  electric shocklike
		Pain along distribution of
		  single nerve or dermatome
			Mononeuropathies:
			Nerve root compression
			Trigeminal neuralgia
			Multiple
			  mononeuropathies:
			Postherpetic neuralgia

Data from Boivie, J. (1999). Central pain. In P.D. Wall & R. Melzack (Eds.). *Textbook of pain* (4th ed., pp. 879-941). New York: Churchill Livingstone; Cousins, M. & Powers, I. (1999). Acute and postoperative pain. In P.D. Wall & R. Melzack (Eds.). *Textbook of pain* (4th ed., pp. 474-491). New York: Churchill Livingstone; Jensen, T.S. & Nikolajsen, L. (1999). Phantom pain and other phenomena after amputation. In P.D. Wall & R. Melzack (Eds.). *Textbook of pain* (4th ed., pp. 799-814). New York: Churchill Livingstone; McCaffery, M. & Pasero, C. (1999). *Pain: Clinical manual* (2nd ed.). St. Louis: Mosby; Scadding, J.W. (1999a). Complex regional pain syndrome. In P.D. Wall & R. Melzack (Eds.). *Textbook of pain* (4th ed., pp. 835-849). New York: Churchill Livingstone; and Scadding, J.W. (1999b). Peripheral neuropathies. In P.D. Wall & R. Melzack (Eds.). *Textbook of pain* (4th ed., pp. 815-834). New York: Churchill Livingstone.

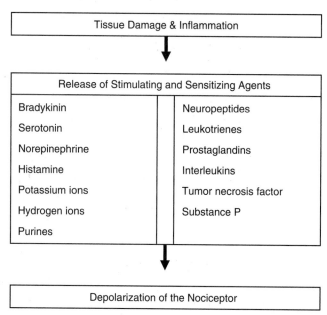

Figure 32-3 Substances involved in nociceptor transduction. (Data from Wilke, D.J. [1995]. Neural mechanisms of pain: A foundation for cancer pain assessment and management. In D.B. McGuire, C.H. Yarbro, & B.R. Ferrell [Eds.]. *Cancer pain management* [2nd ed., pp. 61-87]. Boston: Jones & Bartlett; and Hudspith, M.J., Siddall, P.J., & Munglani, R. [2006]. Physiology of pain. In H.B. Hemmings & P.M. Hopkins [Eds.]. *Foundations of anesthesia: Basic sciences for clinical practice* [2nd ed., pp. 267-285]. St. Louis: Mosby.)

these fibers end. In order to transmit the impulse to dorsal horn neurons, neurotransmitters are required. These neurotransmitters include glutamate, substance P, neurokinin A, and calcitonin gene–related peptide (CGRP). Glutamate plays a major role in nociceptive transmission by binding with α-amino-3-hydroxy-5-methyl-4-isoxazolepropionic acid (AMPA) and *N*-methyl-D-aspartate (NMDA) receptors. AMPA receptors are responsible for fast transmission of nociceptive impulses. Sustained activation of AMPA and/or sustained activation of neurokinin receptors primes the NMDA receptor so that it reaches a state ready for activation. Activation of NMDA receptors causes large and prolonged depolarization; prolonged activation initiates processes that contribute to changes observed in chronic pain states, including central sensitization (Hudspith et al., 2006). Thus, prolonged exposure to nociceptive pain may lead to neuropathic pain.

Once transmitted across the synaptic space in the dorsal horn, the impulse is transmitted through several different ascending pathways to the brainstem, thalamus, and higher brain centers. This ends the transmission phase of nociception and begins the phase of perception. Precisely where pain is perceived in the brain is not clear, but this is thought to occur at several cerebral levels. Processing by the somatosensory cortex allows an individual to localize and characterize the pain. The emotional and behavioral responses to pain occur when the pain stimulus is processed in the limbic system.

The reticular activating system is responsible for the autonomic responses to pain (Hudspith et al., 2006; McCaffery & Pasero, 1999; Wilke, 1995).

The fourth process in nociception is modulation. This involves the descending pathways from the brain to the dorsal horn of the spinal cord. Substances that inhibit the transmission of pain may be released by these descending fibers. Among these substances are endogenous opioids (enkephalin), serotonin, norepinephrine, γ-aminobutyric acid (GABA), α_2-adrenergic substances, acetylcholine, thyrotropin-releasing hormone, and somatostatin (Hudspith et al., 2006).

Neuropathic Pain Processes

As mentioned, neuropathic pain processes are not as clearly understood but involve abnormal processing of sensory input. Peripheral neuropathic pains may be caused by injury to the nerve that causes a spontaneous generation of an action potential (Coderre & Melzack, 1992; Paice, 2003). The pain pathway is typically along a single dermatome, affected nerve, or plexus. Combined motor and sensory involvement is suspected if the individual is found to have altered reflexes, muscle atrophy, or weakness (Paice, 2003). There are three categories of damage that cause neuropathic pain: physical (e.g., surgery, trauma), chemical (e.g., neurotoxic medications, hyperglycemia), and viral (e.g. HIV, herpes zoster).

Centrally generated neuropathic pain may occur as a result of repetitive transmission of nociceptive signals to the dorsal horn, causing changes in the processing of these impulses. Hypersensitivity and hyperexcitability result. As mentioned, prolonged activation of NMDA receptors is likely involved in this process. Prevention and prompt treatment of pain may prevent these dorsal horn changes.

Physiologic Rationale for Pain Medications

Medications used to treat pain are discussed in detail in the "Intervention and Treatment" section of this chapter. It is important to understand the rationale for the use of these medications, which is based on the physiologic characteristics of pain. Most medications used to manage pain function by interrupting transduction or transmission or by enhancing modulation, as summarized in Table 32-2. Nociceptive

TABLE 32-2 ■ The Physiologic Rationale for Pain Medications

Medication Class	Mechanism of Action
Nonsteroidal antiinflammatory drugs	Block production of prostaglandins
Anticonvulsants	Block influx of sodium ions, preventing depolarization and generation of an action potential
Local anesthetics	Block influx of sodium ions, preventing depolarization and generation of an action potential
Corticosteroids	Block production of prostaglandins
Opioids	Bind with opioid receptors and block release of substance P
N-Methyl-D-aspartate receptor antagonists	Inhibit binding of excitatory amino acids, such as glutamate, preventing transmission
Tricyclic antidepressants	Prevent reuptake of serotonin and norepinephrine
GABA agonists	Enhance release of GABA
α-Adrenergic agonists	Inhibit release of substance P

From McCaffery, M. & Pasero, C. (1999). *Pain: Clinical manual* (2nd ed.). St. Louis: Mosby.

pains tend to respond to traditional analgesics, nonopioids, and opioids. The interplay of the inflammatory process in, particularly, the somatic pains indicates that antiinflammatory medications may be helpful. Neuropathic pains are less responsive to traditional analgesics; often an adjuvant medication, such as an antidepressant or an anticonvulsant, is needed alone or in combination with an opioid.

MYTHS AND MISCONCEPTIONS ABOUT PAIN

The treatment of pain is wrought with myths, misconceptions, and erroneous beliefs. Understanding these myths and correcting them are essential to the assessment and treatment of pain. Unfortunately, these issues are quite common among patients, families, health care professionals, and the general public.

Many patients and families hesitate to report pain or use analgesics because of misperceptions, misinformation, and fear. Ward, Goldberg, Miller-McCauley et al. (1993) identified eight barriers:

1. Fear of opioid side effects
2. Fear of addiction
3. Belief that increasing pain signifies disease progression
4. Fear of injections
5. Concern about drug tolerance
6. Belief that "good" patients do not complain about pain
7. Belief that reporting pain may distract the physician from treating or curing the cancer
8. Fatalism, the belief that pain is inevitable with cancer and that it cannot be relieved

Likewise, health care professionals retain erroneous attitudes and beliefs about pain and the use of medications that negatively affect pain assessment and management:

1. *The patient's self-report of pain is not to be believed; health care professionals are the best judge of pain.* The patient's report of pain must be accepted because there are no diagnostic or "objective" tests for pain. Pain is whatever the experiencing person says it is, existing whenever he or she says it does (McCaffrey, 1968).

2. *Addiction to pain medication is common.* When pain medications are used to treat pain and there is no history of substance abuse, addiction is rare (Weissman, Burchman, Dahl et al., 1994). To clear up confusion over the meanings and application of these terms, addiction, tolerance, and physical dependence are defined as follows:

   ■ "*Addiction* is a primary, chronic, neurobiologic disease, with genetic, psychosocial, and environmental factors influencing its development and manifestations. It is characterized by behaviors that include one or more of the following: impaired control over drug use, compulsive use, continued use despite harm, and craving" (American Academy of Pain Medicine, American Pain Society, & American Society of Addiction Medicine, 2001, p. 6).

   ■ "*Tolerance* is a state of adaptation in which exposure to a drug induces changes that result in a diminution of one or more of the drug's effects over time" (American Academy of Pain Medicine et al., 2001, p. 7).

   ■ "*Physical dependence* is a state of adaptation that is manifested by a drug class specific withdrawal syndrome that can be produced by abrupt cessation, rapid dose reduction, decreasing blood level of the drug, and/or administration of an antagonist" (American Academy of Pain Medicine et al., 2001, p. 8).

Tolerance and physical dependence are physiologic responses to prolonged use of many substances and medications, including caffeine (e.g., caffeine withdrawal headache), and are not signs of addiction. Requests for pain medication, "clock watching," and other "drug-seeking" behaviors due to poorly controlled pain are often mistaken for addiction. This is referred to as opioid pseudo-addiction.

■ *Opioid pseudo-addiction* is an iatrogenic (meaning "health care system–acquired") syndrome in which certain behavioral characteristics of psychologic dependence develop as a consequence of inadequate pain treatment (American Academy of Pain Medicine et al., 2001).

3. *Respiratory depression is a frequent, serious complication with opioid use.* Respiratory depression is feared and misunderstood by patients, families, and health care professionals. Tolerance develops rapidly to respiratory depression; thus, it is rarely a problem except in the opioid-naïve patient. Keep in mind that respiratory rate alone is not an indicator of respiratory depression; careful assessment of the whole patient, not just respiratory rate, is required. Most important, adequate pain management does not shorten life or hasten death (Fohr, 1998; Sykes & Thorns, 2003).

There are other barriers to adequate pain management including the "antidrug" culture and perceived regulatory barriers that vary from state to state. Such restrictions include triplicate prescription programs or other systems that monitor prescribing patterns or a lack of laws facilitating pain management in end-stage illness, including partial filling of scheduled medications. Be familiar with the state's nurse practice act, regulations, and controlled substances laws.

ASSESSMENT AND MEASUREMENT

If pain is not assessed, appropriate management is impossible. Pain is a multidimensional human experience and thus requires a comprehensive, holistic evaluation. Each new pain report requires a systematic assessment, appropriate treatment, and follow-up. A complete pain assessment includes the following:

■ *Site:* The patient identifies primary sites as well as sites of radiation on his or her body or a diagram. Remember also that the patient may have several sites of pain; it may be helpful to number pains to organize assessment, interventions, and evaluations.

■ *Character:* Use the patient's own words; a careful description will lead to the diagnosis of pain type and assist in determining appropriate analgesics (i.e., *sharp, shooting* describes neuropathic pain syndromes).

■ *Onset:* When did it start? Did (or does) a specific event trigger the pain? Carefully distinguish between new and preexisting pain (i.e., arthritis, chronic low back pain syndromes).

■ *Duration and frequency:* How long has the pain persisted? Is it constant or intermittent?

- *Intensity*: Intensity is commonly defined on a scale, most frequently of 0 to 10. The 0-to-10 scale has been validated in international populations (Serlin, Mendoza, Nakamura et al., 1995). However, the pain intensity measure must be adapted to the patient. Have an alternate scale available for patients unable or unwilling to use the 0-to-10 scale. For example, some patients prefer a verbal descriptor scale or a modification of a smile-to-sad scale. Find a scale that is meaningful to the patient. Ask patients to rate their pain intensity "now," at its "worst," and at its "least." Note that ratings of pain intensity are the most important pain assessment data to collect if time is short; pain intensity directly correlates with interference with the patient's quality of life.
- *Exacerbating factors*: What times, activities, or other circumstances make the pain worse?
- *Associated symptoms*: What other symptoms occur before, with, or after the pain? Nausea is frequently associated with pain and often attributed to pain medications and not the pain itself. If nausea occurs at the peak of the drug, it may be drug related; if it occurs at the end of the dose, it may be pain related.
- *Alleviating factors*: What makes the pain better? What treatments have been successful in the past? What treatments have been unsuccessful? Remember that treatments that did not work in the past may work now if the previous dose was inappropriate or the type of pain problem is different. Include a thorough medication history, especially for the past 24 hours.
- *Effect on quality of life*: How does the pain affect the patient's ability to perform activities of daily living? How does the pain affect relationships with close others? What does the pain mean to the patient and family? How has this pain affected them? How much do the patient and family know about pain? Do they have the expectation that it can be relieved? Are there emotional or spiritual components to the pain? Does unrelieved pain lead to increased fear or anxiety, or to fears that death is imminent?
- *Patient's goal for relief*: Consider using either a pain intensity score or a functional goal, for example, the ability to walk without pain. What would you like to do that your pain is preventing you from doing? What pain score would allow you to perform that activity?
- *Physical examination*: Observe the site of the pain, and validate with the patient the pain's location. Note skin color, warmth, irritation, integrity, and any other unusual findings (Berry, Eagan, Eighmy et al., 1999).
- *Other effects of pain*: Assess for the presence of depression, anxiety, and other emotional aspects of the pain experience.

There are multiple pain assessment forms and scales available. Figure 32-4, one example, presents a 0-to-10 scale and other alternate scales.

Assessment of the Cognitively Impaired

Assessment of patients who lack verbal skills because of cognitive impairment requires astute observation of behavior. A change in behavior is the gold standard for suspecting pain or discomfort in a cognitively impaired person. Several pain rating scales have been proposed for use with nonverbal patients; most include monitoring for changes in breathing patterns, negative vocalizations, frowning or grimacing, tense body language or agitation, and the ability to console the person (Warden, Hurley, & Volicer, 2003).

INITIAL PAIN ASSESSMENT

LOCATION
Mark site A, B, or C

PATIENT NAME	MEDICAL RECORD NUMBER
DATE	RN SIGNATURE

Pain Intensity Rating Scale:

0 1 2 3 4 5 6 7 8 9 10
No Pain — Worst Possible Pain

Patient's Rating of Pain Intensity:	Site A	Site B	Site C
Scale used: ☐ 0-10 (preferred) ☐ Smile-Sad ☐ Verbal	Present: At Worst: At Best:		
Pain Characteristics Cues: Aching, deep, dull, gnawing, sharp, stabbing Crampy, pressure, squeezing Burning, numb, radiating, shooting, stabbing, tingling, touch sensitive	Describe:	Describe:	Describe:

A

History of pain management:

What relieves pain?

What have you done in the past when you've had pain?

How does the pain affect your day-to-day life and activities?

How do you feel about taking pain medications?

Physical findings at the site of pain:

Present pain medication and effectiveness:

PATIENT'S PAIN CONTROL GOAL
☐ Sleep comfortably
☐ Comfort at rest
☐ Comfort with movement
☐ Total pain control
☐ Stay alert
☐ Perform activity
☐ Other

PATIENT'S PAIN INTENSITY GOAL
0 1 2 3 4 5 6 7 8 9 10

Start Pain Management Flowsheet if:
• Pain score is 5 or greater *or*
• Patient is taking analgesics *or*
• Pain score is greater than patient's goal

Figure 32-4 **A,** Initial pain assessment. (**A,** Adapted from an assessment form developed by Karen Stevenson and Kate Ford Roberts in consultation with the University of Wisconsin Hospital and Clinical Home Health Agency, Madison, Wisc.)

Continued

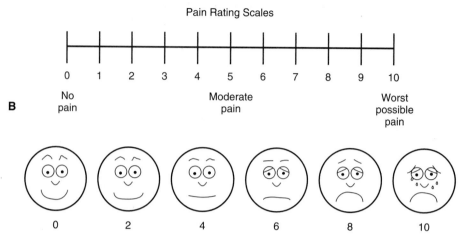

Figure 32-4, cont'd **B**, Wong-Baker, FACES Pain Rating Scale. (**B**, From Hockenberry, M.J., Wilson, D., Winkelstein, M.L.: (Eds.), (2005). *Wong's essentials of nursing* [7th ed.]. [p. 1259], St. Louis, Mosby.)

Kovach, Weissman, Griffie et al. (1999) suggest the following protocol for assessing discomfort in patients with dementia who exhibit a change in behavior:

- Perform a physical assessment for a cause of discomfort and pain. If a cause is found, treatment is initiated.
- Review the patient's history for possible causes of pain through medical records and family members.
- Trial nonpharmacologic interventions appropriate to the circumstances; levels of environmental stimuli should also be evaluated and adjusted for the patient's comfort.
- If the preceding steps are unsuccessful, trial of a nonopioid analgesic is indicated.
- If the nonopioid is unsuccessful, choose a stronger medication, using the World Health Organization (WHO) analgesic ladder as a guide (Figure 32-5); for example, a smaller dose of an opioid in combination with acetaminophen such as hydrocodone (WHO, 1990).

The importance of including a caring approach and the use of nonpharmacologic interventions that enhance the dignity and self-esteem of the individual cannot be overstressed in the care of persons with cognitive impairment.

HISTORY AND PHYSICAL EXAMINATION

Physical examination, appropriate to each identified location of pain, should be performed. Additional history may be suggested by physical findings.

DIAGNOSTICS

Radiologic examinations may be appropriate to direct treatment of the underlying cause of pain within the patient's goals of care. As discussed in the previous chapters,

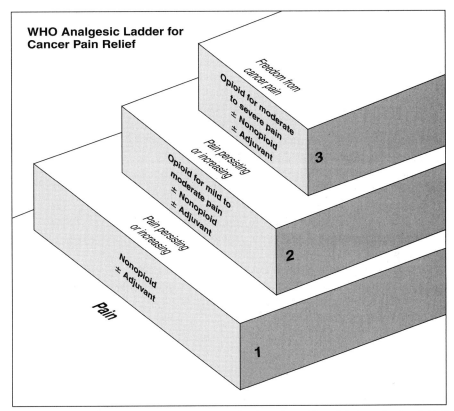

Figure 32-5 The WHO three-step analgesic ladder. (From World Health Organization [1996]. *Cancer pain relief* [2nd ed.]. Geneva: Author.)

decisions to pursue further diagnostics are based on the patient's place on the disease trajectory and the goals of care.

Laboratory evaluation may or may not be appropriate. In any case, the most recent laboratory values should be reviewed. Blood urea nitrogen (BUN) and creatinine levels may be indicated to ascertain renal function before the initiation of opioid therapy if renal insufficiency is suspected. Likewise, liver function tests may be indicated if hepatic insufficiency is suspected.

INTERVENTION AND TREATMENT

Basic Principles of Pain Management

The following principles serve as a guide to the basics of pain management (American Pain Society, 2003; Gordon, Dahl, Miaskowski et al., 2005; National Cancer Institute, 2005; National Comprehensive Cancer Network [NCCN], 2005).

1. Document the pain assessment data so that pain syndrome can be identified and appropriately treated.
2. Match the choice of drug with the intensity and type of pain.

3. Give adequate doses. Titrate to the dose that relieves pain without incurring intolerable side effects.

4. Use the oral route whenever possible. If the patient is unable to swallow oral medications, buccal, sublingual, rectal, and transdermal routes are considered before parenteral routes. The intramuscular route is avoided.

5. Continuous pain requires treatment with a scheduled sustained-release (modi-fied-release) or long-acting opioid and a short-acting medication for break-through pain. Patients and families, however, need to be educated about taking the medication when the pain is first perceived—not when it has become severe or unbearable.

6. Educate patients and families about side effects of opioids to avoid the percep-tion that these are allergic reactions.

7. Use an adequate rescue dose for breakthrough pain: 10% to 20% of the 24-hour dose every 1 to 2 hours is the customary rescue dose.

8. Increase the baseline dose if the patient needs more than three rescue doses in 24 hours.

9. If an increase in the baseline dose is required, it can be done safely every 2 hours with immediate-release preparations, every 12 hours with long-acting prepara-tions, and every 48 hours (2 days) with a fentanyl transdermal patch (Davis, Weissman, & Arnold, 2004).

10. Order only one analgesic for breakthrough pain.

11. Order only one long-acting opioid for constant pain.

12. Increase doses of opioids commensurately with the patient's report of pain:
    ‣ For mild to moderate pain, increase by 25% to 50%.
    ‣ For moderate to severe pain, increase by 50% to 100%, although at higher opioid doses, increases of 20% to 30% are deemed safer.
    ‣ Increases of less than 25% are meaningless.

13. The appearance of analgesic tolerance may require switching to a different opioid. Consider reducing the calculated equianalgesic dose by 25% to 50% to address issues of incomplete cross-tolerance.

14. Use equianalgesic conversions when changing medications or routes.

15. Use adjuvant medications for opioid-resistant neuropathic pain.

16. Nonpharmacologic approaches should always be a part of any pain manage-ment plan.

17. Order an appropriate preventative bowel regimen at the initiation of opioid therapy.

Commonly used analgesics can be found in Tables 32-3, 32-4, 32-5, and 32-6. The following medications should be avoided:

■ Meperidine is short acting with a duration of 2 to 3 hours; active excitatory metabolites accumulate with chronic use.

■ Propoxyphene has modest analgesic efficacy and is biotransformed to potentially toxic central nervous system and cardiac metabolites (Ulens, Daenens, & Tytgat, 1999).

■ Agonist-antagonists (e.g., buprenorphine, butorphanol, nalbuphine, pentazocine) have a ceiling effect (i.e., above a certain dose there is no more gain in analgesia) and can generate an acute withdrawal syndrome if used with opioids.

TABLE 32-3 ■ Commonly Used Nonopioid Analgesics

Chemical Class	Generic Name	Starting Dose (Oral) in Adults	Dosing Schedule	Maximal Daily Dose
p-Aminophenol derivatives	Acetaminophen	325 to 650 mg	Every 4 to 6 hr	4000 mg
Salicylates	Aspirin*	650 mg	Every 4 to 6 hr	4000 mg
	Choline magnesium trisalicylate†	1500 mg × 1, then 1000 mg	Every 12 hr	4000 mg
Proprionic acids	Ibuprofen	200 to 400 mg	Every 4 to 6 hr	3200 mg
	Naproxen	500 mg	Every 8 to 12 hr	1500 mg
Acetic acids	Diclofenac	25 to 50 mg	Every 8 to 12 hr	150 mg
	Nabumentone	1000 mg	Every 24 hr	2000 mg
Pyranocarboxylic acids	Etodolac	200 to 400 mg	Every 6 to 8 hr	1200 mg
Cyclooxygenase-2 inhibitors‡	Celecoxib	100 mg	Every 12 to 24 hr	400 mg

Data from McCaffery, M. & Pascero, C. (1999). *Pain: Clinical manual* (2nd ed.). St. Louis: Mosby; and Hogdson, B.G. & Kizior, R.J. (2004). *Saunders nursing drug handbook 2004.* St. Louis: Saunders.
*Aspirin is not recommended for long-term use due to risk of bleeding and gastrointestinal ulceration.
†Choline magnesium trisalicylate is the only nonsteroidal antiinflammatory drug that does not interfere with platelet aggregation.
‡Cyclooxygenase-2 inhibitors should be used with caution in persons with impaired renal or hepatic functioning.

TABLE 32-4 ■ Formulations of Commonly Used Combination Analgesics

Opioid	Proprietary Name and Combination Agent
Codeine	Tylenol #3 30/300 APAP
	Tylenol #4 60/300 APAP
Hydrocodone	Lorcet HD 5/500 APAP
	Lorcet Plus 7.5/650 APAP
	Vicodin 5/500 APAP
	Vicodin HP 10/650 APAP
	Vicodin ES 7.5/750 APAP
	Vicoprofen 7.5/200 ibuprofen
	Zydone 5/400, 7.5/400, 10/400 APAP
	Co-Gesic 5/500 APAP
	Norco 5/325, 7.5/325, 10/325 APAP
	Lortab 2.5/500, 5/500, 7.5/500, 10/500 APAP
	Lortab ASA 5/500 ASA
Oxycodone	Percocet 5/325, 7.5/325, 10/325, 7.5/500, 10/650 APAP
	Percodan 4.5/325 ASA
	Percodan-Demi 2.25/325 ASA
	Roxicet 5/325, 5/500 APAP
	Roxilox 5/500 APAP
	Roxiprin 4.5/325 ASA
	Endocet 5/325, 7.5/325, 10/325, 7.5/500, 10/650 APAP
	Tylox 5/500 APAP

*Caution: The first number of the dosage listed is the milligram dosage of the opioid; the second is the milligram dosage of the nonopioid analgesic that is used in combination. APAP is the pharmacologic designation for acetaminophen. The acetaminophen dosage should not exceed 4 g/24 hr. ASA is the pharmacologic designation for aspirin.

TABLE 32-5 ■ Formulations of Commonly Used Opioid Analgesics

Opioid	Formulations	Available Dosages
Short-Acting Opioids		
Morphine	Tablet	15, 30 mg
	Solutab	10, 15, 30 mg
	Liquid	10 mg/5 ml, 20 mg/5 ml, 20 mg/ml
	Suppository	5, 10, 20, 30 mg
Oxycodone	Tablet	5, 10 mg
	Liquid	5 mg/5 ml, 20 mg/ml
Hydromorphone	Tablet	2, 4, 8 mg
	Suppository	3 mg
Long-Acting Opioids		
Morphine		
Oramorph SR	Tablet	15, 30, 60, 100 mg every 8 to 12 hr (initial starting interval: 12 hr)
MS Contin	Tablet	15, 30, 60, 100, 200 mg every 8 to 12 hr (initial starting interval: 12 hr)
Kadian	Capsule	20, 50, 100 mg every 12 to 24 hr (starting interval: 24 hr)
Avinza	Capsule	30, 60, 90, 120 mg every 24 hr
Fentanyl		
Duragesic-25, -50, -75, -100 patch	Transdermal	25, 50, 75, 100 mcg/h every 72 hr
Oxycodone		
OxyContin	Tablet	10, 20, 40, 80, 160 mg every 12 hr

Selection of an Opioid Starting Dose

The starting dose of an opioid is determined by the patient's pain intensity and the results of the history and physical examination, including the patient's age, circulatory status, and hepatic and renal function. The WHO analgesic ladder (Figure 32-5) may also be used as a guide. Be aware, however, that successful pain management requires an individualized approach, frequent monitoring, and appropriate dosage escalation (as outlined in "Basic Principles of Pain Management") until the patient is comfortable.

Equianalgesic Conversions

Understanding opioid pharmacodynamics requires an understanding of the concepts of potency and equianalgesia. Refer to an equianalgesic conversion table (Table 32-7) when converting from one route to another or from one opioid to another. Note that 10 mg of parenteral morphine sulfate has the same analgesic effect as 30 mg of oral morphine sulfate. Clinicians should use such tables with caution, in that the dosages stated are not standard starting doses. Starting doses should be based on pain intensity combined with other information from the patient assessment. The doses on the table represent ratios of one drug to another, and one route to another. These ratios do not take into account individual differences in response to various opioids; use these ratios as estimates for a new starting dose and evaluate the patient's response (American Pain Society, 2003). Doses may need to be titrated up or down after the

TABLE 32-6 ■ Adjuvant Analgesics

Class	Uses	Generic Name	Starting Dose in Adults	Dosing Schedule	Titration, Maximal Dose, Comments
Tricyclic antidepressants*	Neuropathic pain	Despiramine Nortriptyline	10 to 25 mg orally	Every 24 hr	Titrate every 3 to 4 days to a maximum of 150 mg/day
Anticonvulsants	Neuropathic pain	Carbamazepine	100 to 200 mg orally	Every 12 hr	Titrate to a maximum of 400 mg every 8 hr; monitor liver function
		Gabapentin	100 mg orally	Every 8 hr	Titrate to effectiveness; reported maximal daily dose of 3600 mg†
		Clonazepam	0.5 mg orally	Every 12 hr	Titrate every 2 to 3 days; maximal dose cited between 2 to 8 mg/day
Corticosteroids	Inflammation not responsive to NSAIDs; increased intracranial pressure; spinal cord compression	Dexamethasone	1 to 10 mg orally‡	Every 6 to 24 hr	Maximum of 96 mg/day; taper dose slowly to lowest effective dose
		Prednisone	5 to 10 mg orally	Every 24 hr in the morning	Taper slowly to lowest effective dose

Continued

Data from American Pain Society. (2003). *Principles of analgesic use in the treatment of acute pain and cancer pain* (5th ed.). Glenview, Ill.: Author; Hogdson, B.G. & Kizior, R.J. (2004). *Saunders nursing drug handbook 2004.* St. Louis: Saunders; Hugel, H., Ellershaw, J.E., & Dickman, A. (2003). Clonazepam as an adjuvant analgesic in patients with cancer-related neuropathic pain. *J Pain Symptom Manage, 26*(6), 1073-1074; and Kuebler, K., Varga, J., & Davis, M.P. (2005). Medications by disorder. In K.K. Kuebler, M.P. Davis, & C.D. Moore (Eds.), *Palliative practices: An interdisciplinary approach* (pp. 418-441). St. Louis: Elsevier.

GABA, Gamma-aminobutyric acid; *NMDA, N-*methyl-D-aspartate; *NSAID,* nonsteroidal antiinflammatory drug.

*All tricyclic antidepressants exhibit anticholinergic properties. Use with caution in the elderly. Desipramine and nortriptyline have the lowest incidence of anticholinergic effects of this class.

†Some specialists titrate gabapentin up to 6000 mg/day.

‡Dexamethasone starting dose is dependent on severity of symptom. Avoid administration late in day as may interfere with sleep.

TABLE 32-6 ■ **Adjuvant Analgesics—cont'd**

Class	Uses	Generic Name	Starting Dose in Adults	Dosing Schedule	Titration, Maximal Dose, Comments
Bisphosphonates	Bone pain associated with hypercalcemia	Pamidronate	60 to 90 mg intravenously over 1 to 2 hr	Every 4 wk	Monitor for hypocalcemia
		Zolendronic acid	3-4 mg intravenously over 15 min	Every 4 wk	Monitor for hypocalcemia Use renal dosing
GABA agonist	Neuropathic pain	Baclofen	5 mg orally	Three times daily	May increase by 15 mg/day at 3-day intervals; maximum dose
NMDA receptor antagonist	Neuropathic pain	Ketamine	100 to 200 mg subcutaneously over 24 hr		Narrow therapeutic index; high risk for psychomimetic effects
Local anesthetics	Neuropathic pain	Lidocaine 5% patch	1 to 3 transdermal patches	12 hr on; 12 hr off	

TABLE 32-7 ■ Approximate Equianalgesic Dosages of Opioids*

Drug[†]	Oral Dose (mg)	Parenteral Dose (mg)	Duration of Action	Comments
Morphine sulfate	30-60	10	3 to 4 hr	Active metabolites M6G and M3G can lead to neurotoxicity—especially in renal insufficiency
Oxycodone	20	NA	3 to 4 hr	Adverse effects milder than morphine
Hydrocodone	30	NA	3 to 4 hr	Not available as single agent
Methadone‡	—	—	4 to 12 hr	Dosage decreases as opiate substituted for increases—see footnotes
Hydromorphone	7.5-8	1.5	4 to 5 hr	Opioid of choice for continuous subcutaneous infusions
Fentanyl [transdermal]	n/a	50 mcg/hr = 100 mg po morphine/ 24 hr	48 to 72 hr	Caution must be used in handling/disposal of patches Absorption affected by changes in body temperature. Also available in transmucosal delivery for breakthrough pain

*Equianalgesic tables are intended to be a guide. Each individual patient must be evaluated for the appropriateness of the opiate dose used based on prior opiate use, comorbidities, and concomitant medications.
†The following drugs are not recommended for analgesic use in palliative care settings:
   -Codeine [intolerance common]
   -Meperidine [neurotoxicity risk]
   -Propoxyphene [long half-life with toxic accumulations of cardiac and CNS metabolites]
‡Use the following guide to calculate the dose for methadone:
   -Calculate 24-hour equivalent dose of oral morphine
      <90 mg, use 4:1 ratio
      91 to 300 mg, use 8:1 ratio
      301 to 600 mg, use 12:1 ratio

initial dose. One dose can be converted to another by following a four-step procedure. Figure 32-6 works through four basic steps for calculating an equianalgesic conversion.

Common Side Effects of Opioids and Their Management

Sedation

Sedation usually clears in 1 to 3 days. If sedation persists, patients may benefit from a slight reduction in the opioid dose and an evaluation for the need to add an adjuvant medication or a stimulant such as methylphenidate. Excessive sedation is often a sign that the pain syndrome is opioid resistant. This assumes that an assessment has ruled out the potential contribution of other patient medications to oversedation.

Constipation

This is a common but preventable side effect. Regularly scheduled laxatives are almost always required; surface wetting agents in addition to a gentle laxative such as senna should be considered as a starting regimen. Start a bowel regimen before initiating an around-the-clock analgesic dosing schedule.

Equianalgesic Calculation Guide

This guide illustrates one method of changing from one opioid or route of administration to another. Clinicians must be able to identify appropriate opioid doses when a patient requires a change of opioid or route of administration. Mastering this skill enables you to determine a dose of a new opioid that is approximately equal in analgesic effect to the dose of a former opioid to ensure continued pain relief

Step 1. Add up the total amount of current drug given in 24 hours. Remember to add in both scheduled and rescue doses. (If two or more different opioids have been taken, they must each be converted to the same drug and route.)

Step 2. Plug numbers into the following proportion:

Go to equianalgesic table—find dose for current drug — Put in 24-hr dose of current drug (from step 1)

Go to equianalgesic table—find dose for new drug — N (24-hr dose of the new drug)

$$\frac{\text{Go to equianalgesic table—find dose for current drug}}{\text{Go to equianalgesic table—find dose for new drug}} = \frac{\text{Put in 24-hr dose of current drug (from step 1)}}{N \text{ (24-hr dose of the new drug)}}$$

Shortcut tip: Look at the left side of the proportion as a fraction. If possible reduce the fraction. This new fraction provides the ratio and applies the relationship between the 24-hr doses and may immediately show you the value of N. If you can see this, skip to step 4.

Step 3. Solve for N by cross-multiplying:

$$\frac{\text{Equianalgesic table dose of current drug}}{\text{Equianalgesic table dose of new drug}} \diagup\!\!\!\!\diagdown \frac{\text{(24-hr dose of the current drug)}}{N}$$

Example: Step 1

Patient is taking 10 mg PO morphine q4h, 6 doses per day:
6 doses at 10 mg = 60 mg per day
Convert to oral hydromorphone:

Step 2

$$\frac{30 \text{ mg morphine}}{7.5 \text{ mg hydromorphone}} = \frac{60 \text{ mg morphine}}{N \text{ (24-hr dose of hydromorphone)}}$$

$$\frac{30 \text{ mg morphine}}{7.5 \text{ mg hydromorphone}} = \frac{4}{1} = \frac{60 \text{ mg morphine}}{N}$$

Step 3

$$\frac{30 \text{ mg morphine}}{7.5 \text{ mg hydromorphone}} = \frac{60 \text{ mg morphine}}{N}$$

B

$$\text{24-hr dose current drug} \times \frac{\text{Equianalgesic table dose new drug}}{\text{current drug}} = \text{Equianalgesic table dose current drug} \times N$$

C

$$\frac{\text{24-hr dose current drug} \times \frac{\text{Equianalgesic table dose new drug}}{\text{current drug}}}{\text{Equianalgesic table dose current drug}} = N$$

D Answer: N will be the 24-hr dose of the new drug.

E Does this answer make sense? Double-check. Plug it into the proportion in step A, and cross-multiply; the numbers should be equal.

4. Look up the duration of action (the dosing interval) of the new drug in the equianalgesic table and determine how many doses the patient should take each day. Divide N by the number of doses per day. This gives the amount for each scheduled dose of the new opioid.

B

$$60 \text{ mg morphine} \times \frac{7.5 \text{ mg hydromorphone}}{30 \text{ mg morphine}} = 30 \text{ mg morphine} \times N$$

C

$$\frac{60 \text{ mg morphine} \times \frac{7.5 \text{ mg hydromorphone}}{30 \text{ mg morphine}}}{} = N$$

D 15 mg hydromorphone = N

E

$$\frac{30 \text{ mg morphine}}{7.5 \text{ mg hydromorphone}} = \frac{60 \text{ mg morphine}}{15 \text{ mg hydromorphone}}$$

4. Hydromorphone can be given every 4 hr, 6 doses per day. To administer 15 mg of hydromorphone in a day, divide the 24-hr dose by 6.

2.5 mg hydromorphone q4h

Because hydromorphone is available in 2-, 4-, and 8-mg tablets, the dose would be rounded up or down, depending on the clinical situation.

Figure 32-6 Equianalgesic Calculation Guide. (From Gordon, D., Stevenson, K., Griffie, J., et al. [1999]. Opioid equianalgesic calculations. J Palliat Med, 2[2], 209-218.)

Nausea

Persons usually become tolerant to the emetic effect after 3 to 5 days. In the interim, use an antiemetic. Persistent nausea requires further assessment for other etiologies.

Confusion and Excitability

Evaluate for the underlying cause. Eliminate nonessential central nervous system (CNS)–acting medications. If analgesia is satisfactory, reduce the dosage of the opioid by 25%. Neurotoxic effects of opioids can be seen in those patients who have impaired renal function and have been on higher dose or prolonged therapy. Symptoms manifest as delirium, myoclonus, agitation, and hyperalgesia. These symptoms may require a change in opioid (Bruera & Kim, 2003).

Less Common Side Effects

Less common side effects include sweating, pruritus, and urinary retention.

Nonsteroidal Antiinflammatory Drugs

The nonsteroidal antiinflammatory drugs (NSAIDs) are believed to inhibit prostaglandin synthesis, ultimately reducing the patient's pain perception. NSAIDs are considered nonopioid analgesics and serve as the first line in the management of somatic pain. When an NSAID alone is not sufficient to control the pain, a medication that combines an NSAID with an opioid is the second step of treatment (see Table 32-4). NSAIDs have the potential of producing gastritis, fluid retention, renal failure, and platelet dysfunction (Chang, 2004; Esper & Heidrich, 2005; NCCN, 2005). They are contraindicated in the following situations:

■ History of gastrointestinal bleeding secondary to NSAIDs
■ History of peptic ulcer disease
■ Active gastrointestinal bleeding
■ Coagulopathies

There are multiple NSAIDs to choose from, and further discussion can be found in many existing resources; some of the more common NSAIDs and dosages are highlighted in Table 32-3.

NSAID choice is determined by availability, cost, patient convenience, adverse effects, and efficacy. The extent of gastrointestinal distress caused by NSAIDs has no relation to the severity of the gastrointestinal symptoms. Concomitant administration of a proton pump inhibitor has been shown to help decrease the risk of gastropathy (American Pain Society, 2003).

Adjuvant Analgesics

An adjuvant analgesic, also called a *coanalgesic,* is a medication that has a primary indication other than analgesia but has also been found to have analgesic properties (McCaffery & Pasero, 1999). Tricyclic antidepressants and anticonvulsants are the two most commonly used classes of adjuvant medications used to treat neuropathic pain. These medications often require titration, starting with a low dose and titrating to pain relief or intolerable side effects. Explain to the patient that complete pain relief will not begin immediately; it takes time to find the right dose and right medication for each person (Bruera & Kim, 2003). If the first choice of a medication is not effective

Box 32-1	Guidelines for the Initiation of Adjuvant Analgesics

- Perform a comprehensive patient evaluation.
- Optimize current regimen.
- Select the drug which best addresses pain syndrome.
- Understand the pharmacologic properties of the adjuvant analgesic selected.
- Evaluate risks of polypharmacy.
- Understand individual variability.
- Educate patients on specific role of adjuvant therapy.
- Utilize adjuvant analgesics as part of the entire pain management regimen.

Data from Lussier, D., Huskey, A.G., & Portenoy, R.K. (2004). Adjuvant analgesics in cancer pain management. *The Oncologist, 9(4)*, 571-591.

or not tolerated after careful titration, consider switching to a different adjuvant analgesic. This continuous monitoring of both analgesia and side effects is an acquired skill that requires a working knowledge of the varied patient responses coupled with medication-specific pharmacokinetics.

Table 32-6 highlights some of the commonly used adjuvant analgesics. There is no "cookbook" approach to prescribing adjuvant analgesics. Individuals respond differently to medications based on their underlying pathophysiologic condition, metabolism, organ function, and physical status. It is important that the clinician assess all of the symptoms that the patient is experiencing and tailor adjuvant analgesics specifically to both the pain syndrome and other symptoms (Box 32-1). Many of the adjuvant analgesics used to treat the various pain syndromes prove useful for other symptoms such as dyspnea, depression, and restlessness.

Corticosteroids

Corticosteroids are useful because of their antiinflammatory effects. They are considered not only for treatment of somatic bone pain but also for both visceral and neuropathic pain syndromes. Corticosteroids are also used in the management of anorexia, depression, nausea, spinal cord compression, superior vena cava syndrome, organ distention, and other conditions (Lussier, Huskey & Portenoy, 2004; National Cancer Institute, 2005). Dosing schedules vary with the disease trajectory and the underlying pathophysiologic condition. The adverse effects of corticosteroids include candidiasis, gastritis, fluid retention, hypertension, hyperglycemia, and mood alterations even to the point of psychosis (Lussier et al., 2004).

Corticosteroid dosage is dependent upon the underlying pathophysiologic condition; doses differ, for example, when treating pain, anorexia, intracranial edema, and spinal cord compression (see individual symptoms). Start with low doses and titrate upward to desired effect.

Bisphosphonates

The bisphosphonate class of medication, although costly, may be considered for the treatment of bone pain due to metastasis when other adjuvants fail. These agents induce apoptosis of osteoclasts, which can lead to tumor shrinkage (Sabino & Mantyh, 2005).

The most commonly used bisphosphonates are pamidronate and zolendronic acid. Both must be used with caution in patients with renal impairment. And, due to the potential for the development of osteonecrosis of the jaw, patients should not have invasive dental procedures done while taking these agents (Ruggiero, Mehrotra, Rosenberg et al., 2004).

Radiopharmaceuticals

Under the direction of a radiation oncologist, the use of medications such as strontium 89 may be considered to relieve bone pain in the active patient with a longer prognosis. This medication is absorbed into areas of high bone turnover and can help reduce pain (Nilsson, Strong, Ginman et al., 2005; Reisfield, Silberstein & Wilson, 2005). Be aware that patients often exhibit a short-term "pain flare" when radiopharmaceuticals are started, requiring additional analgesics for several days. Then, analgesics can be titrated down as pain decreases. Never stop opioid medications abruptly.

Invasive Interventions

Tumor Embolization

A novel means of attempting palliation of symptoms performed by interventional radiologists is to localize tumor blood supply under fluoroscopic guidance and inject alcohol, coils, or other agents to occlude those vessels supplying the tumor. When a large percentage of vessels can be embolized, subsequent tumor shrinkage can provide significant improvement in pain. Patients must be educated regarding the potential for increased pain during the first 24 to 72 hours postprocedure (Kent, Forauer, Esper et al., 2004).

Intraspinal Medication Delivery

Pain that responds poorly to standard pharmacologic and conventional modalities may require more invasive measures. Opioids such as morphine may be delivered intrathecally or epidurally and often involve an implantable pump. Intrathecal morphine is currently the most commonly used analgesic administered by pump but remains in the cerebrospinal fluid for extended periods and can spread to the level of the brainstem, possibly inducing respiratory depression. Fentanyl is taken up more readily into the systemic circulation due to its increased lipid solubility and, as a result, has fewer central nervous system depressive effects. Prior to implanting permanent pumps, opioid trials need to be performed to demonstrate that the patient's pain is opioid responsive. Pumps can be implanted in a permanent fashion if a beneficial response is seen (American Pain Society, 2003; Pappagallo, Dickerson, Varga et al., 2002). Opioids may be administered alone or in combination with other agents such as local anesthetics or clonidine. It is important to consider the variation in systemic absorption between various routes of administration. For example, the approximate equivalent of 30 mg of oral morphine administered on a regular schedule is 10 mg intravenously, 1 mg epidurally, and 100 mcg (0.1 mg) intrathecally (American Pain Society, 2003).

The use of intraspinal delivery systems requires expertise in both insertion and management arenas. It is therefore generally reserved for a select subset of individuals who, under a multidisciplinary review, are deemed appropriate candidates.

Additional Therapeutic Interventions

Radiation Therapy

Tumors involving bone may be exquisitely sensitive to radiation therapy, and the role of this treatment for improving patient functional status and quality of life must be evaluated in correlation to the patient prognosis, anticipated toxicities, and treatment-related burden. It has been reported that radiation therapy can achieve pain relief in this setting for as many as 75% of patients receiving treatment (Rutter & Weissman, 2004). There is good evidence that single-fraction radiation therapy is as effective as multifraction dosing schedules in relieving bone pain (Sze, Shelley, Held et al., 2003).

Neurolytic Blocks

Neurolytic blocks may also provide pain relief in situations where enlarging masses are placing pressure on adjacent structures. The procedure involves the application of a local anesthetic or neurolytic agent as in the case of celiac plexus blocks for the pain associated with pancreatic cancer (NCCN, 2005; Wong, Schroeder, Carns et al., 2004).

At times pain is difficult to treat, even with the means already suggested. Resources for difficult pain management problems should be identified in advance.

Nondrug and Complementary Therapies for Pain

Medications and treatments are not the only effective interventions to alleviate pain and the suffering that may accompany pain. Although not substitutes for analgesics, nondrug and complementary therapies play an important role in managing the total pain experience. Physically, these interventions are believed to decrease stimulation to the sympathetic nervous system, promote muscle relaxation, interfere with pain transmission, and stimulate the release of endogenous pain-relieving substances (e.g., endorphin) (Eshkevari & Heath, 2005). Cognitive and emotional effects of these nondrug interventions include decreased anxiety, restoration of hope, decreased fatigue, improved sleep, and decreased feelings of helplessness and hopelessness. Examples of nondrug and complementary therapies for pain are listed in Table 32-8.

Research data on the effects of nondrug and complementary therapies often show conflicting or inconclusive results (Allard, Maunsell, Labbe et al., 2001; Fellowes, Barnes & Wilkinson, 2004; Mundy, DuHamel, & Montgomery, 2003). This may be due to the heterogeneity of the research populations, small sample sizes, lack of randomization, varying techniques in the application of these interventions, and inconsistent control for confounding variables. In a meta-analysis of psychoeducational interventions for pain, Devine (2003) concluded that there is reasonably strong evidence for relaxation-based cognitive-behavioral interventions, education about analgesic use, and supportive counseling. More research on complementary therapies in the palliative care setting is needed.

PAIN MANAGEMENT IN SUBSTANCE ABUSE

Treating pain in patients with either a current or a past history of substance abuse presents complex psychosocial and physical issues to any clinician. These patients fall into three basic categories (Paice & Fine, 2001):

1. Persons who have used or abused drugs or other substances in the past but are no longer using them

TABLE 32-8 ■ Nondrug and Complementary Therapies for Pain

Type of Intervention	Effects	Examples
Muscle relaxation	Decreases anxiety Promotes vasodilatation	Slow, controlled breathing Progressive muscle relaxation
Cold	Reduces inflammation Relieves muscle spasm	Ice packs Towels soaked in ice water
Heat	Increases blood flow and oxygenation to tissues	Hot water bottles Warm, moist compresses Heating pads Immersion
Massage	Aids relaxation Increases circulation at site	Gentle body massage Therapeutic massage with a licensed therapist
Exercise	Strengthens muscles Mobilizes stiff joints	Walking Gentle stretching
Immobilization/ splinting	Supports painful areas	Canes, walkers Braces, slings, binders
Touch/Energy therapies	Proposed to affect the human energy system	Healing touch Therapeutic touch Reiki therapy
Relaxation	Alters state of consciousness Increase receptivity to suggestion — often used with imagery Decreases anxiety	Music Mindful meditation Deep breathing Hypnosis
Imagery	Aids in relaxation Focuses attention away from pain, or to control pain Decreases powerlessness	Many different images may be used
Distraction	Focuses attention away from pain	Music Pets Art Humor Activities/socialization
Education	Instructs on appropriate reporting and management of pain Addresses fears, concerns, misunderstandings about pain	Individual or group education session Written materials
Support	Decreases powerlessness Improves coping	Structured psychotherapy Facilitated support groups, including those on the internet Peer support groups, including those on the internet
Pastoral counseling	Addresses existential issues contributing to the pain experience	Consultation with chaplain or individual's own clergy Prayer

2. Persons in methadone maintenance programs
3. Persons who are actively abusing drugs

Most clinicians lack even the most basic background in and knowledge of chemical dependency and often struggle with these issues in the treatment of pain in general and certainly in the treatment of pain in patients who have a current or past history of substance abuse. Any patient in a palliative care setting may experience significant pain. The challenge is to offer those who have substance abuse histories the same compassionate, comprehensive care given any patient, recognizing a potential need for some modifications in care and use of additional resources. Many clinicians fear they will be fooled or duped into providing pain medications to individuals who are seeking drugs rather than pain relief. Pain is a subjective symptom, without observable physical signs, and thus in many clinician's mind, its occurrence cannot be confirmed objectively. Keep in mind that if the goal is to relieve pain, the clinician must accept the patient's report of pain.

Although additional epidemiologic studies are needed, substance disorders are believed to be present in as many as 6% to 15% of the U.S. population, although researchers believe that the incidence may be a little higher because of underreporting and institutional biases, including a lack of data from primary care centers and from persons alienated from the health care system (Passik & Kirsh, 2005). While the medical use of opioids has increased markedly, reports of abuse have either decreased or remained constant (Joranson, Ryan, Gilson et al., 2000). Thus, treating pain aggressively with opioids does not appear to contribute to increases in the reported health consequences of opioid analgesic abuse.

Treating a patient with a current or past history of substance abuse requires a comprehensive approach that recognizes and considers the interaction of the biologic, chemical, social, and psychologic and psychiatric aspects of substance abuse and addiction (Passik & Kirsh, 2005). Although the principles and guidelines outlined in the discussion that follows provide a framework for treating the patient who is actively abusing a substance, they also apply to those who are substance free but have used them in the past and those in methadone maintenance programs (Passik & Theobald, 2000).

Involve an interdisciplinary team. Reflect on one's expertise and identify resources that can be accessed for managing this patient and family. A team approach is essential to address the multitude of medical and psychosocial problems presented and to prevent caregiver burnout and fatigue. An ideal team includes a physician with expertise in pain management and palliative care, staff nurses, social workers, and, if possible, a mental health professional versed in addiction medicine.

Set realistic goals for care. Relief of pain and enhancement of quality of life are the goals of care. What is the effect of the patient's past or current history of substance abuse? Is addiction increasing the patient's suffering? Are recovery programs aimed at abstinence appropriate? What should be the focus of the patient's energy and the family's and caregiver's intervention? Be mindful that patients who are seeking pain relief and do not receive it may relapse into abuse patterns to alleviate that pain (Passik & Kirsh, 2005).

Define the problem. What often appears as drug-seeking behavior is, rather, pain relief–seeking behavior. Review the definitions of addiction, tolerance, physical dependence, and pseudo-addiction. Review apparently aberrant drug-taking behaviors: Do they suggest addiction or uncontrolled pain? Recommend including most currently accepted definitions—the joint statement would be a great reference.

Evaluate and treat comorbid psychiatric disorders. Substance abuse is accompanied by a high incidence of other psychiatric disorders, including depression and personality and anxiety disorders. Being mindful of the goals of care, obtain assistance in treating these disorders. Successful treatment may enhance patient comfort and quality of life: the goal of care.

Consider the therapeutic effect of tolerance. Tolerance may or not be a factor in treating the pain in persons with a current or past history of substance abuse; it is highly variable. Higher initial doses may be required along with relatively rapid dose escalation to manage pain. What appears as tolerance may indeed be rapidly advancing disease and thus worsening pain. The principle of titrating to effect applies regardless of the underlying cause of the need to increase dosage.

Apply appropriate pharmacologic principles to treat pain. The principles discussed earlier apply equally to the patient with a current or past history of substance abuse. The principle of titration to effect and the individualization of therapy, including providing the right drug at the right dose, however, is often difficult in this population. Be mindful of the goals of care and the definitions of addiction, tolerance, physical dependence, and pseudo-addiction (Passik & Kirsh, 2005). *Remember that unrelieved pain can lead to the development of aberrant drug-related behavior, including relapse.*

Select drugs and routes of administration for the symptom and setting. Although no data confirm this relationship, among persons with known substance abuse, long-acting medications may not contribute as significantly to aberrant drug-taking behavior as do short-acting drugs (Passik & Kirsh, 2005). Balance the medication choice with the type of pain, goals of care, and patient needs.

Recognize specific drug abuse behavior. Persons with a current or past history of substance abuse, including alcohol abuse, should be observed for actions that suggest substance abuse. If there is a high level of concern about aberrant behavior, the interdisciplinary team may determine and plan a higher level of monitoring, including more frequent visits, interviews with family members, and perhaps urine screening for prescribed and illicit drugs. Keep in mind the goals of care; if more monitoring is indicated, including urine drug screening, patients should be reassured that it will provide a foundation for aggressive symptom-oriented treatment (Passik & Kirsh, 2005).

Use nonpharmacologic approaches as appropriate. Nonpharmacologic approaches should augment pain and symptom management, not replace the use of appropriate pharmacologic therapies. Include educational initiatives (e.g., methods to communicate effectively with staff members about pain and to navigate a complex medical system) and cognitive and behavioral techniques to foster relaxation and enhance coping.

In order to improve the quality of life, and thus the quality of death, clinicians caring for the patient and family should focus on the reduction of suffering—whether the result of the disease process or of the patient's own acts (Passik & Theobald, 2000).

Anyone who provides palliative care must either be familiar with the basic concepts of addiction treatment or have access to readily available resources in this specialty area. Given the impact of either a current or a past substance abuse history on patient suffering and quality of life, identification of resources in advance is essential. Unless a clinician has a background in substance abuse disorders and is conversant with current thought in this area, he or she should not manage such patients and families without the appropriate assistance. The successful outcome of care and the patient's and family's quality of life depend on it.

Rapidly Escalating Pain

Rapidly escalating pain needs to be carefully referenced. When pain is severe and escalating rapidly, frequent increases of the dose of opioid may lead to severe side effects. Excitatory toxicity from large opioid doses can include myoclonus, grand mal seizures, delirium, hallucinations, and hyperalgesia. Management may require dose reduction, opioid rotation, hydration, and additional medications to control symptoms, such as midazolam, barbiturates, and baclofen. Take advantage of the resources available to ensure patient comfort.

PATIENT AND FAMILY EDUCATION

The complete plan of pain management and method for alterations should be fully discussed with the patient and family. Potential opioid side effects should be discussed at the time of the first prescription (information should include the assurance that tolerance develops to most of the side effects of opioids except constipation). A plan for a bowel regimen appropriate to the patient should also be agreed upon.

Many patients confuse addiction with the physical dependence that occurs in all patients over time; concerns for addiction need to be addressed. The emphasis of the education must be on alleviating the fear of addiction, as it is extremely rare in patients who are adequately treated for pain. Patients and families should be instructed not to decrease or stop opioids suddenly except under the direction of the health care professionals and should be informed of when to contact the health care provider about the patient's pain and the frequency of use of as-needed medications. For example, the clinician may tell a patient to call when as-needed medication is used more than three times a day. The following should be provided in written form for the patient and family:

- A list of each medication with directions on when to take it
- Notification as to whether refills can be called in or require an original prescription
- Potential side effects and what to do if they occur
- Telephone numbers (24 hours a day, 7 days a week) of a health care professional for assistance with
  - Problems obtaining or taking medications
  - New pain or unrelieved pain
  - Uncontrolled nausea and vomiting
  - No bowel movement for longer than 2 days
  - Oversedation, confusion, or other neurologic changes
  - Any intolerable side effect

EVALUATION AND PLAN FOR FOLLOW-UP

Evaluation intervals are based on the assessment and achievement of pain management goals. The frequency of follow-up is dependent on the level of pain, planned interventions, and patient response. For example, a patient in a pain crisis may need frequent reassessment, including telephone contact between visits. A patient with stable pain may need only periodic evaluations. Gather information on present pain, the worst the pain has been since the last visit, and the most relief the patient has experienced since the last visit. On the basis of the patient's underlying pathophysiologic condition, the clinician may be able to anticipate and thus assess for new pain syndromes. While caring for a patient with prostate cancer, assessing for the presence of bone pain is wise. Always be mindful of the patient- and family-related barriers to reporting pain and using analgesics discussed at the beginning of the chapter and how they might affect the plan of care.

The management of pain at end-of-life is essential. Uncontrolled pain robs the patient—and family—of quality of life that is so precious and important during these final months.

CASE STUDY

Mrs. W. is a 78-year-old woman with a history of oral pharyngeal cancer. She is known to have widespread metastatic bone disease. She enters the clinic in a wheelchair accompanied by her daughter, saying she is "absolutely miserable."

Mrs. W. reports pain in her neck that has been present for over a year and has slowly increased in intensity. It hinders her ability to turn her head. She reports that it is about a 7 on a scale of 0 to 10 and is fairly constant all the time. She describes it as a dull, achy pain that moves from her neck up to her head. Her mobility has markedly decreased in the past 2 to 3 weeks. She has been taking acetaminophen 500 mg with 5 mg of hydrocodone (Vicodin), one tablet every 3 hours, with no real relief: "At first they helped; now they don't do anything." She expresses concern about becoming addicted to her pain medication.

She denies constipation. Laboratory values are all within normal range. Recent radiologic examinations reveal widespread increase in disease. Mrs. W. is aware of her advancing disease and expresses a desire to be able to feed her cats, enjoy her children and grandchildren, and be as free of pain as possible. She lives alone and, overall, manages well. She is able to swallow oral medications.

Pharmacologic Choices

There are several options for improving the management of Mrs. W.'s pain. Because it is severe (7 on a 0-to-10 scale), it is appropriate to increase her dose of medication by 50% to 100%. (Note that Mrs. W. is already at the maximum safe dosage of acetaminophen per day, or 4 g, so instructing her to take her Vicodin, two tablets every 4 hours, is not an option.) Consider the following:

- Convert Mrs. W. to a sustained-release preparation. Presently Mrs. W. is taking a total of 40 mg of hydrocodone a day. Following the principle of increasing the opioid by 100% because of her severe pain, and using the equianalgesic conversion chart, change her medication to sustained-release morphine, 40 mg orally every 12 hours. Adequate breakthrough medication is also ordered: 10% to 20% of the 24-hour dose, or immediate-release morphine, 12 to 20 mg orally every 1 to 2 hours as needed. If an increase of 50% is more appropriate, the sustained-release morphine dosage would be 30 mg orally every 12 hours with immediate-release morphine, 9 to 15 mg every 1 to 2 hours as needed.
- Add an NSAID, if not contraindicated by Mrs. W.'s history, for the pain secondary to metastatic bone disease.
- Transdermal fentanyl is not an appropriate choice at this time because her pain is not well controlled. Increases in transdermal fentanyl doses are only appropriate every 72 hours.

Because of the severity of her pain Mrs. W. was switched to sustained-release morphine, 40 mg orally every 12 hours, with immediate-release morphine, 12 to 20 mg orally every 1 to 2 hours as needed for breakthrough pain. Daily contact with Mrs. W. and her family was planned, and she was urged to keep a pain diary. She was a little sleepy the first day but rated her pain as 2 on a 0-to-10 scale, stating, "I can turn my head!" She reported taking no breakthrough medications. By the third day she was alert, sleeping all night, and feeding her cats and reported taking 5 mg of her breakthrough medication only once a day. She was instructed to call if she requires more than three doses of breakthrough medication a day.

REFERENCES

Allard P., Maunsell E., Labbe J., et al. (2001). Educational interventions to improve cancer pain control: a systematic review. *J Palliat Med*, 4(2):191-203.

American Academy of Pain Medicine, American Pain Society, & American Society of Addiction Medicine. (2001). *Definitions related to the use of opioids for the treatment of pain*. Retrieved October 31, 2005, from www.ampainsoc.org/advocacy/opioids2.htm

American Pain Society. (2003). *Principles of analgesic use in the treatment of acute pain and cancer pain* (5th ed.). Glenview, Ill.: Author.

Anderson, G., Vestergaard, K., Ingeman-Nielsen, M., et al. (1995). Incidence of central post-stroke pain. *Pain*, 61, 187-193.

Berry, P.H., Eagan, K., Eighmy, J.B., et al. (1999). *Hospice and palliative nurses practice review* (3rd ed.). Dubuque, Iowa: Kendall/Hunt.

Boivie, J. (1999). Central pain. In P.D. Wall & R. Melzack (Eds.). *Textbook of pain* (4th ed., pp. 879-941). New York: Churchill Livingstone.

Breitbart, W. Passik, S.D., & Rosenfeld, H.D. (1999). Cancer, mind and spirit. In P.D. Wall & R. Melzack (Eds.). *Textbook of pain* (4th ed., pp. 1065-1112). New York: Churchill Livingstone.

Bruera, E. & Kim, H.N. (2003). Cancer pain. *JAMA*, 290(18), 2476-2479.

Caraceni, A., Martini, C., Zecca, E., et al.; Working Group of an IASP Task Force on Cancer Pain. (2004). Breakthrough pain characteristics and syndromes in patients with cancer pain: An international study. *Palliat Med*, 18(3), 177-183.

Chang, H.M. (2004). Pain and its management in patients with cancer. *Cancer Invest, 22(5)*, 799-809.

Cherny, N. & Portenoy, R.K. (1999). Cancer pain: Principles of assessment and syndromes. In P.D. Wall & R. Melzack (Eds.). *Textbook of pain* (4th ed., pp. 1017-1064). New York: Churchill Livingstone.

Coderre, T.J. & Melzack, R. (1992). The contribution of excitatory amino acids to central sensitization and persistent nociception after formalin-induced tissue injury. *J Neurosci, 12*, 3671-3675.

Corbett, C.F. (2005). Practical management of patients with painful diabetic neuropathy. *Diabetes Educ, 31(4)*, 523-524, 526-528, 530.

Devine, E.C. (2003). Meta-analysis of the effect of psychoeducational interventions on pain in adults with cancer. *Oncol Nurs Forum, 30(1)*, 75-89.

Eshkevari, L. & Heath, J. (2005), Use of acupuncture for chronic pain: optimizing clinical practice. *Holist Nurs Pract, 19(5)*, 217-221.

Esper, P. & Heidrich, D. (2005). Symptom clusters in advanced illness. *Semin Oncol Nurs, 21(1)*, 20-28.

Fellowes, D., Barnes, K., & Wilkinson, S. (2004). Aromatherapy and massage for symptom relief in patients with cancer. *Cochrane Database Systematic Reviews, (2)*, CD002287.

Fohr, S.A. (1998). The double effect of pain medication: Separating myth from reality. *Journal of Palliative Medicine, 1(4)*, 315-328.

Georgesen, J. & Dungan J.M. (1996). Managing spiritual distress in patients with advanced cancer pain. *Cancer Nurs, 19(5)*, 376-383.

Gordon, D.B., Dahl, J.L., Miaskowski, C., et al. (2005). American pain society recommendations for improving the quality of acute and cancer pain management: American Pain Society Quality of Care Task Force. *Arch Intern Med, 165(14)*, 1574-1580.

Hudspith, M.J., Siddall, P.J., & Munglani, R. (2006). Physiology of pain. In H.B. Hemmings & P.M. Hopkins (Eds.). *Foundations of anesthesia: Basic sciences for clinical practice* (2nd ed., pp. 267-285). St. Louis: Mosby.

International Association for the Study of Pain, Subcommittee on Taxonomy. (1979). Pain terms: A list with definitions and notes on usage. *Pain, 6*, 249-252.

Joranson, D.E., Ryan, K.M., Gilson, A.M., et al. (2000). Trends in medical use and abuse of opioid analgesics. *JAMA, 283*, 1710-1714.

Kent, E.C., Forauer, A., Esper, P., et al. (2004). Palliative embolization of metastases from kidney cancer [Abstract]. *J Clin Oncol, ASCO Annual Meeting Proceedings (Post-Meeting Edition), 22 (July 15 Suppl)*, 14S.

Kovach, C., Weissman, D., Griffie, J., et al.. (1999). Assessment and treatment of discomfort for people with late-stage dementia. *J Pain Symptom Manage, 18*, 412-419.

Leddy, K.M. & Wolosin, R.J. (2005). Patient satisfaction with pain control during hospitalization. *Joint Comm J Qual Patient Safety, 31(9)*, 507-513.

Levenson, J.W., McCarthy, E.P., Lynn, J., et al. (2000). *J Am Geriatr Soc, 48(5 Suppl)*, S101-S109.

Levy, M. (1994). Pharmacologic management of cancer pain. *Semin Oncol, 21(6)*, 718-739.

Lussier, D., Huskey, A.G., & Portenoy, R.K. (2004). Adjuvant analgesics in cancer pain management. *Oncologist, 9(5)*, 571-591.

McCaffery, M. (1968). *Nursing practice theories related to cognition, bodily pain, and man-environment interactions*. Los Angeles: UCLA Student Store.

McCaffery, M. & Pasero, C. (1999). *Pain: Clinical manual* (2nd ed.). St. Louis: Mosby.

McCarthy, M., Lay, M., & Addington-Hall, J. (1996). Dying from heart disease. *J R Coll Physicians Lond, 30(4)*, 325-328.

Mercadante, W. & Portenoy, R.K. (2001). Opioid responsive cancer pain, part 3: Clinical strategies to improve opioid responsiveness. *J Pain Symptom Manage, 21(4)*, 338-354.

Mundy, E.A., DuHamel, K.N., & Montgomery, G.H. (2003). The efficacy of behavioral interventions for cancer treatment-related side effects. *Semin Clin Neuropsychiatry, 8(4)*, 253-275.

National Cancer Institute (NCI). (2005). *Pain (PDQ)—health professional version*. Retrieved August 25, 2005, from www.cancer.gov/cancertopics/pdq/supportivecare/pain/healthprofessional.

National Comprehensive Cancer Network (NCCN). *NCCN clinical practice guidelines in oncology*. Retrieved August 31, 2005, from www.nccn.org/professionals/physician_gls/PDF/pain.pdf.

Nilsson, S., Strang, P., Ginman, C., et al. (2005). Palliation of bone pain in prostate cancer using chemotherapy and strontium-89. A randomized phase II study. *J Pain Symptom Manage, 29(4)*, 352-357.

Ogle, K.S. & Hopper, K. (2005). End-of-life care for older adults. *Primary Care, 32*, 811-828.

Page, G.G. (2005). Surgery-induced immunosuppression and postoperative pain management. *AACN Clin Issues, 16(3)*, 302-309.

Paice, J.A. (2003). Mechanisms and management of neuropathic pain in cancer. *J Support Oncol, 1(2)*, 107-120.

Paice, J.A. & Fine, P.G. (2001). Pain at the end of life. In B.R. Ferrell & N. Coyle (Eds.). *Textbook of palliative nursing* (pp. 76-90). New York: Oxford University Press.

Pappagallo, M., Dickerson, E.D., Varga, J., et al. (2002). Management of neuropathic pain. In K.K. Kuebler & P. Esper (Eds.), *Palliative practices from A to Z for the bedside clinician* (pp. 247, 248, 253). Pittsburgh: ONS Press.

Passik, S.D. & Kirsh, K.L. (2005). Managing pain in patients with aberrant drug-taking behaviors. *J Support Oncol, 3(1)*, 83-86.

Passik, S.D. & Theobald, D.E. (2000). Managing addiction in the advanced cancer patient: Why bother? *J Pain Symptom Manage, 19*, 229-234.

Portenoy, R. & Waldman, S. (1994). Adjuvant analgesics in pain management: Part 1. *J Pain Symptom Manage, 9(6)*, 390-391.

Portenoy, R.K. & Hagen, N.A. (1990). Breakthrough pain: Definition, prevalence, and characteristics. *Pain, 41*, 273-281.

Reisfield, G.M., Silberstein, E.B., & Wilson, G.R. (2005). Radiopharmaceuticals for the palliation of painful bone metastases. *Am J Hospice Palliat Care, 22(1)*, 41-46.

Ruggiero, S.L., Mehrotra, B., Rosenberg, T.J., et al. (2004). Osteonecrosis of the jaws associated with the use of bisphosphonates: A review of 63 cases. *J Oral Maxillofac Surg, 62(5)*, 527-534.

Rutter, C. & Weissman, D.E. (2004). Radiation for palliation—part 2. *J Palliat Med, 7(6)*, 866-867.

Sabino, M.A. & Mantyh, P.W. (2005). Pathophysiology of bone cancer pain. *J Support Oncol, 3(1)*, 15-24.

Sela, R.A., Bruera, E., Conner-Spady, B., et al. (2002). Sensory and affective dimensions of advanced cancer pain. *Psycho-Oncology, 11*, 23-34.

Serlin, R.C., Mendoza, T.R., Nakamura, Y., et al. (1995). When is cancer pain mild, moderate or severe? Grading pain severity by its interference with function. *Pain, 61*, 277-284.

SUPPORT Study Principal Investigators. (1995). A controlled trial to improve care for seriously ill hospitalized patients: A study to understand prognoses and preferences for outcomes and risks of treatments (SUPPORT). *JAMA, 274*, 1591-1598.

Svendsen, K.B., Andersen, S., Arnason, S., et al. (2005). Breakthrough pain in malignant and non-malignant diseases: A review of prevalence, characteristics and mechanisms. *Eur J Pain, 9(2)*, 195-206.

Sykes, N. & Thorns, A. (2003). The use of opioids and sedatives at the end of life. *Lancet Oncol, 4(5)*, 312-318.

Sze, W.M., Shelley, M.D., Held, I., et al. (2003). Palliation of metastatic bone pain: single fraction versus multifraction radiotherapy: A systematic review of randomized trials. *Clin Oncol (R Coll Radiol), 15(6)*, 345-352.

Ulens, C., Daenens, P., & Tytgat, J. (1999). Norpropoxyphene-induced cardiotoxicity is associated with changes in ion-selectivity and gating of HERG currents. *Cardiovasc Res, 44(3)*, 568-578.

Vachon, M.L. (2004). The emotional problems of the patient in palliative medicine. In D. Doyle, G. Hanks, N. Cherny, et al. (Eds.). *Oxford textbook of palliative medicine* (3rd ed.). New York: Oxford University Press.

Ward, S.E., Goldberg, N., Miller-McCauley, V., et al. (1993). Patient-related barriers to management of cancer pain. *Pain, 52*, 319-324.

Warden, V., Hurley, A.C., & Volicer, L. (2003). Development and psychometric evaluation of the Pain Assessment in Advanced Dementia (PAINAD) scale. *J Am Med Dir Assoc, 4(1)*, 9-15.

Wilke, D.J. (1995). Neural mechanisms of pain: A foundation for cancer pain assessment and management. In D.B. McGuire, C.H. Yarbro, & B.R. Ferrell (Eds.). *Cancer pain management* (2nd ed., pp. 61-87). Boston: Jones & Bartlett.

Wong, G.Y., Schroeder, D.R., Carns, P.E., et al. (2004). Effect of neurolytic celiac plexus block on pain relief, quality of life, and survival in patients with unresectable pancreatic cancer. *JAMA, 291(9)*, 1092-1099.

World Health Organization. (1990). *Cancer pain relief and palliative care* (Technical Report Series 804). Geneva: Author.

Zeppetella, G., O'Doherty, C.A., & Collins, S. (2000). Prevalence and characteristics of breakthrough pain in cancer patients admitted to hospice. *J Pain Symptom Manage, 20(2)*, 87-92.

Zeppetella, G., O'Doherty, C.A., & Collins, S. (2001). Prevalence and characteristics of breakthrough pain in patients with non-malignant terminal disease admitted to hospice. *Palliat Med, 15(3)*, 243-246.

CHAPTER 33

PALLIATIVE CARE EMERGENCIES
Roberta Kaplow
■

There are a number of emergent situations that can arise in patients with advanced disease. These can create circumstances that are stressful for the patient and family. It is vital that a multidisciplinary approach of care be developed for patients who are at risk to develop a palliative emergency. In every case, the decision whether to take emergency action must be based on the patient's overall condition, the disease and its prognosis, the patient's and family's wishes, the potential side effects of treatment, and the distress caused by the emergency itself (Wrede-Seaman, 2001). This chapter discusses some common emergencies that can occur in the palliative care setting.

Many palliative emergencies are predictable from the nature and extent of disease. Therapies may be implemented to prevent and manage symptoms or to alleviate suffering. When intervention is inappropriate, prior discussion with patient and family of what may occur may avoid the stress of unexpected developments and the need for urgent decisions (Fowell & Stuart, 2005). The management of any event depends on the distress the symptoms are causing, the patient's condition and quality of life, wishes of the patient and family, and possible treatment side effects (Fowell & Stuart, 2005; Gullatte, Kaplow & Heidrich, 2005; Kaplow & Reid, in press; Shuey & Brant, 2004).

HYPERCALCEMIA OF MALIGNANCY

Definition and Incidence
Hypercalcemia of malignancy (HCM) is defined as a serum calcium level greater than 10.5 mg/dl (Gullatte et al., 2005; Kaplow & Reid, in press).

The reported incidence of HCM is 10% to 40% of patients (Crossno, 2004; Gullatte et al., 2005; National Coalition for Cancer Survivorship [NCCS], 2005; Solimando, 2001).

Etiology and Pathophysiology
Etiologic factors of HCM include specific cancers, treatment modalities, and nonmalignant causes. HCM is most often associated with primary tumors of the breast, lung, head and neck, kidney, esophagus, gastrointestinal (GI) tract, and cervix; lymphomas; leukemia; multiple myeloma; and melanomas (Gullatte et al., 2005; Kaplow & Reid, in press; National Cancer Institute [NCI], 2005).

Cancer treatment modalities such as estrogen, antiestrogen agents, and all-*trans* retinoic acid are associated with the development of HCM (Gullatte et al., 2005).

Non–cancer-related factors associated with HCM development include immobility dehydration, excessive intake of calcium and vitamin D, decreased parathyroid hormone levels, vitamin A intoxication, hyperparathyroidism, and thiazide diuretic or lithium use (Carroll & Schade, 2003; Crossno, 2004; Gullatte et al., 2005; Kaplow, in press; NCI, 2005).

HCM most often results from bone metastasis. This causes osteoclastic bone resorption and release of calcium. Calcium is released from the bone faster than the kidneys can excrete it (Gullatte et al., 2005; Kaplow & Reid, in press). The types of HCM are osteolytic (results from direct bone destruction by a tumor or metastasis) and humoral (results from circulating factors secreted by cancer cells) (Carroll & Schade, 2003; Inzucchi, 2004; Kaplow, in press; NCI, 2005; Solimando, 2001).

History and Physical Examination

Clinical manifestations of HCM vary depending on effects of calcium on the neurologic, GI, renal, and cardiovascular systems; rate of the rise of calcium levels; and patient's stage of disease and overall condition, renal function, and degree of HCM. They are usually related to the effects of calcium on smooth, skeletal, and cardiac muscle (Gullatte et al., 2005). Neurologic symptoms include mental status changes, hallucinations, jumbled speech, depression, and fatigue. Patients may report visual changes. Diminished deep tendon reflexes may be noted (Beckles, Spiro, Colice et al., 2003; Carroll & Schade, 2003; Crossno, 2004; Inzucchi, 2004; Kaplow & Reid, in press; NCI, 2005; NCCS, 2005; Shuey & Brant, 2004; Solimando, 2001).

Several cardiovascular symptoms exist. These include potential electrocardiographic changes such as prolonged PR interval, widened QRS complex, shortened QT interval, shortened or absent ST segments, and widened QT intervals. Patients may present with atrioventricular block bradycardia, bundle-branch block, or cardiac arrest, depending on severity. Hypertension and myocardial irritability may be observed (Beckles et al., 2003; Carroll & Schade, 2003; Crossno, 2004; Inzucchi, 2004; Kaplow & Reid, in press; NCI, 2005; NCCS, 2005; Shuey & Brant, 2004).

GI manifestations may include nausea, vomiting, anorexia, abdominal pain, ileus, constipation, abdominal distention, dry mouth, increased gastric acid production, pancreatitis, or peptic ulcer disease (Beckles et al., 2003; Carroll & Schade, 2003; Crossno, 2004; Inzucchi, 2004; NCI, 2005; NCCS, 2005; Shuey & Brant, 2004; Solimando, 2001).

Renal effects are polyuria, polydipsia, nocturia, renal failure, dehydration, and nephrogenic diabetes insipidus. Calcium phosphate crystals may be present in the renal tubules (Beckles et al., 2003; Carroll & Schade, 2003; Crossno, 2004; Inzucchi, 2004; Kaplow & Reid, in press; NCI, 2005; NCCS, 2005; Shuey & Brant, 2004; Solimando, 2001).

Other symptoms that may manifest in a patient with HCM include osteoporosis, arthritis, pathologic fractures, and pruritus (Beckles et al., 2003; Carroll & Schade, 2003; Crossno, 2004; Inzucchi, 2004; Kaplow & Reid, in press; NCI, 2005; Shuey & Brant, 2004; Solimando, 2001).

Diagnostics

Laboratory findings linked with HCM are abnormal serum creatinine, calcium, electrolytes, magnesium, phosphorus, and possibly elevated alkaline phosphatase (Crossno, 2004; Kaplow & Reid, in press; Shuey & Brant, 2004). The degree of HCM is determined by laboratory measurement of serum calcium in relation to serum albumin levels. Calcium levels should be corrected based on albumin levels, since 40% of calcium is bound to albumin (Gullatte et al., 2005; Kaplow & Reid, in press).

Intervention and Treatment

The primary treatment of HCM is treatment of the causal malignancy. This may require chemotherapy, radiation therapy (RT), hormonal therapy, and/or surgical resection (Gullatte et al., 2005; Kaplow & Reid, in press). Irrespective of severity, management should include treatment of any underlying non–disease-related causes.

Patients with a corrected calcium level less than 12 mg/dl may require only monitoring. Patients with moderate to severe HCM (more than 13 mg/dl) require aggressive treatment (Kaplow & Reid, in press).

Rehydration

Patients should drink 1 to 2 liters of fluid per day if able to tolerate oral fluids (Shuey & Brant, 2004). Patients with moderate to severe HCM may need 5 to 10 liters of fluid to restore extracellular fluid balance. Administration of isotonic saline may be required (Kaplow & Reid, in press). Loop diuretics should be avoided until volume status has been restored (Shuey & Brant, 2004).

Antiresorptive Therapy

Once rehydrated, patients require intravenous bisphosphonates. Bisphosphonates decrease the rate of bone resorption and prevent worsening or recurrence of HCM in patients with bone metastasis (Gullatte et al., 2005; Kaplow & Reid, in press; Ross, Saunders, Edmonds et al., 2004).

Corticosteroids

Patients with HCM due to steroid-responsive tumors may benefit from corticosteroid therapy. Glucocorticoids augment urinary calcium excretion and inhibit GI calcium reabsorption (Kaplow & Reid, in press; NCI, 2005).

Symptom Management

Management of HCM may also require symptom management and increasing mobility, as clinically indicated. If patients have been immobile for long periods of time, collaboration with physical therapy may be indicated (Kaplow & Reid, in press; Shuey & Brant, 2004). Constipation should be evaluated and treated. Bone pain must be managed but nonsteroidal antiinflammatory drugs (NSAIDs) should be avoided in patients using bisphosphonates (Gullatte et al., 2005). Some patients develop clinically significant and distressing mental status changes. Collaboration among physicians, midlevel clinicians, and pharmacy should focus on strategies to manage delirium or other such changes (Kaplow & Reid, in press).

Cardiac, renal, and GI function and electrolyte balance should be monitored during fluid resuscitation. This is especially important for patients who have heart failure or who have received cardiotoxic therapies. Monitoring serum creatinine is vital when receiving bisphosphonates because of the reported deterioration in renal function with these therapies (Gullatte et al., 2005).

Evaluation and Follow-up

The degree of monitoring required will depend on the patient's condition and overall goals of care. Many side effects of treatment can be prevented or managed. Since serum sodium, potassium, calcium, phosphorus, and magnesium levels may decrease, levels should be monitored at least daily. Serum calcium levels will require monitoring, especially during bisphosphonate therapy. The management of symptoms and side effects is essential (NCI, 2005).

Patients treated for HCM will require close follow-up once normal calcium levels have been attained. The underlying malignancy, following its trajectory, may worsen and ongoing HCM management may be required (NCI, 2005; Shuey & Brant, 2004). Frequency of follow-up is also based on the anticipated lasting effect of the treatment modalities used (NCI, 2005).

Patient and Family Education

Patients and families require education regarding what symptoms to observe and the importance of reporting symptoms early. Measures can include preventing dehydration, weight-bearing activities, managing pain, and avoiding thiazide diuretics (Gullatte et al., 2005).

Patients and families should have the sequelae of untreated HCM explained to them; these include loss of consciousness and coma, which may be acceptable outcomes for patients at end-of-life who are suffering or have uncontrollable symptoms or when treatment of the underlying malignancy is no longer feasible (NCI, 2005).

SYNDROME OF INAPPROPRIATE ANTIDIURETIC HORMONE SECRETION

Definition and Incidence

Syndrome of inappropriate antidiuretic hormone secretion (SIADH) is a condition of water intoxication. It is depicted by inappropriate production and secretion of antidiuretic hormone (ADH). This causes increased tubular water reabsorption with subsequent water retention, dilutional hyponatremia, a decreased serum osmolality, and increased urine osmolality (Flounders, 2003; Kaplow & Reid, in press; Shirland, 2001). The secretion of ADH occurs despite adequate circulating fluid volume and urinary sodium excretion and (Beckles et al., 2003; Gullatte et al., 2005).

SIADH occurs in 1% to 14% of patients with malignancy. Patients with small-cell lung cancer (SCLC) have an incidence of up to 10% (Hemphill & Ismach, 2001; Kaplow, 2005; Kaplow & Reid, in press).

Etiology and Pathophysiology

The causes of SIADH are (1) cancer, (2) neurologic disorders, (3) benign lung disease, and (4) drugs (Baylis, 2003; Gullatte et al., 2005). SCLC is the most common cancer associated with the development of SIADH. Other associated malignancies are non–small-cell lung cancer (NSCLC); carcinoid tumors; squamous cell carcinoma of the head and neck; breast, brain, prostate, esophagus, pancreas, colon, thymus, uterus, bladder, ovarian, or duodenal tumors; neuroblastoma; mesothelioma; Hodgkin's and non-Hodgkin's lymphomas; and leukemia. It can also be caused by metastasis to the central nervous system (CNS) (Flounders, 2003; Gullatte et al., 2005; Kaplow & Reid, in press).

Some chemotherapeutic agents place patients at risk to develop SIADH. These include vincristine, vinblastine, cyclophosphamide, ifosfamide, cisplatin, and melphalan. Each of these agents can cause hyponatremia and elevated ADH levels (Gucalp & Dutcher, 2001; Gullatte et al., 2005; Kaplow & Reid, in press; Tan, 2002).

Non–cancer-related etiologic factors for SIADH include medications (e.g., opioids, antidepressants, NSAIDs, thiazide diuretics, barbiturates, and anesthetic agents), CNS disorders (e.g., brain abscess or herniation, hemorrhage, head trauma), and pulmonary disorders (e.g., infection, pneumonia, lung abscess, tuberculosis). Pain, stress, and nicotine have also been identified as causative factors (Flounders, 2003; Kaplow & Reid, in press; Tan, 2002).

Pathophysiology

SIADH results from a tumor secreting a protein similar to ADH. This protein is not responsive to normal body feedback mechanisms. SIADH may also be caused by chemotherapy provoking the posterior pituitary to secrete ADH. Both of these mechanisms cause inappropriate ADH secretion. When ADH is secreted, there is stimulation of water absorption in the distal tubules and collecting ducts. This results in decreased urinary excretion, concentration of urine, dilution of plasma, decreased serum osmolality, and dilutional serum hyponatremia (Kaplow & Reid, in press).

Assessment and Measurement

The symptoms depend on the degree and speed at which hyponatremia develops (Baylis, 2003). The hallmark signs of SIADH are hyponatremia, serum hypo-osmolality, and inappropriately concentrated urine for serum osmolality (Gullatte et al., 2005).

History and Physical Examination

Patients present with a variety of symptoms that may be due to dilutional hyponatremia, hypocalcemia, or hypokalemia. SIADH affects the CNS, GI, renal, musculoskeletal, cardiac, and respiratory systems. CNS symptoms include mental status changes, headache, ataxia hallucinations, agitation, fatigue, malaise, tremors, hyporeflexia, myoclonus, and unexplained seizures (Gullatte et al., 2005). GI symptoms may include nausea, vomiting, diarrhea, anorexia, and abdominal cramping. If the renal system is affected, the patient may manifest thirst, weight gain without edema, and oliguria. Musculoskeletal symptoms are muscle cramps and weakness. Patients may have hypotension or normal blood pressure and heart rate as well as fluid retention. Possible respiratory symptoms include inability to maintain a patent airway and inability to mobilize secretions (Baylis, 2003; Beckles et al., 2003; Flounders, 2003; Gullatte et al., 2005; Kaplow & Reid, in press; Tan, 2002). If a serum sodium level is less than 120 mmol/L and develops acutely, the patient is at risk for the development of cerebral edema (Gullatte et al., 2005; Langfeldt & Cooley, 2003).

Diagnostics

Diagnosis of SIADH is based on laboratory data and through the exclusion of other contributing factors of hyponatremia. The clinician should have a high index of suspicion based on the presence of risk factors in a hyponatremic patient (Gullatte et al., 2005; Janicic & Verbalis, 2003). Laboratory data consistent with a diagnosis of SIADH are a urinary sodium level of greater than 40 mEq/L, urinary osmolality greater than 1000 mOsm/kg, serum hypo-osmolality, and hyponatremia (Kaplow & Reid, in press).

Intervention and Treatment

Continuous monitoring of the patient is important to identify changes in clinical status. Assessment of fluid and electrolyte status and for side effects of treatment is equally essential. Collaboration among the physician, pharmacist, and nurse to manage anxiety and depression will help optimize patient outcomes, as many medications will need to be avoided (Flounders, 2003; Kaplow & Reid, in press).

Treatment of the underlying cause of SIADH may be implemented. Treatment modalities include chemotherapy, RT, and/or corticosteroids (Kaplow & Reid, in press). The foundation of management is fluid restriction to less than 800 to 1000 ml/day until serum sodium improves (Kaplow & Reid, in press; Flounders, 2003). Demeclocycline administration is recommended if fluid restriction alone is not effective (Gullatte et al., 2005; Kaplow & Reid, in press; Flounders, 2003; Tan, 2002).

Patients with acute hyponatremia and severe neurologic symptoms should receive 3% saline at a rate of 300 to 500 ml over 4 to 6 hours until a serum sodium of 125 mg/dl is attained (Crook, 2002). Serum sodium should be corrected at a rate of 0.5 to 2 mEq/h to prevent complications of therapy (Flounders, 2003; Gucalp & Dutcher, 2001; Gullatte et al., 2005; Kaplow & Reid, in press; Kozniewska, Podlecka, & Rafalowska, 2003). Loop diuretics are recommended to decrease urine concentration and promote urinary free water excretion (Gucalp & Dutcher, 2001; Gullatte et al., 2005).

The key to managing SIADH is early detection to prevent complications. Monitoring fluid status may require urine specific gravity, daily weights, serum and urine electrolytes, and strict intake and output (I/O). Patients receiving hypertonic saline require ongoing assessment for overcorrection and/or fluid overload. Neurologic assessment is essential as rapid changes in mental status may signify worsening hyponatremia and rapid changes in sodium (Gullatte et al., 2005).

Evaluation and Follow-Up

SIADH resolves in less than 3 weeks when treatment of the underlying cause has been successful. Symptoms often recur if there is tumor progression (Beckles et al., 2003; Flounders, 2003; Kaplow & Reid, in press). While patients are being treated, serum chemistries may be monitored on a periodic basis (Tan, 2002).

Patient and Family Education

Patients and family members should be taught signs and symptoms to observe for, actions to take, and when to seek medical attention. While the patient is receiving treatment of SIADH, comfort measures such as mouth care and administration of small amounts of ice chips may be given to combat the discomfort of thirst. Family members should also be taught to observe for changes in mental status (Flounders, 2003; Gullatte et al., 2005).

SUPERIOR VENA CAVA SYNDROME

Definition and Incidence

Superior vena cava syndrome (SVCS) results from obstruction of the superior vena cava (SVC). The blockage may be above or below the azygous vein from an intravascular clot, tumor in the right main upper lobe bronchus, or significant mediastinal lymphadenopathy. The obstruction impairs blood flow to the right atrium and venous drainage above the upper thorax. This results in a decreased venous return (Gullatte et al., 2005; Hemann, 2001; Kaplow & Reid, in press; Rowell & Gleeson, 2005; Wudel & Nesbitt, 2001).

An incidence of 2.4% to 21.1% of SVCS in lung cancer patients has been reported (Rowell & Gleeson, 2005).

Etiology and Pathophysiology

Most cases of SVCS are due to malignancy. Of these, 80% are due to NSCLC and non-Hodgkin's lymphoma (Beckles et al., 2003; Kaplow & Reid, in press; Thirlwell & Brock, 2003). In patients with lung cancer, SVCS is usually due to direct extension or lymph node metastasis (Beckles et al., 2003; Kvale, Simoff, & Prakash, 2003). Some cases are due to breast or testicular cancer metastasis. T-cell leukemia causes mediastinal adenopathy and enlargement of the thymus, which can compress the SVC. Rare cases of SVCS are attributed to Kaposi's sarcoma, esophageal cancer, thymoma, mesothelioma, and Hodgkin's disease (Kaplow & Reid, in press).

Nonmalignant causes of SVCS include tuberculosis, indwelling central venous catheters or pacemaker wires, Silastic or dialysis catheters, aneurysm of the aortic arch, or constrictive pericarditis (Gullatte et al., 2005; Kaplow & Reid, in press).

Because of the location of the SVC (it is surrounded by structures that do not compress), the SVC's thin walls, and the low presssure of blood flow in the SVC, when regional lymph nodes or the aorta enlarge, the SVC constricts effortlessly, and thus blood flow becomes sluggish and occlusion frequently occurs (Gullatte et al., 2005).

Assessment and Measurement

The signs and symptoms of SVCS are related to severity and location of the obstruction. It is usually not until the obstruction is complete that clinical manifestations become obvious. This makes the diagnosis of SVCS more challenging.

History and Physical Examination

Symptoms tend to be more severe when the obstruction is below the azygous vein (Rowell & Gleeson, 2005). The respiratory, cardiac, and CNS systems are affected. CNS manifestations include mental status changes, headache, dizziness (especially when leaning forward), blurred vision, and syncope. Respiratory symptoms are shortness of breath, dyspnea, hoarseness, cyanosis, cough, dysphagia, and stridor. Cardiac symptoms may include edema of the face, arm, and upper chest; dilated veins in the upper torso, shoulders, and arms; jugular venous distention; tachycardia; chest pain; and hypotension. Patients may present with erythema of the eyelids, tightness of the neck (Stokes sign), or periorbital edema (Beckles et al., 2003; Gucalp & Dutcher, 2001; Gullatte et al., 2005; Kaplow & Reid, in press).

Diagnostics

Radiology Findings

Both computed tomography (CT) and magnetic resonance imaging (MRI) help to determine the extent of the underlying tumor. A contrast-enhanced spiral CT scan can identify the obstruction site and presence of a thrombus. A venogram may be used to determine if the obstruction is due to stenosis or obstruction and the extent of a thrombus (Kaplow & Reid, in press; Rowell & Gleeson, 2005).

Chest CT can help locate mediastinal lymph nodes (Gucalp & Dutcher, 2001). A Doppler ultrasound can detect SVC obstruction if the patient cannot tolerate CT (Benenstein, Nayar, Rosen et al., 2003; Gullatte et al., 2005; Kaplow & Reid, in press).

Intervention and Treatment

Management of SVCS is designed for symptom management and treatment of the underlying cause. If the patient has adequate collateral circulation and symptoms are minimal, treatment may not be required (Hemann, 2001; Wudel & Nesbitt, 2001).

Patients with SVCS should be maintained with the head of the bed elevated. Oxygen therapy may be needed for dyspnea (Thirlwell & Brock, 2003). The patient should be protected from fluid overload. Upper extremity venous catheters should be avoided (Gullatte et al., 2005).

Routinely, management consists of steroids and either chemotherapy or RT. Steroids are usually given to patients receiving RT due to potential radiation-induced edema. If used, high-dose steroids should be given for a limited time period (Kaplow & Reid, in press; Rowell & Gleeson, 2005).

Radiation Therapy

If the patient develops respiratory distress, immediate RT is indicated. Almost 50% of patients report relief with RT. Positioning patients for RT may be problematic because many will have worsening dyspnea in the supine position (Gullatte et al., 2005).

Chemotherapy

Chemotherapy is indicated for chemosensitive tumors. Patients report symptom relief in 7 to 10 days, and many report complete resolution of symptoms within 2 weeks (Gucalp & Dutcher, 2001; Gullatte et al., 2005; Kaplow & Reid, in press; Thirlwell & Brock, 2003).

Diuretic Therapy

Diuretics may be used in patients with SVCS with airway edema (Kaplow & Reid, in press; Rowell & Gleeson, 2005). Use of diuretics may also decrease right-sided preload, which will decrease pressure on the SVC. Diuretics should be avoided in patients who have a pericardial effusion or cardiac tamponade. Furosemide is used most often (Gullatte et al., 2005).

Endovascular Techniques

Endovascular techniques, such as thrombolysis, angioplasty, or stenting, can be done in conjunction with antineoplastic therapies (Kaplow & Reid, in press). The former should be initiated if the cause of the obstruction is a thrombus. Best results with thrombolytics are seen in patients who are treated within 2 days (Gullatte et al., 2005). Anticoagulation is used in conjunction with thrombolysis (Kaplow & Reid, in press). SVCS related to central catheters warrants catheter removal and anticoagulant therapy (Gullatte et al., 2005; Thirlwell & Brock, 2003). Placement of expandable metallic stents into the SVC has been done to reopen the SVC. This has resulted in return of normal blood flow and resolution of symptoms in most patients (Thirlwell & Brock, 2003). Balloon angioplasty may be used to enlarge a vessel lumen for stent placement (Kvale et al., 2003).

Ongoing monitoring and maintenance of a patent airway are vital for a patient with SVCS. Although rare, it is possible for the patient to develop airway compromise or tracheal obstruction (Gullatte et al., 2005; Kaplow & Reid, in press). Airway management strategies are indicated. Some temporary relief from dyspnea may occur with upright posture and oxygen (Gucalp & Dutcher, 2001; Gullatte et al., 2005; Thirlwell & Brock, 2003). Suction equipment should be readily available at the patient's bedside.

Corticosteroids

Glucocorticoids may decrease edema surrounding the tumor (Thirlwell & Brock, 2003). Dosage should be tapered as symptoms resolve (Gullatte et al., 2005).

Surgery

Surgery is mostly indicated for benign causes of SVCS (Thirlwell & Brock, 2003). It is performed to bypass and relieve the pressure associated with an obstructed SVC (Gullatte et al., 2005).

Patients classically present with anxiety from respiratory distress, poor prognosis, or body image changes. Administration of sedatives that do not act on the CNS and provision of a quiet environment, emotional support, and reassurance may help allay anxiety (Kaplow & Reid, in press).

Evaluation and Follow-Up

Patients are at risk for bleeding from thrombolytic therapy, anticoagulation, perforation, or hematoma from endovascular procedures. Interventions that are indicated for this include monitoring complete blood cell count and coagulation profiles and maintaining bleeding precautions. If possible, avoid use of a blood pressure cuff on the arm (Kaplow & Reid, in press).

Patients are also at risk for infection from antineoplastic therapy, steroids, or endovascular procedures. They should have their white blood cell count monitored and be considered for prophylactic antibiotics. There is also a potential for dehydration, electrolyte imbalance, and hypotension from diuretic therapy. Monitoring fluid and electrolyte balance, vital signs, and strict I/O are essential (Kaplow & Reid, in press).

The 30-month mortality rate of SVCS is 90%. Relief of symptoms is likely within 1 month of the onset of RT (Gullatte et al., 2005).

An 11% recurrence rate has been reported with stent insertion. A low incidence of complications is reported with stents, especially when thrombolytics are used (Kaplow & Reid, in press; Rowell & Gleeson, 2005).

Patient and Family Education

Patient and family education is needed to increase knowledge of subtle signs and symptoms of SVCS. The patient and family should be taught to observe for complications related to stent placement; these include bleeding from vascular injury and thrombosis within the stent (Kvale et al., 2003). Patients and family members should be taught what to report to their physician so that early treatment can be initiated, if indicated.

SPINAL CORD COMPRESSION

Definition and Incidence

Spinal cord compression (SCC) is compression of the thecal sac by a tumor. The compression may be located in the spinal cord or at the level of the cauda equina (Flounders, 2003; Kaplow & Reid, in press; Quinn & DeAngelis, 2000).

Data suggest that 0.2% to 30% of patients with cancer can develop SCC (Crossno, 2004; Kvale et al., 2003; Loblaw, Laperrier, & Mackillop, 2003; Pease, Harris, & Finlay, 2004; Purdue, 2004, Osowski, 2002). There is an incidence of 10%, 70%, and 20% in the cervical, thoracic, and lumbosacral spine, respectively (Crossno, 2004; Kaplow & Reid, in press).

Etiology and Pathophysiology

SCC often results from metastatic tumors. The most frequently reported tumors are lung, breast, and prostate. Others include lymphoma, melanoma, GI cancers, seminoma, neuroblastoma, sarcoma, myeloma, and renal cell carcinoma. Patients with primary cancers of the spinal cord are also at risk (Founders & Ott, 2003; Gucalp & Dutcher, 2001; Gullatte et al., 2005; Kaplow & Reid, in press; Tan, 2002).

SCC is classified as either intramedullary (within the spinal cord), intradural (within the dura mater), extramedullary (outside the spinal cord), or extradural (outside the dura mater) (Kaplow & Reid, in press). The latter is the most common type (Founders & Ott, 2003; Tan, 2002). Tumors usually arise from the anterior vertebral body and extend into the epidural space, compressing the spinal cord and vasculature and leading to ischemic damage to motor and sensory pathways and associated gray matter (Gullatte et al., 2005). The tumor applies pressure on the spinal cord, affecting its blood supply. This can lead to infarction or vertebral collapse. When a tumor spreads to the spinal cord, it breaks up the vertebral body, causing it to collapse. The spinal cord compresses as tumor or particles of bone are pushed into the epidural space (Founders & Ott, 2003; Kaplow & Reid, in press).

Most tumors spread to the spinal cord as an embolic process. CNS cancer can also spread to the cerebrospinal fluid. This results in spread to the subarachnoid space, brain, and spinal cord (Founders & Ott, 2003). As the cancer spreads, edema of the tissues and nerves, ischemia, neural distortion, and tissue death result (Kaplow & Reid, in press; Tan, 2002).

History and Physical Examination

Presentation of SCC varies, depending on location and extent of the compression, cause, blood supply involvement, and rapidity of development. Effects can be sensory, motor, and/or autonomic (Founders & Ott, 2003; Gullatte et al., 2005; Kaplow & Reid, in press).

Motor Symptoms

Patients most frequently report back or neck pain (Crossno, 2004; Founders & Ott, 2003; Kaplow & Reid, in press). Pain may be localized at the site of the tumor and is constant, dull, or aching. Pain may also be radicular or medullary, which may intensify over time and when lying supine (Founders & Ott, 2003; Gullatte et al., 2005). The pain may develop slowly over months before other neurologic symptoms occur or quickly, over hours, before complete, irreversible damage occurs to the spinal cord (Crossno, 2004). Patients may also report pain on coughing or sneezing, a sudden change in pain, or pain that waxes and wanes. Patients may further report unilateral or bilateral radiating leg pain (Kaplow & Reid, in press; Spinal Cord Compression, 2005).

Motor symptoms may also include easy fatigue, gait disturbance, lower extremity weakness, ataxia, loss of coordination, hypotonicity, and hyporeflexia (Founders & Ott, 2003; Kaplow & Reid, in press; Kvale et al., 2003). Weakness usually occurs over some time following pain and begins in the feet and moves proximally (Crossno, 2004; Spinal Cord Compression, 2005). Patients with compression of the cervical spine will have quadriplegia. Patients with compression of the thoracic spine have paraplegia.

Sensory Symptoms

Sensory changes usually begin distally and rise to the level of the compression. When a patient has compression of the cauda equina, there is bilateral sensory loss. Sensory symptoms include paresthesias, severe pain, sensory loss to level of compression, decreased light touch, joint, position sense, and proprioception, numbness, loss of thermal sense, loss of deep pressure sensation, loss of vibration sensation, decrease in strength, and Lhermitte's sign. Sensory changes progress if interventions are not initiated. Weakness and sensory abnormalities are late findings and are frequently irreversible (Founders & Ott, 2003; Gullatte et al., 2005, Kaplow & Reid, in press; Kvale et al., 2003; Tan, 2002).

Autonomic Symptoms

Patients usually experience sensory and motor symptoms prior to autonomic dysfunction. Autonomic symptoms include impotence, changes in bowel and bladder function, hesitancy, urinary retention or incontinence, lack of urge to defecate or bear down, constipation, decreased anal tone, and bladder distention (Founders & Ott, 2003; Gullatte et al., 2005, Kaplow & Reid, in press; Kvale et al., 2003; Tan, 2002).

The most vital data to assist in the diagnosis of SCC are the patient history and clinical evaluation (Arch, Sass, & Abul-Khoudou, 2001). A complete history, physical, and neurologic assessment, as well as evaluation of pain, sensory, motor, and autonomic function are essential. It is vital that reported back or neck pain be meticulously evaluated because the strongest predictor of a patient with SCC is neurologic status upon presentation. A patient's ability to ambulate upon diagnosis will significantly predict ability to ambulate following treatment (Founders & Ott, 2003; Kaplow & Reid, in press).

Patient history should include determination of presence and characteristics of symptoms. Complete examination of the neurologic and musculoskeletal systems is imperative in any patient who is at risk for development of SCC and who is symptomatic.

The patient performs a straight leg raise. If radicular pain is present, it increases with this movement. Sharp pain on dorsiflexion suggests nerve root compression (Founders & Ott, 2003; Kaplow & Reid, in press).

Sensory evaluation should be conducted (Founders & Ott, 2003). The area of sensory loss can determine the level of the compression. Positive sensation is usually one or two levels below the site of the compression (DeMichele & Glick, 2001; Founders & Ott, 2003). The patient will usually report tenderness to percussion at the site of the compressed vertebrae (Crossno, 2004; Kaplow & Reid, in press).

Patients should be evaluated for gait disturbances, muscle strength, involuntary movements, and coordination. A patient's tendon reflexes are increased below the compression, absent at the level of the compression, and normal above the level of the compression (Founders & Ott, 2003; Kaplow & Reid, in press).

Autonomic dysfunction requires further evaluation, as it is a poor prognostic indicator (Gullatte et al., 2005; Kaplow & Reid, in press).

Respiratory distress may occur if the patient has a cervical compression. Evaluation for declining oxygenation and ventilation is pivotal, especially in patients with tumor involvement at the C4 level or above (Kaplow & Reid, in press).

Diagnostics

Radiology Findings

A spinal radiograph is the initial diagnostic study for SCC. It may be normal or may reveal fracture, damage or erosion to vertebrae, and any lesion in up to 85% of the vertebrae (Founders & Ott, 2003; Gullatte et al., 2005; Kaplow & Reid, in press; Spinal Cord Compression, 2005; Spinal Cord Trauma, 2005). It may also detect presence of epidural metastasis (Crossno, 2004). It will not detect early SCC, as 50% of bone must be destroyed for it to be viewed (Founders & Ott, 2003; Kaplow & Reid, in press).

MRI of the spine is used to establish the precise location of the compression, evaluate extent of spinal involvement, and determine the presence of vertebral tumors (Crossno, 2004; Gullatte et al., 2005). It is also useful to visualize soft tissue, the spinal cord, and the cauda equina. The entire spine should be visualized, since metastasis can occur in multiple sites. Either MRI or CT scan may identify the location and extent of spinal cord trauma. It can also be used to assess for bone destruction. A myelogram may be done as well (Founders & Ott, 2003; Kaplow & Reid, in press; Spinal Cord Trauma, 2005).

CT with contrast will detect paraspinal masses and early lesions. It may verify SCC and fully determine the level and extent of the lesion. Positron emission tomography can confirm data received from MRI or CT. Bone scan may show extent of bone involvement and spinal level 20% of the time and detect abnormalities not detected on radiograph (Founders & Ott, 2003; Gullatte et al., 2005; Kaplow & Reid, in press; Levack, Graham, Collie et al., 2002).

Intervention and Treatment

Treatment options include surgery, steroids, RT, and chemotherapy. Goals of therapy are to provide pain relief, restore neurologic function, possibly treat the underlying malignancy, and prevent permanent disability. Management depends on the type of underlying tumor, location, and characteristics (Founders & Ott, 2003; Gullatte et al., 2005; Kaplow & Reid, in press; Osowski, 2002).

Radiation Therapy

RT is the definitive treatment for SCC and is administered in fractionated doses over a 2- to 4-week period (Gullatte et al., 2005; Tan, 2002). The area that is radiated usually extends one or two vertebrae above and below the compression (Founders & Ott, 2003). RT is used to minimize the size of the tumor, to decompress the spinal cord, and to provide pain relief. Around 85% of patients report pain relief with RT (Kaplow & Reid, in press).

Surgery

Surgery should be the first line of therapy in patients with spinal instability, bony compression, or paraplegia on initial presentation. It may be used to alleviate pain and stabilize the spine. Surgery is also indicated for (1) rapidly declining neurologic function, (2) compression occurring in a previously radiated field, (3) progressive neurologic deficits during radiation, (4) when the underlying tumor will not respond to RT, or (5) if the area has already been treated with RT (Bartanusz & Porchet, 2003; Crossno, 2004; Founders & Ott, 2003; Gullatte et al., 2005; Kaplow & Reid, in press; Kvale et al., 2003; Maranzano et al., 2003).

Corticosteroids

Steroids are commonly used initially until treatment of the underlying cause can begin (Crossno, 2004; Founders & Ott, 2003). They are used to decrease edema, inflammation, and pain (Gullatte et al., 2005; Kaplow & Reid, in press). For patients who are not paretic and ambulatory, high-dose steroids and RT are recommended (Kaplow & Reid, in press; Kvale et al., 2003).

Chemotherapy

Patients with chemosensitive tumors may benefit from chemotherapy to treat the underlying malignancy. Chemotherapy may also be used in patients who are not candidates for RT or surgery. Hormonal therapy may help patients with breast or prostate cancer (Gucalp & Dutcher, 2001; Gullatte et al., 2005; Kaplow & Reid, in press).

Evaluation and Follow-Up

When patients with SCC are discharged from the hospital, determination should be made of the need for ambulatory care, visiting nurses, or hospice care (Flounders, 2003). Paralysis or numbness of part of the body is common in patients with SCC. Death is also a possibility if the diaphragm becomes paralyzed (Spinal Cord Trauma, 2005). If a patient has neurologic deterioration or recompresses after undergoing RT, additional RT can be considered. Patients may continue to require physical therapy. Monitoring should include assessment for side effects that can occur with high-dose steroids.

Patient and Family Education

The patient and family must be educated about signs of SCC to report so that treatment can begin when indicated (Loblaw et al., 2003). If the patient is at risk for the development of SCC, the patient and family should be taught to report any new or increase in back pain. The patient and family member should be taught when to call the physician. They should also be taught about side effects of treatment to monitor (Flounders, 2003; Kvale et al., 2003; Osowski, 2002).

Patients with SCC usually have a poor prognosis. The life expectancy may be 3 months or less, but a reasonable quality of life can be attained for that time (Tan, 2002).

HEMORRHAGE

Definition and Incidence

Hemorrhage refers to blood loss that is striking and sudden. The incidence of hemorrhage in the palliative care setting is difficult to quantify, since it depends on the cause. It has been found that 20% of patients with a recurrent cancer will sustain a catastrophic bleed. In the case of advanced head and neck cancer, hemorrhage can account for 11.6% of deaths. In one study, 5% of patients died of a carotid artery rupture (British Association of Head and Neck Oncology Nurses [BAHNON], 2005). In a study of patients with acute myeloid leukemia, 44% of patients in the final phase had episodes of bleeding noted (Stalfelt, Brodin, Pettersson et al., 2003).

Etiology and Pathophysiology

Patients at risk for the development of hemorrhage are those with head and neck cancer, hematologic malignancies, or any malignancy that is adjacent to a major artery, thrombocytopenia, or coagulopathies. Patients with bladder cancer, hepatocellular carcinoma, or cirrhosis are also at risk (Letier, Krige, Lemmer et al., 2000; Shah, Mumtaz, Jafri et al., 2005; Textor, Wilhelm, Strunk et al., 2000; Uemura, Matsusako, Numaguchi et al., 2005). Any patient who has undergone surgery for head and neck cancer in areas adjacent to the carotid artery is a potential candidate (Casey, 1988; Cohen & Rad, 2004; Freeman et al., 2004). Hemorrhage is a complication of a radical neck dissection (Rodriguez, Carmeci, Dalman et al., 2001). This is especially so if the patient has received RT to the area (Cohen & Rad, 2004). RT to the neck is the most common factor leading to carotid artery rupture (Cohen & Rad, 2004; Rodriguez et al., 2001). Patients may also develop carotid artery rupture related to direct tumor invasion leading to damage to the arterial wall (BAHNON, 2005).

With head and neck cancer, hemorrhage may occur either externally from the neck, internally from within the oropharynx, or directly into the airway or tracheostomy (Cohen & Rad, 2004; Lovel, 2000).

There are several pathophysiologic reasons for a patient to develop hemorrhage. These include vessel injury, platelet dysfunction, coagulopathies (e.g., disseminated intravascular coagulation), and changes in viscosity of blood. If a tumor invades a blood vessel, significant and sudden blood loss can occur. Bone marrow failure or tumor invasion into the bone marrow can cause thrombocytopenia. If the patient develops liver failure, bleeding problems may ensue. Several medications can also lead to hemorrhage as a side effect (Heidrich & McKinnon, 2002).

Assessment and Measurement

Patients should be assessed for risk of bleeding based on past medical history. Factors to consider include type and location of malignancy. Patients with head and neck or GI malignancies are at the highest risk for hemorrhage. Patients who have received chemotherapy or RT are at risk due to myelosuppressive toxicities of these therapies. Surgical patients may also be at risk depending on the extent of the procedures. In addition, tumors themselves can disturb vasculature, placing the patient at risk for hemorrhage (Heidrich & McKinnon, 2002).

History and Physical Examination

A complete history may assist the clinician to identify patients at risk for hemorrhage. A patient history should include determination of whether the patient has had bleeding from any site in the past, degree of bleeding, and what interventions were used. The location of tumors, history of antineoplastic therapies and dates of these therapies, any hepatic dysfunction, and the patient's medication profile will all provide clues for the risk of hemorrhage (Heidrich & McKinnon, 2002).

Patients with minor bleeding from a wound, a flap site, a tracheostomy, or the mouth may hemorrhage. This is caused by a small rupture of the intima (BAHNON, 2005). Some patients manifest 'pulsations' from artery or tracheostomy or flap site, or report sternal or high epigastric pain several hours before rupture Some patients develop 'ballooning' of an artery prior to carotid artery rupture (BAHNON, 2005; Lovel, 2000).

Diagnostics

Laboratory tests may provide clues as to the etiology of hemorrhage. These include platelet count, coagulation profile, and liver function tests. Determination of any herbal or over-the-counter remedies that the patient has taken may help identify the cause as well (Heidrich & McKinnon, 2002).

Intervention and Treatment

There are only a small number of alternatives to treat a patient in the palliative care setting who is hemorrhaging (Puetz & Bourhasin, 2002). Much of the data reported are in the form of case studies rather than clinical trials.

The patient's coagulation profile and platelet count should be monitored. If the patient is receiving anticoagulants, these will need to be adjusted. Administration of blood products may be considered, but this can pose a challenge in the home or hospice setting. A case report describes the use of an agent, recombinant factor VIIa, that was effective in the palliative care setting (Puetz & Bourhasin, 2002).

Some patients with head and neck cancer have a particular event to achieve and wish to avoid imminent death. For these patients, additional head and neck surgery may be attempted to decrease the likelihood of a bleed. However, there are risks associated with the surgery that warrant consideration. Ligation of the involved artery to avoid carotid artery rupture carries a mortality risk of 32% to 77%, and 12% to 50% of survivors experienced permanent neurologic defects (BAHNON, 2005). Endovascular embolization of the carotid artery is considered an alternative method to avoid carotid artery rupture. This procedure has a lower (0% to 10%) mortality rate and fewer (10%) patients have neurologic damage (Luo, Chang, Teng et al., 2003). Superselective embolization with a substance, Ethibloc (Ethicon, Inc., Somerville, NJ), has been reported in the literature. This procedure was recommended for use as palliative treatment for select patients with advanced head and neck cancer (Sittel, Gossman, Jungehulsing et al., 2001).

Intraarterial embolization therapy is suggested as a treatment option for patients with urinary bladder hemorrhage from bladder cancer. Intraarterial chemoperfusion with mitoxantrone may also be effective, depending on the acuity of the bleeding (Textor, Wilhelm, Strunk et al., 2000).

Management of GI bleeding is dependent on the source. For the patient with cancer, it may require a multidisciplinary approach with a medical, surgical, and radiation oncologist (Imbesi & Kurtz, 2005). Strategies to control bleeding may include combined treatment of sclerotherapy and octreotide infusion over 48 hours for patients with acute variceal bleeding resulting from cirrhosis, or sclerotherapy alone in patients with acute variceal bleeding from hepatocellular carcinoma (Letier et al., 2000; Shah et al., 2005).

One case report describes relief of pain in a patient with hepatocellular carcinoma with hemorrhagic metastasis. This patient received percutaneous sacroplasty with combined injections of bone cement and n-butyl cyanoacrylate (Uemura et al., 2005).

In the event of hemorrhage, it is essential that a clinician remain with the patient, avoid panicking, and call for help. Towels should be applied to the bleeding site for absorption, if possible. If the patient has a tracheostomy, inflate the cuff to avoid choking. Gentle suctioning to the mouth and tracheostomy site should be applied as necessary to avoid sensation of choking, since this may add greatly to distress (BAHNON, 2005).

Patients should be spoken to gently and calmly, and attempts should be made, if possible, to keep the patient in one place. It is important to be aware of family presence and needs. It is ideal to determine in advance whether the family wishes to stay with the patient and important to be respectful of their wishes. If the family elects to stay with the patient, it is vital to ascertain that support is given (BAHNON, 2005).

The patient experiencing hemorrhage should be sedated. Administration of intravenous midazolam has the most rapid onset. If the patient does not have intravenous access, subcutaneous or intramuscular administration is possible. The dose may then be titrated until the patient is fully sedated (BAHNON, 2005).

Evaluation and Follow-Up

Witnessing a hemorrhage can be very frightening for the family. Families should be referred to a counselor for support following such an episode. In addition, steps to prevent hemorrhage or minimize blood loss should be undertaken (Heidrich & McKinnon, 2002).

Patient and Family Education

Although the risk for major hemorrhage is very rare, the fear is very realistic and present for the patient and family. If the patient is at risk for major hemorrhage, the patient and family must be prepared for this possibility (Feber, 2000). Management of the bleeding and treatment will depend on decisions made between the patient and family. If the patient's life expectancy and quality of life warrants, management of hemorrhage consists of general resuscitative measures, such as volume replacement and specific measures to stop the bleeding. If the patient's goals are palliative, management may include measures to stop bleeding without full resuscitative measures. Comfort measures only may be most appropriate for end-stage patients (Pereira & Phan, 2004).

Medication should be available in event of the emergency. For patients at home, where intravenous access is not possible, families can be taught how to administer injectable midazolam. If family members do not feel able to do this, an alternative is rectal diazepam (BAHNON, 2005).

The family should be advised to have equipment such as dark towels, gloves, and buckets readily available. The patient should be encouraged to wear dark undergarments or pads. Use of green or blue toilet disinfectant is recommended to disguise blood loss (depending on the site of bleeding) if the patient or family is frightened (North Cumbria Palliative Care, 2005).

SEIZURES

Definition and Incidence

A seizure is a symptom of irritation to the CNS resulting in excessive and abnormal neuronal discharges. An acute seizure refers to 5 minutes or more of either continuous seizures or two or more seizures between which there is incomplete return to consciousness (Regional Palliative Care Program [RPCP], 2005).

Etiology and Pathophysiology

Patients at risk for the development of seizures are those with primary or metastatic cerebral tumors. Cancers that metastasize to the brain include breast, lung, melanoma, kidney, leukemia, and lymphoma. Leptomeningeal disease and AIDS have been implicated as well (Fox, 2001; RPCP, 2005; Vaicys & Fried, 2000). Patients with HIV/AIDS may develop seizures secondary to opportunistic infection (Papadakis & McPhee, 2005). Seizures reportedly occur in 25% to 30% of patients with cerebral cancer (RPCP, 2005).

Noncancer causes of seizures include metabolic alterations, infection, medications, drug withdrawal, intracranial hemorrhage, increased intracranial pressure, SIADH, encephalopathy, and hypoxia (Paice, 2001).

A seizure occurs when a large number of neurons discharge in an unusual manner. This results in paroxysmal behavioral changes. The two types of seizures described in the literature are generalized and focal. Generalized seizures involve large portions of the brain, whereas focal seizures involve specific areas of the brain (Paice, 2001).

History and Physical Examination

Patients with a history of seizures or untreated myoclonus are at risk to develop seizures (RPCP, 2005). A review of the medications the patient has received may provide valuable information. Patients should also be questioned regarding use of recreational drugs (Paice, 2001).

A complete history should be taken to determine what symptoms were present upon the start of seizure activity, the type of seizure activity, and presence of an aura before the seizure started (Paice, 2001).

Diagnostics

Laboratory tests should include assessment for hypoglycemia and electrolyte abnormalities. Renal and liver function tests should also be assessed (Papadakis & McPhee, 2005). If the patient is currently receiving anticonvulsants, obtaining serum levels may be indicated to determine if the medication is being absorbed (Paice, 2001).

Electroencephalography can be performed to help classify seizure activity and presence of a seizure disorder. MRI can be done if there are focal neurologic signs or symptoms, focal seizure, or focal electroencephalographic imbalance (Papadakis & McPhee, 2005). If the patient has a brain lesion, evaluation may be accomplished with either MRI or CT scanning (Paice, 2001).

Intervention and Treatment

Prophylactic measures are usually recommended in patients who have had a seizure. Phenytoin and phenobarbital are the most commonly used anticonvulsants. Valproic acid is the second most common medication used. Management of actual seizures includes administration of medications. A benzodiazepine or phenytoin may be used. If patients are unable to tolerate oral medications, phenobarbital may be administered subcutaneously. Although rare, if seizures persist, a continuous subcutaneous midazolam infusion may be used (RPCP, 2005).

While having a seizure, the patient should be protected from self-injury, turned on the side, and provided with oxygen if applicable. If hypoglycemia is the cause of the seizure, the patient should receive intravenous glucose (RPCP, 2005).

Evaluation and Follow-Up

If the patient develops medication side effects before reaching therapeutic levels of the agent, it is recommended that the dosage be decreased or an alternative agent be tried. If the patient continues to have seizures and is free of side effects but has a high serum concentration of the agent, a higher dose of medication should be administered (RPCP, 2005).

Patient and Family Education

If a patient is at risk for the development of seizures, the patient and family should be informed of this likelihood. They should be taught what to observe for and expect and interventions that can be implemented (RPCP, 2005). Like the sight of blood, seizures can be very frightening, but they can be managed at home by family members who can be taught to give the patient medication. Family members should also be taught that a seizure is brief and self-limited and that it is rarely the patient's cause of death. Family should be instructed to call the physician once the seizure activity has stopped (RPCP, 2005).

Family members should be taught to remove items that might cause harm to the patient during the seizure and the placement of pillows in strategic places to prevent trauma. They can also be shown ways to protect the patient's airway during the seizure and to refrain from giving the patient anything orally until full consciousness is restored after the seizure (Paice, 2001).

Patients may benefit from an environment low in stimulation while recovering from the seizure. They should be spoken to softly and with reassurance (Paice, 2001).

CONCLUSION

In the case of palliative emergencies, management includes making the patient comfortable, preventing suffering, thinking of the needs of family members observing the event, explaining what is happening and management strategies being taken, and communicating reassurance to the patient and the family. Emergent interventions are determined on an individual basis.

CASE STUDY

L.C. is a 53-year-old woman who presents with dull, aching back and neck pain present for the past 2 weeks. She attributes it to "sleeping funny." The pain has been constant but tolerable up until now. The patient's past medical history includes breast cancer for which she underwent a modified radical mastectomy and chemotherapy 3 years ago. Six weeks ago she learned that the cancer had recurred and that additional therapy was required. The patient is receiving additional doxorubicin and cyclophosphamide.

Physical examination by the clinician reveals fatigue and weakness. A detailed neurologic examination was negative for leg pain, gait disturbance, loss of coordination, paresthesias, changes in proprioception, loss of thermal sense, loss of deep pressure sensation, loss of strength, and autonomic symptoms. Reflexes are normal.

Results of serum chemistries and coagulation profile are within normal limits. Complete blood cell count is significant for mild pancytopenia; white blood cells = 3.1, hemoglobin/hematocrit = 10.2/31, platelets = 103.

Spinal radiograph shows damage to T5-6 vertebrae. MRI revealed compression and presence of a tumor at the level of the fourth thoracic vertebra.

In collaboration with the oncologist and radiation oncologist, 4000 cGy of RT in fractionated doses is delivered over 4 weeks with the result of good pain relief. She is also given a loading dose of dexamethasone with subsequent tapering. Given the metastatic nature of her cancer and the poor prognosis of spinal cord compression (SCC), the patient did not opt for surgery to relieve the compression and decided not to continue chemotherapy. She is satisfied with her pain relief and has requested hospice care. She is ambulatory upon discharge from the hospital.

This case illustrates the clinician detecting a sign of SCC. The patient was given a comprehensive neurologic examination because of her medical history. It is essential to evaluate back and neck pain in any patient at risk for SCC, even if pain is the only presenting symptom. The prompt assessment and intervention by the NP allowed the patient to obtain pain relief and sustain no additional disabilities from the compression. She was discharged to hospice care, as requested.

REFERENCES

Arch, D., Sass, P., & Abul-Khoudou, H. (2001). Recognizing spinal cord emergencies. *Am Fam Physician,* *64(4)*, 631-638.

Bartanusz, V. & Porchet, F. (2003). Current strategies in the management of spinal metastatic disease. *Swiss Surg, 9(2)*, 55-62.

Baylis, P.H. (2003). The syndrome of inappropriate antidiuretic hormone secretion. *Int J Biochem Cell Biol, 35(11)*, 1495-1499.

Beckles, M.A., Spiro, S.G., Colice, G.L., et al. (2003). Initial evaluation of the patient with lung cancer: Symptoms, signs, laboratory tests, and paraneoplastic syndromes. *Chest, 123(1)*, 97S-104S.

Benenstein, R., Nayar, A.C., Rosen, R., et al. (2003). Doppler diagnosis of acute occlusion of the superior vena cava. *Echocardiography, 20(1)*, 97-98.

British Association of Head and Neck Oncology Nurses [BAHNON]. (2005). The management of carotid artery rupture related to the terminal care of the head and neck cancer patient. Retrieved July 1, 2005, from www.bahnon.org.uk/Professional%20Guidelines/CAR%20guidelines%20revised%20March%2005.doc.

Carroll, M.F. & Schade, D.S. (2003). A practical approach to hypercalcemia. *Am Fam Physician, 67(9)*, 1959-1966.

Cohen, J. & Rad, I. (2004). Contemporary management of carotid blowout. *Curr Opin Otolaryngol Head Neck Surg, 12*, 110-115.

Crook, N. (2002). Vasopressin V receptor antagonists. *J Clin Pathol, 53*, 883.

Crossno, R.J. (2004). Dying in the emergency department: What emergency physicians should know about palliative medicine. *Top Emerg Med, 26(1)*, 19-28.

DeMichele, A. & Glick, J. (2001). Cancer-related emergencies. In R. Lenhard, R. Osteen, & T. Gansler (Eds.). *Clinical oncology* (pp. 733-764). Atlanta: American Cancer Society.

Feber, T. (2000). *Head and neck oncology nursing* (pp. 245-252). London: Whurr Publishers Ltd.

Flounders, J.A. (2003a). Syndrome of inappropriate antidiuretic hormone. *Oncol Nurs Forum, 30(3)*, E63-E68.

Flounders, J.A. (2003b). Oncology emergencies modules: Spinal cord compression. *Oncol Nurs Forum, 30(1)*, E17-E21.

Fowell, A. & Stuart, N.S. (2005). Emergencies in palliative medicine. *Palliat Care, 32(4)*, 17-23.

Fox, G.N. (2001). Hyponatremic seizures after ultrasonic imaging. *J Am Board Fam Pract, 14(3)*, 229.

Gucalp, R. & Dutcher, J. (2001). Oncologic emergencies. In E. Braunwald, A.S. Fauci, & D.L. Kasper (Eds.). *Harrison's principles of internal medicine* (15th ed., pp. 642-650). New York: McGraw-Hill.

Gullatte, M.M., Kaplow, R., & Heidrich, D. (2005). Oncology. In K.K. Kuebler, M.P. Davis, & C.D. Moore (Eds.). *Palliative practices: An interdisciplinary approach* (pp. 197-245). St. Louis: Elsevier.

Heidrich, D.E. & McKinnon, S. (2002). Palliative care emergencies. In K.K. Kuebler, P.H. Berry, & D.E. Heidrich (Eds.). *End-of-life care. Clinical practice guidelines* (pp. 383-408). Philadelphia: Saunders.

Hemann, R. (2001). Superior vena cava syndrome. *Clin Excell Nurse Pract, 5(2)*, 85-87.

Hemphill, R.R. & Ismach, R.B. (2001). Oncologic emergencies: Diagnosis, triage, and management. *Emerg Med Rep, 22(15)*, 1-11.

Imbesi, J.J. & Kurtz, R.C. (2005). A multidisciplinary approach to gastrointestinal bleeding in cancer patients. *J Support Oncol, 3(2)*, 111-112.

Inzucchi, S.E. (2004). Understanding hypercalcemia. Its metabolic basis, signs, and symptoms. *Postgrad Med, 115(4)*, 69-76.

Janicic, N. & Verbalis, J.G. (2003). Evaluation and management of hypo-osmolality in hospitalized patients. *Endocrinol Metab Clin North Am, 32(2)*, 459-481.

Kaplow, R. (in press). Oncologic emergencies. In American Association of Critical Care Nurses (Ed.), *AACN advanced acute and critical care nursing*. Philadelphia: Saunders.

Kaplow, R. & Reid, M. (in press). Oncologic emergencies. In H.M. Schell & K.A. Puntillo (Eds.), *Critical care nursing secrets*. Philadelphia: Hanley & Belfus.

Kozniewska, E., Podlecka, A., & Rafalowska, J. (2003). Hyponatremic encephalopathy: Some experimental and clinical findings. *Folia Neuropathol, 41(1)*, 41-45.

Kvale, P.A., Simoff, M., & Prakash, V.B. (2003). Palliative care. *Chest, 123(1)*, *Suppl*, 284S-311S.

Langfeldt, L.A. & Cooley, M.E. (2003). Syndrome of inappropriate antidiuretic hormone secretion in malignancy: Review and implications for nursing management. *Clin J Oncol Nurs, 7(4)*, 425-430.

Leiomyosarcoma. (2005). Retrieved July 2, 2005, from www.leiomyosarcoma.info.

Letier, M.H., Krige, J.E., Lemmer, E.R., et al. (2000). Injection sclerotherapy for variceal bleeding in patients with irresectable hepatocellular carcinoma. *Hepato-Gastroenterol, 47(36)*, 1680-1684.

Levack, P., Graham, J., Collie, D., et al.; Scottish Cord Compression Study Group. (2002). Don't wait for a sensory level—Listen to the symptoms: A prospective audit of the delays in the diagnosis of malignant cord compression. *Clin Oncol, 14(6)*, 472-480.

Loblaw, D.A., Laperriere, N.J., & Mackillop, W.J. (2003). A population-based study of malignant spinal cord compression in Ontario. *Clin Oncol, 13(4)*, 211-217.

Lovel, T. (2000). Palliative care and head and neck cancer [Editorial]. *Br J Oral Maxillofac Surg, 38*, 253-254.

Luo, C.B., Chang, F.C., Teng, M.M., et al. (2003). Endovascular treatment of the carotid artery rupture with massive haemorrhage. *J Chin Med Assoc, 66*, 140-147.

National Cancer Institute (NCI). (2005). *Hypercalcemia*. Retrieved April 19, 2005, from http://cancernet. nci.nih.gov/cancertopics/pdq/supportivecare/hypercalcemia/healthprofessional

National Coalition for Cancer Survivorship (NCCS). (2005). *Hypercalcemia*. Retrieved April 19, 2005, from http://cancer.nccs.drtango.com/411.asp?article=bone_hypercalcemia&type=tnpv&style=default.css&nav Type=1&lid=&otherParams=.

North Cumbria Palliative Care. (2005). *Hemorrhage*. Retrieved June 28, 2005, from www.northcumbriahealth.nhs.uk/palliativecareat.

Osowski, M. (2002). Spinal cord compression. An obstructive oncologic emergency. *Top Adv Pract Nurs, 2(4)*.

Paice, J.A. (2001). Neurological disorders. In B.R. Ferrell & N. Coyle. *Textbook of palliative nursing* (pp. 262-268). New York: Oxford University Press.

Papadakis, M.A. & McPhee, S.J. (2005). *Current consult: Medicine* (pp. 54, 368). New York: McGraw Hill.

Pease, N.J., Harris, R.J., & Finlay, I.G. (2004). Development and audit of a care pathway for the management of patients with suspected malignant spinal cord compression. *Physiotherapy, 90(1)*, 27-34.

Pereira, J. & Phan, T. (2004). Management of bleeding in patients with advanced cancer. *Oncologist, 9*, 561-570.

Puetz, J.J. & Bourhasin, J.D. (2002). Use of recombinant factor VIIa to control bleeding in an adolescent male with severe hemophilia A, HIV thrombocytopenia, hepatitis C, and end-stage liver disease. *Am J Hospice Palliat Care, 19(4)*, 277-282.

Purdue, C. (2004). Clinical diagnosis and treatment of malignant spinal cord compression. *Nurs Times, 100(38)*, 38-41.

Quinn, J. & DeAngelis, L. (2000). Neurologic emergencies in the cancer patient. *Semin Oncol, 27*, 311-321.

Regional Palliative Care Program. (2005). Retrieved July 1, 2005, from www.palliative.org/clinicalinfo.

Rodriguez, F., Carmeci, C., Dalman, R.L., et al. (2001) Spontaneous late carotid-cutaneous fistula following radical neck dissection—A case report. *Vasc Surg, 35(5)*.

Ross, J.R., Saunders, Y., Edmonds, P.M., et al. (2004). A systematic review of the role of bisphosphonates in metastatic disease. *Health Technol Assess, 8(4)*, 1-176.

Rowell, N.P. & Gleeson, F.V. (2005). Steroids, radiotherapy, chemotherapy, and stents for superior vena caval obstruction in carcinoma of the bronchus. *Cochrane Database of Systematic Reviews, 1*.

Shah, H.A., Mumtaz, K., Jafri, W., et al. (2005). Sclerotherapy plus octreotide versus sclerotherapy alone in the management of oesophageal variceal hemorrhage. *J Ayub Med Coll Abbottabad, 17(1)*, 10-14.

Shirland, L. (2001). SIADH: A case review. *Neonatal Network J Neonatal Nurs, 20(1)*, 25-32.

Shuey, K.M. & Brant, J.M. (2004). Hypercalcemia of malignancy: Part II. *Clin J Oncol Nurs, 8(3)*, 321-323.

Sittel, C., Gossman, A., Jungehulsing, M., et al. (2001). Superselective embolization as palliative treatment of recurrent hemorrhage in advanced carcinoma of the head and neck. *Ann Otol Rhinol Laryngol, 110(12)*, 1126-1128.

Solimando, D.A. (2001). Overview of hypercalcemia of malignancy. *Am J Health-Syst Pharm, 58*, S4-S7.

Spinal Cord Compression. (2005). *A palliative care emergency*. Retrieved April 19, 2005, from www.palliative.org/pc/clinicalinfo/nursesnotes/spinalcordcompression.html.

Spinal Cord Trauma. (2005). Retrieved April 19, 2005, from www.nlm.nih.gov/medlineplus/spinalcordinjuries.html.

Stalfelt, A.M., Brodin, H., Pettersson, S., et al. (2003). The final phase in acute myeloid leukaemia (AML). A study on bleeding, infection and pain. *Leukotriene Res, 27(6)*, 481-488.

Tan, S. (2002). Recognition and treatment of oncologic emergencies. *J Infus Nurs, 25(3)*, 182-188.

Textor, H.J., Wilhelm, K., Strunk, H., et al. (2000). Locoregional chemoperfusion with mitoxantrone for palliative therapy in bleeding bladder cancer compared with embolization [in German]. *RoFo, 172(5)*, 462-466.

Thirlwell, C. & Brock, C.S. (2003). Emergencies in oncology. *Clin Med, 3(4)*, 306-310.

Uemura, A., Matsusako, M., Numaguchi, Y., et al. (2005). Percutaneous sacroplasty for hemorrhagic metastases from hepatocellular carcinoma. *AJNR Am J Neuroradiol, 26(3)*, 493-495.

Vaicys, C. & Fried, A. (2000). Transient hyponatremia complicated by seizures after endoscopic third ventriculostomy. *Minim Invasive Neurosurg, 43(4)*, 190-191.

Wedin, R. (2001). Surgical treatment for pathologic fracture. *Acta Orthoped Scand, 302*, 3-29.

Wrede-Seaman, L.D. (2001). Management of emergent conditions in palliative care. *Primary Care, 28(2)*, 317-328.

Wudel, L.J. & Nesbitt, J.C. (2001). Superior vena cava syndrome. *Curr Treat Options Oncol, 2(1)*, 77-91.

CHAPTER 34

PRURITUS

Carol L. Scot

■

The overall prevalence of significant pruritus in palliative care patients is low, probably no more than 2% to 3%, despite the facts that the palliative care population is predominantly elderly and that pruritus increases with age. The prevalence of pruritus within the palliative care population with certain diseases, such as renal or liver failure, is much higher.

Because of the overall low prevalence of pruritus in the palliative care population, pruritus is not always included in the list of distressing symptoms to be addressed with palliation, but its relief matters greatly to the few people who have it. Severe pruritus can destroy sleep and diminish quality of life.

DEFINITION AND INCIDENCE

Pruritus, or itching, is the unpleasant sensation that provokes an urge to scratch. It generally involves a complex series of interactions among the skin, inflammatory processes, cutaneous nerves, and the central nervous system (Fleischer, 2000). Because minor or short-lived itching episodes rarely come to medical notice, the incidence of itching in the general population is not known. The lifetime experience of itching probably approaches 100%.

Researchers have attempted to assess the incidence and prevalence of itching in some subsets of patients. Pruritus occurs in about 30% of patients with psoriasis (Levine & Levine, 2004). Approximately 50% to 70% of patients with primary biliary cirrhosis experience pruritus (Talwalkar, Souto, Jorgensen et al., 2003). The fact that intractable pruritus can be an indication for liver transplantation demonstrates how severely pruritus can affect the quality of a person's life (Terg, Coronel, Sorda et al., 2002). The prevalence of renal itch among patients on dialysis is estimated to be between 22% and 48% (Manenti, Vaglio, Costantino et al., 2005). In survivors of severe burns, the incidence of pruritus is as high as 87% (Field, Peck, Hernandez-Reif et al., 2000).

Even though much of the physiological basis of pruritus has been described, it is not completely understood, with the consequence that no specific antipruritic drug is available. "This is particularly unfortunate as, although itching is popularly perceived as a minor social or even humorous disability, it is frequently so severe and intractable as to cause the sufferer abject misery or even suicidal inclination" (Greaves & Wall, 1999, p. 487).

When itching is a major symptom in patients with far-advanced illness, all efforts need to be made to alleviate the discomfort, whether or not a precise cause is known.

ETIOLOGY AND PATHOPHYSIOLOGY

The sensation of itching appears to be the same in conditions as diverse as renal failure, insect bites, fungal infections, lymphoma, dry skin, liver failure, multiple sclerosis, and healing wounds, yet its pathophysiology in these conditions is not all the same, and treatments that work for some fail for others.

Itch can be cutaneous, neuropathic, neurogenic, mixed, or psychogenic.

In the skin, unmyelinated nerve fibers—C-fibers—mediate both cutaneous itch and pain. The C-fibers that mediate cutaneous itch cannot be differentiated anatomically from the ones that mediate pain, but they can be differentiated functionally (Fleischer, 2000; Twycross, Greaves, Handwerker et al., 2003). "The afferent C-fibres subserving this type of itch are a functionally distinct subset: they respond to histamine, acetylcholine and other pruritogens, but are insensitive to mechanical stimuli" (Twycross et al., 2003, p. 8).

Such C-fibers comprise about 5% of the C-fibers in human skin. Differentiation of the sensations of pain and itch may also depend on the specific anatomy and physiology of the person experiencing it. Acetylcholine causes itching in the skin of atopic patients, but when it is injected into the skin of nonatopic persons, it causes pain (Twycross et al., 2003).

Another similarity in the physiology of pain and itch is the phenomenon of severe pain or pruritus sensitizing an area around it. With pain, this is called allodynia, in which the skin interprets benign touch as pain. The area around an intensely pruritic area can similarly be sensitized to interpret light touch as intense itch (allokinesis) (Twycross et al., 2003).

Histamine plays a primary role in the pruritus of many commonly occurring itchy conditions such as insect bites, drug reactions, urticaria, and wound healing, but not in other conditions. Histamine receptors H_1 and H_2 are found in the skin.

Serotonin is less pruritogenic in the skin than histamine, but in some types of itch, such as cholestasis-related itching, it seems to play a major role (Fleischer, 2000). Serotonin can cause itch via both peripheral and central mechanisms. In the skin, it releases histamine from mast cells. The central mechanism is inferred because ondansetron (Zofran), a specific $5\text{-}HT_3$ receptor antagonist, relieves the itch associated with exogenous opioids, and no $5\text{-}HT_3$ receptors have been found in the skin (Twycross et al., 2003).

Many other naturally occurring chemicals cause local itch when injected into the skin. These include amines, proteases, growth factors, neuropeptides, opioids, eicosanoids, and cytokines. Some produce itch by causing histamine release from mast cells and/or by sensitizing C-fibers. Some stimulate the nerve endings directly (Twycross et al., 2003).

Neuropathic itch can originate from damage to the nervous system, such as with postherpetic neuralgia, notalgia paresthetica (nerve entrapment of spinal nerve roots), and HIV infection. Paroxysmal itch can occur in multiple sclerosis, whereas unilateral pruritus occurs in brain damage, such as with tumors, infections, or stroke (Twycross et al., 2003).

Neurogenic itch is induced centrally without nerve damage and is associated with increased endogenous or exogenous opioids.

Psychogenic itching is a diagnosis of exclusion when itching occurs in association with neuropsychiatric disease and other causes of itching have been ruled out. No systemic disease is found, and no primary skin lesions are found. Secondary lesions of excoriations and lichenification are found on the parts of the body that can be reached by the fingernails, usually sparing the upper back. Some patients deny they scratch despite witnessed scratching and bleeding excoriations (Fleischer, 2000).

CONDITIONS AND MECHANISMS OF ITCHING

Localized

Atopic eczema (or atopic dermatitis) results from an abnormality of T helper type 2 cells resulting in increased transepidermal water loss. Patients usually have had this condition intermittently all their lives. They often have other atopic conditions such as asthma or hayfever and a family history of atopy (Levine & Levine, 2004).

With bites and infestations, scabies, chiggers, lice, and fleas release histamine into the skin.

Brachioradial pruritus is one of the rare forms of persistent localized itching in normal skin, occurring on the lateral aspect of the arms. It occurs most commonly in fair-skinned persons with significant sun exposure but has also had nerve root damage suggested as a cause (Bueller, Bernhard, & Dubroff, 1999; Winhoven, Coulson & Bottomley, 2004).

Burn pruritus is a frequently reported complication in burn survivors, persisting past the active healing phase. It is believed to be mediated by persistent increased mast cells and histamine release (Hettrick, O'Brien, Laznick et al., 2004).

Contact dermatitis (dermatitis venenata; contact eczema) is caused by irritants, which are substances that can damage cells in anyone if given enough exposure (e.g., soaps), or by a type IV hypersensitivity reaction affecting only sensitized persons. Other variants are contact urticarial, which may be immunological, and photocontact variant, where light transforms substances into irritants or antigens (Levine & Levine, 2004).

Fungal infection with *Candida albicans* causes candidiasis (moniliasis) of the mouth, vagina, skin, and nails, and in immunocompromised persons, it can cause infections of the esophagus, lungs, and blood (Hall, 2000). Tinea pedis is usually caused by *Epidermophyton floccosum*, *Tricophyton rubrum*, or *T. mentagrophytes*. Tinea cruris has the same causative agents as tinea pedis.

"Virtually anything that itches may create a self-perpetuating itch-scratch cycle" (Fleischer, 2000, p. 90). Lichen simplex chronicus (localized neurodermatitis, lichenified dermatitis) and prurigo nodularis are forms of neurodermatitis. "To understand the importance of lichenification and the symptoms which make patients scratch or rub repeatedly, the reader must understand that it takes over 100,000 scratches to make significant lichenification" (Fleischer, 2000, p. 89).

Nummular eczema (nummular dermatitis; discoid eczema) is associated with xerosis, atopy, and venous stasis.

Pruritus ani is an embarrassing proctologic condition affecting about 5% of the population, characterized by intense itching localized in the anus and perianal skin.

Local irritants and psychosomatic factors have been suggested as causes but not proved to be of relevance (Lysy, Sistiery-Ittah, Israelit et al., 2003). Urticaria (hives) are caused by allergic and nonallergic mechanisms, with the final common pathway consisting of histamine and other mediator release from mast cells (Levine & Levine, 2004).

Generalized

"It can be stated almost without exception that any drug systemically administered is capable of causing a skin eruption" (Hall, 2000, p. 82). Enteral or parenteral drugs must always be suspected in a generalized skin eruption.

Essential pruritus is the rarest form of generalized pruritus, and is a diagnosis of exclusion only after drug reactions, uremia, malignancy, liver disease, bullous pemphigoid, AIDS, and intestinal parasites have been ruled out (Hall, 2000).

Liver diseases may precipitate pruritus, especially those with cholestasis. Pruritus occurs in approximately 50% to 70% of patients with primary biliary cirrhosis (Talwalkar et al., 2003).

Itching may occur with any malignancy, and the etiology of paraneoplastic itching is poorly understood. Peripheral T-cell lymphoma and other cutaneous lymphomas are notoriously pruritic. Itch has the highest reported prevalence in Hodgkin's disease, at 10% to 30% (Fleischer, 2000).

Psoriasis occurs most commonly on the scalp, elbows, and the knees but can occur anywhere. The condition is marked by increased proliferation of epidermal keratinocytes associated with an infiltrate of neutrophils and lymphocytes. Erythematous papulosquamous lesions vary in size and shape and usually have a thick, silvery scale. About 30% of these patients itch (Hall, 2000).

Senile pruritus of the elderly occurs year round, mostly in the scalp, shoulders, sacral areas, and the legs and not necessarily associated with dry skin. It may involve a disorder of keratinization (Hall, 2000).

Uremic pruritus is most often paroxysmal, frequently affecting the forearms and back. It may involve unidentified pruritogenic substances accumulating in dialysis patients as a result of molecular size; other theories implicate xerosis, hyperparathyroidism, hypercalcemia, hyperphosphatemia, elevated plasma histamine levels, and uremic neuropathy (Levine & Levine, 2004). The confusion of etiology can be seen in the statements of other reviewers, who state that for the last 20 years various causes of the pruritus of uremia have been explored, and promising mechanisms have been found to be undependable. Some primary culprits of causation have been touted and eliminated, including excessive parathyroid hormone and calcium phosphate crystals. And "it remains to be established whether the opioidergic system plays a significant role in the pathophysiology of uraemic pruritus" (Mettang, Pauli-Magnus & Alscher, 2002, p. 1561).

Water-induced itching or aquagenic pruritus is pruritus that occurs after contact with water or with sudden temperature changes. It may occur alone or in conjunction with polycythemia vera. Aquagenic pruritus is characterized by itching with a pricking sensation that lasts 15 to 60 minutes. Elevated histamine levels are found in the skin during attacks (Fleischer, 2000; Levine & Levine, 2004).

Winter pruritus (pruritus hiemalis) is most common in the elderly and most prominent on the legs and is due to low humidity in heated air (Hall, 2000).

ASSESSMENT AND MEASUREMENT

Like pain, pruritus is by definition an unmeasurable, subjective sensation. If the itch occurs in conjunction with an observable skin condition, the skin abnormality can be described and measured. But the pruritus itself must be reported by the patient or, if not reported, inferred from a patient's scratching behavior. Most advanced practice nurses assess a patient's degree of pruritus by the patient's report that the itch is minor, moderate, or "driving me crazy."

In a typical pruritus research study, subjects kept a weekly diary, quantifying the amount of itch they were experiencing and their overall well-being on 5-point scales (Browning, Combes & Mayo, 2003). Another commonly used research tool is the visual analogue scale consisting of a 10-cm line marked 0 (no itch) at one end and 10 (maximum itch) at the other end. This is used to measure pruritus at one point in time (Manenti et al., 2005).

Itch in Normal Skin

Itch occurring without visible abnormalities of the skin is usually generalized. The scratching associated with generalized itch can produce the secondary lesions of excoriations.

For patients already known to have conditions that cause generalized pruritus (e.g., malignancy, renal failure, or cholestatic liver disease), efforts can move directly to treatment for relief.

Whether patients with generalized itch who do not have a probable cause will be subjected to an intense search for occult disease or treated empirically depends on the functional status of the patient and his or her desires.

Itch with Localized Abnormality of the Skin

When pruritus is associated with abnormalities of the skin, the abnormality should be carefully assessed and described. The size of the afflicted area, the types of lesions, and their distribution should all be noted.

A short review of the proper terms and descriptions for primary and secondary lesions of the skin follows (Hall, 2000).

Primary and secondary lesions of the skin often occur together in itchy conditions. Secondary lesions may obscure distinctive primary lesions, but a careful examination usually identifies both the primary and the secondary lesions.

Primary Skin Lesions

- *Macules* range up to 1 cm and are round, flat discolorations of the skin.
- *Patches* are larger than 1 cm, flat discolorations of the skin, like vitiligo and senile freckles.
- *Papules* range up to 1 cm in size and are circumscribed elevated superficial solid lesions. A *wheal* is a type of papule that is edematous and transitory (present less than 24 hours), like hives and some insect bites.
- *Plaques* are larger than 1 cm and are circumscribed, elevated, superficial, solid lesions.
- *Nodules* range up to 1 cm and are solid lesions with depth; they may be above, level with, or beneath the skin surface.

- *Tumors* are larger than 1 cm and are solid lesions with depth; they may be above, level with, or beneath the skin surface.
- *Vesicles* range up to 1 cm and are circumscribed elevations of the skin containing serous fluid.
- *Bullae* are larger than 1 cm and are circumscribed elevations that containing serous fluid (e.g., pemphigoid, second-degree burns).
- *Pustules* vary in size and are circumscribed elevations of the skin that contain purulent fluid.
- *Petechiae* range to 1 cm and are circumscribed deposits of blood or blood pigments in the skin.
- *Purpura* is larger than 1 cm and is a circumscribed deposit of blood or blood pigments in the skin.
- *Burrows* are tunnels in the epidermis caused by insects or larvae, such as in scabies or cutaneous larva migrans.

Secondary Skin Lesions

- *Scales* are shedding dead epidermal cells that may be dry (e.g., psoriasis) or greasy (e.g., dandruff).
- *Crusts* are variously colored masses of skin exudates such as seen in impetigo or infected dermatitis.
- *Excoriations* are abrasions of the skin, usually superficial and traumatic.
- *Fissures* are linear breaks in the skin, sharply defined with abrupt walls.
- *Ulcers* are irregularly sized and shaped excavations of the skin extending into the dermis or deeper.
- *Scars* are formations of connective tissue replacing tissue lost through injury or disease.
- *Keloids* are hypertrophic scars beyond the borders of the original injury.
- *Lichenification* is a diffuse area of thickening and scaling with resultant increase in the skin lines and markings (Hall, 2000, pp. 14-17).

HISTORY AND PHYSICAL EXAMINATION

History

In the ideal medical interview, the patient describes his or her symptoms freely and spontaneously and stops when what needs to be communicated has been expressed. The clinician then repeats any information that needs clarification and asks any indicated further questions. When the current problems have been discussed, the clinician then asks questions to uncover any additional problems.

A person suffering from itch may fail to communicate that fact. A patient with intermittent itch may forget to mention it, and even a patient with constant itch may put it out of mind to discuss more urgent matters. If a patient is observed scratching, questions about itch obviously need to be asked. For others, the symptom of itch may be uncovered with general dermatologic questions: Any skin problems? Any lumps, bumps, rashes, itching?

When any symptom, such as itch, is positive, it needs to be further characterized. Has this been a lifelong problem, a recurrent one, or a new one? If new, when did it start?

Is the itching localized or general, constant or intermittent? When does it occur (if intermittent), or when is it worst (if constant)? (For a patient who is bothered by itch only at night, morning treatment is unnecessary.) What makes it better; what makes it worse? What treatments have been tried, and with what effect?

The ideal medical interview will always include a careful and complete drug history that includes all prescription, over-the-counter, and recreational drugs. This is especially important for persons troubled by pruritus.

Physical Examination

The physical examination must include the entire skin surface, with particular attention to those areas the patient has indicated as itchy. All abnormalities of the skin and mucous membranes should be described and recorded using standard dermatologic terminology, with careful measurements of areas involved.

The negative finding of no rash or lesions is equally important.

DIAGNOSTICS

Localized Pruritus

When the findings of the history and physical examination have identified a likely diagnosis with an easily used treatment, a presumptive diagnosis and therapeutic trial are warranted. For instance, if the inflamed itchy areas coincide with areas of tape applied to the skin, an acquired tape sensitivity is likely. When the measures of avoidance of tape, oral antihistamines, locally applied antihistamine cream, or possibly mild steroid cream resolve the problem, the diagnosis is confirmed.

Infestations and fungal infections may also be treated presumptively or may be confirmed with microscopic examination.

Occasionally, a localized outbreak defies identification and treatment and must be referred to a dermatologist. A skin biopsy with special stains may be required for a definitive diagnosis (Hall, 2000).

Generalized Pruritus

As stated, a patient with known renal failure, malignancy, or bile duct obstruction probably needs no further investigation into the cause of generalized pruritus. An elderly patient may certainly be treated for a presumptive diagnosis of senile pruritus or winter pruritus (Hall, 2000). For others, simple laboratory tests can identify or rule out kidney, liver, or endocrine disorders. The search for an occult malignancy is much more difficult, and whether it is undertaken should be decided by the patient.

In a sense, all routine medical care is a search for occult disease, especially malignancy, but when a person presents with generalized persistent pruritus and wants an answer, the search has more intensity. It starts with the complete history and physical examination, including a rectal examination and, for women, a pelvic examination. A chest radiograph or computed tomography scan is warranted, especially for smokers. Stool studies for parasites and occult blood should be done. Older patients who have not had a recent colonoscopy should have one performed (Hall, 2000). If no other cause is found, a skin biopsy of normal skin may find occult pemphigoid (Greaves & Wall, 1999).

If that is also normal, one of the diagnoses of exclusion—psychogenic pruritus or essential pruritus—may be made, with treatment as described later.

INTERVENTION AND TREATMENT

General Measures

"Improved understanding of the pathophysiology of itch has led to modest advances in treatment. No doubt in time this progress will lead to selective topical antipruritics. Topical corticosteroids are not direct antipruritics and should not be used as such, although they effectively relieve itching secondary to inflammatory skin disease" (Yosipovitch, Greaves, & Schmelz, 2003, p. 693).

All of the following suggested measures may or may not be effective and to varying degrees. Individual responses to treatment must be carefully followed. When success occurs, that treatment should be continued, even if a reason for the success is not known.

Itch is usually intensified by heat, so cooling measures may be helpful for any patient with pruritus. Cool clothes, a cool but not dry ambient temperature, and tepid showers or baths may help (Twycross et al., 2003).

Because histamine is the known pruritogen responsible for all or some of the itching in most pruritic conditions, antihistamines remain a mainstay of pruritus treatment. Antihistamine medication is available in both oral and topical forms. The sedation of first-generation antihistamines may be part of the relief provided and is especially helpful and acceptable for nocturnal pruritus.

Antihistamines come from various chemical classes (Table 34-1) (Werth, 2004, p. 2457), and sometimes an antihistamine from one class may have more effect and fewer side effects than one from a different chemical class for a particular patient. Many patients will already know which antihistamines work well for them. If a patient does not know and a search needs to be made for a more effective, better tolerated antihistamine, it makes sense to try one from an untried chemical class.

Specific Measures

Aquagenic Pruritus

Treatments include photochemotherapy, ultraviolet B (UVB) phototherapy, first-generation antihistamines, alkalinization of bath water, and intramuscular triamcinalone (Levine & Levine, 2004). If associated with polycythemia vera, the first treatment is aspirin 300 mg as needed, which is usually effective for 12 to 24 hours. If a patient is receiving interferon α (Intron-A) as treatment for polycythemia vera, the itch is usually improved. Paroxetine (Paxil) has also been shown to be effective (Twycross et al., 2003).

Atopic Dermatitis

Doxepin (Sinequan) is a tricyclic compound with high potency as an antihistamine. It is available in a cream (Zonalon) and is effective in suppressing the pruritus of atopic eczema. However, it is absorbed through the skin and, like other antihistamines, can be sedating (Yosipovitch et al., 2003).

Standard treatments include intermediate potency topical corticosteroids, such as Cutivate, Valisone, Diprosone, or oral prednisone (Orapred, Deltasone) for temporary

TABLE 34-1 ■ Groups of Antihistamines

Antihistamine Group	Generic Name
First-Generation H₁-Type Antihistamines	
Alkylamine	Brompheniramine (Dimetapp)
	Chorpheniramine (Chlor-Trimeton)
Aminoalkyl ether (ethanolamine)	Clemastine fumarate
	Diphenhydramine (Benadryl)
Ethylenediamine	Pyrilamine (Triaminic)
Phenothiazine	Promethazine (Phenergan)
	Trimeprazine (Temaril)
Piperidine	Azatadine
	Cyproheptadine
	Diphenylpyraline
Piperazine	Chlorcyclizine
	Hydroxyzine (Atarax)
Second-Generation H₁-Type Antihistamines	
Alkylamine	Acrivastine (combined with pseudoephedrine in allergy medication)
Piperidine	Astemizole (Hismanal)
	Loratidine (Claritin)
	Fexofenadine (Allegra)
Piperazine	Cetirizine (Zyrtec)
H₂-Type Antihistamines	Cimetidine (Tagamet)
	Ranitidine (Zantac)
	Famotidine
	Nizatidine
H₁- and H₂-Type Antihistamines	Doxepin (Sinequan)

From Goldman, L. & Ausiello, D. (Eds.). (2004). *Cecil textbook of medicine* (22nd ed., p. 2455). Philadelphia: Saunders.

therapy of severe flares; azathioprine (Imuran); cyclosporine (Neoral); first-generation antihistamines for nighttime sedation; UVB phototherapy; photochemotherapy (PUVA); evening primrose oil; Chinese herbs; and emollients applied at least twice daily, particularly during the winter months (Smith, 2000; Tofte & Hanifin, 2001).

Capsaicin cream 0.025% to 0.075% is effective but can cause irritation at first. The irritation can be reduced by using the topical anesthetic eutectic mixture of local anesthetics (EMLA) cream (Yosipovitch et al., 2003).

Brachioradial Pruritus

This rare condition responds poorly to the usual treatments of topical or oral corticosteroids and antihistamines or to spinal manipulation and capsaicin. Early reports have found good response with gabapentin (Neurontin) (Bueller et al., 1999; Winhoven et al., 2004).

Burn Pruritus

The standard treatment is to use oral antihistamines and topical lotions such as Revive (Dermalife, Albuquerque, N.M.) lotion or Corrective Concepts (Corrective Concepts Co., Dallas, Tex.) in the attempt to prevent the rubbing or scratching that can damage healed and grafted skin. Research into additional measures when the standard treatment is insufficient has shown benefit from massage (Field et al., 2000), transcutaneous electrical nerve stimulation treatment (Hettrick et al., 2004), and scheduled rather than as-needed dosage of H_1 and H_2 blockers (Baker, Zeller, Klein et al., 2001).

Cholestatic Pruritus

Practice guidelines from the American Association for the Study of Liver Disease list treatments for cholestatic pruritus as, first, bile acid–binding resins like cholestyramine, a treatment that is at least partly effective but unpalatable and that can interfere with other medications, and, second, rifampicin (rifampin), which may help pruritus but can cause further liver damage (Heathcote, 2000). All other treatments, including naltrexone (Depade), phenobarbitol and propofol (Diprivan), antihistamines, S-adenosylmethionine (SAMe, a dietary supplement), phototherapy, anticonvulsants, ondansetron (Zofran), and plasmaphersis, are considered experimental (Heathcote, 2000).

A later study showed significant relief of cholestatic pruritus in 9 of 20 patients treated with naltrexone. (Note that naltrexone *cannot* be used for patients who require opioids for pain control.) In patients without pain and with severe pruritus, this opioid antagonist may help. One study determined that side effects occurred in the first 48 hours and were consistent with opioid withdrawal. They resolved spontaneously within 2 days of treatment, and the authors concluded, "Naltrexone can be considered as an alternate option to treat pruritus of cholestasis" (Terg et al., 2002).

A serendipitous report of patients treated with sertraline (Zoloft) for depression who had improvement of their cholestatic pruritus led to a study that showed improvement in the cholestatic pruritus of nondepressed patients as well (Browning et al., 2003).

Drug Eruptions

The most important first step is to attempt to identify the causative drug and stop it. If several drugs seem equally likely, all of them should be discontinued. If the patient's reaction is mild and subsides when the drugs are stopped, no other treatment may be necessary. If the reaction is severe, systemic corticosteroids may be required to quiet it. Antihistamines (unless an antihistamine is the inciting medication) can be given for relief of pruritus in either case (Hall, 2000).

If some of the discontinued drugs are considered essential, they can cautiously be resumed, one at a time, after the reaction is controlled.

Dry Skin

Even for patients with other probable causes of itching, the use of an emollient cream may eliminate the portion of itch caused by dry skin. Bathing should be limited, and soap substitutes such as bath gels should be used. Sedating first-generation antihistamines help with nighttime sleep (Levine & Levine, 2004).

Essential Pruritus

This diagnosis (of exclusion) of generalized pruritus in normal-appearing skin is treated in the same manner as senile and winter pruritus (Hall, 2000).

Malignancies

"Paraneoplastic itch associated with solid tumors is not eased by corticosteroids or cimetidine. However, paroxetine (Paxil) is almost always beneficial, often within 24 hours" (Twycross et al., 2003).

For Hodgkin's disease, the usual treatments of radiotherapy and/or chemotherapy will relieve itch if otherwise effective. Corticosteroids usually relieve itch in late-stage disease (Twycross et al., 2003).

Neurodermatitis

Locally circumscribed neurodermatitis (lichen simplex chronicus) is an itchy dermatitis with a prolonged course and is most common in Asians. The usual treatment is steroid creams. For persons in whom that was not sufficiently helpful, the application of an aspirin-dichloromethane solution reduced pruritus and improved healing (Yosipovitch, Sugeng, Chan et al., 2001).

Thalidomide reduced the signs and symptoms of prurigo nodularis in HIV-infected patients, although one-third of the study subjects developed a degree of thalidomide peripheral neuropathy (Maurer, Poncelet, & Berger, 2004).

Pruritus Ani

Pruritus ani with dermatosis may be treated for up to 1 month with mild steroid cream (Lysy et al., 2003). "When pruritus ani has no demonstrable aetiology, it is often described as idiopathic, and advice regarding hygiene and drying methods is usually given, with poor results" (p. 1323). Some patients, however, do respond to conservative measures: gentle cleansing with an emulsifying ointment and drying (preferably with a hair dryer) and avoidance of underwear that traps sweat such as nylon and acrylic (Lysy et al., 2003). In their study, Lysy and colleagues treated patients with dilute capsaicin cream (0.006% or 0.012%). It was far more effective than placebo menthol cream for 31 of the 44 patients in the study, and long-term follow-up showed it continued to be, with few side effects (Lysy et al., 2003).

Senile Pruritus

The treatment of senile pruritus is the same as that for winter pruritus (see p. 514). In addition to the treatment recommendations for winter pruritus, two or three injections of triamcinalone acetonide suspension 30 mg (Kenalog-40) intramuscularly every 4 to 6 weeks can be beneficial (Hall, 2000).

Uremic Pruritus

Because the itch associated with chronic uremia has been recognized for over 100 years, it must be assumed to be due to uremia and not just dialysis. In fact, the incidence of uremic pruritus has fallen. In the early 1970s, when dialysis was new, the incidence of pruritus was reported as 85%. By the late 1980s it fell to 50% to 60%, and now the prevalence of renal itch among patients on dialysis is estimated at between 22% and 48% (Manenti et al., 2005).

The physiology of uremic pruritus is complex and not well understood, and many treatments have been tried, with varying success. "Most of the success stories have turned into reports of failure" (Mettang et al., 2002). One such story involved ondansetron (Zofran), where early reports of success were followed by a controlled trial that showed no difference between it and placebo (Murphy, Reaich, Pai et al., 2003). "Whenever a new treatment option is reported to be effective, some time elapses before conflicting results are published; in the meantime, the mood of patients and physicians changes from euphoria to disillusionment. This happened with erythropoi-etin and naltrexone" (Mettang et al., 2002). Other researchers still believe that naltrex-one is helpful in a subset of patients and "might be considered as a second-line treatment" (Legroux-Crespel, Cledes, & Misery, 2004).

Other researchers state, "Pruritus is the most distressing symptom in haemodialy-sis (HD) patients. Its aetiology has not yet been delineated, and thus there are no good therapeutical options" (Weisshaar, Dunker, Rohl et al., 2004). Their study concluded that 5-HT$_3$ receptor blockers such as tropisetron and ondansetron (Zofran) and the antihistamine cetirizine (Zyrtec) do not reduce itching in hemodialysis patients.

Two studies of gabapentin treatment have had positive conclusions.

"[O]ur data suggest that gabapentin could be considered an effective and safe alternative treatment for uremic pruritus" (Manenti et al., 2005). "Our study shows that gabapentin is safe and effective for treating uraemic pruritus in haemodialysis patients" (Gunal, Ozalp, Yoldas et al., 2004).

The nondrug treatment of UVB therapy has been used with some success (Gilchrest, Rowe, Brown et al., 1997). Levine and Levine (2004) mark it as a clear treatment of choice. Their other listed possible treatments are cholestyramine 4 g orally twice daily, activated charcoal 6 g orally daily divided into four to six doses, first-generation anti-histamines, emollients, acupuncture, or naltrexone 50 mg orally daily (Levine & Levine, 2004). Naltrexone should never be given to patients requiring opioids for pain control.

Capsaicin use in uremic pruritus received a weak endorsement as a possible co-medication (Weisshaar, Dunker & Gallnick, 2003).

Thalidomide is also recommended, although it is teratogenic and must not be used in women who may become pregnant (Twycross et al., 2003).

Urticaria

Chronic idiopathic urticaria is the most common type of chronic urticaria, and pruritus is its most prominent symptom. Antihistamines are effective, but the side effects of first-generation antihistamines for persons who need constant suppressive treatment can limit their use. Some promising second-generation nonsedating antihis-tamines (terfenadine and astemizole) were taken off the market in 1998 and 1999 because of the rare occurrence of a potentially fatal cardiac arrhythmia, torsades de pointes. Other second-generation antihistamines on the market do not have this danger and have been shown to be effective for urticaria, with few side effects (Brown & Roberts, 2001; Ring, Hein, Gauger et al., 2001).

Winter Pruritus

"Treatment of winter pruritus consists of the following:
1. Bathing should involve as cool water … and as little soap as possible.
2. A bland soap such as Dove, Oilatum, Cetaphil, or Basis is used sparingly.
3. An oil is added to the bath water, such as Lubath, RoBathol, Nivea, or Alpha-Keri. (The patient should be warned to avoid slipping in the tub.)

4. Emollient lotions are beneficial, such as Complex 15, Pen-Kera, or Mosturel. Alpha-hydroxy acid preparations include LactiCare, Lac-Hydrin, and Eucerin Plus. Urea products that are beneficial include Aquacare HP, Carmol, and Eucerin Plus. These lubricants should be applied immediately after bathing.
5. A low-potency corticosteroid ointment applied twice-daily is effective.
6. Oral antihistamines are sometimes effective, such as chlorpheniramine (Chlor-Trimeton), 4 mg hs or qid, or diphenhydramine (Benedryl), 50 mg hs" (Hall, 2000, p. 98).

EDUCATION, EVALUATION, AND PLAN FOR FOLLOW-UP

The conversation about a patient's problem with itching begins with the first mention of it by the patient, a family member or friend, or the clinician and continues until either the problem is completely resolved or the patient dies. A part of this communication is the mutual education of the patient by the clinician and of the clinician by the patient.

The clinician will attempt to communicate everything he or she knows about the cause, treatment, and amelioration of itch, including the preventative measures that are especially important in contact allergies, winter pruritus, and dry skin pruritus.

When the patient has a specific diagnosis, particularly if it is a relatively rare one, the clinician may want to share his or her research with the patient and family. Of course, today many patients and families are doing their own research on the Internet. Some information from the Internet is credible; some is not.

Communication with the patient involves careful listening to determine the patient and family's understanding of the cause and treatment of the patient's pruritus. As long as the symptoms persist, the communication will include a continuing careful review of what the patient and family have used or done, or not used or done, and why.

The patient may have difficulties with treatments prescribed by the clinician and be reluctant to admit this. Problems with the cost, side effects, or inconvenience of a treatment may prevent a patient from following the clinician's advice. The clinician needs to elicit this information and take it into account while making further plans with the patient.

On the other hand, a clinician may have little choice but to continue to follow a patient who is relying on dubious authorities and using expensive useless (or harmful) treatments. Over time, these treatments will work or not work. If they do, that is great. If not, the patient and family may once again be willing to try other recommendations.

CASE STUDY   Mrs. D. is a 78-year-old widowed European American woman referred for hospice care by her case manager at an acute care hospital. The hospice receives the referral on April 12, with the information that her terminal diagnosis is end-stage liver disease. The patient's family wavers about accepting and agreeing to end-of-life care, and her admission to inpatient hospice care is delayed until April 25.

Mrs. D. had been hospitalized 3 months earlier with upper gastrointestinal bleeding, which was found to be due principally to a bleeding duodenal ulcer. She also had mild gastritis and small esophageal varices. She was discharged to a long-term care facility for rehabilitation but hospitalized again on April 7 with upper and lower gastrointestinal bleeding. Laboratory values at the time showed thrombocytopenia with a platelet count of 84,000 (normal, 130,000 to 280,000), blood urea nitrogen of 85 ng/dl (normal, 6 to 23 ng/dl), creatinine of 1.2 mg/dl (normal, 0.5 to 1.2 mg/dl), ammonia of 120 mcg/dl (normal 19 to 87 mcg/dl), amylase of 189 U/L (normal, 23 to 100 U/L), and lipase of 79 U/L (normal, 16 to 63 U/L). All hepatitis markers were negative. Total bilirubin was 1.1 mg/dl (normal, 0 to 1.0 mg/dl), direct bilirubin was 0.4 mg/dl (normal, 0 to 0.3 mg/dl), alkaline phosphatase was 69 U/L (normal, 35 to 117 U/L), SGOT was 77 U/L (normal, 35 to 46 U/L), SGPT was 25 U/L (normal, 13 to 50 U/L), and albumin was 2.7 g/dl (normal, 3.4 to 4.8 g/dl). In 2 days, SGPT rose to 59 U/L and albumin fell to 2.2 g/dl.

Her other medical problems are heart failure, a systolic ejection murmur, osteoporosis, Parkinson's disease, and asthmatic chronic obstructive pulmonary disease.

Her surgical history includes cholecystectomy, appendectomy, removal of a left ankle tumor, and bilateral venous stripping.

She is allergic to aspirin, iodine, sulfa, and codeine.

On her April 7 admission to the acute care hospital, her home medications were continued, the following being ordered: Os-Cal, ferrous sulfate, Klor-Con, carbidopa, levodopa, Primidone, Keflex, Advair, Xopenex, omeprazole, Evista, folic acid, Lasix, and Zaroxolyn. Medication records from the hospital add Inderal, Bentyl, Chronulac, Insulin, Flovent, Serevent, Tylenol, Demerol started April 9, Benadryl started April 9 for nausea, Mephyton from April 11 to 13, Risperdal started April 13, morphine started April 14, and Reglan and Duragesic 25 mcg patch started on April 24.

When she arrives at the hospice, the staff is surprised that her most pressing problems are rash and pruritus, which were not mentioned in her written records or verbal report.

Mrs. D.'s only complaint is itching all over. She has a bright red, confluent macular-papular rash of her arms, neck, chest, and thighs. She has 0.5- to 1-cm blisters of her inner left knee, perhaps where her latex catheter tube has been lying. She also has a fungal-appearing rash of her groin and axillae.

Although she has compromised liver and renal function, it is unlikely her pruritus is associated with either condition. Cholestatic and uremic itching occur in normal-appearing skin, and she has a rash. Because this is pruritus in abnormal skin, the differential diagnosis includes drug reaction, contact dermatitis, and candidiasis.

A drug reaction seems likely from the appearance, extent, and severity of the rash and the fact that a woman known to be allergic to four medications has received approximately 28 different medications in the previous 17 days, some of them new to her. Contact dermatitis also seems possible. The adhesive of Duragesic patches can cause contact dermatitis, and she may have developed a latex sensitivity. With the wide distribution of her skin reaction, she might also have an allergy to something like the hospital sheets or the soap with which they are washed.

None of her previously given medications are continued. The fentanyl patch is removed, and her indwelling catheter is changed to a silicone one. Paper sheets are not yet changed; the clinician will wait to see if other measures are sufficient. To treat the probable drug reaction, we start oral dexamethasone (Decadron) 4 mg orally three times daily and hydroxazine (Atarax) 50 mg orally three times daily. In hospice, essential oils are also used for symptom control, so a spritzer of dilute lavender oil to spray on the itchy places as needed is given to the patient.

Her rash and pruritus fade with the first doses of medication and come under good control within 36 hours. The medications are continued without change to consolidate the improvement.

On April 28, she is noted to have a vaginal discharge. She is given fluconazole (Diflucan) one 150-mg pill only, for vaginal candidiasis. The vaginal discharge and groin and axillary rash resolve completely over the next few days.

On May 9, her skin is normal but dry, and she is able to tolerate and enjoy the application of lavender oil to the skin.

On May 10, the Atarax order is changed from "routine three times daily" to "three times daily only as needed for itch," and she takes no more of it.

On May 17, the Decadron is reduced to 4 mg twice daily, with no ill effects.

By May 19, she is having trouble swallowing, oral medications are discontinued, and the Decadron is changed to 4 mg per rectum every 24 hours.

On May 20, she has an upper gastrointestinal hemorrhage and dies.

The exact cause of this patient's severe rash and pruritus will never be known. However, rapid empiric measures (removal of possible offending substances, systemic steroids, and a first-generation antihistamine) relieved the problems and gave her 3 weeks of comfortable good time with her family before her death.

REFERENCES

Baker, R.A.U., Zeller, R.A., Klein, R.L., et al. (2001). Burn wound itch control using H1 and H2 antagonists. *J Burn Care Rehabil, 22(4)*, 263-268.

Brown, N.J. & Roberts, L.J., II (2001). Histamine, bradykinin, and their antagonists. In J.G. Hardman, L.E. Limbird, & A.G. Gilman (Eds.). *Goodman & Gilman's the pharmacological basis of therapeutics* (10th ed.). New York: McGraw-Hill.

Browning, J., Combes, B., & Mayo, M.J. (2003). Long-term efficacy of sertaline as a treatment for cholestatic pruritus in patients with primary biliary cirrhosis. *Am J Gastroenterol, 98(12)*, 2736-2741.

Bueller, H.A., Bernhard, J.D., & Dubroff, L.M. (1999). Gabapentin treatment for brachioradial pruritus. *J Eur Acad Dermatol Venereol, 13*, 227-228.

Field, T., Peck II, M., Hernandez-Reif, M., et al. (2000). Postburn itching, pain, and psychological symptoms are reduced with massage therapy. *J Burn Care Rehabil, 21(3)*:189-193, May-June.

Fleischer, A.B. (2000). *The clinical management of itching*. New York: Parthenon Publishing Group.

Gilchrest, B.A., Rowe, J.W., Brown, R.S., et al. (1977). Relief of uremic pruritus with ultraviolet phototherapy. *N Engl J Med, 297,* 136-138.

Greaves, M.W. & Wall, P.D. (1999). Pathophysiology and clinical aspects of pruritus. In I.M. Freedberg, A.Z. Eisen, K. Wolff, et al. (Eds.). *Fitzpatrick's dermatology in general medicine* (5th ed.). Hightstown, N.J.: McGraw-Hill.

Gunal, A.I., Ozalp, G., Yoldas, T.K., et al. (2004). Gabapentin therapy for pruritus in haemodialysis patients: A randomized, placebo-controlled, double-blind trial. *Nephrol Dial Transplant, 19,* 3137-3139.

Hall, J.C. (2000). *Sauer's manual of skin diseases.* Philadelphia: Lippincott Williams & Wilkins.

Heathcote, E.J. (2000). Management of primary biliary cirrhosis. *Hepatology, 31,* 1005-1009.

Hettrick, H., O'Brien, K., Laznick, H., et al. (2004). Effect of transcutaneous electrical nerve stimulation for the management of burn pruritus. *J Burn Care Rehabil, 25(3),* 236-240.

Legroux-Crespel, E., Cledes, J., & Misery, L. (2004). A comparative study on the effects of naltrexone and loratadine on uremic pruritus. *Dermatology, 208(4, Health Module),* 326-330.

Levine, N. & Levine, C.C. (2004). *Dermatology therapy: A to Z essentials.* Berlin: Springer-Verlag.

Lysy, J., Sistiery-Ittah, M., Israelit, Y., et al. (2003). Topical capsaicin—A novel and effective treatment for idiopathic intractable pruritus ani. *Gut, 52,* 1323-1326.

Manenti, L., Vaglio, A., Costantino, E., et al. (2005). Gabapentin in the treatment of uremic itch. *J Nephrol, 18,* 86-91.

Maurer, T., Poncelet, A., & Berger, T. (2004). Thalidomide treatment for prurigo nodularis in human immunodeficiency virus-infected subjects. *Arch Dermatol, 140,* 845-849.

Mettang, T., Pauli-Magnus, C., & Alscher, D.M. (2002). Uraemic pruritus: New perspectives and insights from recent trials. *Nephrol Dial Transplant, 17,* 1558-1563.

Murphy, M., Reaich, D., Pai, P., et al. (2003). A randomized, placebo-controlled, double-blind trial of ondansetron in renal itch. *Br J Dermatol, 148,* 314-317.

Ring, J., Hein, R., Gauger, A., et al. (2001). Once-daily desloratadine improves the signs and symptoms of chronic idiopathic urticaria. *Int J Dermatol, 40,* 72-76.

Smith, C.H. (2000). New approaches to topical therapy. *Clin Exp Dermatol, 25,* 567-574.

Talwalkar, J.A., Souto, E., Jorgensen, R.A., et al. (2003). Natural history of pruritus in primary biliary cirrhosis. *Clin Gastroenterol Hepatol, 1,*297-302.

Terg, R., Coronel, E., Sorda, J., et al. (2002). Efficacy and safety of oral naltrexone treatment for pruritus of cholestasis: A crossover, double blind, placebo-controlled study. *J Hepatol, 37,* 717-722.

Tofte, S.J. & Hanifin, J.M. (2001). Current management and therapy of atopic dermatitis. *J Am Acad Dermatol, 44(1 suppl),* S13-S16.

Twycross, R., Greaves, M.W., Handwerker, H., et al. (2003). Itch: scratching more than the surface. *Q J Med, 96,* 7-26.

Weisshaar, E., Dunker, N., & Gallnick, H. (2003). Topical capsaicin therapy in humans with hemodialysis-related pruritus. *Neurosci Let, 345,* 192-194.

Weisshaar, E., Dunker, N., Rohl, F.-W., et al. (2004). Antipruritic effects of two different 5-HT3 receptor antagonists and an antihistamine in haemodialysis patients. *Exp Dermatol, 13,* 298-304.

Werth, V.P. (2004). Principles of therapy. In L. Goldman & D. Ausiello (Eds.). *Cecil textbook of medicine* (22nd ed., pp. 2455-2458). Philadelphia: Saunders.

Winhoven, S.M., Coulson, I.H., & Bottomley, W.W. (2004). Brachioradial pruritus: Response to treatment with gabapentin. *Br J Dermatol, 150,* 786-787.

Yosipovitch, G., Greaves, M.W., & Schmelz, M. (2003). Itch. *Lancet, 361,* 690-694.

Yosipovitch, G., Sugeng, M.W., Chan, Y.H., et al. (2001). The effect of topically applied aspirin on localized circumscribed neurodermatitis. *J Am Acad Dermatol, 45,* 910-913.

CHAPTER 35

ULCERATIVE LESIONS

Elizabeth A. Ayello and Joy E. Schank

■

DEFINITION AND INCIDENCE

Persons at end-of-life are at risk for skin injury and ulcerations due to immobility, inadequate nutrition, incontinence, and underlying disease processes. In particular, pressure ulcers, skin tears, and malignant cutaneous wounds (MCWs) create physical and psychoemotional challenges for patients.

Palliative wound care is an emerging concept. It takes a holistic approach to improving the quality of life and relieving suffering for persons with chronic wounds. Because wound treatment goals and priorities are based on the person's changing health status, the aims of interventions may shift from wound closure to wound stabilization and prevention of wound deterioration and infection (Ferris, Khateib et al., 2004) (Table 35-1).

Both pressure ulcers and MCWs can have devastating physical and psychosocial effects. These wounds can be a source of pain, anemia, and infection. These sometimes unsightly and foul-smelling lesions can cause self-concept disturbance, social isolation due to shame or embarrassment, anxiety, fear, and depression (Foltz, 1980; Goodman, Ladd, & Purl, 1993; Miller, 1998; Waller & Caroline, 2000). The family of a patient receiving palliative care at home may not be aware of how to prevent and treat pressure ulcers; therefore, a palliative patient may have to be admitted to the hospital against his or her wishes.

ETIOLOGY AND PATHOPHYSIOLOGY

Pressure Ulcers

Pressure ulcers are wounds caused by "unrelieved pressure resulting in damage of underlying tissue" (National Pressure Ulcer Advisory Panel [NPUAP] et al., 2001). Usually located over bony prominences (e.g., sacrum, heels), pressure ulcers develop when the soft tissue is compressed between a bony prominence and an external surface, disrupting the blood supply and resulting in cellular death. Risk factors for the development of pressure ulcers include immobility, incontinence, inadequate nutrition, friction and shearing forces, and altered level of consciousness (Agency for Healthcare Research and Quality [AHRQ] [formerly the Agency for Health Care Policy and Research], 1992), as well as a previous healed pressure ulcer.

The author would like to acknowledge Debra Heidrich for her contributions that remain unchanged from the first edition of this textbook.

TABLE 35-1 ■ **Malignant Cutaneous Wound Staging System**

	Staging Classification				
	Stage 1	Stage 1N	Stage 2	Stage 3	Stage 4
Wound					
Closed wound/intact skin	X				
Closed wound/superficially open to drain then close/hard and fibrous		X			
Open wound/dermis and epidermis tissue involved			X		
Open wound/full thickness skin loss involving subcutaneous tissue				X	
Open wound/invasive to deep anatomic tissues and structures					X
Predominant Color					
Red/pink	X	X	X		
Red/pink/yellow				X	X
Hydration					
Dry	X				
Both moist and dry		X			
Moist			X	X	X
Drainage					
None	X				
Clear/purulent		X			
Serosanguineous/bleeding			X		
Purulent/serosanguineous				X	
Serosanguineous/bleeding/purulent					X
Pain					
No	X				
Pain possible		X	X	X	
Yes					X
Odor					
No	X	X			
Yes			X	X	X
Tunneling/Undermining					
No	X	X	X	X	
Yes					X

From Haisfield-Wolfe, M.E., & Baxendale-Cox, L.M. (1999). Staging of malignant cutaneous wounds: A pilot study. *Oncol Nurs Forum, 26*, 1055-1064.

The incidence of pressure ulcers in any particular practice setting is somewhat difficult to determine, since study designs vary significantly. For example, some studies include stage I pressure ulcers and some do not, and as a result study outcomes vary greatly. In the acute care setting, the incidence of pressure ulcers ranges from 0.4% to 38%, with increased incidence in higher-risk groups, such as the elderly and persons with paralysis. The incidence of pressure ulcers in the nursing home setting is 2.2% to 23.9%. Beginning data from home care studies provide a range of 0% to 17% (NPUAP, Cuddigan, Ayello et al., 2001).

Malignant Cutaneous Wounds

MCWs are ulcerating skin lesions that develop when malignant cells infiltrate the epithelium (Foltz, 1980). MCWs may occur as single lesions or in groups

(Haisfield-Wolfe & Baxendale-Cox, 1999). Approximately 5% to 10% of persons with metastatic malignancies have MCWs, usually during the last 3 to 6 months of life (Crosby, 1998; Foltz, 1980; Thiers, 1986; Waller & Caroline, 2000). The malignant processes associated with the development of cutaneous metastases include breast cancer, malignant melanoma, lung cancer, and colorectal cancer (Crosby, 1998). These wounds are sometimes called *fungating tumor wounds*, which refers to the tendency of these wounds to both ulcerate and proliferate (Mortimer, 1998).

MCWs may result from primary skin lesions or metastasis from other malignant processes. As mentioned, breast cancer is the most common cause of MCWs; up to 25% of persons with breast cancer experience skin metastasis (Waller & Caroline, 2000). The malignancies associated with the development of MCWs are listed in Box 35-1.

The initial appearance of a primary skin malignancy may be a sore that does not heal. Metastatic MCWs may begin as hard dermal or subcutaneous nodules and may be fixed to underlying tissue (Crosby, 1998; Thiers, 1986). These lesions occur most commonly in the vicinity of the primary tumor (Crosby, 1998). However, MCWs are also seen at a secondary site related to metastatic disease (Goodman et al., 1993; Miller, 1998). They may vary in color from flesh-toned to red and are usually asymptomatic at early stages (Crosby, 1998).

Malignancies spread to the cutaneous tissues via direct extension or embolization into the vascular or lymph channels (Goodman et al., 1993; Mortimer, 1998). Eventually these

Box 35-1	**Tumors Associated with Malignant Cutaneous Wounds**

PRIMARY SKIN MALIGNANCIES

Untreated basal cell carcinoma
Untreated squamous cell carcinoma
Malignant melanoma

METASTATIC SPREAD FROM PRIMARY MALIGNANCY

Breast
Head and neck
Lung
Stomach
Kidney
Uterine
Ovarian
Colon
Bladder
Lymphoma
Melanoma

Data from Mortimer, P.S. (1998). Management of skin problems: Medical aspects. In D. Doyle, G.W.C. Hanks, & N. MacDonald (Eds.). *Oxford textbook of palliative medicine* (2nd ed., pp. 617-627). New York: Oxford University Press; Crosby, D.L. (1998). Treatment and tumor-related skin disorders. In A.M. Berger, R.K. Portenoy, & D.E. Weissman (Eds.). *Principles and practice of supportive oncology* (pp. 251-264). Philadelphia: Lippincott-Raven; and Waller, A. & Caroline, N.L. (2000). *Handbook of palliative care in cancer*. Boston: Butterworth-Heinemann.

lesions infiltrate the epithelium and supporting lymph and blood vessels, interfering with blood flow and the supply of oxygen and nutrients to the tissues, leading to ulceration (Haisfield-Wolfe & Baxendale-Cox, 1999; Mortimer, 1998). Capillary rupture, necrosis, and infection are common, leading to a purulent, friable, and malodorous ulceration (Foltz, 1980; Mortimer, 1998).

Infections in MCWs may be caused by both anaerobic and aerobic pathogens. Anaerobic organisms proliferate in necrotic tissue. The foul-smelling odor of many of the MCWs is due to the release of malodorous volatile fatty acids as metabolic end-products of anaerobic activity (Mortimer, 1998). These wounds can readily become infected with aerobic organisms and produce yellow to green purulent discharge.

Skin Tears

Skin tears are acute traumatic wounds that occur when the epidermis separates from the dermis (Malone, Rozario, Gavinski et al., 1991). Most skin tears are found on the arms and legs, especially over areas of senile purpura (areas where blood vessels become more purple as an individual ages) (Malone et al., 1991; McGough-Csarny & Kopac, 1998; Payne & Martin, 1990). Skin tears can be very distressing for the patient. This can occur from something as simple as tape used to hold an intravenous line. With age, the subcutaneous tissue decreases and leaves the skin very thin and easy to tear. The main concern is often pain control.

ASSESSMENT AND MEASUREMENT

Risk Assessment

Two validated risk assessment tools that are used in the United States to identify persons at risk for the development of pressure ulcers are the Braden Scale (www.braden-scale.com/braden.pdf) and the Norton Scale (AHRQ, 1992). Although the onset of risk score differs, both scales produce risk scores based on known risk factors, such as mobility, mental status, and moisture. The Centers for Medicaid and Medicare Services (CMS) (2004) also advises that prevention strategies must be implemented for persons with low scores in any risk assessment subscale. These risk scales are readily available in the published guidelines from the AHRQ as well as the newer pressure ulcer guidelines from the Wound Ostomy and Continence Nurses Society (WOCN) (2003). It is important to reassess risk on admission and at intervals, especially in the palliative care setting, where declining functional status and nutritional impairment are anticipated.

Skin Assessment

Do not confuse a skin assessment with a wound assessment. The CMS has provided clinicians with a minimal standard for skin assessment in the recently revised guidance to surveyors for long-term care facilities, Tag F 314 (CMS, 2004). This includes assessing the skin for temperature, color, moisture, turgor, and integrity. Skin assessment should be done on admission, discharge, and weekly. Skin tears and stage I ulcers may be in places that cannot be seen on quick assessment and can be missed. It is important not only to look at the patient's skin but also to assess pressure areas related to, for example, the wheelchair, bed, linens, stockings, and so on.

Wound Assessment

When any type of ulceration is present, documentation of the degree of tissue destruction is an important aspect of wound assessment. Pressure ulcers, MCWs, and skin tears each have their own classification systems. The current staging system for pressure ulcers from the NPUAP 2001) is as follows:

- *Stage I:* Observable, pressure-related alteration of intact skin whose indicators as compared to an adjacent or opposite area on the body may include changes in one or more of the following parameters: skin temperature (warmth or coolness), tissue consistency (firm or boggy feel), and sensation (pain, itching). The ulcer appears as a defined area of persistent redness in lightly pigmented skin; in darker skin tones, the ulcer may appear with persistent red, blue, or purple hues.
- *Stage II:* Partial-thickness skin loss involving epidermis and/or dermis. The ulcer is superficial and presents clinically as an abrasion, a blister, or a shallow crater.
- *Stage III:* Full-thickness skin loss involving damage or necrosis of subcutaneous tissue that may extend down to, but not through, underlying fascia. The ulcer presents clinically as a deep crater with or without undermining of adjacent tissue.
- *Stage IV:* Full-thickness skin loss with extensive destruction, tissue necrosis, or damage to muscle, bone, or supporting structures (e.g., tendon or joint capsules). Undermining and sinus tracts also may be associated with stage IV pressure ulcers.

Because the depth of tissue destruction cannot be seen in necrotic pressure ulcers, these wounds are categorized as "unstageable" in acute or home care. CMS requires necrotic pressure ulcers to be documented as stage IV in long term care (CMS, 2004).

NPUAP raised the issue of problems with the stage I and II definitions at their 2005 consensus conference (Ankrom, Bennett, Sprigle et al., 2005). At present, NPUAP recommends that a new type of pressure ulcer, deep tissue injury (DTI), does not fit into the current staging system and is working on how best to stage it (Black & NPUAP, 2005). The NPUAP Website (www.npuap.org) provides up-to-date information about DTI.

A special type of pressure ulcer that is seen during the last few weeks of life and signals impending death is called the Kennedy terminal ulcer (Kennedy, 1989). Based on research findings, it is pear shaped with irregular borders; the tissue is red, yellow, or black; onset is sudden; it is usually found on the coccyx or sacrum; and death is imminent (occurring within 2 weeks to several months) (Kennedy, 1989; www.kennedyterminalulcer.com).

Staging of Malignant Cutaneous Wounds

Recognizing that the staging system for pressure ulcers does not necessarily apply to assessment of MCWs, Haisfield-Wolfe and Baxendale-Cox (1999) developed and tested a specific staging system for these lesions, which is presented in Table 35-1. The purpose of this scale is to clarify communication among health care professionals to improve patient care, consultation, and comparison of research results. Haisfield-Wolfe and Baxendale-Cox (1999) used digital photography as an adjunct to observation to assess and record the MCW accurately on initial assessment and follow-up.

Classifying Skin Tears

Skin tears have a separate classification system that has three categories based on the amount of tissue lost. In category I skin tears, there is no loss of the epidermal flap.

Category II skin tears have partial loss of the epidermal flap, while in category III there is complete loss of the epidermal skin flap (Payne & Martin, 1990, 1993).

Wound Assessment Variables

Staging or classification of wounds is only one part of wound assessment. Photographic documentation may be helpful in assessing and monitoring all types of ulcerative lesions (Miller, 1998). In addition to the stage of pressure ulcer, CMS (2004) requires the following minimal assessment of the wound:

- Location
- Size of the wound
  - Length and width are measured, using established landmarks for measurement.
  - Depth is noted at the deepest point. This is measured by inserting a sterile applicator into the deepest area, holding or marking the applicator stick at the skin surface level, and measuring from the tip of the stick to the mark.
- Exudate
  - Color and consistency of the drainage are documented. Drainage may be serous, sanguineous, serosanguineous, or purulent.
  - Amount of drainage is noted. It may be described (1) verbally, as scant, moderate, large, or copious; (2) in terms of the number of soaked dressings; or (3) by weight of the dressings.
- Pain
  - Pain at the site may indicate infection, tissue destruction, or vascular insufficiency. The absence of pain may indicate nerve damage (Hess, 1999).
- Color and type of wound bed tissue
  - Red or pink color generally indicates clean, healthy granulation tissue.
  - Yellow may be the result of infection-related exudate or necrotic slough.
  - Black tissue indicates eschar from necrosis.
  - Some wounds have mixed colors. Clinicians use one of two approaches in documenting the color of mixed wounds: (1) use the least desirable color or (2) estimate the percentage of each color within the wound (Hess, 1999). For clear communication, the palliative care team should adopt one of these two approaches as a standard.
- Description of wound edges and surrounding tissue
  - Color and condition of the skin surrounding the pressure ulcer are noted (Hess, 1999).
  - Temperature of the intact skin is also noted. Heat is a sign of pressure ulcer formation and can also indicate an underlying infection (Hess, 1999).

Some clinicians go beyond these minimal documentation requirements and include the following additional wound characteristics:

- Tunneling, which is tissue destruction under intact skin, is also noted and measured. It is measured by inserting a sterile applicator into tunneled areas, holding or marking the applicator stick at the wound edge, and measuring from the tip of the stick to the mark.
- Odor is also noted. Wound odor may be described as pungent, strong, foul, fecal, or musty.

HISTORY AND PHYSICAL EXAMINATION

Medical history identifies those persons who have diseases that create skin integrity risks, such as heart disease, peripheral vascular disease, diabetes, and cancer. Past treatments that may affect skin integrity and wound healing, such as radiation therapy or extensive surgery, are also important aspects of the patient's history. In addition, the advanced practice nurse (APN) assesses the patient's activity level, mobility, level of consciousness, nutritional status, and hydration status. Many of these factors are included in the risk assessment tools described.

The routine skin inspection includes observing for any areas of discomfort, redness, edema, or ulceration, paying special attention to bony prominences, heels (Figure 35-1), and elbows. Some patients with cancer can have a dehiscence of their wound. In addition, for persons at risk for MCWs, the skin is inspected for the presence of any new nodules, especially in the same general region as the primary tumor. The presence of incontinence or excessive diaphoresis must also be noted for all patients.

When an ulcerative lesion is present at initial assessment, a history of the lesion is important, including how long it has been present, previous treatments for the lesion, the effectiveness of these treatments, and the psychosocial effect of the lesion on the patient and family (Miller, 1998).

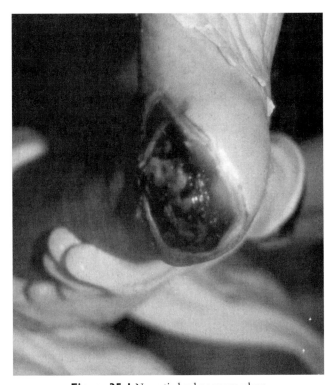

Figure 35-1 Necrotic heel pressure ulcer.

DIAGNOSTICS

On occasion, wound cultures may be appropriate to determine the exact organism causing an infection, to guide subsequent more-specific interventions. Orders must be written to obtain cultures for both aerobic and anaerobic organisms. It is often appropriate to forgo cultures and treat the likely infection on the basis of the appearance and odor of the exudate as recommended in the Clinical Signs and Symptoms checklist developed to identify infection in chronic wounds (Gardner, Frantz, Troia et al., 2001).

INTERVENTION AND TREATMENT

At a CMS meeting (www.cms.hhs.gov/transmittals/downloads/R4SOM.pdf), it was recommended that the usual care of chronic wounds include the following elements:
1. Debridement
2. Cleansing
3. Dressings
4. Compression (venous ulcers only)
5. Antibiotics
6. Pressure redistribution and offloading
7. Team care
8. Nutrition

Prevention of Pressure Ulcers

- Document the risk assessment and initiate prevention protocols based on levels of risk (Ayello & Braden, 2002).
- Assess skin routinely; the frequency depends on the risk assessment. For persons who are relatively inactive, daily inspection by the nurse and/or primary caregiver is recommended.
- Keep the skin clean and free of excessive external moisture:
- Use mild cleansers that minimize irritation and dryness.
- Treat dry skin with moisturizers.
- If there is incontinence, perspiration, or drainage, use padding or dressing materials that whisk moisture away from skin rather than keeping the moisture against the skin, causing maceration (WOCN, 2003).
- Use skin barriers (creams, ointments, pastes, films, hydrocolloids, and film-forming products) to protect and maintain the skin's integrity (WOCN, 2003).
- Prevent friction and shear injuries:
  - Use proper positioning and careful transfer and turning techniques. Two-person lifts using the bed sheets or a pad for turning and lifting are very helpful. Overhead trapezes can also be of assistance if the patient is able to use this device.
  - Friction can also be reduced by using lubricants, such as corn starch or petroleum jelly, polyurethane thin film dressings, or hydrocolloids, over heels and elbows or protective padding, such as sleeves and heel or elbow protectors.
- Encourage dietary intake with sufficient protein, calories, vitamins, minerals, and fluids. Vitamin and zinc supplements are indicated when a deficiency is present.

- Encourage mobility or range-of-motion exercise as appropriate for the patient's physical condition.
- Reduce pressure on tissues:
  ▶ Teach the patient and caregiver the importance of turning and repositioning at least every 2 hours. Pain management may be an important part of getting a patient to turn and reposition. If a patient and/or caregivers decide that turning and repositioning cause too much discomfort for the patient, it should be clearly explained to them the consequences to the skin with pressure ulcer formation. An understanding of this by the patient and family needs to be documented.
  ▶ Active or passive range-of-motion exercises can also be used to relieve pressure and to maintain muscle tone.
  ▶ Prevent positioning on the trochanter.
  ▶ Use supports, such as wedges, pillows, and heel supports.
  ▶ Persons who are at high risk may benefit from using a special pressure-redistributing device, such as air-filled overlays, alternating air-filled mattress overlays, foam-, gel- or water-filled mattress overlays, and specialty mattresses and beds (AHRQ, 1992; Hess, 1999).
  ▶ Prevent the pressure of chair sitting by teaching patients to shift their weight every 15 minutes, if they are able, or by instructing caregivers to reposition the patient in the chair at least every hour. Pressure-reducing devices, such as foam, gel, or air chair pads, may also be used.
  ▶ Instruct caregivers not to use doughnut-type devices.
- Prevent other mechanical tissue damage. Evidence suggests that massage over bony prominences may actually lead to deep tissue trauma and increase the risk of pressure ulcers (AHRQ, 1992). All caregivers need to be instructed not to massage any reddened areas.

Preventing and Treating Skin Tears

There is no universal protocol for preventing skin tears (Baranoski, 2000, 2001). Clinicians (Baranoski, 2000, 2001; Baranoski & Ayello, 2004) have suggested the following interventions to help prevent skin tears:

- Have patient wear long sleeves and pants to protect the skin over these at-risk areas.
- Pad the chair arm and wheelchair leg supports.
- Use the least potentially disruptive method of securing a dressing or drain to a person's skin. This might include paper tape or nonadherent dressings, gauze wrap, and tube securing devices.
- Avoid rubbing or scrubbing the skin during bathing and cleansing activities.
- Use no-rinse bathing products with emollients; limit use of nonemollient soap and alcohol products on the skin.
- Pat the skin dry rather than rubbing the skin dry.
- Apply moisturizing products to treat xerosis (dry) skin.
- Gently handle skin when turning and positioning patients; lift rather than drag skin.

Skin tears can be painful. Various treatments are used for skin tears, including the following:

- Initially the tear is cleansed with normal saline, wound cleanser or other solution, then patted dry.

■ The edges of the tear are approximated if possible. Some clinicians choose thin hydrocolloid or film dressings, when there is minimal exudate. If there is increased exudate, hydrofiber or calcium alginate dressings may be first applied to the skin tear and then covered with the thin hydrocolloid or film. Other choices include composite dressings if there is increased exudate; these come with adhesive or nonadhesive borders. Some of the adhesive dressings are designed for fragile skin. These dressings, as well as the hydrocolloid and composite dressings, may stay in place up to 7 days. The film dressings may stay in place for 3 to 5 days. It is best to check the package inserts for specific directions regarding the products. Any dressing should be changed when loose or leaking or when there is an odor. Clinicians are encouraged to use adhesive remover wipes when using any adhesive products; this lessens the chance of additional skin damage and often decreases the pain of dressing removal.

■ Another approach to skin tears includes applying hydrogel to minimally exuding wounds. Sometimes health care providers cover this with an Adaptic (nonadhering dressing; Johnson & Johnson)-type product, to decrease chances of the wound adhering to the dressing. This can also decrease pain. Others top the hydrogel with gauze if there is no worry of further skin damage. Telfa (nonadhering dressing; Kendall)-type products have also been used, often in conjunction with antibiotic ointment or hydrogel. At times, Telfa is the only treatment. If there is increased drainage, hydrofiber or calcium alginate dressings have been used and topped with gauze. Dressings are usually changed daily with these approaches and more often if necessary.

Treatment of Malignant Cutaneous Wounds

An ulceration that is confined to local recurrence may be treated by one or a combination of the following: surgery, radiation therapy, chemotherapy, or hyperthermia. However, lesions that recur only locally are rare in end-of-life care; most skin ulcerations are a manifestation of a disseminated disease. Hormonal manipulation may shrink some lesions associated with metastatic breast cancer. Most often, the care is directed to minimizing infection, bleeding, and odor (Foltz, 1980; Goodman et al., 1993; Miller, 1998).

Care and Dressing of Ulcerations

All ulcerative lesion treatment plans include instructions for the cleansing solution, frequency of cleansing, type of dressing materials, and frequency of dressing changes. In addition, each includes a time frame for reevaluation (Hess, 1999). Consultation with a wound, ostomy, continence nurse (formerly known as an enterostomal therapist) is helpful when treating particularly challenging wounds.

■ Irrigate the wound to flush out cellular debris and drainage. Wounds are irrigated at time of dressing changes.

▶ Use normal saline solution or water for a wound with no signs of infection. A 35-ml syringe with a 19-gauge needle or angiocatheter delivers adequate pressure. Bulb syringe, gravity drip through intravenous tubing, or piston syringe with rubber catheter attached may be used but may not deliver adequate pressure for thorough irrigation.

- The type of dressing often guides the frequency. For example, hydrocolloid dressings may be changed only once a week. Infected or draining wounds may require more frequent dressing changes.
- Use one of the following for short-term treatment of infected and foul-smelling wounds. All of these solutions are toxic to fibroblasts, inhibiting wound healing (Hess, 1999). The solutions must be rinsed from the wound with normal saline solution. Use these solutions for infected wounds only and discontinue after infection is adequately treated:
  - Acetic acid solution is effective for *Pseudomonas* infection (Hess, 1999). This solution can be made from equal parts of vinegar and water (Foltz, 1980).
  - Hydrogen peroxide works for mechanical cleansing, helping to dissolve and remove crusted exudate.
  - Povidone-iodine can be used for its broad-spectrum antimicrobial action (Hess, 1999).
  - Sodium hypochlorite solution (Dakin's solution) is effective for staphylo-coccal and streptococcal infections (Hess, 1999). It may also be helpful for managing odor. This solution can be made by using one part of household bleach to nine parts of water (Foltz, 1980).

- Debridement is performed to remove necrotic tissue and promote healing (Walker, 1996; Hess, 1999). When healing is anticipated, this is a necessary step. The clinician must, of course, be cautious of the wound with poor arterial flow and consult a vascular surgeon as appropriate. In the palliative care setting, complete healing of a pressure ulcer is not always possible, and healing of an MCW is next to impossible. Consider the purpose and potential outcomes of debridement for each individual. When removal of necrotic tissue will decrease infection, reduce inflammation, and improve comfort, debridement is appropriate. If the debridement procedure itself causes significant discomfort, the removal of the "protective" layer of eschar causes prolonged pain or active bleeding, or the patient is not likely to live long enough to derive benefit, debridement may not be appropriate. Different types of debridement are available, and often a combination of them is used to achieve adequate wound debridement and wound bed preparation.
  - Surgical debridement is the quickest method but may be the most uncomfortable. It may require general anesthesia. Pain management is an important issue.
  - Mechanical debridement includes the use of wet-to-dry dressings to pull necrotic tissue from the wound. It may be helpful for removing encrusted, purulent materials. The disadvantage of this method is that it is nonselective: healthy tissue is also removed with the dry dressings and it is painful. Hydrotherapy and wound irrigation are other examples of mechanical debridement.
  - Enzymatic debridement is the use of topical enzymes to digest necrotic tissue. These products can be very effective. Some enzymes are selective and are specific to collagen, whereas others are nonselective and will break down many types of proteins. These medications can be expensive, so the ability of the family to pay for the prescription may be a consideration. Enzymes that have been used for this purpose include collagenase (Santyl) and papain-urea ointments (Accuzyme [also available as a spray], Gladase, Kovia, and others). It is important to read

the manufacturer's directions specific to each type of enzyme for correct method and frequency of application (Ayello & Cuddigan, 2004).

▶ Autolytic debridement is the use of the body's enzymes and white blood cells to remove the necrotic tissue. Many dressings are designed to promote this process (Ayello & Cuddigan, 2004; Hess, 1999; Walker, 1996), including transparent films, hydrocolloids, semipermeable polyurethane foams, and hydrogels.

▶ Maggot debridement therapy (MDT) has been revived as a debridement option after being out of use for many years. Beginning evidence points to better patient outcomes when free-range technique rather than contained maggots are used (Steenvoorde, Jacobi & Oskam, 2005).

■ Clean the skin around the wound with normal saline solution or plain water.

■ Pack deep wounds, being careful not to pack too tightly; the dressing needs to be flexible enough to touch all wound surfaces:

▶ Any solution used on the packing materials must be nontoxic to cells. A possible exception is the use of wet-to-dry dressings moistened with Dakin's solution for infection and odor control. However, as mentioned, both the procedure and the solution are cytotoxic and its use should be limited (CMS, 2004).

▶ Wounds that require packing or fillers of any kind generally require a secondary dressing.

■ Select a dressing that promotes a moist, but not wet, environment. The wound characteristics (stage, depth, location, and the amount of drainage) help guide the selection of the appropriate dressing:

▶ Use moisture-retentive dressings for wounds that have light to moderate drainage. Examples for stage I or II ulcers include polyurethane transparent film dressings, hydrocolloids, and foam. Hydrofiber or calcium alginate may be used under these dressings to control moderate exudate. For stage III and IV ulcers, both a primary and a secondary dressing are often required. The primary dressing comes in contact with the wound first. Hydrogels may be used for the dry wound, whereas hydrofiber and calcium alginate are used to absorb exudate from the draining wound. These are then topped with the secondary dressing, which may be a hydrocolloid, foam, composite, or other type of cover dressing. Gauze or abdominal pad dressings are also used as the secondary dressing.

▶ Use absorbent dressings such as foam, calcium alginates, or hydrofiber for wounds with moderate to heavy drainage. There are many excellent products on the market, both absorbent wound fillers and absorbent dressings:

• If wound drainage is less than 50 ml/day, an absorbent dressing may be sufficient.

• If wound drainage is greater than 50 ml/day, a wound drainage bag or pouch may be helpful. Use of a drainage collection system allows accurate measurement of drainage, decreases dressing changes, decreases contamination, improves comfort, and protects surrounding skin (Hess, 1999). A good seal around any appliance used to collect drainage is important. Stomahesive paste or a similar product may be helpful to fill in creases or indentations in the skin and improve the seal (Miller, 1998). Pouching is an effective way of managing patients who develop fistulas. A WOCN nurse can provide insight about the most cost-effective type of drainage bag and sealant to use.

- Keep in mind that sterile absorbent dressings are more expensive than clean absorbent materials. Sanitary pads and disposable diapers are made to be absorbent and may be used as secondary dressings when the APN determines that a clean dressing is sufficient (Goodman et al., 1993).
  - ▶ Dry wounds may benefit from use of one of the many hydrogels available. Most are amphorous gels and others are available as sheets of dressing materials.
  - ▶ A new method of wound dressing is the wound vacuum-assisted closure. This is intended for pressure ulcers, flaps, diabetic ulcers, and chronic wounds. It is not appropriate for MCWs. The purpose of this device is to promote wound closure by exerting a continuous and/or intermittent negative pressure on the wound. This pressure is typically kept on 22 of 24 hours each day (KCI, 2005).
- Protect surrounding skin.
  - ▶ Remove all dressings carefully to prevent damage to surrounding tissue. An acetone-free adhesive remover or baby oil may be helpful in removing old adherent dressings.
  - ▶ When significant drainage necessitates frequent dressing changes, avoid using tape to secure dressings if possible. Options include gauze wrap bandages, flexible netting or stretch elastic bands (e.g., tube tops), and Montgomery straps. Another option is to place strips of hydrocolloid strategically around the wound and tape to the hydrocolloid rather than to the patient's skin.
  - ▶ Skin sealants, petroleum-based products, and other water-resistant products such as protective barrier ointments may be used to protect the surrounding skin from wound drainage.
- Control bleeding. MCWs are especially prone to bleeding as a result of the disruption of the capillary bed. The selection of an intervention depends on the degree of oozing and patient tolerance.
  - ▶ Reduce any trauma to the tissue by keeping the wound moist and using nonadherent dressings if needed. If dressings become too dry, it may be helpful to moisten with saline solution before removal (Goodman et al., 1993). Another option may be to have the patient shower in order to loosen the dressing. Calcium alginate and hydrofiber dressings may be effective in stopping minor bleeding. Wet-to-dry dressings should be avoided.
  - ▶ Pressure may be applied to visible bleeding vessels, but only if the underlying structures can support the force (Foltz, 1980; Waller & Caroline, 2000).
  - ▶ Silver nitrate sticks can be used for pinpoint capillary oozing (Foltz, 1980).
  - ▶ Gauze soaked in 1:1000 epinephrine can be applied over areas of bleeding (Waller & Caroline, 2000).
  - ▶ Coagulant dressings, such as absorbable gelatin (Gelfoam), or QR Powder (www.biolife.com) are helpful for multiple areas of oozing.
  - ▶ Sucralfate paste is another option for widespread oozing. Crush a 1-g sucralfate tablet and mix with 2 to 3 ml of water or soluble gel (Waller & Caroline, 2000).
  - ▶ Radiation therapy is also an option for some patients (Mortimer, 1998).
- Control odor, which is often a problem with MCWs. This is most likely caused by infection in necrotic tissue and can be minimized if the lesion can be adequately cleansed and debrided or the infection treated with a bacteriostatic agent.

Additional measures that filter or mask the odor are beneficial when other interventions do not eliminate it:

▶ Topical metronidazole is active against anaerobic bacterial infections and has been demonstrated to be helpful in controlling wound odor (Finlay, Bowszyc, Ramlau et al, 1996; Poteete, 1993; Rice, 1992). Most studies use metronidazole 0.75% to 0.8% gel. Some practitioners report that use of metronidazole (parenteral) solution to irrigate wounds controls odor well (McMullen, 1992). Metronidazole irrigation has not been studied to compare its effectiveness and cost with those of topical gel.

▶ Sodium hypochlorite solution can be used for its debriding and bacteriostatic properties, either in irrigation or on wet-to-dry dressings (Foltz, 1980; Hess, 1999). Use with caution, however, as it is very irritating to healthy tissues (both in and around the wound) and interferes with blood clotting.

▶ A chlorophyll-containing ointment applied to the wound or chlorophyll tablets taken orally may be helpful (Goodman et al., 1993), although no studies have compared the effectiveness of this intervention with that of the others discussed.

▶ Some dressings are designed to filter odors with a carbon-and-charcoal layer. Some products on the market are combination dressings, with both absorptive and carbon-filtering layers. Until comparative studies are available, the APN must determine the best product with respect to amount of drainage, size of wound, ease of use, and cost. The following are dressings with carbon layers (Hess, 1999):
  • Lyofoam C Polyurethane Foam Dressing with Activated Carbon (ConvaTec) is designed to neutralize odors on wounds with light or moderate exudate.
  • CarboFlex Odor Control (ConvaTec) is designed for odor control on wounds with light or moderate exudate.
  • Odor-Absorbent Dressing (Hollister) is designed for odor control on dry wounds or as a secondary dressing over an absorbent dressing if there is exudate.

▶ Home remedies for controlling odor include honey, sugar, yogurt, or buttermilk in wounds (Goodman et al., 1993; Miller, 1998). No studies have evaluated the effectiveness of these treatments.

▶ Deodorizers can be used to mask odors. These often have odors of their own, which may or may not be desirable to the patient:
  • Some deodorizers (e.g., Banish, Hexon) can be used sparingly on dressings.
  • Room deodorizers, including commercial products, scented candles, and scented oils (e.g., spirit of wintergreen), may be used.
  • Some clinicians report using pans of charcoal briquettes under the bed to assist in absorbing room odor. No studies have reported on the effectiveness of this approach.

▶ Treat pain. Depending on the severity of the pain, the APN may select a local treatment, a systemic analgesic, or a combination of several interventions.
  • Aluminum hydroxide–magnesium hydroxide suspension (Maalox) or yogurt applied to the wound may relieve burning sensations (Waller & Caroline, 2000). However, Maalox can be drying, and yogurt can be messy and require frequent dressing and linen changes. The reports of using these interventions are anecdotal; no research has documented their effectiveness.

- Topical morphine made with 5 mg of morphine solution in 5 ml of neutral gel is an option for severe wound pain (Waller & Caroline, 2000).
- Since some of the pain is due to inflammation, systemic nonsteroidal anti-inflammatory drugs (NSAIDs) are appropriate. For moderate to severe pain, an opioid analgesic may be required.

PATIENT AND FAMILY EDUCATION

The patient and family require instruction in the prevention and management of ulcerative lesions (Tomaselli, 2005). A comprehensive teaching plan includes the following:
- Teach general assessment and skin care measures:
  - Inspect the skin daily for redness, irritation, or breakdown.
  - Keep the skin clean and prevent excessive dryness:
    - Avoid hot water, use a mild cleanser, and minimize force and friction on skin (AHRQ, 1992).
    - Keep air humidified.
    - Use a moisturizer on the skin.
    - Clean the patient as soon as possible if there is urinary or bowel incontinence.
  - Avoid massage over bony prominences.
  - Keep the bed and bed clothing clean and dry. Use incontinence pads as necessary.
- Teach measures to reduce pressure and friction:
  - Use heel and elbow protectors.
  - Use a recommended special mattress and overlay.
  - Position the patient to prevent pressure, using pillows, wedges, or other padding. Prevent positioning of the patient on the trochanter.
  - Keep the head of the bed at its lowest comfortable position to prevent shearing that can occur when the patient slides down in bed.
  - Use good technique when lifting, using two-person lifts whenever possible. Use lift pads instead of dragging the patient. Add an overhead trapeze to the bed when feasible.
- Teach appropriate wound cleansing and dressing techniques for those situations in which the family will be providing some of the wound care. Teaching should include demonstration, verbal instruction, and return demonstration. Ensure that the caregiver is comfortable with the procedure. Issues to be addressed in the teaching plan include the following:
  - Preparation and storage of cleansing solution
  - Cleansing techniques for wound and surrounding skin
  - Use of all dressing products, including fillers and secondary dressings
  - Appropriate disposal of soiled dressing materials
- Teach the patient and family to report any changes to their health care team:
  - Changes in wound size, color, drainage, or odor
  - Changes in the appearance of surrounding skin
  - Signs of discomfort

EVALUATION AND PLAN FOR FOLLOW-UP

The APN monitors for changes in any of the wound assessment variables from the baseline and changes the intervention plan accordingly. For pressure ulcers, the Pressure Ulcer Scale for Healing (PUSH) (www.novartisnutrition.com/pdfs/us/moreproduct-info/PUSH_Tool_03.pdf) can be a way of monitoring wound progress. The goal of care is determined by the underlying cause and the patient's overall condition. It may not be appropriate to expect wound healing because of the poor nutritional status and impaired circulation many patients have at end-of-life. Under these circumstances, the goals may be to prevent or minimize progression and to prevent infection. For patients with MCWs in end-of-life care, the goal is to promote physical and psychoemotional comfort by managing pain, drainage, infection, and odor.

The entire team is involved in the planning, intervention, and evaluation process. Support from the physical therapist, occupational therapist, pharmacist, social workers/counselors, home health aides, clergy, and volunteers is required to address the many needs of the patient and family. Consultation with a certified wound specialist is extremely helpful when facing particularly challenging wounds.

CASE STUDY

Mrs. J. is 83 years old and has a diagnosis of metastatic breast cancer. She has an extensive fungating tumor wound covering most of the right side of her chest. The skin is reddish purple from the clavicle to the bottom of the rib cage and from the axilla to the sternum, and there are multiple raised, hard nodules across the chest. There are multiple areas where the skin appears to have surface abrasions, and there is an open wound located about 5 cm from the sternum and 15 cm from the clavicle that measures 10 cm across and 8 cm down. The wound bed is light red around the edges, but about 60% of the wound is covered by a yellowish, stringy, purulent material. The wound is deepest at the sternal margin and measures 1.5 cm. No tunneling is observed and there is no bleeding. The patient reports that the wound is not painful, but the foul odor is "driving her and her family crazy." She has been cleaning the wound with soap and water using a gauze pad and covering it with a gauze dressing. There is a moderate amount of serosanguineous drainage noted. Mrs. J. reports the gauze gets soaked and needs to be changed four or five times each day. She also says that the surface abrasions surrounding the wound were caused by the tape.

The clinician determines that this is a stage III MCW. She recommends initially using Dakin's solution for infection control followed by rinsing with normal saline solution for 3 days. After the first 3 days, saline solution only is to be used for wound cleansing. The surrounding skin is cleaned with normal saline solution and a protective skin barrier is applied around the wound to protect the skin from drainage. Metronidazole 0.75% gel is applied topically to the wound bed. A wet-to-damp gauze dressing is selected, and saline solution is used to wet the gauze, which is then fluffed to fill the wound lightly. This dressing is covered with a gauze pad, which is reinforced with a sanitary napkin. An elastic "tube top" is used to secure the dressing in place to prevent tape from touching the sensitive skin.

After 1 week the clinician reassesses the wound and finds that only about 20% of it shows signs of slough and the odor has decreased. The padding has been sufficient to control the drainage during the day, but the dressing is sometimes soaked through by morning. The cleansing and dressing procedures are continued and additional padding by sanitary napkins used at night. After another week, the metronidazole gel is discontinued as the wound odor is no longer a problem. The clinician changes the dressing procedure to cleansing with normal saline solution, filling the wound bed with an alginate because of the amount of exudate, covering the alginate with a gauze pad to fit the wound, and covering the gauze with a pad. The dressing is secured with the tube top, and the caregiver is instructed to change the dressing every 3 days or when there are signs of moisture on the pad. (If the surrounding tissue was healthy and could tolerate the adhesive, a hydrocolloid wound filler and dressing might have been selected at this point. This type of dressing might allow for more time between dressing changes.)

A month later the wound is larger, now measuring 11 cm by 8.5 cm. The wound bed is 90% pink and drainage is moderate. The dressing requires changing every 2 days, but these procedures are becoming more difficult because Mrs. J. is weaker and maneuvering the tube top for dressing changes requires much effort by both Mrs. J. and her caregiver. To make securing the dressing easier, the clinician applies four 2 × 5-cm strips of hydrocolloid dressing wafers to the healthy skin at the four corners of the wound and tapes the dressing in place, using the hydrocolloid wafer as the tape anchor.

REFERENCES

Agency for Healthcare Research and Quality (AHRQ). (1992). *Pressure ulcers in adults: Prediction and prevention: Clinical practice guideline number 3.* Rockville, Md.: Author.

Ankrom, M., Bennett, R., Sprigle, S., et al.; National Pressure Ulcer Advisory Panel. (2005). Pressure-related deep tissue injury under intact skin and the current ulcer staging systems. *Adv Skin Wound Care, 18(1),* 35-42.

Ayello, E.A. & Braden, B. (2002). How and why to do pressure ulcer risk assessment. *Adv Wound Care, 15(3),* 125-131.

Ayello, E.A. & Cuddigan, J.E. (2004). Conquer chronic wounds with wound bed preparation. *Nurse Pract, 29(3),* 8-25.

Baranoski, S. (2000). Skin tears: The enemy of frail skin. *Adv Skin Wound Care, 13(3),* 123-126.

Baranoski, S. (2001). Skin tears: Guard against this enemy of frail skin. *Nurs Manage, 32(8),* 25-31.

Baranoski, S. & Ayello, E.A. (2004). *Wound care essentials: Practice principles.* Springhouse, Pa.: Lippincott Williams & Wilkins.

Black, J. & National Pressure Ulcer Advisory Panel. (2005). Moving toward consensus on deep tissue injury and pressure ulcer staging. *Adv Skin Wound Care, 18(8),* 415-421.

Centers for Medicare and Medicaid Services (CMS). (2004). *CMS manual for guidance to surveyors for long term care facilities, Tag F 314.* Retrieved August 10, 2006, from www.cms.hhs.gov/mcd/viewmcac.asp?where=&what=&from=&mid=28&basketitem=mcac:28: Usual%20Care%20of%20Chronic%20Wounds:3/29/2005.

Crosby, D.L. (1998). Treatment and tumor-related skin disorders. In A.M. Berger, R.K. Portenoy, & D.E. Weissman (Eds.). *Principles and practice of supportive oncology* (pp. 251-264). Philadelphia: Lippincott-Raven.

Ferris, F. D., Khateib, A.A.A., et al. (2004). *Palliative wound care: managing chronic wounds across life's continuum.* A consensus statement from the International Palliative Wound Care Initiative.

Finlay, I.G., Bowszyc, J., Ramlau, C., et al. (1996). The effect of topical 0.75% metronidazole gel on malodorous cutaneous ulcers. *J Pain Symptom Manage, 11,* 158-162.

Foltz, A.T. (1980). Nursing care of ulcerating metastatic lesions. *Oncol Nurs Forum, 7(2),* 8-13.

Gardner, S.E., Frantz, RA., Troia, C., et al. (2001). A tool to assess clinical signs and symptoms of localized chronic wound infection: Development and reliability. *Ostomy Wound Manage, 47(1),* 40-47.

Goodman, M., Ladd, L.A., & Purl, S. (1993). Integumentary and mucous membrane alterations. In S.L. Groenwald, M.H. Frogge, M. Goodman, et al. (Eds.), *Cancer nursing: Principles and practice.* Boston: Jones & Bartlett.

Haisfield-Wolfe, M.E. & Baxendale-Cox, L.M. (1999). Staging of malignant cutaneous wounds: A pilot study. *Oncol Nurs Forum, 26,* 1055-1064.

Hess, C.T. (1999). *Clinical guide: Wound care* (3rd ed.). Springhouse, Pa.: Springhouse Corporation.

KCI. (2005). *How V.A.C. therapy works.* Retrieved July 25, 2006, from www.kci1.com/82.asp.

Kennedy, K.L. (1989). The prevalence of pressure ulcers in an intermediate care facility. *Decubitus, 2(2),* 44-45.

Malone, M.L., Rozario, N., Gavinski, M., et al. (1991). The epidemiology of skin tears in the institutionalized elderly. *J Am Geriatr Soc, 39(6),* 591-595.

McGough-Csarny, J. & Kopac, C.A. (1998). Skin tears in institutionalized elderly: An epidemiological study. *Ostomy Wound Manage, 44(3A suppl),* 14S-24S.

McMullen, D. (1992). Topical metronidazole: Part 2. *Ostomy Wound Manage, 38(3),* 42-46.

Miller, C. (1998). Skin problems in palliative care: Nursing aspects. In D. Doyle, G.W.C. Hanks & N. MacDonald (Eds.), *Oxford textbook of palliative medicine* (2nd ed., pp. 642-656). New York: Oxford University Press.

Mortimer, P.S. (1998). Management of skin problems: Medical aspects. In D. Doyle, G.W.C. Hanks & N. MacDonald (Eds.). *Oxford textbook of palliative medicine* (2nd ed., pp. 617-627). New York: Oxford University Press.

National Pressure Ulcer Advisory Panel (NPUAP), Cuddigan, J., Ayello, E.A., et al. (Eds.). (2001). *Pressure ulcers in America: Prevalence, incidence, and implications for the future.* Reston, Va.: Author.

Payne, R.L. & Martin, M.L. (1990). The epidemiology and management of skin tears in older adults. *Ostomy Wound Manage, 26(1),* 26-37.

Payne, R.L. & Martin, M.L. (1993). Defining and classifying skin tears: Need for a common language. *Ostomy Wound Manage, 39(5),* 16-20, 22-24, 26.

Poteete, V. (1993). Case study: Eliminating odors from wounds. *Decubitus, 6(4),* 43-46.

Rice, T.T. (1992). Metronidazole use in malodorous skin lesions. *Rehabil Nurs, 17,* 244-245, 255.

Steenvoorde, P., Jacobi, C.E. & Oskam, J. (2005). Maggot debridement therapy: Free-range or contained? An in-vivo study. *Adv Skin Wound Care, 18(8),* 430- 435.

Thiers, B.H. (1986). Dermatologic manifestations of cancer. *CA: Cancer J Clin, 36,* 130-148.

Tomaselli, N.L. (2005). Teaching the patient with chronic wound. *Adv Skin Wound Care, 18(7),* 379-387.

Walker, D. (1996). Choosing the correct wound dressing. *Am J Nurs, 96(9),* 35-39.

Waller, A. & Caroline, N. L. (2000). *Handbook of palliative care in cancer.* Boston: Butterworth-Heinemann.

Wound Ostomy and Continence Nurses Society (WOCN). (2003). *Guideline for prevention and management of pressure ulcers.* Number 2 WOCN Clinical Practice Guideline Series. Glenview, Ill.: Author.

CAREGIVER RESOURCES
Crystal Dea Moore
■

National Family Caregivers Association, 537
Other Caregiver Organizations and Websites, 537
Resources to Assist in the Caring for Elders, 538
End-of-Life Planning, Hospice, and Bereavement Information, 538
Financial Help for Health Insurance and Prescription Drugs, 538
Advocacy Assistance for Caregivers, 539
Respite Resources for Caregivers, 540
Books for Caregivers, 540

The list of associations for caregivers was adapted from the Website of The National Family Caregivers Association (NFCA). NFCA serves as a public voice for family caregivers to the press, to the U.S. Congress, and to the general public.

National Family Caregivers Association
   800-896-3650
   www.thefamilycaregiver.org

OTHER CAREGIVER ORGANIZATIONS AND WEBSITES

Children of Aging Parents (CAPS)
   800-227-7294
   www.caps4caregivers.org
   Assists caregivers with information, referrals, and a network of support groups.
Friends' Health Connection
   800-483-7436
   www.48friend.org
   Links persons with others experiencing the same challenges.
National Alliance for Caregiving
   www.caregiving.org
   Videos, pamphlets, etc. reviewed and approved as providing solid information.
Rosalynn Carter Institute for Human Development (RCI)
   229-928-1234
   www.rci.gsw.edu
   Provides educational programs and information and conducts research.
Well Spouse Foundation
   800-838-0879
   www.wellspouse.org
   Gives support to husbands, wives, and partners of the chronically ill and/or disabled.

RESOURCES TO ASSIST IN THE CARING FOR ELDERS

The county office of senior services or elder affairs, area adult day centers, and/or local social service agencies; all provide services to the elderly.

AARP
> 800-424-3410
> www.aarp.org
> Supplies information about caregiving, long-term care, and aging.

Eldercare Locator, National Association of Area Agencies on Aging
> 800-677-1116
> www.n4a.org or www.eldercare.gov
> Provides referrals to Area Agencies on Aging via ZIP code locations.

The National Association of Professional Geriatric Care Managers (GCMs)
> 520-881-8008
> www.caremanager.org

U.S. Administration on Aging
> 202-619-0724
> www.aoa.gov

END-OF-LIFE PLANNING, HOSPICE, AND BEREAVEMENT INFORMATION

Aging with Dignity
> 888-5-WISHES (594-7437)
> www.agingwithdignity.org
> Publishes the Five Wishes Living Will document for advance care planning.

Hospice Foundation of America
> 800-854-3402
> www.hospicefoundation.org

Last Acts
> www.lastacts.org
> Focused on affecting medical and public education, legislation, and more.

National Hospice and Palliative Care Organization
> 800-658-8898
> www.nhpco.org

FINANCIAL HELP FOR HEALTH INSURANCE AND PRESCRIPTION DRUGS

Contact the local Department of Health and Human Services or area social service agencies (e.g., Catholic Charities, Association of Jewish Family and Children's Agencies, local chapters of voluntary health agencies) to find out if they offer any financial support programs and how to apply for them.

Benefits Check-Up and Benefits Check-Up RX
www.benefitscheckup.org
Helps people over 55 find programs that may pay for some medical care and/or prescription costs.

HealthInsurance.com
800-942-9019
www.healthinsurance.com
Provides consumers and small businesses with quotes for health insurance, and may help those who have lost their health insurance find an affordable alternative.

Hill-Burton Free Medical Care Program
800-638-0742
www.hrsa.gov/osp/dfcr
Gives a list of participating facilities that provide some free or below-cost health care services as well as information on eligibility.

Medicine Program
573-996-7300
www.themedicineprogram.com
For persons who do not have insurance for outpatient prescription drugs and who cannot afford to purchase medications at retail prices.

ADVOCACY ASSISTANCE FOR CAREGIVERS

Homecare Agencies, Assisted Living, and Nursing Homes

Consumer Consortium on Assisted Living
703-533-8121:
www.ccal.org

Medicare Rights Center
888-HMO-9050
www.medicarerights.org

National Association for Home Care and Hospice
202-547-7424
www.nahc.org

National Citizens' Coalition for Nursing Home Reform
202-332-2275
www.nccnhr.org

New LifeStyles
800-869-9549
www.NewLifeStyles.com
Publishes free regional directories of nursing homes, assisted living, and retirement communities.

Patient Advocate Foundation
800-532-5274
www.patientadvocate.org
Serves as a liaison between patients and their insurer, employer, and/or creditors to resolve insurance, job retention, and/or debt crisis matters relating to a patient's condition.

Visiting Nurse Associations of America
617-737-3200
www.vnaa.org
Promotes community-based home health care.

RESPITE RESOURCES FOR CAREGIVERS

Easter Seals
800-221-6827
www.easter-seals.org
Provides a variety of services for children and adults with disabilities.

Faith in Action
877-324-8411
www.fiavolunteers.org
Makes grants to local groups representing many faiths who volunteer to work together
to care for their neighbors who have long-term health needs.

National Adult Day Services Association, Inc
866-890-7357
www.nadsa.org

National Respite Locator Service
800-473-1727, ext. 222
www.respitelocator.org/index.htm

Shepherd's Centers of America
800-547-7073
www.shepherdcenters.org
Provides respite care; telephone, in-home, and nursing home visitors; home health
aides; support groups; adult day care; and information and referrals.

BOOKS FOR CAREGIVERS

Houts, P., Bucher, J., & Nezu, A. (2000). *Caregiving: A step-by-step resource for caring for people with cancer at home.* Atlanta: American Cancer Society.

Johnson, A. & Rejnis, R. (1998). *The cost of caring: Money skills for caregivers.* New York: John Wiley and Sons.

Lieberman, T. (2000). *Consumer Reports complete guide to health services for seniors.* New York: Three Rivers Press.

Mace, N. & Rabins, P. (2001). *The 36-hour day: Family guide to caring for persons with Alzheimer's disease and relating dementing illnesses and memory loss in later life* (Revised), New York: Warner Books.

Meyer, M. (2002). *The comfort of home: An illustrated step-by-step guide for caregivers* (2nd ed.). Portland, Ore.: Caretrust Publications.

Mintz, S. (2002). *Love, honor & value.* Sterling, Va.: Capital Books Inc.
A moving book by the president and cofounder of the National Family Caregivers Association that discusses her caregiving experiences and provides valuable resources.

Schacht, M. (2004). *A caregiver's challenge: Living, loving, letting go* (2nd ed.). Santa Rosa, Calif.: Feterson Press.
Offers information and support needed to navigate the stages from initial diagnosis to planning a memorial. Rich with resources, helpful exercises, and questions to explore.

CLINICIAN RESOURCES AND ASSESSMENT TOOLS

Marilyn O'Mallon

■

Resources, 541
Assesment Tools, 546
   Spiritual Well Being Scale, 546
   The Edmonton Labeled Visual Information System (ELVIS), 547
   Memorial Delirium Assessment Scale (MDAS), 548

RESOURCES

Aging with Dignity
   888-5-WISHES
   www.agingwithdignity.org
   National nonprofit organization that promotes human dignity as America ages, with emphasis on improved care for those near the end of life; distributes *Five Wishes*, an easy-to-use advance directive that over 1 million American families have used to discuss how they want to be treated during times of serious illness; has new project to promote *Five Wishes* in the workplace.

American Academy of Hospice and Palliative Medicine
   www.aahpm.org
   An organization of physicians and other health professionals dedicated to the advancement of the practice, research, and education of hospice and palliative medicine.

American Alliance of Cancer Pain Initiatives
   www.aacpi.org
   State-based initiatives and their participants provide education, training, information, and organizational support to health care providers, cancer patients, and their families. The site includes links to all state initiatives, information, e-mail addresses, and a list of professional and patient educational materials available from AACPI and other organizations.

American Hospice Foundation
   202-223-0204
   www.americanhospice.org
   Educational and training materials for schools, the workplace, faith communities, and hospices, including Grief-at-School, Grief-at-Work, Talking about Hospice: Tips for Physicians, Tips for Nurses, and Hospice & Alzheimer's Disease; offers on-site, full-day training workshops for managers, employee assistance professionals, educators, bereavement counselors, and mental health professionals.

American Pain Foundation
www.painfoundation.org
A nonprofit organization representing patients with pain; includes extensive resources for patients, families, and health care professionals regarding pain management and current issues.

American Pain Society
847-375-4715
www.ampainsoc.org
Advances pain-related research, education, treatment, and professional practice; maintains database of pain treatment centers and an Internet resource list for pain professionals.

Americans for Better Care of the Dying
202-895-9485
www.abcd-caring.org
Dedicated to social, professional, and policy reform to improve care for patients with serious illness and their families.

Beth Israel Medical Center: MAYDAY Resource Center for Pain Medicine and Palliative Care
877-620-9999
www.stoppain.org
Serves as a clearinghouse for the dissemination of educational materials in pain medicine and palliative care and as a nucleus of scholarship for physicians, nurses, pharmacists, psychosocial professionals, patients, and family caregivers.

Center to Advance Palliative Care
212-241-7885
www.capcmssm.org
Provides technical assistance to hospital and health systems interested in planning and establishing palliative care services.

City of Hope Pain/Palliative Care Resource Center
626-359-8111, ext 63829
www.prc.coh.org
Serves as a clearinghouse for the dissemination of information on resources that enable individuals and institutions to improve the quality of pain management. The center is a central source for collecting a variety of materials, including pain assessment tools, patient education materials, quality assurance materials, research instruments, and other resources.

Community-State Partnerships Program
816-842-7110
www.midbio.org/npo-about.htm
Promotes broad-based policy reform at the state and community level. Publications include *Making Our Voices Heard: A Guide to Public Engagement*, an 85-page manual; *State Initiatives in End-of-Life Care*, a policy brief series on various topics; and *Media Tactics*, a newsletter. See also the "Pathways Project" on this site.

Compassion Sabbath
816-221-1100

www.midbio.org/cs/index.htm

Interfaith initiative to provide clergy and religious leaders with tools for addressing the spiritual needs of dying people and their families. Resources include the *Compassion Sabbath Resource Kit*, consultation, faculty, networking, and peer contact information.

Decisions Near the End of Life at the Education Development Center (EDC), Inc.
617-969-7100 Ext. 2388

www.edc.org/CAE/Decisions/dnel.html

An institution-based, multidisciplinary quality improvement program in use in over 225 U.S. health care institutions; includes extensive curriculum resources, a needs assessment survey tool, and annotated bibliographies on major topics in end-of-life care. National leadership conferences are held annually for new teams.

Edmonton Regional Palliative Care Program
Edmonton, Alberta, Canada

www.palliative.org

Clinical information including reviews on palliative care topics, listings of publications, a journal watch, palliative care tips for primary care physicians and nurses, and tools for clinical assessment. A patient and family section provides basic information on death, dying, grief, and bereavement.

Education for Physicians on End-of-Life Care
877-524-EPEC (toll free)

www.epec.net

Educates physicians and other members of the interdisciplinary team through its core curriculum on essential clinical competencies required to provide quality end-of-life care. The core curriculum teaches fundamental skills in communication, ethical decision making, palliative care, psychosocial considerations, and pain and symptom management.

End-of-Life Nursing Education Consortium
202-463-6930

www.aacn.nche.edu/elnec

A comprehensive national education program instituted to develop a core of expert nursing educators and to coordinate national nursing efforts in end-of-life care.

End-of-Life Physician Education Resource Center
414-805-4607

www.eperc.mcw.edu

Assists physician educators and others in locating high-quality, peer-reviewed training materials. Search materials are indexed by end-of-life care topics and educational formats.

Family Caregiver Alliance
www.caregiver.org

A nonprofit organization providing support and information for caregivers, including an online support group and specialized information on Alzheimer's disease, stroke, traumatic brain injury, Parkinson's disease, amyotrophic lateral sclerosis, and similar illnesses. Extensive information is also available on every conceivable aspect of caregiving, including end-of-life decision-making conservatorship, and evaluation of research findings. Many resources are available in Spanish and Chinese.

Growth House

www.growthhouse.org

Includes a search engine that offers access to the Internet's most comprehensive collection of reviewed resources for end-of-life care. The Inter-Institutional Collaborating Network (IICN) on end-of-life care links health care organizations through a shared network.

Hospice Foundation of America

202-638-5419

www.hospicefoundation.org

A nonprofit, grassroots foundation promoting the hospice philosophy of care, informing the public about end-of-life options, and training health care workers and the families they serve in issues related to loss, spirituality, and psychosocial issues, including the annual National Living with Grief Teleconference.

Hospice & Palliative Nurses Association

412-361-2470

www.hpna.org

Provides convenient access to current information in the areas of hospice and palliative nursing, including information on conferences and certification of hospice and palliative nurses.

Innovations in End-of-Life Care

www.edc.org/lastacts

An international online journal featuring peer-reviewed examples of promising practices in end-of-life care. Each bimonthly issue focuses on a different theme.

Institute for Healthcare Improvement

www.ihi.org

An independent, nonprofit organization offering resources and services to help health care organizations make long-lasting improvements that enhance clinical outcomes and reduce cost.

International Association for Hospice and Palliative Care

www.hospicecare.com

A nonprofit organization whose mission is to increase the availability and access to high-quality hospice and palliative care worldwide through promoting communication; facilitating and providing education; and providing information for patients, professionals, health care providers, and policy makers.

Last Acts

www.lastacts.org

A national coalition to improve care and caring near end-of-life. The goals of the coalition are to bring death-related issues out in the open and to help individuals and organizations pursue better ways of caring for the dying.

Mayday Pain Project

906-343-6545

www.painandhealth.org

Increases awareness and provides objective information concerning the treatment of pain. The Website is set up as an index for visitors and contains carefully chosen Internet links and resources.

National Hospice and Palliative Care Organization (NHPCO)

703-837-1500

www.nhpco.org

The largest nonprofit membership organization representing U.S. hospice and palliative care programs and professionals. The NHPCO develops public and professional educational programs and materials, convenes meetings and symposia on emerging issues, provides technical informational resources to members, conducts research, monitors congressional and regulatory activities, and works closely with other organizations interested in end-of-life care.

National Institute for Healthcare Research (NIHR)

www.nihr.org

Encourages professional collaboration to advance the understanding of spirituality and health. As an educational, medical, and social science research organization, the NIHR develops world-class educational programs, conducts research on the spirituality-health interface, and reviews and disseminates research findings.

Pain and Policy Studies Group (PPSG)

608-263-7662

www.medsch.wisc.edu/painpolicy

Facilitates public access to domestic and international information about pain relief and public policy. Intended audiences include patients, the public, and professionals in medicine, pharmacy, nursing, palliative care, cancer care, law, and other related disciplines.

Partnership for Caring: America's Voices for the Dying

800-989-9455

www.partnershipforcaring.org

A national nonprofit organization devoted to raising consumer expectations and demand for excellent end-of-life care; offers resources for talking about end-of-life choices, the process of health care, and state-specific advance directives.

Project on Death in America (PDIA)

212-548-0600

www.soros.org/death

PDIA's mission is to understand and transform the culture and experience of dying and bereavement through initiatives in research, scholarship, humanities, and arts and to foster innovations in the provision of care, public education, professional education, and public policy.

Promoting Excellence in End-of-Life Care

406-243-6668

www.promotingexcellence.org

Manages 22 grant-funded projects designed to demonstrate excellence in end-of-life care in institutional settings. Promoting Excellence in End-of-Life Care also facilitates a network of peer workgroups that comprise innovators and emerging leaders across the spectrum of palliative care.

Safe Crossings

www.providence.org/safecrossings

Designed to meet the needs of children up to age 18 facing the loss of a loved one. The Website is designed to provide activities and resources for kids, families, and professionals.

Supportive Care of the Dying
503-215-5053
www.careofdying.org
Develops and tests innovative projects with individuals and organizations working to improve delivery of care to those facing the end of life. Print and video products are available on many end-of-life issues, including the improvement of physician communication with patients and families.

ASSESSMENT TOOLS

Spiritual Well Being Scale

For each of the following statements circle the choice that best indicates the extent of your agreement or disagreement as it describes your personal experience:

SA	=	Strongly Agree	D	=	Disagree
MA	=	Moderately Agree	MD	=	Moderately Disagree
A	=	Agree	SD	=	Strongly Disagree

1. I don't find much satisfaction in private prayer with God.	SA	MA	A	D	MD	SD
2. I don't know who I am, where I came from, or where I am going.	SA	MA	A	D	MD	SD
3. I believe that God loves me and cares about me.	SA	MA	A	D	MD	SD
4. I feel that life is a positive experience.	SA	MA	A	D	MD	SD
5. I believe that God is impersonal and not interested in my daily situations.	SA	MA	A	D	MD	SD
6. I feel unsettled about my future.	SA	MA	A	D	MD	SD
7. I have a personally meaningful relationship with God.	SA	MA	A	D	MD	SD
8. I feel very fulfilled and satisfied with life.	SA	MA	A	D	MD	SD
9. I don't get much personal strength and support from my God.	SA	MA	A	D	MD	SD
10. I feel a sense of well-being about the direction my life is headed in.	SA	MA	A	D	MD	SD
11. I believe that God is concerned about my problems.	SA	MA	A	D	MD	SD
12. I don't enjoy much about life.	SA	MA	A	D	MD	SD
13. I don't have a personally satisfying relationship with God.	SA	MA	A	D	MD	SD
14. I feel good about my future.	SA	MA	A	D	MD	SD
15. My relationship with God helps me not to feel lonely.	SA	MA	A	D	MD	SD
16. I feel that life is full of conflict and unhappiness.	SA	MA	A	D	MD	SD
17. I feel most fulfilled when I'm in close communion with God.	SA	MA	A	D	MD	SD
18. Life doesn't have much meaning.	SA	MA	A	D	MD	SD
19. My relationship with God contributes to my sense of well being.	SA	MA	A	D	MD	SD
20. I believe there is some real purpose for my life.	SA	MA	A	D	MD	SD

Paloutzian, R., & Ellison, C.W. (1991). Spiritual Well Being Scale. In R.K. Bufford, R.F., Paloutzain & C.W. Ellison (Eds.). Norms for the Spiritual Well Being Scale. *J Psychol Theol,* 19, 56-70.

Author contact information: Raymond Paloutzian, PhD, at paloutz@westmont.edu and Craig W. Ellison, PhD, at www.lifeadvance.com

The Edmonton Labeled Visual Information System (ELVIS)

= Tumor, \\\\ = Resection, ☐ = Radiotherapy

Cancer Diagnosis: _____

Age: _____

Date Form Completed: _____

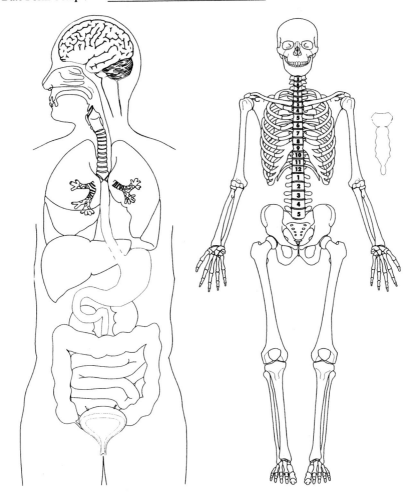

From Walker P, Nordell C, Neumann CM, et al. (2001). Impact of the Edmonton Labeled Visual Information System on physician recall of metastatic cancer patient histories: A randomized controlled trial. *J Pain Symptom Manage, 21*(1): 4-11.

Memorial Delirium Assessment Scale (MDAS)[1996]

Subject # _____   Rater _____   TOTAL SCORE:_____
Date   _____   Time _____

INSTRUCTIONS

Rate the severity of the following symptoms of delirium based on current interaction with subject or assessment of his/her behavior or experience over past several hours (as indicated in each time).

ITEM 1: REDUCED LEVEL OF CONSCIOUSNESS (AWARENESS)

Rate the patient's current awareness of and interaction with the environment (interviewer, other people/objects in the room; e.g., ask patients to describe their surroundings).

____ **0 None** (patient spontaneously fully aware of environment and interacts appropriately)

____ **1 Mild** (patient is unaware of some elements in the environment, or not spontaneously interacting appropriately with the interviewer; becomes fully aware and appropriately interactive when prodded strongly; interview is prolonged but not seriously disrupted)

____ **2 Moderate** (patient is unaware of some or all elements in the environment, or not spontaneously interacting with the interviewer; becomes incompletely aware and inappropriately interactive when prodded strongly; interview is prolonged but not seriously disrupted)

____ **3 Severe** (patient is unaware of all elements in the environment with no spontaneous interaction or awareness of the interviewer, so that the interview is difficult-to-impossible, even with maximal prodding)

ITEM 2: DISORIENTATION

Rate current state by asking the following 10 orientation items: date, month, day, year, season, floor, name of hospital, city, state, country.

____ **0 None** (patient knows 9 to 10 items)

____ **1 Mild** (patient knows 7 to 8 items)

____ **2 Moderate** (patient knows 5 to 6 items)

____ **3 Severe** (patient knows no more than 4 items)

ITEM 3: SHORT-TERM MEMORY IMPAIRMENT

Rate current state by using repetition and delayed recall of three words. (Patient must immediately repeat and recall words 5 minutes later after an intervening task. Use alternate sets of three words for successive evaluations [e.g., apple, table, tomorrow; sky, cigar, justice].)

____ **0 None** (all 3 words repeated and recalled)

____ **1 Mild** (all 3 repeated, patient fails to recall 1)

____ **2 Moderate** (all 3 repeated, patient fails to recall 2-3)

____ **3 Severe** (patient fails to repeat 1 or more words)

ITEM 4: IMPAIRED DIGIT SPAN

Rate current performance by asking subjects to repeat first 3, then 4, then 5 digits forward and then 3, then 4 backwards; continue to the next step only if patient succeeds at the previous one.

____ **0 None** (patient can do at least 5 numbers forward and 4 backward)

____ **1 Mild** (patient can do at least 5 numbers forward, 3 backward)

____ **2 Moderate** (patient can do 4-5 numbers forward, cannot do 3 backward)

____ **3 Severe** (patient can do no more than 3 numbers forward)

ITEM 5: REDUCED ABILITY TO MAINTAIN AND SHIFT ATTENTION

As indicated during the interview by questions needing to be rephrased and/or repeated because patient's attention wanders, patient loses track, patient is distracted by outside stimuli or over-absorbed in a task.

___ **0 None** (none of the above; patient maintains and shifts attention normally)
___ **1 Mild** (above attentional problems occur once or twice without prolonging the interview)
___ **2 Moderate** (above attentional problems occur often, prolonging the interview without seriously disrupting it)
___ **3 Severe** (above attentional problems occur constantly, disrupting and making the interview difficult-to-impossible)

ITEM 6: DISORGANIZED THINKING

As indicated during the interview by rambling, irrelevant, or incoherent speech, or by tangential, circumstantial or faulty reasoning. Ask patient a somewhat complex question (e.g., Describe your current medical condition.).

___ **0 None** (patient's speech is coherent and goal-directed)
___ **1 Mild** (patient's speech is slightly difficult to follow; responses to questions are slightly off target but not so much as to prolong the interview)
___ **2 Moderate** (disorganized thoughts or speech are clearly present, such that interview is prolonged but not disrupted)
___ **3 Severe** (examination is very difficult or impossible due to disorganized thinking or speech)

ITEM 7: PERCEPTUAL DISTURBANCE

Misperceptions, illusions, hallucinations inferred from inappropriate behavior during the interview or admitted by subject, as well as those elicited from nurse/family/chart accounts of the past several hours or of the time since last examination:

___ **0 None** (no misperceptions, illusions, or hallucinations)
___ **1 Mild** (misperceptions or illusions related to sleep, fleeting hallucinations on 1 or 2 occasions without inappropriate behavior)
___ **2 Moderate** (hallucinations or frequent illusions on several occasions with minimal inappropriate behavior that does not disrupt the interview)
___ **3 Severe** (frequent or intense illusions or hallucinations with persistent inappropriate behavior that disrupts the interview or interferes with medical care)

ITEM 8: DELUSIONS

Rate delusions inferred from inappropriate behavior during the interview or admitted by the patient, as well as delusions elicited from nurse/family/chart accounts of the past several hours or of the time since the previous examination.

___ **0 None** (no evidence of misinterpretations or delusions)
___ **1 Mild** (misinterpretations or suspiciousness without clear delusional ideas or inappropriate behavior)
___ **2 Moderate** (delusions admitted by the patient or evidenced by his/her behavior that do not or only marginally disrupt the interview or interfere with medical care)
___ **3 Severe** (persistent and/or intense delusions resulting in inappropriate behavior, disrupting the interview, or seriously interfering with medical care)

ITEM 9: DECREASED OR INCREASED PSYCHOMOTOR ACTIVITY

Rate activity over past several hours, as well as activity during interview, by circling
    a: Hypoactive   **b:** Hyperactive   **c:** Elements of both present

a	b	c	0	**None** (normal psychomotor activity)
a	b	c	1	**Mild** (Hypoactivity is barely noticeable, expressed as slightly slowing of movement. Hyperactivity is barely noticeable or appears as simple restlessness.)
a	b	c	2	**Moderate** (Hypoactivity is undeniable, with marked reduction in the number of movements or marked slowness of movement; subject rarely spontaneously moves or speaks. Hyperactivity is undeniable, subject moves almost constantly; in both cases, exam in prolonged as a consequence.)
a	b	c	3	**Severe** (Hypoactivity is severe; patient does not move or speak without prodding or is catatonic. Hyperactivity is severe; patient is constantly moving, overreacts to stimuli, requires surveillance and/or restraint; Getting through the exam is difficult or impossible.)

ITEM 10: SLEEP-WAKE CYCLE DISTURBANCE (DISORDER OF AROUSAL)

Rate patient's ability to either sleep or stay awake at the appropriate times. Utilize direct observation during the interview, as well as reports from nurses, family, patient or charts describing sleep-wake cycle disturbance over the past several hours or since last examination. Use observations of the previous night for morning evaluations only.

___ **0 None** (at night, sleeps well; during the day, has no trouble staying awake)

___ **1 Mild** (mild deviation from appropriate sleepfulness and wakefulness states: at night, difficulty falling asleep or transient night awakenings, needs medication to sleep well; during the day, reports periods of drowsiness or, during the interview, is drowsy but can easily fully awaken him/herself)

___ **2 Moderate** (moderate deviations from appropriate sleepfulness and wakefulness states: at night, repeated and prolonged night awakening; during the day, reports of frequent and prolonged napping or, during the interview, can only be roused to complete wakefulness by strong stimuli)

___ **3 Severe** (severe deviations from appropriate sleepfulness and wakefulness states: at night, sleeplessness; during the day, patient spends most of the time sleeping or, during the interview, cannot be roused to full wakefulness by any stimuli)

From Breitbart, W., Rosenfeld, B., Roth, A., et al. (1997). The Memorial Delirium Assessment Scale. *J Pain Symptom Manage, 13(3)*:128-137.
Author contact information: William Breitbart, MD, Chief Psychiatric Services, at Memorial Sloan-Kettering Cancer Center at breitbaw@mskcc.org.

INDEX

A

Abstract thinking, tests of, 338b
Acetaminophen toxicity
causes of, 186-187
liver failure due to, 186
Acetic acids, dosing information, 461t
Acetylcholinesterase inhibitors for Alzheimer's disease, 203
Acquired immune deficiency syndrome. *See* HIV/AIDS
Active listening, advance care planning and, 50-51
Addiction to pain medications, 454
Adhesions with malignant bowel obstruction, 269
Adrenal glands, metastasis to, 223
Advance care planning, 49-54
challenges in, 50
communication strategies for, 50-52, 52b
defined, 49
in HIV/AIDS, 241
psychological barriers in, 50
suggested questions for, 55b
values clarification/goal setting in, 53-54
Advance directives, 54-58, 65
documentation of, timing of, 66
ethical issues in, 66
forms of, 56
legislation pertaining to, 56-57
planning discussions for, 55b, 56
Advanced practice nurse, 3-18
certification of, 9
direct reimbursement to, 13
in diverse settings, 9-10
educational background, 3

Page numbers followed by b, f, and t indicate boxes, figures, and tables, respectively.

Advanced practice nurse *(Continued)*
in interdisciplinary team, 9
Macmillan nurse and, 7-8
roles of, 3-4
differentiating, 4-7
Adverse drug reactions
age and, 105-106
polypharmacy and, 108
Agency for Healthcare Research and Quality, website for, 17b
Agency for Healthcare Research and Quality National Guideline Clearinghouse, website for, 17b
Aging, medication implications of, 105-106
Agitation, dehydration and, 317
Agonist-antagonists, contraindication to, 460
Agonists, pharmacodynamics of, 103
AIDS. *See* HIV/AIDS
Airway diseases, obstructive and restrictive, differentiating among, 173-174
Albuterol sulfate for dyspnea, 387t
Alcohol use, medications and, 107
Allodynia, 504
Allokinesis, 504
α-Adrenergic agonists, mechanism of action, 453t
Alprazolam for anxiety, dosage, routes, half-life, 253t
Alzheimer's disease, 202-203
Ambien. *See* Zolpidem (Ambien)
American Academy of Nurse Practitioners, website for, 12, 17b
American College of Nurse Practitioners, website for, 17b
American Nurses Credentialing Center, 9
p-Aminophenol derivatives, dosing information, 461t

Amitriptyline (Elavil)
dosage and effects, 354t
dose and half-life, 124t
Amyotrophic lateral sclerosis
etiology and pathophysiology, 204
symptoms, 204
treatment, 204-205
ANA Social Policy Statement, 10-11
Analgesics
adjuvant
indications and dosing information, 463t-464t
initiation of, 469b
formulations of, 461t
nonopioid, dosing information, 461t
sleep-impairing properties of, 120t
Anemia
dyspnea due to, management of, 384t
fatigue due to, 398
Anesthetics, local
indications and dosing information, 464t
mechanism of action, 453t
Angiotensin-converting enzyme inhibitors
cough associated with, 301, 306
characteristics and symptoms, 307t
pharmacological treatment of, 308t
for heart failure, 164, 167
Ankylosing spondylitis, characteristics of, 175
Anorexia. *See also* Cachexia
in advanced cancer, 222
versus cachexia, 131
case study, 283-285
in HIV/AIDS, 239t
weight loss due to, 131
Antagonists, pharmacodynamics of, 104
Antibiotics for chronic renal failure, 196t
Anticholinergic activity, medications with, 337b

551

Anticholinergics
constipation and, 288
for COPD, 178
dehydration associated
with, 316
for dyspnea, 388t
Anticonvulsants
indications and dosing
information, 463t
mechanism of action, 453t
titration of, 468
Antidepressants
classes of, 353
dosage and effects, 354t-355t
dose and half-life, 124t
for fatigue, 403
sleep-impairing properties
of, 120t
titration of, 468
Antidiuretic hormone,
inappropriate secretion
of. See Syndrome of
inappropriate antidiuretic
hormone secretion
Antiemetics
for nausea/vomiting,
440-441, 441t
sleep-impairing properties
of, 120t
Antihistamines
for anxiety, 254
dosage, routes, half-life,
253t
classification and generic
names, 511t
dose and half-life, 125t
for nausea/vomiting, 441t
Antihypertensives, sleep-
impairing properties of,
120t
Antipsychotic agents for
delirium, 341
Antisecretory agents for
nausea/vomiting, 441t
Anxiety, 245-257
assessment and
measurement, 248-249,
249t
coping skills in, 251-252
definition and incidence,
245-246
with delirium, 330
diagnostics, 250
diarrhea associated with,
364t

Anxiety (Continued)
etiology and
pathophysiology,
246-248, 247b
evaluation and follow-up,
255
history and physical
examination, 249-250
in HIV/AIDS, 240t
intervention and treatment,
250-254
levels of, 249t
medication-related, 246
patient and family education
about, 254-255
pharmacological
interventions, 252,
253t, 254
physical causes of, 250
prevalence of, 245
sleep disorders and, 117-118
Anxiety disorders, DSM-IV
diagnoses, 245
Anxiolytics
for anxiety, 252, 253t, 254
for COPD, 180
for dyspnea, 385-386
sleep-impairing properties
of, 120t
Apnea, defined, 113b
Appetite, loss of
interventions for, 136-137
pharmacologic options for,
143t
Aprepitant (Emend) for
nausea/vomiting, 441t
Arousal, defined, 113b
Arrhythmias in heart failure,
164-165
Arteriosclerosis, defined, 153
Ascites, 259-268
assessment and
measurement, 260
case study, 265-266
definition and incidence, 259
diagnostics, 262
dyspnea due to, management
of, 384t
effects of, 260
etiology and
pathophysiology,
259-260
evaluation and follow-up, 265
history and physical
examination, 261

Ascites (Continued)
intervention and treatment,
262-265
with sodium restriction
and diuretics, 262
patient and family
education, 265
Asthenia, signs of, 37
Asthma
characteristics of, 174
versus COPD, 177
cough in
characteristics and
symptoms, 307t
pharmacological
treatment of, 308t
dyspnea due to, management
of, 384t
Atherosclerosis, defined, 153
Atherothrombotic disease,
pathophysiology of,
153-154
Athetoid movements, in
Huntington's disease,
205
Atopic dermatitis, intervention
and treatment, 510-511
Atrial fibrillation in heart
failure, 160
Attention, tests of, 338b

B

Baclofen for hiccups, 414t
Baseline Dyspnea Index, 381
BEARS Assessment System,
121, 121t
Beck Depression Inventory, 351
Beneficence, defined, 64
Benzodiazepine hypnotics, dose
and half-life, 124t
Benzodiazepines
for anxiety, 252
dosage, routes, half-life,
253t
contraindications to, 252
for delirium, 341-342
for dyspnea, 385
for nausea/vomiting, 441t
Benzonatate for cough, 309
Bereaved, care of, 42-43, 44t
Best interests standard, 59
β-agonists for COPD,
178-179
β-blockers for heart failure,
167

Bile salt malabsorption, diarrhea due to, treatment of, 371
Biliary obstruction, diarrhea associated with, 362t
Bioavailability, drug, 89
Bisphosphonates
for hypercalcemia of malignancy, 483
indications and dosing information, 464t
indications for, 469-470
Bites, pruritus due to, 505
Bloating
in ascites, 259
interventions for, 135
Boards of nursing, guidelines of, 12
Bone, metastasis to, 223
interventions for, 225-226
Bonica, J., 21
Bowel, pseudo-obstruction of, causes of, 270
Bowel obstruction, 269-277
assessment and measurement, 270-271
case study, 275-276
versus constipation, 291
definition and incidence, 269
diagnostics, 272
diarrhea associated with, 362t
etiology and pathophysiology, 269-270
evaluation and follow-up, 274
history and physical examination, 271-272
interventions and treatment, 272-274
malignant. See Malignant bowel obstruction
nonmalignant, 269
patient and family education, 274
Brain, metastasis to, 223
interventions for, 226
Breast cancer
epidemiology of, 219
ER- and PR- positive/ negative tumors in, 219-220
hiccups in patient with, case study, 415
metastatic, 218t, 219-220
lymphedema and, 427-429
ulcerative lesion in, case study, 534-535

Breathing, normal control of, 378
Breathing patterns during dying process, 39
Breathing techniques
for cough, 309
for dyspnea, 389
Breathlessness. See Dyspnea
Bromocriptin for chronic kidney disease symptoms, 198t
Bronchial obstruction, dyspnea due to, management of, 384t
Bronchiectasis, cough in characteristics and symptoms, 307t
pharmacological treatment of, 308t
Bronchitis
chronic, characteristics of, 174
cough in, 306
characteristics and symptoms, 307t
pharmacological treatment of, 308t
Bronchodilators
for dyspnea, 386-388, 387t
sleep-impairing properties of, 120t
Bronchospasm, cough characteristics in, 306
Bulk-forming laxatives, 293
Buprenorphine, contraindication to, 460
Bupropion (Wellbutrin), dosage and effects, 355t
Burns, pruritus due to, 505
treatment of, 511-512
Buspirone for anxiety, 252, 254
dosage, routes, half-life, 253t
Butorphanol, contraindication to, 460

C

Cachexia, 279-286. See also Anorexia
in advanced cancer, 222
versus anorexia, 131
assessment and measurement, 280
cardiac, in heart failure, 163
cause of, 132
definition and incidence, 279
diagnostics, 281

Cachexia (Continued)
etiology and pathophysiology, 279-280
evaluation and follow-up, 283
fatigue and, 398-399
history and physical examination, 280-281
in HIV/AIDS, 239t
intervention and treatment, 281-283
metabolic abnormalities of, 132-133
patient and family education, 283
prevention of, 281
weight loss due to, 131-132
Cancer. See also Malignancies; specific types
advanced, symptoms of, 222
cachexia in, 132-133, 279
cough in, characteristics and symptoms, 307t
deaths from, 24
diarrhea associated with, 361, 362t
dying trajectory in, 215-216, 216f
epidemiology of, 215
familial, 217
fatigue and, 395-396
functional decline in, 33
mortality rates for, 215
pain management for, history of, 20-21
survival of, 216
symptom profile in, 216
Cannabinoids
for cachexia, 282
for nausea/vomiting, 441t
for stimulating appetite, 143
CAPC. See Center to Advance Palliative Care
Capsaicin for atopic dermatitis, 511
Carbamazepine for hiccups, 414t
Carbidopa-levodopa for chronic kidney disease symptoms, 198t
Carcinoid syndrome, treatment of, 373
Cardiac tamponade
conditions associated with, 303
cough in, 303

Cardiomyopathies, pathophysiology of, 154-155

Cardiovascular disease, 153-169
  definition and incidence, 156-157
  device therapy for, 164-168
  diagnosis of, 158
  etiology and pathophysiology, 153-156
  history of, 158-159
  interventions for, 163
  management of, 163-164
  pathophysiology of, 157
  physical examination for, 159-160
  signs and symptoms of, 160-163
  staging of, 157-158

Caregivers, caring for, 40-41

Carnitine for chronic kidney disease symptoms, 198t

Catheters for ascites, 264

Celexa. See Citalopram HBr (Celexa)

Celiac plexus block, diarrhea associated with, 364t

Center to Advance Palliative Care, 26, 27

Centers for Medicare and Medicaid Services, collaboration defined by, 12-13

Cerebrovascular accidents
  etiology and pathophysiology, 201-202
  risk factors for, 201
  symptoms, 202
  treatments, 202

C-fibers in mediation of itch versus pain, 504

Chemoreceptor trigger zone, 431-432
  nausea/vomiting receptors and neurotransmitters in, 433t

Chemotherapy
  diarrhea due to, 362t, 373
  emetic risk of, 437b-438b
  intracavitary, for ascites, 263-264
  for spinal cord compression, 493
  for superior vena cava syndrome, 488

Chlordiazepoxide for anxiety, dosage, routes, half-life, 253t

Chlorpromazine (Thorazine)
  for anxiety, dosage, routes, half-life, 253t
  for dyspnea, 385-386
  for hiccups, 414t
  for nausea/vomiting, 441t
  for terminal sedation, 342

Cholestatic pruritus, treatment of, 512

Cholinergic system, delirium-related changes in, 334t

Choreiform movements in Huntington's disease, 205

Chronic and restrictive airway diseases, characteristics of, 175

Chronic illness, sleep disorders and, 118

Chronic kidney disease, 191-199. See also End-stage renal disease
  causes of, 192
  defined, 191
  diagnostics, 195
  etiology and pathophysiology, 192-193
  history and physical examination, 193, 195
  interventions, 192, 195-197
  medication modifications in, 196t
  mortality rate for, 191
  risk factors for, 191-192
  stages of, 191, 191t
  symptoms, 193

Chronic obstructive pulmonary disease, 175
  versus asthma, 177
  cough in, 301
  definition of, 172
  diagnosis of, 171, 173, 177
  dyspnea due to, management of, 384t
  etiology and pathophysiology of, 173-175
  history of, 175-176, 176t
  mortality rates for, 171
  patient with, 172-173
  pharmacologic interventions for, 177-180
  with anticholinergics, 178

Chronic obstructive pulmonary disease (Continued)
  with anxiolytics, 180
  with β-agonists, 178-179
  with corticosteroids, 179
  with opioids, 180
  with theophylline, 179-180
  physical examination for, 177

Chronic upper airway congestion syndrome, cough in, pharmacological treatment of, 308t

Circadian rhythm, defined, 113b

Circulation during dying process, 38

Cirrhosis, causes of, 185-186

Citalopram HBr (Celexa), dosage and effects, 354t

Cleveland Clinic palliative medicine program, 26-27

Clinical decision making, guidelines and protocols in, 11-12

Clinical nurse specialist
  credentialing of, 5-6
  educational background, 3
  role-delineation study of, 3
  scope of practice, 5-6

Clonazepam
  for anxiety, dosage, routes, half-life, 253t
  for chronic kidney disease symptoms, 198t
  for dyspnea, 386

Clonidine
  for chronic kidney disease symptoms, 198t
  for diarrhea, 373

Clorazepate, contraindications to, 252

CMS. See Centers for Medicare and Medicaid Services

Codeine
  for controlling diarrhea, 372
  effects of renal failure/dialysis on, 98t
  formulations of, 461t

Cognitive function, tests for, 338b

Cognitive impairment
  in delirium, 328-329
  pain assessment and, 456, 458

Cognitive impairment during
dying process, 38
Cognitive-behavioral therapy
for fatigue, 404-405
Cold therapy, effects of, 472t
Colitis, pseudomembranous,
diarrhea associated
with, 365
Collaborative practice
agreement, 12-13
sample of, 14f
Collagen disease, characteristics
of, 175
Colon cancer
bowel obstruction in, case
study, 275-276
fatigue and, case study,
405-406
Colorectal cancer, metastasis
of, 218t, 219
Common cold, cough in,
pharmacological
treatment of, 308t
Communication
ALS and, 205
ethical issues in, 70-71
nonverbal, self-awareness of,
50-51
Communication strategies
advance care planning and,
50-52
balancing hope and honesty
in, 52
rapport-enhancing, 52b
Compassion and Choices, Web
site for, 56
Complementary therapies in
pain management, 471
Complete decongestive
therapy
adapting for palliative care,
425t
for lymphedema, 422-426
Confusion
acute. See Delirium/acute
confusion
dehydration and, 317
opioid-related, 468
Confusion Assessment Method,
335
Congenital heart disease,
pathophysiology of, 155
Congestive heart failure
cachexia in, 279
cough in, 301

Congestive heart failure
(Continued)
characteristics and
symptoms, 307t
Connecticut Hospice, 28
Consciousness, disturbance of,
in delirium, 328
Constipation, 287-300
in ascites, 259
assessment and
measurement, 290
bowel obstruction and,
269-270
case study, 298-299
definition and incidence, 287
diagnostics, 291
etiology and
pathophysiology,
287-289
evaluation and follow-up, 298
history and physical
examination, 290-291
in HIV/AIDS, 240t
interventions for, 134-135,
292-296
versus obstruction, 291
opioid-related, 465
patient and family education,
134-135, 296-298
pharmacologic options for,
143t
prophylactic interventions, 292
treatment, 292-296
Contact dermatitis, 505
COPD. See Chronic obstructive
pulmonary disease
Coronary artery disease,
pathophysiology of, 154
Corticosteroids
for atopic dermatitis, 510-511
for cachexia, 282
for COPD, 179
for dyspnea, 386
for fatigue, 404
for hypercalcemia of
malignancy, 483
indications and dosing
information, 463t
indications for, 469
mechanism of action, 453t
sleep-impairing properties
of, 120t
for spinal cord compression,
493
for stimulating appetite, 143

Corticosteroids (Continued)
for superior vena cava
syndrome, 489
titration of, 469
Cough, 301-313
assessment and
measurement, 303-304
assessment and physical
exam, 304-305
case study, 311
characteristics and associated
symptoms, 307t
definition and incidence, 301
diagnostics, 305-306
emergent conditions
associated with, 303
etiologies and complications,
302-303, 302t, 303b
evaluation and follow-up,
311
history, 304
in HIV/AIDS, 240t
intervention and treatment,
306, 308-310
pathophysiology, 301-302
patient and family
education, 310-311
progressive diseases
associated with, 301
protective function of,
301, 306
treatment
nonpharmacological,
309-310
pharmacological, 306,
308-309, 308t
of underlying cause, 306
tumor-induced, intervention
for, 310
Cough diary, 310
Creatine clearance, Cockcroft-
Gault formula for, 106
Credentialing for CNS
practice, 5-6
Cruzan, N., 54
Cryptosporidiosis, diarrhea
due to, 363t, 365, 367
treatment of, 371
Cultural competence, 76-77
cultural versus specific, 77
defined, 75, 76
Cultural issues, 75-84
Culture, defined, 75
Cushing's syndrome, lung
cancer and, 218

Cyclooxygenase-2 inhibitors, dosing information, 461t
Cylert. *See* Pemoline (Cylert)
Cyproheptadine (Periactin) for stimulating appetite, 143
Cystic fibrosis, cough in, interventions for, 310
Cytochrome P450 enzymes, drug metabolism and, 100, 101t
Cytokines
in depression, 350
fatigue and, 398
proinflammatory, in cachexia, 279-280
Cytomegalovirus, diarrhea due to, 367
treatment of, 371

D

Death
arrangements following, 41
awareness of, 40
care at time of, 41-42
care of bereaved after, 42-43, 44t
care of body after, 41-42
good, defined, 63
leading causes of, 19
legal notification of, 42
Debridement of ulcerative lesions, 529-530
Decision making
choosing surrogates for, 55b, 57-58
clinical, 11-12
ethical, 63. *See also* Ethical issues
Decisional capacity. *See also* Cognitive impairment
ethical issues in, 65
Decubitus ulcers. *See also* Ulcerative lesions
in HIV/AIDS, 240t
Dehydration, 315-325
assessment and measurement, 318
case study, 323-324
controversy about, 315
definition and incidence, 315-316
diagnostics, 319-320
etiology and pathophysiology, 316-317

Dehydration *(Continued)*
evaluation and follow-up, 323
from high-volume emesis, 271
history and physical examination, 318-319
in HIV/AIDS, 240t
hypernatremia and, 315
hypodermoclysis for, 322b
intervention and treatment, 320-322
medication-related, 316
patient and family education, 323
signs and symptoms, 315-319, 318b
Delirium Index, 336
Delirium Observation Screening Scale, 335
Delirium Rating Scale—Revised-98, 335-336
Delirium/acute confusion, 327-348
acute onset/fluctuating course, 329
assessment and measurement, 333-336
case study, 344-345
cognitive changes in, 328-329
definition and incidence, 327-331, 328b
diagnostics, 339
disturbance of consciousness in, 328
DSM-IV-TR criteria for, 327, 328b
emotional disturbance in, 330
etiology and pathophysiology, 331, 332b-333b
evaluation and follow-up, 343
history, 337
intervention and treatment, 339-342
nonpharmacological, 340-341
pharmacological, 341-342
for underlying causes, 340
neurochemical changes in, 334t
patient and family education, 342-343

Delirium/acute confusion *(Continued)*
physical examination, 338-339
prevalence and outcomes, 331
prodromal/subsyndromal signs of, 330-331
psychomotor activity in, 330
reversibility of, 327
risk factors for, 332b-333b
sleep-wake disturbances in, 329-330
subsyndromal, 330
terminology for, 327
underlying causes of, management of, 340
Dementia. *See* Alzheimer's disease
Depression, 349-359
in Alzheimer's disease, 203
assessment and measurement, 351-352
case study, 357-358
cytokine-mediated, 350
definition and incidence, 349
etiology and pathophysiology, 350
evaluation and follow-up, 357
fatigue and, 399-400
history and physical examination, 352-353
in HIV/AIDS, 240t
in Huntington's disease, 207
intervention and treatment, 353
nonpharmacological, 353
pharmacological, 353, 354t-355t, 356
patient and family education, 356
risk factors for, 350
stroke-related, 202
Dermatitis
atopic, intervention and treatment, 510-511
contact, 505
Dermatolymphangioadenitis, 424
Desipramine (Norpramin), dosage and effects, 354t
Desyrel. *See* Trazodone (Desyrel)
Dexamethasone (Decadron)
for dyspnea, 386
for nausea/vomiting, 441t

Diabetes, chronic kidney
disease and, 192-193
Dialysis, 196-197
effect on opioids, 98t
withdrawal of, 197, 197b
Diarrhea, 361-376
assessment and
measurement,
367-369
cancer-treatment-related,
mechanisms,
descriptors, treatment,
362t-363t
case study, 374-375
control of, 372-373
definition and incidence,
361
diagnostics, 369
discomfort due to, 372
etiology and
pathophysiology, 361,
365-367
evaluation and follow-up,
374
exudative, 366-367
in HIV/AIDS, 240t, 367
hypermotility-related, 366
intervention and treatment,
135-136, 370-373
for underlying cause,
370-371
osmotic, 365-366
patient and family
education, 373-374
secretory, 365
toxicity criteria for, 367t
Diazepam
for anxiety, dosage, routes,
half-life, 253t
contraindications to, 252
for dyspnea, 386
lipid solubility of, 96
Diet
for altered sense of
taste/smell, 137
for bloating, 135
constipation and, 134-135,
288, 292
for diarrhea, 135-136
for dry mouth/thick saliva,
137-138
for GERD, 310
for HIV/AIDS patient, 237
for nausea/vomiting, 139
for poor appetite, 136-137

Diet (Continued)
for sore mouth/throat,
138-139
Diffuse interstitial pulmonary
fibrosis, characteristics
of, 175
Diphenhydramine (Benadryl)
for nausea/vomiting,
441t
Diphenoxylate for controlling
diarrhea, 372
Disorientation with delirium,
328-329
Distraction in pain
management, effects of,
472t
Distress Thermometer, 352
Diuretics
for ascites, 262
dehydration associated
with, 316
for superior vena cava
syndrome, 488
Dopamine antagonists for
nausea/vomiting, 441t
Dopamine system, delirium-
related changes in,
334t
Double effect, principle of,
69-70
Doxepin (Sinequan)
for atopic dermatitis, 510
dosage and effects, 354t
Dronabinol (Marinol)
for nausea/vomiting, 441t
for stimulating appetite,
143
Drug monitoring, therapeutic,
102
Drug therapy, key factors in,
108
Drugs
absorption of, factors
affecting, 88b
aging and, 105-106
agonist, 103
antagonist, 104
clearance of, 93-94, 97-99
hepatic, 98-99, 99t
renal, 97-98, 98t
disease state and, 107
dosing intervals for, 93
efficacy of, 104
elimination of, 94, 95f
ethnicity and, 107

Drugs (Continued)
gender and, 106-107
hypnotic/sedating,
124t-125t
ionization of, 96-97
lipid solubility of, 96-97
loading doses of, 91-92
metabolism of, 99-100
cytochrome system in,
100, 101t
multiple compartment
distribution of, 94
pharmacodynamics of. See
Pharmacodynamics
pharmacokinetics of.
See Pharmacokinetics
potency of, 104
protein binding of, 94-96
routes of administration, 86,
87t-88t, 89
sleep-impairing properties
of, 120t
smoking/alcohol
consumption and,
107
steady state of, 93
therapeutic window of,
92
volume of distribution/
half-life of, 91t, 92,
92f
Dry mouth
in cancer patients, 317
interventions for, 137-138
pharmacologic options
for, 143t
Durable power of attorney,
56, 58
Dying process, 33-45. See also
End-of-life
awareness of, 40
imminent, signs and
symptoms of, 37-40
patient's experience
with, 55b
patient's familiarity with,
54
psychosocial symptoms
in, 35
symptom changes in, 33,
34t, 35
Dyspepsia Quality-of-Life
Questionnaire, 303
Dysphagia, feeding patient
with, 310

Dyspnea, 377-394
in ALS, 205
assessment and
measurement, 379-381
case study, 391-392
cognitive factors in, 379
conditions associated with,
379, 380t
cough, and sputum scale, 303
defined, 377
diagnostics, 382-383
etiology and pathophysiology,
377-379
in heart failure, 162
history and physical
examination, 381-382
in HIV/AIDS, 239t
interventions and treatment,
383-390
with anxiolytics, 385-386
with breathing techniques,
389
with bronchodilators,
386-388, 387t-388t
for correctable causes, 384t
with corticosteroids, 386
environmental
adjustments, 390
exercise, 390
with opioids, 384-385
with oxygen, 388-389
positioning in, 390
relaxation techniques, 390
with theophylline, 388
mechanisms leading to,
378-379
patient and family
education, 391
prevalence, 377

E

Eaton-Lambert syndrome, lung
cancer and, 218
Echocardiography for
confirming heart
failure, 158
Eczema
atopic, 505
nummular, 505
Edema. *See also* Lymphedema
in heart failure, 160, 161
Effexor. *See* Venlafaxine (Effexor)
Eicosapentaenoic acid for
cachexia, 132-133
Elavil. *See* Amitriptyline (Elavil)
Electronic Orange Book, The, 89

Embolization, tumor, 470
Emergencies, 481-501
case study, 499
hemorrhage, 494-497
hypercalcemia of
malignancy, 481-484
seizures, 497-498
spinal cord compression,
490-494
superior vena cava
syndrome, 487-490
syndrome of inappropriate
antidiuretic hormone
secretion, 484-486
Emesis, high-volume,
dehydration from, 271
Emollients, 294
Emotional disturbance with
delirium, 330
Emphysema, characteristics of,
174
Endocrine disorders, fatigue
and, 399
End-of-life
care at, 36-40
for asthenia, 37
for breathing pattern
changes, 39
for changes in sensory
perception, 40
for circulatory changes, 38
for decreased food intake,
39-40
for decreased urine
output, 38-39
for dehydration, 37
for inability to close
eyes, 40
medications in, 36
for mentation changes, 38
for nearing death
awareness, 40
for pain, 37-38
decision making and, 58-60
forgiveness/acceptance issues
and, 82-83
nutritional issues in, 144-145
pain at, neglect of, 448-449
symptom changes in, 33,
34t, 35
End-of-life care
APN's role in, 6
current trends in, 19-20
defining, 23-24
future of, 30
for heart failure, 167-168

End-of-life care *(Continued)*
hospice and, 28-30
versus palliative care, 27
pre-World War II, 20
Endovascular techniques for
superior vena cava
syndrome, 488-489
End-stage renal disease
interventions, 196
mortality rate for, 191
Energy therapies in pain
management, effects of,
472t
Enteral nutrition support, 140,
141t, 142
in cachexia, 282
contraindications to, 140
diarrhea associated with,
364t, 366
Enzymes, cytochrome P450, in
drug metabolism, 100,
101t
EPA. *See* Eicosapentaenoic acid
Epinephrine for dyspnea, 387t
Erythropoietin for fatigue, 404
Estazolam (ProSom), dose and
half-life, 124t
Eszopiclone (Lunesta), dose
and half-life, 124t
Ethical issues, 63-74
in advance directives, 66
in clinical leadership, 69
in communication/
mediation, 70-71
decisional capacity, 65
in disagreements about
treatment goals, 63
framework for, 63
justice and, 71-72
medical futility and, 68
in patient self-
determination/informed
consent, 64
in patient-health care
professional
relationship, 64-65
and principle of double
effect, 69-70
in surrogate decision
making, 65-66
in weighing
benefits/burdens, 67-68
in withholding/withdrawing
treatment, 66-67
Ethics, virtue, 64-65
Ethnicity, medications and, 107

Ethylnorepinephrine for dyspnea, 387t
European Society of Medical Oncology, core principles of, 28, 28b
Evangelism, note on, 80b
Excitability, opioid-related, 468
Exercise intolerance in heart failure, 162
Exercise therapy
　for dyspnea, 390
　effects of, 472t
　for fatigue, 402-403
Eyes, inability to close, 40

F

FACES pain rating scale, 458f
Faith, defined, 75
Family
　caring for, 40-41
　surrogate decision-making and, 58-59. *See also* Surrogates, decision-making
Fat malabsorption, diarrhea due to, treatment of, 371
Fatigue, 395-409
　assessment and measurement, 400-401, 400t
　cancer-related, 395-396
　case study, 405-406
　conditions associated with, 387
　definition and incidence, 395-396
　diagnostics, 401-402
　etiology and pathophysiology, 396-400
　evaluation and follow-up, 405
　in heart failure, 162
　history and physical examination, 401
　in HIV/AIDS, 239t
　intervention and treatment, 402-405
　complementary, 404-405
　pharmacological, 403-404
　measures of, 400t
　patient and family education, 405
　sleep disorders and, 118-119
Fecal impaction, diarrhea due to, 364t, 370
Federal Register, rules/updates for, 17b

Fentanyl
　effects of renal failure/dialysis on, 98t
　equianalgesic dosage of, 465t
　formulations of, 462t
Fever in HIV/AIDS, 239t
Fiber supplements for constipation, 134-135
Fluid deficit
　defined, 316
　versus dehydration, 316
　isotonic, 316
Fluid intake, constipation and, 288, 292
Fluid retention in heart failure, 161
Fluoxetine (Prozac), dosage and effects, 354t
Flurazepam, contraindications to, 252
Food intake, decreased, at end-of-life, 39-40
Forgiveness, assessment and interventions, 82-83
Formoterol for dyspnea, 387t
Frank, A., 63
Fungal infection, pruritus due to, 505
Futile treatment, 68

G

GABA, delirium-related changes in, 334t
GABA agonists
　indications and dosing information, 464t
　mechanism of action, 453t
Gabapentin
　for chronic kidney disease symptoms, 198t
　for hiccups, 414t
Gastrectomy, diarrhea associated with, 363t
Gastroesophageal reflux disease
　cough in
　characteristics and symptoms, 307t
　pharmacological treatment of, 308t
　lifestyle changes for, 310
Gastrointestinal symptoms in heart failure, 163
Gastrointestinal tract
　innervation changes in, constipation and, 289
　neurotransmitters in, 433t

Geriatric Depression Scale, 351
Glycopyrrolate for cough, 309
Goals
　discussing, 53-54
　ethical issues and, 63
　patient, 55b
Good death, defined, 63
Grief, manifestations of, 42, 43b
Guaifenesin for cough, 306, 308

H

HAART regimen for HIV/AIDS, 237-238
Halcion. *See* Triazolam (Halcion)
Half-life, drug, 91t, 92, 92f
Hallucinations with delirium, 329
Haloperidol (Haldol)
　for anxiety, dosage, routes, half-life, 253t
　for delirium/acute confusion, 341
　for hiccups, 414t
　for nausea/vomiting, 441t
Harry R. Horvitz Center for Palliative Medicine, 26
Health care
　costs of, 19
　justice issues in, 71-72
Health care proxy, appointment of, 57
Health Insurance Portability and Accountability Act of 1996, 15
Heart failure
　chronic, 156
　management of, 163-164
　classification of, 155t, 157
　comorbidities with, 166
　cough characteristics in, 306
　definition and incidence of, 156-157
　device therapy for, 164-165
　diagnosis of, 158
　dyspnea due to, management of, 384t
　history of, 158-159
　interventions for, 163
　pathophysiology of, 157
　physical examination for, 159-160
　signs and symptoms of, 160-163
　staging of, 157-158
Heart sounds, auscultation of, 159

Heat therapy, effects of, 472t
Hemorrhage, etiology, pathophysiology, diagnosis, management, 494-497
Hepatic disease, 185-190. *See also* Cirrhosis
ascites in, 259-260. *See also* Ascites
diagnostics, 188
end-stage, symptoms, 187
etiology and pathophysiology, 185-187
history and physical examination, 188
Hepatic failure, acetaminophen and, 186
Hiccups, 411-416
assessment and measurement, 412
case study, 415
definition and incidence, 411
diagnostics, 412
etiology and pathophysiology, 411-412
evaluation and follow-up, 413-414
history and physical examination, 412
intervention and treatment, 413, 414t
patient and family education, 413
HIPAA. *See* Health Insurance Portability and Accountability Act of 1996
Histamine in pruritus, 504
HIV/AIDS, 233-242
advance care planning, 241
cachexia in, 279
CD4 count in, 235
CD8 count in, 235
cough in, 301
diagnostics and assessment, 235-237
diarrhea and, 367
treatment of, 371
epidemiology, 233-234
infection prophylaxis in, 236t
interventions, 236t, 237-238
palliative care, 22-23, 238-239
pathophysiology and nomenclature, 234-235

HIV/AIDS *(Continued)*
symptom management and treatment, 233, 239, 239t-240t
trajectory and associated symptoms, 235
Hope, assessment and interventions for, 80-81
Hormone therapy for breast cancer, 220
Hospice care
admission to, requirements for, 16
cancer patients in, 215
defining, 23-24, 28-29
end-of-life care and, 28-30
goal of, 29
hydration practice of, 315
Medicare benefit for, 29
volunteers for, 29
Hospital Anxiety and Depression scale, 351
Houde, R., 21
Human immunodeficiency virus. *See* HIV/AIDS
Huntington's disease
etiology and pathology, 205-206
juvenile-onset, 206-207
symptoms, 206-207
treatment, 207
Hydration
artificial, at end-of-life, 144
benefits/risks of, 320
constipation and, 288
controversy about, 315
enteral, 320-321
goal of, 323
intravenous, 321
via hypodermoclysis, 321-322
via proctoclysis, 321
Hydrocodone
for cough, 309
equianalgesic dosage of, 465t
formulations of, 461t
Hydromorphone
effects of renal failure/dialysis on, 98t
equianalgesic dosage of, 465t
formulations of, 462t
renal failure and, 108t
Hydroxyzine (Vistaril)
for anxiety, dosage, routes, half-life, 253t
for nausea/vomiting, 441t
Hyoscyamine for cough, 309

Hypercalcemia
constipation and, 288
lung cancer and, 218
Hypercalcemia of malignancy, etiology, pathophysiology, diagnosis, management, 481-484
Hypernatremia, dehydration and, 315
Hypersensitivity pneumonitis, characteristics of, 175
Hypertension, chronic kidney disease and, 192-193
Hypnotics
dose/half-life, 124t-125t
sleep-impairing properties of, 120t
Hypodermoclysis
characteristics and advantages/disadvantages, 321
initiating, 322b
Hypokalemia, constipation and, 288-289
Hypotension, orthostatic, drug-induced, 106
Hypothalamic-pituitary-adrenal axis, depression and, 350
Hypoxemia with chronic lung disease, cachexia in, 279
Hypoxia, dyspnea due to, management of, 384t

I

ICD. *See* Implantable cardioverter-defibrillator
IDT. *See* Interdisciplinary team
Ileal resection, diarrhea associated with, 363t
Illness
assessing impact on patient and family, 60
hope and, 80-81
patient's experience with, 55b
patient's understanding of, 55b
searching for meaning in, 79-80
spiritual growth and, 78-79
Imagery in pain management, effects of, 472t
Imipramine (Tofranil), dosage and effects, 354t
Immobility
constipation and, 288

Immobility *(Continued)*
  reducing, 341
Immobilization in pain
  management, effects of,
  472t
Imodium. *See* Loperamide
  (Imodium)
Implantable cardioverter-
  defibrillator for heart
  failure, 164-165
Infection
  artificial hydration and, 320
  cough associated with
    characteristics and
    symptoms, 307t
    pharmacological
    treatment of, 308t
  diarrhea due to, 363t,
    370-371
  dyspnea due to, management
    of, 384t
  fungal, pruritus due to, 505
  in HIV/AIDS, prophylaxis
    of, 236t
  lymphedema and, 424
Influenza vaccine for COPD, 181
Informed consent, ethical
  issues in, 64
Informed proxy, 59
Insomnia
  defined, 113b
  in HIV/AIDS, 240t
Interdisciplinary team, APN in, 9
Interstitial disease,
  characteristics of, 175
Interventions. *See* Treatment
Intestines, compression of,
  constipation due to, 289
Ipratropium bromide for
  dyspnea, 388t
Irritability with delirium, 330
Ischemia in stroke, 201-202
Isospora belli sp., diarrhea due
  to, treatment of, 371
Isoproterenol for dyspnea, 387t
Itching. *See* Pruritus

J

Joint Commission on
  Accreditation of
  Healthcare
  Organizations, treatment
  of community-acquired
  pneumonia and, 305-306
Jugular venous pressure,
  measurement of, 159

Justice, health care decisions
  and, 71-72

K

K complex, defined, 113b
Ketotifen for chronic kidney
  disease symptoms, 198t
Kidney disease, chronic. *See*
  Chronic kidney disease
Kidneys, homeostatic functions
  of, 192-193, 192t
Kübler-Ross, E., 83

L

Lactose intolerance, diarrhea
  associated with, 366
Laryngitis, cough in,
  characteristics and
  symptoms, 307t
Last Acts Palliative Care Task
  Force, 26
Laxatives, 292-296
  bulk-forming, 293
  combination, 295
  emollients/surfactants, 294
  guidelines for, 296
  lubricant, 293
  macrogol osmotic, 294-295
  medications with effects of,
    295-296
  overuse, diarrhea due to, 364t
  saccharine, 294
  saline osmotic, 294
  selection of, 292-293
  stimulant osmotic, 295
Leadership, ethical issues in, 69
Legal issues for death
  notification, 42
Legislation on advance
  directives, 56-57
Leicester Cough Questionnaire,
  303-304
Lethal dose 50%, 105
Lidocaine
  for chronic kidney disease
    symptoms, 198t
  for cough, 309
Lifestyle
  changes in, for reducing
    cough, 310
  in HIV/AIDS, 237
  sleep disorders and, 117
Life-sustaining treatments,
  types of, 66-67
Listening, active, 50-51

Liver, metastasis to, 223
  interventions for, 227
Liver disease, pruritus in, 506
  case study, 515-517
Liver failure, 186
Living will, provisions of, 57, 66
Local anesthetics
  indications and dosing
    information, 464t
  mechanism of action, 453t
Loperamide (Imodium) for
  controlling diarrhea, 372
Lorazepam (Ativan)
  for anxiety, dosage, routes,
    half-life, 253t
  for delirium, 342
  for dyspnea, 386
  for nausea/vomiting, 441t
Lou Gehrig's disease. *See*
  Amyotrophic lateral
  sclerosis
Lubricant laxatives, 293
Ludiomil. *See* Maprotiline
  (Ludiomil)
Lunesta. *See* Eszopiclone
  (Lunesta)
Lung cancer
  constipation with, case study,
    298-299
  cough in, 301, 303
    case study, 311
  metastasis of, 217-219, 218t
Lung Cancer Cough
  Questionnaire, 304
Lung tumors
  cough associated with,
    pharmacological
    treatment of, 308t
  metastasis of, 223
Lymph nodes, metastasis to,
  223
Lymph system, normal
  functioning of, 417-418
Lymphadenopathy,
  compression/
  obstruction from,
  interventions for, 228
Lymphangitis carcinomatosa
  characteristics of, 175
  dyspnea due to, management
    of, 384t
Lymphedema, 417-430
  before and after treatment,
    423f
  assessment and measurement,
    418-421, 419t

Lymphedema *(Continued)*
assessment checklist, 419t
case study, 427-429
conditions associated with, 418t
definition and incidence, 417
diagnostics, 422
etiologies, causes, examples, 418t
etiology and pathophysiology, 417-418
evaluation and follow-up, 426
history and physical examination, 421-422
intervention and treatment, 422, 424-426, 426t
objective signs, 420-421
patient and family education, 426, 426t
subjective symptoms, 420
Lymphoma, cough in, 303

M

M. D. Anderson Cancer Center, 27
Macmillan nurse, role of, 7-8
Macrogol osmotic laxatives, 294-295
Major Depressive Disorder. *See also* Depression
DSM-IV criteria for, 349, 350b
Malignancies, 215-231. *See also* Cancer; specific types
ascites in, 260
diagnostics, 225
etiology and pathophysiology, 217-222
breast cancer, 219-220
colorectal cancer, 219
lung cancer, 217-219
non-Hodgkin's lymphoma, 222
pancreatic cancer, 221-222
prostate cancer, 220-221
history and physical examination, 224-225
hypercalcemia of, etiology, pathophysiology, diagnosis, management, 481-484
metastatic, interventions for, 225-228
pruritus associated with, treatment of, 513
symptoms, 222-223

Malignant bowel obstruction
prevalence of, 269
surgery for
contraindications to, 273b
morbidity/mortality rate, 272
types of, 269
Malignant cutaneous wounds
assessment for, 523
variables in, 524
effects of, 519
etiology and pathophysiology, 520-522
odor due to, 531-532
staging of, 520t, 523
treatment, 528
tumors associated with, 521b
Malnutrition, fatigue and, 398-399
Maprotiline (Ludiomil), dosage and effects, 355t
Marinol. *See* Dronabinol (Marinol)
Maslow, A., 78
Massage, effects of, 472t
Meaning, search for, assessment and interventions for, 79-80
Mediastinal obstruction, dyspnea due to, management of, 384t
Mediation, ethical issues in, 70-71
Medical futility, ethical issues in, 68
Medical Research Council dyspnea scale, 381
Medicare, hospice benefit of, 29
Medicare Prescription Bill. *See* Medicare Prescription Drug Improvement and Modernization Act
Medicare Prescription Drug Improvement and Modernization Act, NP practice and, 16
Medicare services, APN reimbursement for, 13, 15
Medications. *See also* Drugs; specific medications
absorption of, 88b
administration routes, 87t-88t
for Alzheimer's disease, 203

Medications *(Continued)*
for amyotrophic lateral sclerosis, 204-205
for ascites, 263-264
for chronic kidney disease, 196t
constipation and, 288, 292
diarrhea and, 364t, 365, 366, 372-373
fatigue and, 398, 403
for heart failure, 167
with high anticholinergic activity, 337b
with laxative effects, 295-296
for nutrition impact symptoms, 142-144, 143t
pain. *See also* Pain management, pharmacological
fear of addiction to, 454-455
physiologic rationale for, 453-454, 453t
pruritus due to, 506
treatment of, 512
for sleep disorders, 124, 124t-125t, 126
sleep disorders and, 119
Megace. *See* Megestrol acetate (Megace)
Megestrol acetate (Megace) for stimulating appetite, 143-144
Melanoma, metastatic, depression in, case study of, 357-358
Memorial Delirium Assessment Scale, 336
Memorial Sloan-Kettering, 21-22
Memory, tests of, 338b
Memory deficits with delirium, 328-329
Meperidine, contraindication to, 460
Metabolic disorders, fatigue and, 399
Metastasis
defined, 217
interventions for, 225-228
in bone, 225-226
in brain, 226
in compression/obstruction from tumor/lymphadenopathy, 228

Metastasis *(Continued)*
    in liver, 227
    pleural effusions, 227
    sites of, 217
Metclopramide (Reglan) for
    nausea/vomiting, 441t
Methadone
    effects of renal failure/
        dialysis on, 98t
    equianalgesic dosage of, 465t
    renal failure and, 108t
Methylphenidate (Ritalin)
    for chronic kidney disease
        symptoms, 198t
    for fatigue, 403-404
    for hiccups, 414t
Methylxanthines for dyspnea,
    388t
Metoclopramide
    for bowel obstruction,
        272-273
    for hiccups, 414t
Midazolam
    for anxiety, dosage, routes,
        half-life, 253t
    for delirium, 342
    for dyspnea, 386
    for terminal sedation, 342
Midodrine for chronic kidney
    disease symptoms, 198t
Mini-Mental State Examination
    for assessing delirium,
    334-335
Mirtazapine (Remeron), dosage
    and effects, 355t
Modafinil for fatigue, 404
Morphine
    for dyspnea, 385
    effects of renal
        failure/dialysis on, 98t
    equianalgesic dosage of, 465t
    formulations of, 462t
    metabolism of, 99
    renal failure and, 107t
Mouth, sore
    interventions for, 138-139
    pharmacologic options for,
    143t
Multiple sclerosis
    clinical courses in, 207
    etiology and
        pathophysiology, 208
    symptoms, 208
    treatments, 208
Muscle cramps in ALS, 205

Muscle relaxation, effects of,
    472t
Myocardial infarction, 154

N

Nalbuphine, contraindication
    to, 460
National Association of Clinical
    Nurse Specialists,
    website for, 17b
National Hospice and Palliative
    Care Organization, 28-29
National Institute for Clinical
    Excellence, guidelines
    for supportive/palliative
    care, 24, 24b
National provider identifier,
    13, 15-16
    application process for, 15-16
Nausea/vomiting, 431-445
    in ascites, 259
    assessment and measurement,
        433-434, 436, 438
    case study, 443-444
    causes, 435b
    definition and incidence, 431
    diagnostics, 439-440
    etiology and pathophysiology,
        431-432
    evaluation and follow-up, 443
    history and physical
        examination, 438-439
    in HIV/AIDS, 239t
    intervention and treatment,
        139, 440-442
        nonpharmacological,
        441-442
        pharmacological, 440-441,
        441t
    mechanisms and
        neuroreceptors of, 433t
    multidimensional effects, 432f
    opioid-related, 468
    patient and family
        education, 442-443
    pharmacologic options for,
        143t
    risk factors for
        disease-related, 434
        therapy-related, 434, 436,
        437b-438b
    self-care activities for, 442b
Nearing death awareness, 40
NEECHAM Confusion Scale for
    assessing delirium, 335

Nefazodone (Serzone), dosage
    and effects, 355t
Neurodermatitis, treatment
    of, 513
Neuroleptics for anxiety, 252
    dosage, routes, half-life, 253t
Neurological diseases, 201-214
    Alzheimer's disease, 202-203
    amyotrophic lateral sclerosis,
        204-205
    cerebrovascular accidents,
        201-202
    diagnostics, 211
    history of, 209-210
    Huntington's disease, 205-207
    multiple sclerosis, 207-208
    Parkinson's disease, 208-209
    physical assessment for,
        210-211
    psychosocial considerations,
        211-212
Neurological dysfunction,
    fatigue and, 399
Neurolytic blocks for pain, 471
Neuromuscular disorders
    dyspnea in, 379, 380t
    respiratory effects of, 175
Nociception
    phases of, 449-450, 452-453
    substances involved in,
        450, 452f
Non-Hodgkin's lymphoma
    epidemiology, 222
    metastasis of, 218t
    symptoms and treatment, 222
Nonmaleficence, defined, 64
Nonsteroidal antiinflammatory
    drugs
    contraindications to, 468
    mechanism of action,
        453t, 468
Norepinephrine/dopamine
    reuptake inhibitors,
    dosage and effects, 355t
Norpramin. *See* Desipramine
    (Norpramin)
Nortriptyline (Pamelor),
    dosage and effects, 354t
NPI. *See* National provider
    identifier
Nummular eczema, 505
Nurse practitioner
    educational background, 3
    oncology, 10
    patient populations of, 6

Nurse practitioner *(Continued)*
    role-delineation study of, 3
    scope of practice, 6-7, 6b
Nurse Practitioner Central,
    website for, 17b
Nursing, boards of, guidelines
    of, 12
Nursing Delirium Screening
    Scale, 335
Nursing practice, ANA essential
    features of, 10-11
Nutrition, 131-150
    cachexia and, 132-133
    definitions in, 131
    measurement instruments
        for, 146
    pathophysiology and,
        131-132
    patient outcomes and,
        145-146
    professional competencies
        in, 146
Nutrition impact symptoms,
    management of, 133-
    140, 141t, 142-145, 143t
    in end-of-life care setting,
        144-145
    with enteral nutrition
        support, 140, 141t, 142
    with parenteral nutrition
        support, 142
    pharmacologic, 142-144,
        143t

O

Obstructive and restrictive
    airway diseases,
    differentiating among,
    173-174
Octreotide (Sandostatin)
    for bowel obstruction,
        272-273
    for controlling diarrhea,
        372-373
    for nausea/vomiting, 441t
Olanzapine
    for anxiety, dosage, routes,
        half-life, 253t
    for delirium/acute
        confusion, 341
Omega-3 fatty acids for
    cachexia, 132-133
Oncology, pre-World War II, 20
Oncology nurse practitioner,
    10

Ondansetron for chronic
    kidney disease
    symptoms, 198t
Open-ended questions, 50-51
Opioid pseudo-addiction, 455
Opioids
    administration of, 460
    constipation and, 288
    for controlling diarrhea, 372
    for COPD, 180
    dehydration associated with,
        316
    for dyspnea, 384-385
    effects of renal
        failure/dialysis on, 98t
    equianalgesic conversions of,
        462, 465, 465t
        calculation guide,
            466f-467f
    formulations of, 462t
    for heart failure, 167
    mechanism of action, 453t
    in pain management, 21-22,
        462, 462t, 465, 468
    renal failure and, 108t
    respiratory depression and,
        455
    selecting starting dose, 462
Orientation
    providing clues to, 341
    tests of, 338b
Orthostatic hypotension,
    drug-induced, 106
Osmotic laxatives, 294-295
Ovarian cancer, diarrhea with,
    case study, 374-375
Overexertion, fatigue and,
    399
Oxycodone
    effects of renal
        failure/dialysis on, 98t
    equianalgesic dosage of,
        465t
    formulations of, 461t, 462t
    metabolism of, 100
    renal failure and, 108t
Oxygen therapy
    for COPD, 181
    for dyspnea, 388-389

P

Pacemakers for heart failure,
    164
Pain, 447-479
    acute, 447

Pain *(Continued)*
    assessment and
        measurement, 455-458
    in cognitively impaired,
        456, 458
    tools for, 457f-458f
    from bowel obstruction,
        270-271
    breakthrough, 447
    case study, 476-477
    chronic, 447
    classification and examples,
        451t
    definition and incidence,
        447-449
    diagnostics, 458-459
    during dying process, 37-38
    etiology and
        pathophysiology,
        449-454
    evaluation and follow-up, 476
    history and physical
        examination, 458
    in HIV/AIDS, 240t
    incident, 448
    intervention and treatment.
        See Pain management
    medications for, physiologic
        rationale for, 453-454,
        453t
    myths and misconceptions
        about, 454-455
    neuropathic, 448, 449, 453
        descriptors and examples,
            451t
    nociceptive, 448-450, 449,
        452-453
        descriptors and examples,
            451t
        substances involved in,
            450, 452f
    patient and family
        education, 475
    referred, 449, 450f
    sleep disorders and, 118
    substances in nociceptor
        transduction of, 452f
    types of, 448f
        based on inferred
            pathophysiology,
            448-449
    uncontrolled, effects of, 449
Pain management, 459-475
    at end-of-life, 37-38
    myths about, 21

Pain management *(Continued)*
neglect of, 448-449
nondrug/complementary, 471, 472t
nutrition symptoms and, 140
pharmacological
adjuvant analgesics in, 463t-464t, 468-469
bisphosphonates in, 469-470
for cancer, history of, 20-21
combination analgesics in, 461t
corticosteroids in, 469
equianalgesic conversions in, 462, 465t, 466f-467f
intraspinal medication delivery in, 470
neurolytic blocks in, 471
nonopioid analgesics in, 461t
NSAIDs in, 468
opioids in, 21-22, 462, 462t, 465, 468
physiologic rationale for, 453-454, 453t
and principle of double effect, 69-70
in substance abuse, 471, 473-475
principles of, 459-460
radiation therapy in, 471
radiopharmaceuticals in, 470
of rapidly escalating pain, 475
tumor embolization in, 470
for ulcerative lesions, 532-533
WHO three-step analgesic ladder in, 459f
Palliative care
advanced practice nurse in. *See* Advanced practice nurse
in chronic nonmalignant disease, 20
current trends in, 19-20, 23
evaluation of, 27
future of, 30
for heart failure, 165-167
historical perspectives on, 20-21
for HIV/AIDS, 238
integration into traditional medicine, 27

Palliative care *(Continued)*
National Institute for Clinical Excellent guidelines for, 24, 24b
in palliative medicine, 25-26
programs in, 26-27
reconciliation and, 81
sleep disorder interventions in, 122-125, 123t, 124t, 125t
sleep disturbances and, 116
WHO definition of, 25
WHO revised definition of, 23
Palliative care clinician, skills of, 4
Palliative medicine
challenges to, 23
versus end-of-life care, 27
palliative care in, 25-26
skill sets in, 25
as subspecialty, 22
Pamelor. *See* Nortriptyline (Pamelor)
Pancreatic cancer
epidemiology of, 221
metastasis of, 218t
treatment and metastasis, 221-222
Pancreatic obstruction, diarrhea associated with, 362t
Paracentesis
for ascites, 263
complications of, 263
Parenteral nutrition support, 142
in cachexia, 282
Parkinson's disease, etiology, symptoms, treatment, 208-209
Paroxetine (Paxil), dosage and effects, 354t
Pastoral counseling in pain management, effects of, 472t
Patient, values and goals of, 53-54
Patient self-determination, 56-57
ethical issues in, 64
Patient Self-Determination Act, 54, 56
Patient–health care professional relationship, ethical issues in, 64-65

Paxil. *See* Paroxetine (Paxil)
Pemoline (Cylert) for fatigue, 404
Pentazocine, contraindication to, 460
Perception, tests of, 338b
Perceptual disturbances with delirium, 329
Pergolide for chronic kidney disease symptoms, 198t
Periactin. *See* Cyproheptadine (Periactin)
Pericardial effusion, dyspnea due to, management of, 384t
Pericardiocentesis for cough, 310
Periodic limb movement disorder, defined, 113b
Personal identification number, 13
Pharmacodynamics, 86f, 102-104
cellular, 102-104
of agonists, 103
of antagonists, 104
organism, 104
population, 105
principles of, 85, 86f
properties of, 105-107
Pharmacogenomics, focus of, 85
Pharmacokinetics, 86f
aging and, 105-106
bioavailability, 89, 90f
clearance, 93-94
dosing intervals, 93
half-life, 92
ionization, 96-97
linear, 94, 95f
lipid solubility, 96
loading doses, 91-92
in multiple compartment distribution, 94
nonlinear, 102
parameters of, 86-97
principles of, 85, 86f
properties of, 105-107
protein binding, 94-96
routes of administration, 86, 87t-88t, 88b, 89
steady state, 93
therapeutic range, 89-90
volume of distribution, 90, 91t

Pharmacology, 85-109
Pharyngeal cancer, pain
management in, case
study, 476-477
Phenobarbital
for delirium, 342
for terminal sedation, 342
Phenothiazines for dyspnea,
385-386
Physician Orders for Life
Sustaining Treatment,
58
Physiotherapy for cough, 309
Plasmapheresis for chronic
kidney disease
symptoms, 198t
Pleural effusion
characteristics of, 175
cough characteristics in, 306
dyspnea due to, management
of, 384t
in heart failure, 161
metastasis-related,
interventions for, 227
Pneumococcal vaccine for
COPD, 181
Pneumonia
community-acquired,
JCAHO treatment
regulations and, 305-306
cough in, characteristics and
symptoms, 306, 307t
diagnosis of, sputum analysis
in, 306
Pneumonitis, hypersensitivity,
characteristics of, 175
Pneumothorax, characteristics
of, 175
POLST, 58
Polycythemia vera, treatment
of, 510
Polypharmacy, definition
of, 108
Polysomnogram, defined, 113b
Postgastectomy pumping
syndrome, treatment of,
373
Postnasal drip, cough in,
characteristics and
symptoms, 307t
Power of attorney. *See* Durable
power of attorney
Practice guidelines
in clinical decision making,
11-12

Practice guidelines *(Continued)*
defining, 10-11
state practice, 12-13
Prednisolone for dyspnea, 386
Prednisone for cough, 309
Prescriptive authority,
delegation of, 13
Pressure ulcers
etiology and pathophysiology,
519-520
of heel, 525f
prevention of, 526-527
Pressure ulcers effects of, 519
Prochlorperazine (Compazine)
for nausea/vomiting, 441t
Proctoclysis, characteristics and
disadvantages, 321
Progestational agents for
cachexia, 282
Prokinetic agents
for cachexia, 282
for nausea/vomiting, 441t
Promethazine (Phenergan)
for anxiety, dosage, routes,
half-life, 253t
for dyspnea, 386
for nausea/vomiting, 441t
Propofol
for delirium, 342
for terminal sedation, 342
Propoxyphene,
contraindication to, 460
Proprionic acids, dosing
information, 461t
ProSom. *See* Estazolam
(ProSom)
Prostaglandin inhibitors for
controlling diarrhea, 372
Prostate cancer
anorexia in, case study,
283-285
dehydration in, case study,
323
epidemiology and treatment,
220-221
metastasis of, 218t, 221
nausea/vomiting in, case
study, 443-444
Protocols
in clinical decision making,
11-12
defining, 11
Proxy, informed, 59
Prozac. *See* Fluoxetine (Prozac)
Pruritus, 503-518

Pruritus *(Continued)*
aquagenic, 506
intervention and treatment,
510
assessment and
measurement, 507-508
brachioradial, 506
treatment of, 511
burn, 506
treatment of, 511-512
case study, 515-517
cholestatic, treatment of, 512
definition and incidence, 503
diagnostics, 509-510
education and follow-up,
515
essential, treatment of, 512
etiology and
pathophysiology,
504-505
generalized, 506, 509-510
history and physical
examination, 508-509
intervention and treatment,
510-515
antihistamines in, 511t
for aquagenic pruritus,
510
for atopic pruritus,
510-511
for brachioradial pruritus,
511
for burn pruritus, 511-512
for cholestatic pruritus,
512
for drug eruptions, 512
for dry skin, 512
for essential pruritus, 512
general measures, 510
in malignancies, 513
for neurodermatitis, 513
for pruritus ani, 513
for senile pruritus, 513
for uremic pruritus,
513-514
for urticaria, 514
for winter pruritus,
514-515
localized, 505-506, 507-509
neurogenic, 504
neuropathic, 504
psychogenic, 505
senile, 506
treatment of, 513
uremic, 506

Pruritus *(Continued)*
    treatment of, 513-514
Pruritus ani, 505-506
    treatment of, 513
Pseudomembranous colitis,
    diarrhea associated
    with, 365
Pseudo-obstruction, bowel,
    causes of, 270
Psoriasis, 506
Psychological issues in advance
    care planning, 50
Psychomotor disturbances with
    delirium, 330
Psychosocial factors
    in constipation, 289
    in HIV/AIDS, 237
    in neurological diseases,
        211-212
    sleep disorders and,
        117-118
Psychosocial symptoms, APN
    management of, 35-36
Psychostimulants
    for depression, 356
    for fatigue, 403
Pulmonary disease, 171-183.
        See also Chronic
        obstructive pulmonary
        disease
    dyspnea in, 379, 380t
Pulmonary edema in heart
    failure, 161
Pulmonary embolism, dyspnea
    due to, management
    of, 384t
Pulmonary fibrosis, diffuse
    interstitial,
    characteristics of, 175
Pulmonary function tests
    for assessing dyspnea,
        383
Pulse, assessment of, 159-160
Pyranocarboxylic acids, dosing
    information, 461t

Q

Quality of life, patient's
    definition of, 53-54
Questions, open-ended, 50-51
Quetiapine for delirium/acute
    confusion, 341
Quinine for chronic kidney
    disease symptoms, 198t
Quinlan, K. A., 54

R

Radiation therapy
    diarrhea associated with,
        363t
    emetic risk of, 438b
    for pain, 471
    for spinal cord compression,
        493
    for superior vena cava
        syndrome, 488
Radiopharmaceuticals, 470
Rapport, building, 52, 52b
Reconciliation, approach to, 81
Reimbursement
    for APN, 17b
    issues in, 13, 16
Relaxation techniques
    for dyspnea, 390
    in pain management, 472t
Religion. *See also* Spirituality
    defined, 75
    forgiveness and, 82-83
    treatment decisions and, 71
Remelteon (Rozerem), dose
    and half-life, 124t
Remeron. *See* Mirtazapine
    (Remeron)
Renal cell cancer, delirium in,
    case study, 344-345
Renal disease
    chronic. *See* Chronic kidney
        disease
    end-stage. *See* End-stage
        renal disease
Renal failure
    effect on opioids, 98t
    opioid administration and,
        108t
Respiratory depression, opioids
    and, 455
Restless legs syndrome,
    defined, 113b
Restlessness
    dehydration and, 317
    with delirium, 330
Restoril. *See* Tamezepam
    (Restoril)
Retching, defined, 431
Riluzole (Rilutek) for
    ALS, 204
Risperidone
    for anxiety, dosage, routes,
        half-life, 253t
    for delirium/acute
        confusion, 341

Ritalin. *See* Methylphenidate
    (Ritalin)
Rozerem. *See* Remelteon
    (Rozerem)

S

Saccharine laxatives, 294
St. Christopher's Hospice, 22
St. George's Respiratory
    Questionnaire, 381
St. Joseph's Hospice, 21-22
Salicylates, dosing information,
    461t
Saline osmotic laxatives, 294
Saliva, thick
    interventions for, 137-138
    pharmacologic options for,
        143t
Salmeterol xinofoate for
    dyspnea, 387t
Salmonella spp., diarrhea due
    to, treatment of, 371
Sarcoidosis, characteristics of,
    175
Sartre, J.-P., 81b
Saunders, C., 21, 22, 28, 33
Schiavo, T., 54
Scoliosis, respiratory effects of,
    175
Scopolamine (Transderm-
    Scop) for
    nausea/vomiting, 441t
Sedation, terminal, 342
Sedatives, dose/half-life,
    124t-125t
Seizures, etiology,
    pathophysiology,
    diagnosis, management,
    497-498
Selective serotonin reuptake
    inhibitors
    dosage and effects,
        354t-355t
    dose and half-life, 124t-125t
Self-actualization, assessment
    and interventions, 78-
    79
Self-determination, patient. *See*
    Patient self-
    determination
Sensory perception, changes
    in, 40
Serotonin antagonists for
    nausea/vomiting, 441t
Serotonin in pruritus, 504

Serotonin system, delirium-
    related changes in, 334t
Sertraline
    for chronic kidney disease
        symptoms, 198t
    dosage and effects, 354t
Serzone. *See* Nefazodone
        (Serzone)
Short bowel syndrome,
        diarrhea associated
        with, 363t
Shunts for ascites, 264
Sinequan. *See* Doxepin
        (Sinequan)
Skin
    dry, treatment of, 512
    normal, itch in, 507
    risk assessment for ulcerative
        lesions of, 522
Skin tears
    classifying, 523-524
    etiology and
        pathophysiology, 522
    prevention of, 527-528
Sleep, 111-129
    assessment of, 119-122, 121t
    function of, 114-115
    impaired
        drugs causing, 120t
        effects of, 116
    non-REM, 111-112, 112f
    normal, 111-115, 121
    promoting healthy practices
        for, 122, 123t
    rapid eye movement,
        111-112, 112f
    regulation of, 115
    slow-wave, defined, 114b
    terms related to, 113b-114b
Sleep apnea syndrome, defined,
        113b
Sleep cycle, 111-112, 112f
Sleep debt, defined, 113b
Sleep deprivation, defined, 113b
Sleep disorders
    chronic illness and, 111
    defined, 114b
    demographic factors in, 117
    disease-related factors in,
        118-119
    interventions for, 122-125,
        123t, 124t-125t
    lifestyle factors in, 117
    in palliative care setting, 116
    primary, 116-119

Sleep disorders *(Continued)*
    psychosocial factors in,
        117-118
    resources for, 125b
    treatment-related factors in,
        119
    Web sites for, 121-122
Sleep disruption, fatigue and,
        399
Sleep efficiency, defined, 114b
Sleep fragmentation, defined,
        114b
Sleep latency, defined, 114b
Sleep-wake disturbances, with
        delirium, 329-330
Sleepiness, daytime, 122
Smell, altered sense of, 137
Smoking
    COPD and, 174, 178
    medications and, 107
Smoking cessation
    COPD and, 178, 180-181
    for reducing cough, 310
Sodium restriction for ascites,
        262
Sonata. *See* Zaleplon (Sonata)
Spinal cord compression
    case study, 499
    etiology, pathophysiology,
        diagnosis, management,
        490-494
Spiritual care
    cultural issues in, 75-84
    definitions and concepts,
        75-76
    factors enhancing, 76-83
    in HIV/AIDS, 237
Spiritual care competence
    defined, 75
    generic *versus* specific, 77
Spiritual distress in HIV/AIDS,
        240t
Spiritual relatedness,
        assessment and
        interventions for, 82
Spirituality
    advance care planning and,
        56b
    defined, 75
    dying process and, 54
Spirometry for assessing
        dyspnea, 383
Sputum
    analysis of, in diagnosis of
        cough, 306, 307t

Sputum *(Continued)*
    clearing techniques for,
        309
    "Starvation," misconceptions
        about, 144
Stimulant laxatives, 295
Stool osmolality anion gap,
        calculating, 369
Stroke. *See* Cerebrovascular
        accidents
Substance abuse, pain
        management in, 471,
        473-475
Substance P/neurokinin-1
        antagonist for
        nausea/vomiting, 441t
Substituted judgment, 65
Substituted judgment
        standards, 59
Suicide risk
    assessment of, 352
    supervision and, 353
Superior vena cava syndrome
    cough due to, 303
    etiology, pathophysiology,
        diagnosis, management,
        487-490
SUPPORT study, 56, 70
Supportive care
    defining, 24-25
    National Institute for
        Clinical Excellent
        guidelines for, 24, 24b
Surfactants, 294
Surgery
    diarrhea associated with,
        363t
    postanesthesia emetic risk of,
        438b
Surrogate decision making,
        ethical issues in, 65-66
Surrogates, decision-making,
        55b, 57-58
Symptom management, 35
Syndrome of inappropriate
        antidiuretic hormone
        secretion
    etiology, pathophysiology,
        diagnosis, management,
        484-486
    lung cancer and, 218

T

Tachycardia, assessment of,
        159-160

Tamezepam (Restoril), dose and half-life, 124t
Taste, altered sense of, 137
Terminal condition, defined, 66
Terminal illness, hope and, 80-81
Theophylline
  for COPD, 179-180
  for dyspnea, 388, 388t
Therapeutic index, 105
Therapeutic range, defined, 89-90
Thiethylperazine (Torecan) for nausea/vomiting, 441t
Thirst
  in cancer patients, 317
  decreased sense of, 317
Thoracentesis for cough, 310
Throat, sore, interventions for, 138-139
Thrombosis
  artificial hydration and, 320
  defined, 153
  in stroke, 201
Tiotropium bromide for dyspnea, 388t
Tofranil. *See* Imipramine (Tofranil)
Touch therapies in pain management, effects of, 472t
Transcendence, assessment and interventions, 83
Transition Dyspnea Index, 381
Trazodone (Desyrel)
  dosage and effects, 355t
  dose and half-life, 124t
Treatment
  care-enhancing, 77-78
  futile, 68
  hypercalcemia of malignancy associated with, 481
  life-sustaining, types of, 66-67
  patient's right to refuse, 54-55
  religious influences and, 71
  sleep disorders and, 119
  weighing benefits and burdens of, ethical issues in, 67-68
  withholding/withdrawing, ethical issues in, 66-67, 68
Triazolam (Halcion), dose and half-life, 124t

Tricyclic antidepressants
  dosage and effects, 354t
  indications and dosing information, 463t
  mechanism of action, 453t
Tube feeding, withholding/withdrawing, 67
Tuberculosis, cough in, characteristics and symptoms, 307t
Tumor embolization, 470
Tumors
  diarrhea associated with, 365
  endocrine-producing, diarrhea associated with, 362t
  malignant cutaneous wounds and, 521b

U

Ulcerative lesions, 519-536
  assessment and measurement, 522-524
  care and dressing of, 528-533
  case study, 534-535
  definition and incidence, 519
  diagnostics, 526
  etiology and pathophysiology, 519-522
  evaluation and follow-up, 534
  of heel, 525f
  history and physical examination, 525
  intervention and treatment, 526-533
  patient and family education, 533
  risk assessment for, 522
Ulcers, pressure. *See* Pressure ulcers
Universal provider identification number, 13
Uremic pruritus, 506
  treatment of, 513-514
Uremic syndrome, manifestations of, 194t
Urinary incontinence in HIV/AIDS, 240t

Urine output during dying process, 38-39
Urticaria, treatment of, 514

V

Values, patient, 55b
Values clarification, 53-54
Valvular heart disease, pathophysiology of, 155
Vascular endothelial growth factor, ascites and, 260
Venlafaxine (Effexor), dosage and effects, 355t
Ventricular arrhythmias, 165
Vestibular apparatus, neurotransmitters in, 433t
Viral load in HIV/AIDS, 236
Virtue ethics, 64-65
Volume depletion
  versus dehydration, 316
  isotonic, 317
Volume of distribution, 90, 91t
Vomiting. *See* Nausea/vomiting
Vomiting center, 431-432
  neurotransmitters in, 433t

W

Wald, F., 28
Wasting syndromes. *See also* Anorexia; Cachexia
  types of, 279
Weight loss
  anorexia-related, 131
  cachexia-related, 131-132
Wellbutrin. *See* Bupropion (Wellbutrin)
Winter pruritus, 506
  treatment of, 514-515
World Health Organization
  analgesic ladder for, 459f
  demonstration project of, 26
  palliative care defined by, 25

X

Xerostomia, interventions for, 137-138

Z

Zaleplon (Sonata), dose and half-life, 124t
Zolpidem (Ambien), dose and half-life, 124t

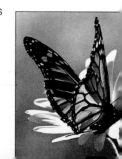